Essentials of
General Surgery

Associate Editors
J. Roland Folse, M.D.
Professor and Chairman
Department of Surgery
Southern Illinois University School of Medicine
Springfield, Illinois

Mitchell H. Goldman, M.D.
Professor of Surgery
University of Tennessee Medical Center
Knoxville, Tennessee

James M. Hassett, Jr., M.D.
Associate Professor of Surgery
State University of New York at Buffalo
Coordinator for Undergraduate Surgical Education
Buffalo, New York

Carol Laputz, R.N., B.S.N.
Instructor
Southern Illinois University School of Medicine
Springfield, Illinois

Patricia J. Numann, M.D.
Associate Professor of Surgery
State University of New York
Health Sciences Center
Syracuse, New York

Jack R. Pickleman, M.D.
Professor and Chief
Division of General Surgery
Loyola University of Chicago Stritch School of Medicine
Maywood, Illinois

Marsha Prater, R.N., M.Ed.
Assistant Professor,
Southern Illinois University School of Medicine
Springfield, Illinois

Richard M. Stillman, M.D.
Associate Professor of Surgery
Director of Student Education
State University of New York
Health Science Center
Director of General Vascular Surgery
Kings County Medical Center
Brooklyn, New York

Illustrated by Lydia Kibiuk

Essentials of General Surgery

Senior Editor

Peter F. Lawrence, M.D.
Associate Professor of Surgery
University of Utah School of Medicine
Salt Lake City, Utah

Editors

Marcia Bilbao, M.D.
Chief of Radiology
Veterans Administration Medical Center
Professor of Radiology
University of Utah School of Medicine
Salt Lake City, Utah

Richard M. Bell, M.D.
Professor of Surgery
Department of Surgery
University of South Carolina
School of Medicine
Columbia, South Carolina

Meril T. Dayton, M.D.
Assistant Professor of Surgery
Department of Surgery
University of Utah School of Medicine
Salt Lake City, Utah

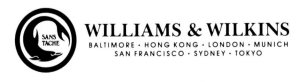

WILLIAMS & WILKINS
BALTIMORE · HONG KONG · LONDON · MUNICH
SAN FRANCISCO · SYDNEY · TOKYO

Editor: Kimberly Kist
Associate Editor: Victoria M. Vaughn
Copy Editors: Elizabeth M. Cowley, Robert Glasgow
Design: JoAnne Janowiak
Illustration Planning: Joanne Och
Production: Raymond E. Reter
Cover Design: Mike Kotarba

Copyright © 1988
Williams & Wilkins
428 East Preston Street
Baltimore, Maryland 21202, USA

Cover painting by Thomas Eakins (1875), *The Gross Clinic,* reproduced by permission of Jefferson Medical College, Thomas Jefferson University, Philadelphia, Pennsylvania.

Accurate indications, adverse reactions, and dosage schedules for drugs are provided in this book, but it is possible that they may change. The reader is urged to review the package information data of the manufacturers of the medications mentioned.

Printed in the United States of America

Library of Congress Cataloging-in-Publication Data

Essentials of general surgery.
  Includes bibliographies and index.
  1. Surgery. I. Lawrence, Peter F. II. Bell,
Richard M. [DNLM: 1. Surgery. WO 100 E783]
RD31.E747 1988   617   87-27999
ISBN 0-683-04893-7

90 91 92
5 6 7 8 9 10

To Karen,
my closest friend, advisor, and supporter,
as well as my wife.

Preface

Do we really need another textbook on surgery? The Association for Surgical Education and the authors of this book obviously believe we do. There are many textbooks that can be used to teach medical students on the surgical clerkship. Unfortunately, the audience for these texts is usually very broad, including surgical residents and practicing surgeons, as well as students. This inclusiveness often means that the material is too comprehensive to be adequately covered during a surgical clerkship, and it may be more detailed and difficult than is necessary for most medical students. Furthermore, much of the existing surgical education material has been developed without first determining what students actually need to know. Medical education has therefore tended to concentrate more on the interests of surgical faculty than on the interests of medical students.

In addition, little coordination of educational material has been attempted. Although excellent texts, audiovisual materials, and computer software are available, they are not integrated into an entire educational package; sometimes information taught by a text is contradicted or refuted in other teaching material. Finally, available standardized examinations, such as the surgical section of National Boards, do not test a specific body of knowledge nor respond to an established set of objectives. Because of these deficiencies in our educational planning, the Association for Surgical Education believes an integrated educational package written solely for the medical student is needed.

The Multi-Media Package for Surgical Clerkships

The text that you are reading is part of an educational package designed to transmit different kinds of information by a multi-media (e.g., computer, videotapes) approach. The educational package includes a text to teach surgical knowledge, videotapes to teach certain surgical procedures and skills, computer problems to teach clinical decision making, a bank of examinations (both oral and written) to test the information that has been learned, and a 35-mm slide set for instructor use. The components of the education package have been developed simultaneously so that they are integrated but not redundant. However, each part of the educational package can also function independently. Although some educators may want to use only certain components of the entire educational package in developing their own surgical curriculum, the complete educational package offers significant pedagogical advantages. The material that is learned in the text can be reinforced and practiced in other parts of the package. A brief description of each component follows.

The Surgical Textbook

The *Essentials of General Surgery* textbook is arranged by organ system (e.g., diseases of the stomach as a chapter). Because the textbook is to be used by students on surgical clerkships, it is designed to be relatively short, so that it can be read in its entirety during the clerkship. One of the major complaints of medical students is that the available surgical textbooks are either *(1)* so lengthy that they cannot be read within the surgical clerkship or *(2)* so brief that students cannot get the information that is necessary to perform adequately while on the surgical clerkship. Our solution to this problem is to emphasize *concepts,* such as pathophysiology of disease, *treatment* of disease (medical and surgical), and outcomes of the *common* surgical disorders, in some detail, and not to attempt to cover obscure surgical diseases. Thus the surgical textbook is not a reference book or encyclopedia of surgical diseases—rather it attempts to teach important surgical diseases in enough depth so that students do not merely memorize information, but understand concepts. Other excellent surgical textbooks are frequently referenced for the student who needs to investigate an uncommon disease or a common disease in greater depth.

Surgical Skill Videotapes

Currently the method of learning technical skills is by trial and error, since there is little educational material available to teach surgical skills. The Association for Surgical Education supports the concept of teaching surgical skills to students before they practice on patients, in order to avoid an extremely stressful situation for both student and patient. The videotapes depict the skills that students must use on patients and present indications for performance of each skill; these videotapes show the equipment that is necessary for successful completion of the task at the patient's bedside and actually demonstrate alternative techniques of performing the skill. We are interested in presenting only those skills that all physicians should know, skills that do not require extensive manual dexterity. Examples of the skills that might be discussed or presented in a videotape are the placement of a nasogastric tube and dressing changes.

Patient Management Problems

Clinical decision making is one crucial area of undergraduate surgical education that has been underemphasized. Frequently students learn problem solving in their encounters with patients as a hit-or-miss process. Because only a small percentage of problems arise in a surgical clerkship, students are not always taught how to approach common surgical problems. The emphasis of this component of the educational package is on teaching students how to deal with problems as they present to the clinician. This section uses a microcomputer to question and teach students in a format called patient management problems. In addition to teaching the students problem solving, the computer can keep track of the student's score and give feedback about performance. The patient management problems stress differential diagnosis, the ability to select the appropriate tests to determine the diagnosis, and the appropriate treatment.

Test Bank of Examinations

We believe that methods should be available to determine whether students have accomplished their educational objectives and have learned the material that is included in the educational package. There are two types of examinations to test learning.

Question Bank. A series of 1100 questions, each related to an organ system and running parallel to the chapters of the textbook, has been placed on computer software. An examination of competency can be generated for each student, keyed to the material that has been taught. The questions are multiple choice, with one correct answer; the questions address the major teaching points in each chapter.

Oral Examination Questions. In addition to the multiple-choice questions, we have also developed questions for an oral examination, based on the contents of the entire education package. The questions draw from each chapter of the surgical textbook as well as all other aspects of the educational package. Oral examination questions differ from multiple-choice questions in that they rely less on a student's ability to recall a specific fact and more on a student's ability to put facts together and plan an approach to a patient problem. Although students need to have certain facts at hand to solve the problems, an oral examination tends to assess the logic and strategy students use to evaluate a problem and come to a valid therapeutic or diagnostic endpoint. In addition, oral examinations assess noncognitive factors such as honesty and self-awareness and provide greater flexibility in the examination process, so that different approaches may be taken by the student and still be judged correct. The oral examination questions are highly structured and are accompanied by instructions for the examiners to improve validity.

35-mm Slide Set

A supplementary set of 35-mm slides has been developed for instructor use to enhance concepts presented in the student textbook. These 198 slides include both line art and radiographs from the textbook to augment lecture and group discussion.

The editors and authors of this package believe that comprehensive educational material will improve the students' experience during their required clerkship and also free the faculty to spend their time guiding observing students. We will be studying the impact of this approach on surgical education programs and will be interested in feedback from students and faculty on its strengths and weaknesses.

Peter F. Lawrence, M.D.

Acknowledgments

This project was nurtured by many members of the Association of Surgical Education (ASE), whose advice and expertise I would like to acknowledge. At its annual meetings the ASE provided an excellent forum for discussion and testing of ideas about the content of the surgical curriculum. In addition, the Curriculum Committee and Testing and Evaluation Committee were responsible for helping to write the objectives for each organ system and developing both oral and written examination questions. My thanks go as well to Laurie Schweikle and Chellie Averett for their meticulous typing and editing throughout the project, and to Vicki Vaughn and Kim Kist, our indefatigable editors at Williams and Wilkins. Finally, I owe thanks to the many medical students at the University of Utah School of Medicine who took time to review videotapes and patient management problems, offering valuable suggestions for improvement.

About the Cover

"Portrait of Professor Gross," also called "The Gross Clinic," was painted by Thomas Eakins in 1875. Eakins had attended lectures at Jefferson Medical College during Samuel David Gross' tenure as Chairman of Surgery. Eakins' students and friends posed as spectators of the operation, and a self-portrait of Eakins himself sketching the procedure (removal of a piece of bone diseased by osteomyelitis) can be found at the center right of the painting. The law at that time required the presence of a relative for surgery on a charity patient *(note woman at lower left)*, a situation permitted by doctors who even then wished to avoid malpractice suits. This nearly life-size painting has hung at Jefferson Medical College since 1879.

(Courtesy of Jefferson Medical College, Thomas Jefferson University, Philadelphia, Pennsylvania.)

Contributors

Adel S. Al-Jurf, M.D.
Professor of Surgery
University of Iowa Hospitals and Clinics
Department of Surgery
College of Medicine
Iowa City, Iowa

Glen F. Baker, M.D.
Professor of Pathology & Dermatology
University of Arkansas for Medical Sciences
Little Rock, Arkansas

Paddy M. Bell, C.S.T.
Certified Surgical Technologist
Columbia, South Carolina

Richard M. Bell, M.D.
Professor of Surgery
Department of Surgery
University of South Carolina School of Medicine
Columbia, South Carolina

Richard A. Bomberger, M.D.
Associate Professor of Surgery
University of Nevada School of Medicine
Reno, Nevada

Anthony Borzotta, M.D.
Assistant Professor of Surgery
Department of Surgery
Case Western Reserve University School of Medicine
Assistant Chief of Surgical Service
Veterans Administration Medical Center
Cleveland, Ohio

Talmadge A. Bowden, Jr., M.D.
Professor of Surgery
Chief, Section of Gastrointestinal Surgery
Medical College of Georgia
Augusta, Georgia

Jay Jeffrey Brown, M.D.
Assistant Professor of Surgery
University of South Carolina School of Medicine
Columbia, South Carolina

Kenneth W. Burchard, M.D.
Associate Professor
Department of Surgery
Brown University
Director, Surgical Intensive Care Unit
Rhode Island Hospital
Providence, Rhode Island

Judith G. Calhoun, Ph.D.
Associate Director
Office of Medical Center Marketing
University of Michigan Medical Center
Adjunct Associate Professor
Office of Educational Resources and Research
Department of Postgraduate Medicine and Health
Professions Education
Ann Arbor, Michigan

Roger L. Christian, M.D.
Assistant Professor of Surgery
Harvard Medical School
Brigham and Women's Hospital
Boston, Massachusetts

Frank Clingan, M.D.
Professor and Chairman
Department of Surgery
University of Oklahoma
Tulsa Medical School
Tulsa, Oklahoma

Charles T. Cloutier, M.D.
Assistant Professor of Surgery
Ohio State University College of Medicine
Columbus, Ohio

James A. Coil, Jr., M.D.
Director of Surgery Education
Iowa Methodist Medical Center
Des Moines, Iowa

James E. Colberg, M.D.
Associate Professor
Department of Surgery
Jefferson Medical College
Philadelphia, Pennsylvania

Rudolph G. Danzinger, M.D.
Head, Department of Surgery
St. Boniface General Hospital
Professor of Surgery
Faculty of Medicine
University of Manitoba
Winnipeg, Manitoba
Canada

Debra A. DaRosa, Ph.D.
Associate Professor
Assistant to the Chairman on Educational Affairs
Department of Surgery

Southern Illinois University School of Medicine
Springfield, Illinois

John Mihran Davis, M.D.
Associate Professor of Surgery
Cornell University School of Medicine
New York, New York

Merril T. Dayton, M.D.
Assistant Professor of Surgery
Department of Surgery
University of Utah School of Medicine
Salt Lake City, Utah

Russell D. Degges, M.D.
Chief Resident, Surgery
University of Arkansas for Medical Sciences
Little Rock, Arkansas

Jeffrey E. Doty, M.D.
Assistant Professor of Surgery
University of California at Los Angeles
Center for the Health Sciences
Los Angeles, California

A. Craig Eddy, M.D.
Acting Instructor of Surgery
University of Washington School of Medicine
Seattle, Washington

E. Christopher Ellison, M.D.
Clinical Assistant Professor of Surgery
Ohio State University College of Medicine
Columbus, Ohio

Dan C. English, M.D.
Former Chairman
Department of Surgery
Michigan State University
College of Human Medicine
East Lansing, Michigan

Douglas B. Evans, M.D.
Instructor-in-Surgery
Dartmouth Medical School
Hanover, New Hampshire

James T. Evans, M.D.
Professor and Chairman
Department of Surgery
Mercer University School of Medicine
Macon, Georgia

William B. Farrar, M.D.
Acting Chief, Division of Surgical Oncology
Assistant Professor of Surgery
Department of Surgery
Ohio State University College of Medicine
Columbus, Ohio

Roger S. Foster, Jr., M.D.
Professor of Surgery
Director, Vermont Regional Cancer Center
University of Vermont School of Medicine
Burlington, Vermont

Donald E. Fry, M.D.
Professor and Chairman
Department of Surgery

University of New Mexico
School of Medicine
Albuquerque, New Mexico

Richard N. Garrison, M.D.
Associate Professor of Surgery
University of Louisville School of Medicine
Louisville, Kentucky

Bruce L. Gewertz, M.D.
Associate Professor of Surgery
Director, Surgical Education
University of Chicago School of Medicine
Chicago, Illinois

Mitchell H. Goldman, M.D.
Professor of Surgery
University of Tennessee Medical Center
Knoxville, Tennessee

Alan M. Graham, M.D.
Assistant Professor of Surgery
McGill University
Royal Victoria Hospital
Montreal, Quebec
Canada

Richard Gusberg, M.D.
Professor of Surgery
Yale University School of Medicine
New Haven, Connecticut

James C. Hebert, M.D.
Assistant Professor of Surgery
University of Vermont
College of Medicine
Burlington, Vermont

David M. Heimbach, M.D.
Professor of Surgery
Director, University of Washington Burn Center
University of Washington School of Medicine
Seattle, Washington

Charles W. Huang, M.D.
Department of Surgery
Veterans Administration Medical Center
Detroit, Michigan

Philip J. Huber, Jr., M.D.
Associate Professor of Surgery
Southwestern Medical School
University of Texas
Southwestern Medical Center at Dallas
Dallas, Texas

Janet K. Ihde, M.D.
Assistant Professor of Surgery
Loma Linda University School of Medicine
Loma Linda, California

Anthony L. Imbembo, M.D.
Vice Chairman and Professor
Department of Surgery
Case Western Reserve University School of Medicine
Director, Department of Surgery
Cleveland Metropolitan General Hospital
Cleveland, Ohio

Edwin C. James, M.D.
Professor and Chairman
Department of Surgery
University of North Dakota School of Medicine
Grand Forks, North Dakota

Bruce Jarrell, M.D.
Associate Professor of Surgery
Jefferson Medical College
Director, Department of Transplantation
Thomas Jefferson University Hospital
Philadelphia, Pennsylvania

Raymond J. Joehl, M.D.
Associate Professor of Surgery
Department of Surgery,
Northwestern University Medical School
Chief, Surgical Service
VA Lakeside Medical Center
Chicago, Illinois

Pardon R. Kenney, M.D.
Assistant Professor of Surgery
Brown University
Providence, Rhode Island

Nicholas P. Lang, M.D.
Associate Professor of Surgery
University of Arkansas for Medical Sciences
Little Rock, Arkansas

Peter F. Lawrence, M.D.
Associate Professor of Surgery
University of Utah School of Medicine
Salt Lake City, Utah

Royce Laycock, M.D.
Professor of Surgery
Southwestern Medical School
University of Texas Health Science Center
Dallas, Texas

Stephen B. Leapman, M.D.
Professor of Surgery
Indiana University Medical Center
Indianapolis, Indiana

Guy Legros, M.D.
General Surgeon
Department of Surgery
University of Montreal
Maisonneuve Hospital
Montreal, Quebec
Canada

E. Stan Lennard, M.D.
Clinical Associate Professor of Surgery
University of Washington School of Medicine
Seattle, Washington

James F. Lind, M.D.
Professor and Chairman
Department of Surgery
Eastern Virginia Medical School
Norfolk, Virginia

Bernard S. Linn, M.D.
Professor of Surgery
University of Miami School of Medicine
Associate Chief of Staff for Education
Veterans Administration Medical Center
Miami, Florida

Bruce V. MacFadyen, Jr., M.D.
Associate Professor
Department of Surgery
University of Texas Medical School
Houston, Texas

Arlie R. Mansberger, Jr., M.D.
Professor and Chairman
Department of Surgery
Medical College of Georgia
Augusta, Georgia

Louis F. Martin, M.D.
Assistant Professor of Surgery & Physiology
University Hospital
Penn State College of Medicine
Milton S. Hershey Medical Center
Hershey, Pennsylvania

Martin H. Max, M.D.
Professor of Surgery
Director, Metabolic Support Services
Chief, Surgical Endoscopy
Loyola University Medical Center
Maywood, Illinois

Mary McCarthy, M.D.
Assistant Professor of Surgery
Indiana University Medical Center
Indianapolis, Indiana

D. Byron McGregor, M.D.
Associate Professor of Surgery
University of Nevada School of Medicine
Chief, Surgical Services
Veterans Administration Medical Center
Reno, Nevada

Hollis W. Merrick III, M.D.
Associate Professor of Surgery
Medical College of Ohio
Toledo, Ohio

Thomas A. Miller, M.D.
Professor of Surgery
University of Texas Health Science Center
Houston, Texas

Ernest E. Moore, M.D.
Professor and Vice Chairman
Department of Surgery
University of Colorado Health Science Center
Chief, Department of Surgery
Denver General Hospital
Denver, Colorado

Arthur Naitove, M.D.
Professor of Surgery
Dartmouth Medical School
Hanover, New Hampshire

Staff Surgeon
Veterans Administration Hospital
White River Junction, Vermont

Patricia J. Numann, M.D.
Associate Professor of Surgery
State University of New York Health Sciences Center
Syracuse, New York

J. Patrick O'Leary, M.D.
Seeger Chair-in-Surgery
Department of Surgery
Baylor University Medical Center
Dallas, Texas

James W. Pate, M.D.
Professor and Chairman
Department of Surgery
University of Tennessee School of Medicine
Memphis, Tennessee

L. Beaty Pemberton, M.D.
Professor and Chairman
Department of Surgery
Truman Medical Center
Kansas, Missouri

James B. Peoples, M.D.
Associate Professor
Department of Surgery
Wright State University School of Medicine
Dayton, Ohio

Thomas G. Peters, M.D.
Professor of Surgery
University of Tennessee Medical School
Staff, General Surgeon
Veterans Administration Medical Center
Memphis, Tennessee

Hiram C. Polk, Jr., M.D.
Professor and Chairman
Department of Surgery
University of Louisville School of Medicine
Louisville, Kentucky

John L. Provan, M.D.
Professor of Surgery
University of Toronto
Toronto, Ontario
Canada

Talmadge J. Raine, M.D.
Assistant Professor of Surgery
Division of Plastic Surgery
University of Chicago
Attending Surgeon
Michael Reese Hospital
Chicago, Illinois

William M. Rambo, M.D.
Professor of Surgery
Medical University of South Carolina
Chief, Surgical Services
Charleston Memorial Hospital
Charleston, South Carolina

Layton F. Rikkers, M.D.
Professor and Chairman
Department of Surgery
University of Nebraska Medical Center
Omaha, Nebraska

Martin C. Robson, M.D.
Truman G. Blocker Professor of Surgery
Chief, Division of Plastic Surgery
University of Texas Medical Branch
Galveston, Texas

Pamela A. Rowland-Morin, Ph.D.
Clinical Instructor
Brown University Program in Medicine
Communications Specialist
Department of Surgery
Rhode Island Hospital
Providence, Rhode Island
Assistant Professor
University of Rhode Island
Kingston, Rhode Island

Steven T. Ruby, M.D.
Assistant Professor of Surgery
University of Connecticut School of Medicine
Chief, Vascular Section
John Dempsey Hospital
Farmington, Connecticut

Ajit K. Sachdeva, M.D.
Assistant Professor of Surgery
Medical College of Pennsylvania
Associate Chief, Surgical Services
Philadelphia, Pennsylvania

Jeffrey T. Schouten, M.D.
Kaiser-Permanente
Waikiki, Hawaii

David J. Smith, Jr., M.D.
Associate Professor of Surgery
Section Head, Plastic Surgery
University of Michigan Medical Center
Ann Arbor, Michigan

Mary R. Smith, M.D.
Associate Professor of Medicine & Pathology
Medical College of Ohio
Toledo, Ohio

J. Michael Stair, M.D.
Private Practice
Little Rock, Arkansas

Gordon L. Telford, M.D.
Assistant Professor
Department of Surgery
Medical College of Wisconsin
Milwaukee, Wisconsin

Carolyn Thompson, Ph.D.
Associate Professor, Biometry
University of Arkansas for Medical Sciences
Little Rock, Arkansas

Jon Thompson, M.D.
Associate Professor
Department of Surgery
University of Nebraska
Omaha, Nebraska

Enrique Vazquez-Quintana, M.D.
Professor and Chairman
Department of Surgery
University of Puerto Rico
San Juan, Puerto Rico

Kent C. Westbrook, M.D.
Professor of Surgery
University of Arkansas for Medical Sciences
Little Rock, Arkansas

Robert F. Wilson, M.D.
Professor of Surgery
Director of Thoracic and Cardiovascular Surgery
Wayne State University Medical Center
Chief of Surgery
Detroit Receiving Hospital
Detroit, Michigan

Christopher K. Zarins, M.D.
Professor of Surgery
University of Chicago School of Medicine
Chicago, Illinois

Contents

1

HEALTH CARE ISSUES

Bernard S. Linn, M.D.

ASSUMPTIONS

The student has fundamental knowledge in basic sciences and some prior exposure to problems and issues in medical care.

The student may not have had prior clinical rotations but has a desire to learn more about health care issues to apply the knowledge to the clinical experiences in the clerkship.

The student recognizes the need to further understand current issues in health care as well as his or her own role in shaping the direction of medical practice.

OBJECTIVES

1. List and define the types of programs that have been implemented for cost containment of medical care.
2. Describe how cost containment programs can affect surgical practice.
3. Describe the magnitude of the problem of providing medical care to an aging population.
4. Describe considerations that need to be taken into account in operating on elderly patients.
5. Describe the physician's role in caring for the terminally ill patient.
6. List the major areas in medical ethics.
7. Describe how medical ethics affect surgery.
8. Describe the interaction between cost containment and quality care.

Background

Surgeons do not practice in a vacuum isolated from other physicians. Patients are referred to them; they refer patients to colleagues. Surgeons are consulted by other physicians, and surgeons seek consultation. This is true because patients rarely have a single clear surgical disease. Hence whatever is happening in medical practice at large will affect the way surgeons practice. Those embarking on careers in medicine today face more challenges than ever before. Not only must they keep abreast of their chosen field, a goal requiring a lifetime of study, but they must gear their practice to fit within a medical environment that is in an unprec-

edented state of change. The entire milieu and method of medical practice in this country is in a process of radical change that most likely is not yet over and most certainly is not fully predictable.

The topics covered in this chapter are generic to medicine. They affect surgeons as well as other practitioners. They represent ever expanding areas that need to be included in medical education. Students who understand such issues will find it easier to communicate with hospital personnel and will be able to place their clinical rotation into the larger picture of future practice. The topics covered represent only the tips of the icebergs. This in itself illustrates one of the dilemmas that is the result of an explosion of knowledge that cannot be covered in depth in the time allotted for undergraduate medical education. It emphasizes the need for students to develop self-directed learning as the primary means for incorporating new and important information that often cannot be included in a busy clerkship. The topics cover cost containment, the growing population of elderly, medical ethics, and quality of care. These areas may seem diverse but are highly interactive. Only summaries of issues can be addressed. The reader is directed to other sources that allow for fuller exploration of the issues.

Cost Containment

The transformation of medical care began in 1965. Medicare and Medicaid were soon to become the largest purchasers of health care in the country. Without built-in cost control, health care costs escalated. In 1965 the total expenditure for health care was about $5 billion. By 1984, 10% of the gross national product ($156 billion) was being spent on hospital costs alone. Efforts to control costs began in for-profit institutions that evolved into large scale, often corporate-like, provider organizations. By 1984, hospital chains, such as Humana, Hospital Corporation of America, and others, had grown until they controlled 90% of the investor-owned, multihospital system. These chains gained a reputation for cost containment, and some of their techniques were adopted by not-for-profit hospitals. Soon it was hard to distinguish between profit and nonprofit institutions. For example, a chain might own a for-profit specialty hospital, a nonprofit general hospital, a nursing home, and an ambulatory care clinic. In the process of change, the hospital, as the primary place where care was given, is rapidly being replaced by other forms of community medical centers, such as ambulatory surgical centers, outpatient rehabilitation facilities, emergency care centers, and dialysis facilities. Fee-for-service structure is also being replaced by other methods of reimbursement. The term *contract medicine* refers to systems where medical services are regulated by contractual agreements between the provider and consumer. Because of the rapid escalation of health care costs these organizations have achieved phenomenal growth.

Health Maintenance Organizations (HMOs)

HMOs include a benefit package that covers care given in physicians' offices (many standard insurance contracts do not), hospitalization, out-of-area services, emergency care, and some include drugs. Most HMOs do not cover psychiatric services or cosmetic surgery. HMOs vary considerably; however, benefits are provided on a prepaid basis, which means the provider guarantees to give care for a prefixed amount. Everyone pays the same amount. Some of the newer programs require the patient to pay a deductible or copayment. HMOs use one of two models. One is a staff model, where a group of physicians is employed by an organized group of consumers. Medical care is limited to those physicians and the hospitals where they practice. The other model is a group model, where groups of physicians organize their own HMO with the idea of drawing in a large number of patients. Both models fit into what is known as a "closed panel" system, where any care provided outside the HMO must be approved before payment can be made. The "open panel" system has become known as the Independent Practice Association (IPA). IPAs often are formed by the county medical societies. Patients have the option of going to any participating physician but are still restricted from going to nonparticipating providers.

HMOs are one of the older models of alternate types of care that has had a strong influence on shaping medical practice. By 1984, 15 million individuals had enrolled in HMOs and 40 million are expected by 1990. The growth of HMOs is attributed to the fact that costs of most insurance carriers have risen substantially, while HMOs have kept their costs down. It is less expensive to enroll in an HMO than to carry the usual health insurance coverage. HMOs generate fewer hospital days by tying physicians to cost-saving incentives. In many HMO plans the physician is at risk for specialty care as well as hospital expenses. The effect on hospitals is fewer admissions and services, and the effect on specialists is fewer referrals.

Preferred Provider Organizations (PPOs)

PPOs are organizations that offer discounts to groups of individuals for using certain providers or facilities. Most PPOs allow patients to select their own provider but offer financial incentives, such as reduced deductible and lower copayments, to induce patients to use the PPO. A small number of PPOs have lock-in provisions called Exclusive Provider Organizations (EPOs) requiring patients to use preferred providers or lose coverage. The majority of PPOs, however, are of the no lock-in variety. PPOs often use diverse groups of unrelated hospitals and physicians that are joined with insurance companies. In PPOs, physicians are paid on a case-by-case basis, with the fee agreed on in advance of surgery, as opposed to HMOs, where the surgeons are generally salaried and are paid regardless of whether they actually deliver services. Some chains, such as Humana Care Plus, have acquired insurance companies to sell coverage at low rates for care provided in their own hospitals.

PPOs led to promotion of Primary Care Networks (PCNs), or what has come to be called the gatekeeper concept. One physician, usually a primary care physician, becomes the gatekeeper responsible for the care of a given patient. Cost of care is reduced because the gatekeeper is expected to be able to handle the majority of the patient's problems.

Prospective Payment System (PPS)

Because Medicare is one of the largest purchasers of care, any change in its policies will have repercussions in other areas of health payments. The PPS had this effect and is perhaps the most dramatic reform in federal financing of health care since Medicare and Medicaid. Traditionally, hospitals were reimbursed by Medicare on the basis of their costs. If they spent more, they received more. There were no built-in controls on expenditures; therefore health care costs could, and did, escalate. PPS was initiated in 1983 and phased in over a period of time ending in 1988.

In essence, reimbursement is based on a fixed price per admission classified by 468 Diagnostic-Related Groups (DRGs). Each DRG has a price that reflects historical variation in the average cost of caring for patients within that DRG. Some adjustments are possible, based on higher costs in teaching hospitals or higher wages paid in some parts of the country. The system of DRGs puts hospitals at risk for cost of care. Increased cost over DRGs has to be absorbed by the hospital. Furthermore, savings in costs can be retained by hospitals, thus providing strong incentives to reduce length of stay and service provided. Although hospitals can control costs to some extent, there is concern that admissions for minor problems will erode any savings accrued. Utilization review was instituted to provide a mechanism for monitoring admissions.

Utilization Review (UR)

In 1970 the Professional Standards Review Organization (PSRO) was established as a means for monitoring care. This was an era when quality of care measurements were developed for internal or external review of medical records using process (lists for adequate care) or patient outcome (morbidity/mortality) criteria. Hospital committees were not very effective, and reviews did not usually influence physician behavior, nor were they cost effective. In 1982 the PSRO·was disbanded and Peer Review Organizations (PROs) were established, with the primary purpose of controlling hospital admissions. UR includes profiling patients, physicians, hospitals, and even drugs, and reviewing the appropriateness of both ambulatory and acute care. Utilization statistics are a way of saying to consumers that dollars spent have not been wasted and that they were spent appropriately. In certain states a speciality panel determines whether surgery was necessary for procedures such as cholecystectomy, hysterectomy, or pacemaker insertion. Other methods, such as preadmission certification, second surgical opinions, and use of outpatient clinics for surgery, have been adopted. The consequence of DRGs and UR has been a sharp drop in average length of stay (up to 12%), which has resulted in closing wards and laying off hospital staff.

Cost Containment and Surgery

The change to prospective payment for health care has resulted in incentives to hospitals and physicians to reduce costs. In the future there will be more patient admissions on the day before or day of surgery, with earlier discharges after surgery. Patients scheduled for elective surgery will have workups done on an outpatient basis, and for elective and emergency procedures, patients will receive more of their postoperative care as outpatients. Thus surgeons will have increasing involvement in outpatient settings. There is a danger that control over patient management will be lost in the outpatient setting. There could also be more confusion, with poor communication between the surgeon and the patient.

On the other hand, surgicenters for minor surgery could reduce costs and improve quality of care at the same time. Advantages are high patient acceptance (no waiting and easy access), procedures that are not "bumped" for emergency operations, and inclusive fees (operating room time, drugs, use of recovery room). The major concerns are pain control and early postoperative voiding problems.

There is always a potential that the influence of DRGs could lead to unnecessary surgery, because some DRGs provide more money for surgical than for nonsurgical treatments. For example, ceseren section is profitable, vaginal delivery is not. Under these circumstances, hospital administrators could urge physicians to perform more surgery than they would otherwise. Some surgeons also may choose to specialize in profitable DRG areas, such as breast surgery. There is no easy solution to this difficult ethical problem; however, quality assurance programs are intended to look for these types of abuse. In addition, the consumer generally will not tolerate poor care and therefore the free enterprise system should be on the side of the competent practitioner.

The Growing Elderly Population

Caring for the Elderly

Today the elderly comprise about 11% of the population of the United States. By the year 2030 the projection is that this number will reach 21%, with 64.5 million individuals over 65 and nearly half of these over age 75. There is already the prediction that Medicare will be bankrupt in the next decade, and such predictions have led to many of the alternate forms of health care for the elderly but does not provide benefits for extended long-term care in nursing homes or at home. Medicaid, which provides short-term care for many poor, is the primary source for long-term institutional care of the elderly. As a result of overlapping responsibilities, neither the poor nor the elderly are served adequately. Little has been done to train physicians to meet the needs of an expanding elderly population. Much has been written about the need to prepare medical students to treat the elderly and deal effectively with their medical problems. The Institute of Medicine, after a comprehensive study, recommended that medical education in geriatrics be integrated throughout the curriculum. There have been isolated attempts to meet those objectives. However, only 2.2% of the medical students graduating in 1984 had had any geriatric training in their third or fourth year, even though these are the years when they interact with older patients. A body of knowledge has developed about surgery in the elderly and attitudes about operating on older people.

A half century ago, most surgeons were cautious about operating on the elderly in the belief that older age per se carried increased surgical risk. However, even in the late 1930s, some surgeons had begun to question whether this opinion was entirely justified. Age is still a factor in the surgical decision process, and operative risk in the elderly is complex. Emergency surgery for all ages carries a greater risk than operating electively for the same disease. In addition, coexisting disease increases with age. Thus increased surgical risk with age can be attributed in part to multiple pathology, more advanced diseases, and more frequent emergency surgery. At the same time, biologic variability increases with age. Functions of various organs change at differing rates in different individuals. There are indications that many individuals who live into extreme old age are biologically elite and have more physical resistance to illness. Age does, however, take its toll, and some physiologic changes occur with normal aging, such as renal function, glucose tolerance, vital capacity of the lungs, lean muscle mass, and cellular immunity. Many other functions do not change. For example, laboratory results for hematocrit, serum electrolytes, and urinalysis are not influenced by age in important ways. A treatable disease may be overlooked if an abnormal finding on such a test is attributed to age alone.

A positive factor for surgery in the elderly is often age, in that older patients are survivors. Some might assume that once a person reached life expectancy that little needs to be done to extend life. Survival to advanced age, however, predicts more survival. Life expectancy at birth is 71.9 years, and even at 80, it is 7.6 years. Anyone who escapes the killer diseases of middle and early old age has demonstrated durability. Numerous studies in surgery suggest that good results can be obtained in operating on the elderly when they are properly managed.

At the same time that surgeons should not be reluctant to operate on the elderly when indicated, heroic measures to extend life through surgery for patients who are terminally ill is a different issue. Sometimes this is done without enough thought as to whether the result will enhance the overall quality of life left to the individual. Surgery may, in fact, make the time left less rewarding. Operations in the elderly can be classified as those expected to result in complete restoration of health, those aimed at diminishing disability, and those aimed at achieving a limited postponement of inevitable death. When considering questions that postpone inevitable death, one should evaluate carefully the chance of improving quality of life as well as survival.

Principles of good surgical care are not specific to the elderly. Careful preoperative assessment and planning can help avoid later problems. Assessment of the older patient should include treating systems that can be improved before surgery or preventing and correcting problems that might lead to an emergency operation later, keeping the patient mobile and out of bed as much as possible, and preparing the patient for postoperative events. In the operative management stage there is less to do that is influenced by age of the patient. The surgeon needs to work closely with the anesthesiologist to plan the operation. Care in handling the tissue is always important, but even more so in older patients who have reduced vascular supply and diminished ability to heal. The postoperative time can be a time of increased risk. The surgeon may be intent on getting the older patient through surgery safely, and then relax attention. During the postoperative stage, vital signs of the older patient need to be checked frequently, extremes of therapy should be avoided, signs of mental confusion monitored, and activity and rehabilitation initiated early.

Thus geriatric patients can do very well with all types of surgical procedures. However, they tolerate complications relatively poorly and are at risk when surgery is done on an emergency basis. With the increased pressure of PROs to reduce admissions, unnecessary surgery, and hospital expenditures, there is some danger that the elderly may suffer in regard to quality care.

Caring for the Dying

Worchester, in his elegant book *The Care of the Aged, the Dying and the Dead*, wrote that ''one of my medical school professors was Oliver Wendell Holmes. I have not forgotten his insistence that, while one of the physician's functions is to assist at the coming-in, another is to assist at the going-out.'' The physician plays a central role in the emotional as well as the physical care of the dying patient. The importance of the doctor in caring for the terminally ill was recognized long ago by Osler. Traditionally it was the family physician who helped the patient make the transition between life and death, while offering support and comfort to the patient's family as well. However, the technological advances in medicine, including the development of hospitals and nursing homes, as well as changes in the family structure, have resulted in patients sometimes being isolated from others in their last few weeks of life. Patients are now more likely to die in hospitals than at home, and medicine in highly specialized hospitals sometimes focuses more on cure than care.

Specific measures to help the dying must be tailored to meet each patient's needs. The physician must often decide whether to tell the patient about expected impending death. Even when the dying person suspects that death might occur, the pronouncement itself is unsettling. There is no hard and fast rule that all patients must be told: some want to know; others do not. The clue generally comes from the patient. Does the patient ask about what is expected? Does the patient persist in questioning what is going to happen? If so, the patient probably wants to know.

At the same time it should be recognized that the physician is not omniscient. Even though there may be little doubt that a condition is fatal, it is difficult (if not impossible) to predict how long a person will live. Therefore some uncertainty about time of death and some hope for life can be maintained, even in the face of dying. Just because a patient does not ask about impending death does not mean he or she is unaware about what is happening.

Listening with empathy may be all that is required. For a busy physician, no more than this may realistically be possible. It does not require firsthand knowledge of an experience to share another person's feelings. One may never have gone around the world, but it is not difficult to celebrate the anticipation of such a venture with another person. In a similar way, one can empathize with sorrow, depression, fear, expectation, or any other emotion expressed by the dying. It is the human contact and the relationship that matters most, and it is wrong to close off avenues for listening or discussing feelings by telling patients that they should not feel as they do or trying to reassure them that they are not dying.

When dying takes some time, there is a tendency to isolate the person as if he or she were already dead. Nurses and attendants may answer calls more slowly and less time is spent with the patient. Physicians and nurses sometimes talk in the presence of the patient as if he or she could not hear or understand. Even families may visit less often, becoming more involved in putting their life together, as if the dying relative were already gone. Although the family must do this eventually, the tendency to initiate the process before the person dies, because it excludes the dying, may be seen by the patient as abandonment.

Lastly, communicating without words is always possible. A touch and a smile from the physician can mean a lot to the patient. Sometimes simply sitting by the patient without talking is supportive. Talk may not be necessary—the comfort of having someone who cares nearby cannot be overestimated. Touching the patient lightly on the arm should convey one's feelings and reassure the person that he or she is touchable and that communication and understanding exist, even at this most basic level.

Being prepared to care for the dying is part of the physician's role. There is a delicate balance between doing this and the ethical questions facing the medical profession today concerning choice of expensive treatments and extension of life through mechanical or resuscitative efforts.

Bioethics

Institutional Ethics Committees (IECs)

Advances in medical technology, in combination with economics, force hard decisions on physicians and consumers of health care. Political, legal, and public policy factors interact in decisions. Forces like cost containment, fear of malpractice suits, concern over access to health care (in particular, for the poor and uninsured), and the aging of the population have opened up areas of concern. Although ethical decisions are not new problems, there are new and changing ones to be addressed. IECs have been established to help with the increasing number of bioethical considerations. IECs are usually composed of a multidisciplinary group of health care professionals who address ethical dilemmas that occur in an institution. The advantages of IECs have been cited as providing education, a forum for sharing concerns, and a place for more rapid and sensitive responses than found in judicial reviews. Some concerns have been expressed that IECs could become burdensome, act as rubber stamps, engender privacy and liability problems, and cause procedural issues related to who convenes and attends meetings or selects cases for review. Surgeons, particularly cardiac, neurologic, and pediatric surgeons, are faced with ethical dilemmas. Transplant surgery was one of the first treatments to raise ethical concerns. The issues of informed consent, incompetent patients, and emergency situations where decisions must be made quickly are some of the difficult areas that accompany the practice of surgery.

Informed Consent

Informed consent for clinical studies and surgical informed consent have been of increasing interest over the past few decades. A number of issues have arisen. It is well recognized and accepted that patients need a full explanation of what is to be done and the possible adverse effects from their participation in a project or from their acceptance of a surgical procedure. To protect the patient's rights, most institutions have established a human rights committee that reviews all research proposals involving humans to determine if the patients have been advised adequately of the details of the study, the risks involved, alternate treatments, and any potential benefits. The review committees are composed of both professional (medicine, law, clergy, or health care providers) and lay representatives. The question of whether a patient's relatives can sign for the patient has been debated and is still not resolved completely from a legal standpoint. In surgical consent, the urgency of the need for surgery may dictate that someone else sign the informed consent when the patient cannot. The issue of legal competency can enter into the determination when the patient appears to be confused. If the confusion is a result of some acute process, the decision about competency may be less well defined than when a patient has a diagnosis of dementia or when a court-appointed guardian is available. Even with a diagnosis of dementia or other psychiatric disorder, the degree of confusion and cognitive ability are not easy to assess without a psychiatric consultation. Therefore, in the absence of a legal guardian, the diagnosis alone is not enough to establish competency. Another problem that can arise concerns patients who object to certain procedures or to receiving blood because of religious beliefs. Usually the surgeon and the patient can reach some agreement. There is more of an issue when parents object about a possible lifesaving operation on a child and no agreement can be reached. It has sometimes been necessary to involve the court in such decisions.

Experiments in Surgery

Sometimes it is difficult to distinguish between medical research and human experimentation. Some would agree that all research involves experimentation. The artificial heart program, the transplantation of a baboon heart, and the implantation of an unauthorized artificial heart have caused controversies related to surgical experimentation. Fetal surgery raises a number of ethical questions related to the ambiguous status of the fetus and the fact that performing surgery on the fetus goes through the mother as well. Concerns have been raised about the quality of informed consents and whether the experiments were subjected to review by an IEC. As vague as the distinctions are between research and therapy, voluntary informed consent should be sought for both. Whether an innovative treatment is research or therapy, disclosure to the patient is necessary. Risks and benefits are explained and patients informed of alternate therapies. If the proposed procedure departs even slightly from a standard procedure, the patient needs to know. If the physician has a good relationship with the patient, the patient will have confidence in the doctor and is not likely to refuse. Surgeons and their patients benefit from taking a scientific approach to new surgical techniques. If there is conformity to high standards, there is a better chance of avoiding ethical problems.

Access to Care

Medical and surgical care in the United States has been judged by the society and Federal Government to frequently be overused and overly expensive. Cost containment is the ultimate goal of the regulatory pressures imposed on hospitals, physicians, and finally the patients. The closing of hospitals and reduction in beds is not a byproduct of the system, but the intent. With the closure of beds as a target, some consumers will ultimately be turned away. It is hoped that this pressure will also reduce the length of stay (LOS) for patients by hospitals increasing their efficiency. There are already questions about operations for the elderly, with suggestions that one-third of the procedures may be unnecessary, and therefore second opinions could be recommended for any operations on the elderly. Death, of course, is the ultimate economy. The longer patients survive, the more costly their care. Surgeons often find ways of prolonging life. The patient comes to the surgeon believing that the surgeon has no hidden agenda. The patient is entitled to a professional opinion that is independent of cost containment problems or the hospital's need to reduce the days of care.

Obligation to Treat

AIDS represents a problem traditional to medicine. It raises questions about the obligations of physicians and surgeons to deal with an epidemic disease. Many health care professionals fear they will be at risk. There are also value-related issues concerning morality and drug abuse. In some cases, physicians and nurses have refused to care for AIDS patients. Medical history reveals a similar situation related to treatment of plague victims. There was a strong belief that physicians had an obligation to care for patients, even at the risk of their own lives. Yet, even then, many physicians left their profession or country to avoid being involved. Some of the prestige associated with medicine came from public perception that physicians and surgeons were willing to risk their lives to care for the sick. This problem has not been faced to any extent by physicians in recent years until the emergence of AIDS. There is a strong cultural obligation in this country to help those who need help, particularly among those who have identified themselves with a helping profession. AIDS is an ethical problem that is as old as medicine itself.

Guidelines for the Terminally Ill

Medical science and technology have increased life expectancy. Machines are capable of keeping hearts and respiratory functions going after destruction of the brain. Death can now be defined. Deliberate decisions can be made about death. This has generated interest in patients' desires about dying and control of their own destiny. Death with dignity is frequently mentioned, but the law regarding death and dying has failed to provide the answers. Ethical issues about limiting treatment often focus on technical interventions, such as mechanical ventilation. Many less dramatic therapies are considered routine, and ethical aspects of their use may be less closely examined. Nutritional support can be important in frail elderly patients, yet

appropriate use of nutritional therapy must consider the circumstances of the patient. Where severe underlying illnesses cannot be reversed, technical means of providing nutrition can represent extraordinary rather than ordinary means of prolonging life. In regard to issues in medical care, physicians need to be aware of their obligations and the patients' rights under state judicial decisions and natural death acts. Some guidelines have been suggested. Physicians may wish to implement steps to shield themselves from liability while respecting the wishes of their patients. It is important to discuss treatment choices that may arise in an illness with patients at the outset of treatment while they can understand and communicate a choice. If there is a question of a patient's capacity to make an informed decision, a psychiatric consultation may be needed. All discussions with patients regarding their treatment should be recorded. If the patient is not competent to make decisions, family can assist in arriving at consensus about treatment. Also, IECs can help in resolution of the issues.

Obligation to Resuscitate

The use of cost containment criteria for health policies may push decisions that are economically attractive but ethically unacceptable. Two major reasons are often given for do-not-resuscitate (DNR). One is futility and the other is the patient's wishes. There may also be another underlying economic reason that implies that certain patients or classes of patients may not be worth the cost. Resuscitation usually means efforts to save an individual from death. It carries some uncertainty about its success. There is clearly no question about intervening when a patient in a restaurant is choking. However, there may be a question about attempting resuscitation of a patient with massive cerebrovascular accidents. Some guidelines can be set. The wishes of the patient should be respected and sought out ahead of time if possible. Economics cannot be the basis for a decision. Age or other demographics should not be the determining factor. The wishes of the patient and the possibility of successful outcome should guide decisions.

Quality of Care

Providing quality care is the physician's primary ethical obligation. Quality is difficult to measure, and measurements are often challenged as to their precision and application. Probably the most important indicator of quality is patient outcome. One cannot simply compare patient outcomes between different hospitals or systems of care, however, because patient outcomes result from the interaction between severity of illness and quality of care. Therefore, unless one first adjusts for the effect of differences in severity of illness between groups being compared, the differences in outcome will not truly reflect differences in quality of care alone.

There is a greater need than ever before to monitor and preserve quality of care as cost containment procedures reduce the health care costs. Pressures to change delivery and financing of care could have adverse effects, because it is unlikely that higher quality will be obtained for less cost. Cost containment means fewer services. Cutting back on some services may not result in poor quality of care; in some instances care might even be improved. However, some types of reductions could lower quality.

The role of students in providing surgical care is related to the question of quality. Students need to be involved in the surgical care of patients as part of the learning process. Students should be members of the surgical team. Having students participate as part of the surgical team has been shown to improve patient satisfaction with care and the overall quality of care. This is probably because students have more time to spend with the patient and can be an advocate for the patient. It is also likely to be related to the fact that the rest of the team is called on to teach and review aspects of care that might not otherwise be done. One person, usually the attending surgeon, is in charge of the patient and responsible to see that no one on the team does anything that is not within his or her ability. The ratio of learning to doing is greater for the student than for other members of the team. With each succeeding year of training, the amount and extent of procedures performed are greater than the year before. The range of surgical skills performed by students can vary to some degree between students and within different hospitals and is often related to the philosophy of the clerkship and its objective within an institution. Some basic skills are important for all students to understand and be able to perform. Most clerkships make these skills explicit to students at the beginning of the clerkship, and students are observed as to whether they can perform these tasks. Students often say that they do too much "scut work," such as holding retractors or changing dressings. This is sometimes true, and a balance between repeating less challenging tasks and learning new level skills must be achieved. Also, it is generally believed that students do more with nonprivate patients than they do with private patients. This also may be true; however, students should never do more than they are trained to do. The physician in charge of the patient is the one who must decide on the limits of what each member of the team can do.

Because cost is part of quality, students should learn the cost of various tests and procedures. They need to know that only those tests that make a difference in care should be ordered. Unnecessary tests add to the cost of care and often to the discomfort of the patient. If the results of the test can change the process of care or establish the diagnosis, then the test can be justified. Ordering tests as a routine without thinking about how the results will be used is unwarranted.

The surgical service has been a leader in quality of care with their morbidity and mortality conferences. Long before peer review procedures became an established routine, all patients with adverse outcomes (complications or deaths) were reviewed by the surgical staff in conferences usually held on a monthly basis. The objective of the conferences is to critically review the process of care, determine preventable or avoidable problems, and learn from these. These ongoing reviews have done much to advance the practice of surgery. The conferences are a central part of the learning process for students, who are helped to focus on patient outcome as the end result of care. Students can also contribute to the conference because, as members of the team, they often see the patient from a slightly different perspective than other members of the team.

Closely related to quality is the possible deterioration in the doctor-patient relationship. Patient satisfaction has always been one indicator of quality. If physicians increase their involvement in organized groups, there could be conflict between commitment to an organization and allegiance to the patient. There is a danger that physicians' obligations to organized groups will not be compatible with preserving patient trust. Patients may lose faith in the relationship that has traditionally existed, and this would influence quality of care.

The emphasis on quality of surgical care at this time is on utilization review more than quality review based on outcome. Contract medicine will reduce the number of elective surgical procedures. Studies have already shown reductions up to 25%. Furthermore, patterns of postoperative care will be influenced further by hospital bed utilization, with length of stays reduced, even after major procedures. There is the chance for increased postoperative morbidity and mortality. Surgeons may see more complications as a result of delayed surgical procedures. Decreases in elective cholecystectomies could increase common duct explorations, or delayed hernia repair could lead to more strangulated hernias.

It has always been important to monitor quality of care to ensure that care provided meets expected standards. Surgeons can be justifiably proud that they lead all other physicians in recognizing the importance of such monitoring. In the face of a changing health care environment, monitoring quality of care becomes even more important than ever before in the history of medicine.

SUGGESTED READINGS

Abramowitz KS: *The Future of Health Care Delivery in America.* New York, Stanford C Bernstein & Co, 1985.

Cope RDT, Coe RM, Rossman I (ed): *Fundamentals of Geriatric Medicine.* New York, Raven Press, 1983.

Dickey NW: Withholding or withdrawing treatment. *JAMA* 256:471, 1986.

Ginzberg E: The destabilization of health care. *N Engl J Med* 315:757–761, 1986.

Gray B (ed): *For-Profit Enterprise in Health Care.* Washington, DC, National Academy of Sciences Press, 1986.

Weisman AD: *On Dying and Denying.* New York, Behavioral Publication, 1972.

Skills _____

Translate the following:

1. Since initiation of PPS, hospitals have reduced LOS because of DRGs. Furthermore, their admissions are controlled by UR using PRO.

2. In the competitive medical market, HMOs (staff and group with open and closed panel systems) have proliferated.

3. PPOs have lock-in EPOs as well as no lock-in features and PCNs are the gatekeepers.

4. If DNR orders are not followed, the IEC may question the management.

Study Questions _____

1. What led to the sharp escalation of health care costs in the United States?

2. Explain the PPS approach to cost containment.

3. What organization is responsible for monitoring physician behavior in regard to hospital admissions, necessary operations, and quality of care?

4. Why is care of the elderly an issue in cost containment?

5. What are the considerations in the decision to operate on elderly patients?

6. What are the guidelines that could help you decide if a patient should be told he or she is dying, and what are some of the ways in which physicians can help a dying patient?

7. What is the role of IECs?

8. Why is AIDS an ethical issue?

9. In what ways are surgeons involved in ethical issues?

10. In what ways do cost containment methods threaten the quality of care?

2

Evaluation of Surgical Patients

Richard M. Bell, M.D.
Paddy M. Bell, C.S.T.
Pamela A. Rowland-Morin, Ph.D.
Kenneth W. Burchard, M.D.

ASSUMPTIONS

The student has successfully completed a basic course in physical diagnosis.

OBJECTIVES

1. Discuss the importance of adequate history and physical examination of surgical patients.
2. List and discuss the essential elements of a patient's medical history in a surgical emergency.
3. Name the four categories of postoperative changes in pulmonary function and discuss their clinical significance in assessing patient risk.
4. Discuss at least 10 factors that predispose patients to pulmonary complications, including recognition and management of each.
5. Describe at least four types of pulmonary function tests, including their limitations in quantifying postoperative pulmonary risk.
6. List and discuss the factors in a patient's medical history that might indicate heart disease.
7. Contrast the uses and limitations of Goldman's classification system in evaluating perioperative risk for cardiac patients.
8. Describe preoperative preparation of patients with a history of rheumatic fever.
9. Name five metabolic abnormalities that can change the surgical approach or preoperative preparation of a patient. Discuss risk factors associated with the problems and appropriate management for each.
10. List at least six sequelae of chronic renal failure and describe preoperative evaluation and preparation methods designed to minimize operative risk to the chronic renal failure patient.

The most important and frequently used physician skill is the ability to extract an adequate history from the patient and perform a thorough physical examination. The importance of this skill is not only the diagnosis of the surgical disease but also the determination of the risk of surgical intervention. Surgical judgment is based on an analysis of the risk-benefit ratio, and this analysis begins with an accurate data base. As the age of the population increases, many surgical patients have coexisting medical problems that may complicate their care. More importantly, many of these coexisting problems have a direct bearing on morbidity and mortality. Surgery and anesthesia profoundly alter normal physiologic and metabolic states, and the patient's ability to respond appropriately to these changes should be the physician's primary concern. More often than not, perioperative complications are the result of failure in the preoperative period to identify underlying medical problems or failure to take adequate preventive measures. Complications are best prevented rather than treated; therefore it is the responsibility of the physician to minimize the risks that the patient assumes. Such preventive foresight begins with information gleaned from a careful history and physical examination. Sophisticated laboratory studies or specialized testing are no substitute, as these diagnostic tools have merit mainly in confirming clinical suspicions.

The inexperienced medical student who is first encountering surgical diseases must develop an understanding of what is normal and the normal variants. These skills are learned through careful observation and repeated exposure. Each patient represents a unique situation for study of the normal and abnormal responses to the stress of illness and surgery. Attention to detail will help the student build the foundation for a keen diagnostic mind and prepare the patient for the physiologic insult that attends the illness and its treatment.

This chapter is not a complete review of how to perform a history and physical examination. It is assumed that the student has completed a course in physical diagnosis. This discussion is instead a review of those elements in a patient's history or finding on the physical examination that may influence operative risk. Such analysis forms the basis of surgical judgment, i.e., weighing the pros and cons of anticipated therapy. The student is referred to other chapters for the signs and symptoms of specific surgical diagnosis.

Improving Communications

The doctor-patient relationship is an essential part of quality care as it relates to patient satisfaction. Good interviewing techniques can help to establish a good doctor-patient relationship. Students need to learn interviewing skills early in their medical careers. Part of good interviewing comes from a general concern about people. Part of good interviewing relies on skills that can also be learned. Effective interviewing can be challenging to the surgeon because of the variety of settings in which interviews can occur. These can be the operating room, the surgical intensive care unit, private offices, hospital bedsides, emergency rooms, and outpatient clinics. Each setting has its own peculiar requirements to achieve quality communication. For good doctor-patient relationships, surgeons must adjust their styles to their environment as well as to the personalities and requirements of the patients. Some basic rules are common to all professional interviews. These include paying attention to personal appearance so that you present a professional image that inspires confidence; establishing eye contact; communicating interest, warmth, and understanding; being nonjudgmental and accepting of the individual as a person; and helping the person feel comfortable in talking with you.

When the patient is seen in an ambulatory setting, the first few minutes should be concentrated on greeting the patient; using his or her formal name; shaking hands; introducing yourself and explaining your role; attending to privacy; adjusting conversational skill and level of vocabulary; eliciting attitude about coming to the clinic; finding out what the patient does for work; and determining what the patient knows about the nature of his problem. The next step involves exploring the problem and moves from more open-ended to closed-ended questions that help to focus the interview. The use of transitions, specific clear questions, and restating the problem for verification are important. Determine, at this point, if there are any questions that the patient may want answered. In the closing phase of the interview, the patient should be told what the next step will be and when the surgeon will examine the individual. Lastly, see that the patient is comfortable.

Most of the techniques used in the ambulatory setting are also appropriate for inpatient encounters. Usually, more time is spent with the patient in the initial and subsequent interviews than in an outpatient setting. Patients are more likely to be in pain, worried about financial problems, concerned about lack of privacy or unpleasant diets, and may have had difficulty sleeping. They may also be fearful about treatment or feel helpless. It is important to communicate the purpose of the interview and how long it will take. Remember that the patient is not only listening to you but also observing your behavior and how you look. Be aware of how the setting affects the interview. A cramped, noisy, crowded environment can influence the quality of communication. Patients may develop negative feelings from insensitivities such as speaking to patients from the doorway, giving or taking personal information in a crowded room, speaking about a patient in the elevator, or speaking to patients without drawing the curtain in a ward.

Although the same interviewing principles apply in the emergency room as in the outpatient and inpatient setting, the emergency room encounter is tremendously condensed. The role of the student in the emergency room is to discover the chief medical complaint, perform a physical examination, and present the findings to the resident or faculty member. Interviewing in the emergency room requires communicating to the patient who you are and how you fit into the team. Ask the patient or family member to briefly describe the problem; ask the patient to concur; focus on the primary medical problem; move from general to specific questions; provide a narrative for the patient; attend to privacy; and be very careful about expressing nonverbal attitudes about the patient or his or her behavior. As you finish the examination, explain what will happen next and approximately how long the patient will have to wait; discuss the patient with the resident or faculty member in a location where the patient cannot hear you or observe nonverbal clues; and guard against any nonprofessional discussion in the emergency room.

Communication with patients is greatly influenced by both verbal and nonverbal behavior. Attention to the techniques outlined can serve to enhance the surgical student's communication skills and will have a profound influence on quality of surgical care, particularly that perceived by patients.

History

A careful history derived from probing questioning of the patient will lead to at least a differential diagnosis in nearly three-fourths of the patients. This underscores the requirement for the student-physician to have a working knowledge of the natural history of surgical disease. The average physician can arrive at the correct diagnosis. The superior physician can determine the preexisting conditions that may complicate management plans. A careful review of systems is essential. Although this chapter does not describe in detail the elements of history taking, those systems whose physiology is directly affected by anesthesia and surgery are considered, so that the student may begin to develop the foundation necessary for accurately assessing operative risk.

Surgical Emergencies

Many surgical emergencies do not provide for the leisurely interrogation of the patient for analysis of the nuances of the medical history. The urgency of the situation should not preclude the obtaining of the essential information. An emergency situation forces the physician to focus on the critical aspects of a history. An ''AMPLE'' history provides the most important elements that may immediately influence surgical care (Table 2-1).

Table 2.1.
AMPLE Medical History

A—allergies
M—medications (current)
P—past medical history
L—last meal
E—events preceding the emergency

For the emergency surgical patient, as well as the elective surgical patient, known sensitivity to drugs is important. The injudicious use of antibiotics or narcotics without an attempt to determine drug sensitivity is ill-advised and has medicolegal implications. Many surgical emergencies, both traumatic and nontraumatic in origin, occur in patients with preexisting medical disease. Many of these (e.g., coronary artery disease, chronic obstructive pulmonary disease, and diabetes) decrease a patient's physiologic reserve and are adversely affected by surgery. Most patients with significant medical problems are under treatment with medications that may have important implications in the perioperative care of the surgical patient. Some drugs adversely interact with anesthetic agents or alter the normal physiologic response to illness, injury, or the stress of surgery. Consider, for example, the hypertensive patient taking an antihypertensive drug that depletes the inherent body stores of catecholamines (e.g., reserpine). This may not only blunt the physiologic response to trauma (increased sympathetic activity) but may seriously limit the pharmacologic support of the patient's blood pressure while under anesthesia.

Because the normal response to the stress of illness or trauma is one of hyperglycemia, this may exacerbate diabetes or make chemical diabetes a condition of clinical significance. Patients with prosthetic heart valves or a history of rheumatic fever *must* be offered antibiotic protection to prevent valve infection or the development of endocarditis. Those individuals with chronic congestive heart failure (CHF) or renal insufficiency must have meticulous attention to fluid and electrolyte imbalance.

Of particular concern to the anesthesiologist is the time of the patient's last meal. A full stomach predisposes to the danger of aspiration of gastric contents during the induction of anesthesia and increases the risk of postoperative pulmonary complications. The history of recent ingestion of food or drink may force significant modifications of the anesthetic technique used, require steps to decompress the stomach, or in some cases postpone surgical intervention until gastric emptying has occurred.

A history of the events preceding the accident or onset of illness may give important clues as to the etiology of the problem, as well as uncovering occult injury or disease. Consider a 48-year-old truck driver who noted the onset of severe substernal chest pain *before* his vehicle struck a bridge abutment. The hypotension exhibited in the emergency department may be related to acute cardiac decompensation from his myocardial infarction, as well as the blood loss associated with his pelvic fracture and midshaft femur fracture. Such a situation might require insertion of a right heart catheter for accurate hemodynamic monitoring and volume restoration, as well as close monitoring in the intensive care unit. Additionally, it should alert the physician to the need for careful monitoring and prophylaxis for cardiac arrhythmia.

Consider the 63-year-old diabetic female who took her usual dose of morning insulin but failed to eat breakfast because of an early appointment in town. At 11:30 AM she collapses while attempting to board a bus, sustaining an intertrochanteric fracture of her right femur. Appropriate resuscitation in this situation requires metabolic support of her hypoglycemia as well as blood volume restoration in preparation for her orthopedic surgical procedure.

Such scenarios, while sounding extreme, are frequently encountered in emergency departments on a daily basis. These historical elements add significantly to the physician's ability to provide optimal care for the patient and therefore must not be overlooked.

Elective Surgical Patients

Fortunately, in most situations the student on a surgical clerkship will have an adequate opportunity for a careful review of systems. This is an opportunity that should be maximized for the sake of the student's education as well as for patient care. Frequently the patient cannot provide details, and the serious investigator must utilize every available resource (e.g., family, friends, emergency medical personnel) to provide the details necessary to solve the riddle.

The evaluation of the elective preoperative patient should include a specific review of the systems, with special emphasis on the patient's ability to respond to the stress of surgery. Clinical suspicions should be investigated by appropriate laboratory or special diagnostic studies. When necessary, specialty consultation should be requested to delineate the degree of medical illness. Such help from our colleagues can provide important information concerning the risk-benefit ratio of a given surgical procedure or suggest therapeutics to minimize perioperative risk. It is foolish to assume that our medical colleagues can "clear" a patient for surgery. The best that can be achieved is an accurate assessment of operative risk. Once accomplished, it is the responsibility of the surgical team in conjunction with the patient and/or the patient's family to determine the advisability of the planned therapeutic approach to the illness.

Because the alterations in normal physiology attendant to surgery and anesthesia are of such importance in the care of the surgical patient and because such information is vital to the assessment of operative risk, these alterations are discussed in detail under specific organ systems. Where applicable, special consideration is given to methods used pre- and postoperatively to minimize complications.

Pulmonary Evaluation

To effectively assess pulmonary function in the surgical patient it is helpful to understand the changes that occur in the patient who undergoes anesthesia. Numerous efforts have been made to quantitate the risk of postoperative pulmonary complications, based on specific abnormalities of spirometry, in the individual with compromised pulmonary function. Unfortunately there is no single predictor of increased risk. The experienced physician makes judgments based on a variety of parameters, including an evaluation of the patient's exercise tolerance, physical findings, and, when indicated, specialized pulmonary function testing.

Postoperative changes in pulmonary function can be classified into four broad categories: 1) changes in lung volumes, 2) changes in ventilatory patterns, 3) changes in gas exchange, and 4) changes in the defense mechanisms of the lung. An understanding of normal physiology is essential to appreciate the effect of anesthesia and surgery. The student is referred to any number of excellent discussions of normal pulmonary physiology if such a foundation is deficient.

A decrease in total lung capacity (TLC) is noted after all surgical procedures on the abdomen. Vital capacity decreases from 25% to 50% (mean 45%) within one to two days postoperatively. The change in vital capacity is greater for upper abdominal and thoracic procedures (55%), compared with those on the lower abdomen (40%). Reserve volume falls by approximately 13% and functional residual capacity (FRC) declines by an average of 20% in the immediate postoperative period. Expiratory reserve volume (ERV) falls by an average of one-third from preoperative levels: 65% in upper abdominal procedures, and 25% in those on the lower abdomen. Coupled with the changes in closing volume that may be present in the patient with already compromised pulmonary function (e.g., obesity or a history of cigarette smoking), the stage is set for postoperative pulmonary dysfunction. Fortunately the changes described are reversible and, as a rule, return to baseline values within one or two weeks postoperatively.

Changes in ventilatory patterns are also pronounced. Within 24 hours tidal volume is decreased by 20%, but respiratory rate is increased by 25%. The net effect for the patient with normal pulmonary function is essentially no change in minute ventilation. Each of these changes generally returns to normal within one to two weeks. Significant changes in pulmonary compliance occur and may be reduced as much as 33%. Normally the average male sighs (a deep inspiratory effort) 10 times per hour. The female sighs about 9 times per hour. This effort normally hyperinflates alveoli and prevents atelectasis. Observations in the animal laboratory and in human clinical experience suggest that FRC falls by 10% when hyperinflation by deep breathing is discontinued. This is thought to be due to small airway closure, especially in lung segments that are in dependent positions of the thorax. Additionally, postoperative ventilatory patterns are altered by sedatives and narcotics used to control pain. Oversedation can depress respiration, centrally ablate the ability to cough and clear secretions, and may promote alveolar collapse.

Gas exchange is directly affected. Arterial saturation and a decline in PaO_2 are seen due to changes in po-

sition and a change in ventilation-perfusion (V/Q) relationship. Areas of the lung with V/Q relationships less than 1 predispose to hypoxemia. In the most dependent portions, particularly in patients who lie supine for long periods, the V/Q relationship in the posterobasal segments may approach 0 secondary to airway closure. Even patients with normal pulmonary function preoperatively may have a decrease in PaO_2 of as much as 33%. The extent of the depression in arterial saturation is related to intrapulmonary shunting, while radiographs of the chest may be normal in this situation. High levels of inspired oxygen contribute to this effect. Filling alveoli with gas mixtures that deplete nitrogen and increase the relative concentration of gases that are actively transported (e.g., oxygen) contributes to atelectasis and physiologic shunting by lowering FRC. This is especially true in segments with small airway collapse or obstruction. The process has been termed *absorption atelectasis*; the end result of this process is perfusion of unventilated pulmonary segments and a return of unoxygenated blood to the left heart, i.e., physiologic shunting (right to left). Our understanding of this phenomenon is not new. As early as 1896, Sachur identified the concept of increased venous admixture and developed the shunt equation to explain hypoxemia, even in the face of a normal $PaCO_2$.

The fourth category of alterations includes those that depress the normal clearing mechanism of the tracheobronchial tree. The cough mechanism is primarily responsible for clearing the upper airway of mucus and inhaled particulate matter. Patients do not cough under anesthesia, and postoperative sedation additionally depresses respiratory drive and inhibits coughing. The lasting effects of neuromuscular blockade weakens the coughing effort. Patients with abdominal or thoracic incisions do not want to cough because it hurts. Normally, mucociliary action clears the lower airway segments, and this mechanism is likewise depressed by anesthetic agents. The drying effect of anticholinergic drugs may change the composition of the mucus itself and make it less effective and difficult to expectorate.

Considering the above changes, one may wonder why every patient who is subjected to a general anesthetic does not develop pulmonary problems in the postoperative period. It is tempting to assume that regional anesthesia would obviate these problems, and that may be true for minor procedures on extremities or those that can be done with very specific regional blockade, e.g., axillary block. Unfortunately, spinal anesthesia is also associated with postoperative pulmonary problems. As a rule, it is not the type of anesthetic agent employed but the circumstances to which patients are exposed, e.g., abdominal procedures, loss of periodic hyperinflation by sighing. Positioning, pain, and sedation are not factors that are alleviated by spinal anesthesia alone.

Overall, the risk of pulmonary complications varies from about 3% to 70% and, as expected, is higher for procedures on the upper abdomen and thorax. Improvements in anesthetic technique and attention to improving pulmonary function pre- and postoperatively have reduced the incidence of respiratory problems, but as much as one-third of all postoperative mortality may still be related directly or indirectly to pulmonary insufficiency. In general, the problems include those of infectious and noninfectious etiology. Pneumonia, exacerbation of chronic bronchitis, and empyema are examples of infectious complications. Atelectasis and pneumonitis secondary to the aspiration of gastric contents are examples of noninfectious complications. Perhaps a third group could be added, those with elements of both, which do not fall clearly into one or the other categories. The etiology is multifactorial. Examples include the adult respiratory distress syndrome (ARDS), a complication that may have infectious components as well as alterations in the basic mechanics of gas exchange at the capillary-alveolar membrane; acute congestive heart failure, related to acute volume overload in a patient with compromised cardiac reserve; or the fat embolism syndrome, an acute pulmonary insult whose etiology remains obscure.

Pulmonary problems can be minimized, and the prudent physician will identify those individuals at increased risk. In general, patients who have obstruction to expiratory flow for any reason are those in greatest jeopardy. They may need specialized pulmonary function studies preoperatively and vigorous preoperative and postoperative pulmonary care for prophylaxis. Table 2-2 lists the categories of conditions known to predispose to both infectious and noninfectious perioperative deterioration of respiratory function.

Cigarette smoking is the leading etiologic agent in chronic bronchitis. Particulate deposition in small airways in addition to the reduced effectiveness of the mucociliary transport mechanism complicate airway cleansing. Smokers also have increased pulmonary secretions secondary to bronchiolar irritation. An eight pack year history appears to be the point at which chronic bronchitis becomes an important component. Smokers also have a closing volume that is higher than normal. It can fall above the end tidal point, and this promotes atelectasis. Because smokers have a relative danger of pulmonary complications 2–6 times greater than the nonsmoker, it is suggested that patients stop smoking at least six weeks before an elective procedure. Evidence suggests that improvements in pulmonary clearance and improvements in small airway disease can be detected at two or four weeks after the cessation of smoking. An immediate effect is the clearance of carboxyhemoglobin, which should improve oxygen transport. Patient compliance with this advice, however, is rare.

Chronic obstructive pulmonary disease (COPD) increases perioperative risk by several factors. As one might expect, hazards are increased based on the severity of the disease. Increased pulmonary secretions, small airway obstruction secondary to mucous plugging, inefficient clearing of secretions, and a general lack of pulmonary reserve predispose the patient to atelectasis and superimposed infection. The patient who is unable to climb one flight of steps without dyspnea or blow out a match at eight inches from the mouth without pursing the lips is a candidate for more sophisticated pulmonary function screening. Another useful bedside test is the loose cough test. A rattle heard through the stethoscope when the patient forcibly coughs is a reliable indicator of underlying pulmonary pathology and warrants investigation.

The asthmatic deserves special attention to prevent bronchospasm. Perioperative stress and many medications, including anesthetic agents, induce bronchoconstriction. It is wise to prepare the asthmatic carefully, ensuring therapeutic levels of bronchodilators preoperatively. Aggressive pulmonary toilet is also indicated.

Patients with a history of occupational exposure to known pulmonary irritants (e.g., silicone, asbestos, textile components) may have significant restrictive disease and a marked reduction in respiratory reserve. Patients who cannot cough or even breathe deeply for any reason (i.e., an altered level of consciousness, neuromuscular disease, paraplegia, weakness from malnutrition) are also at a substantial risk based on the alterations discussed above.

Tracheal intubation promotes direct colonization of the upper airway by Gram-negative organisms and sets the stage for infection. Iatrogenic induction of nosocomial organisms into the tracheobronchial tree by suction catheters passed without attention to aseptic technique are responsible for a significant portion of hospital-acquired infections. The general metabolic derangements listed in Table 2-2 also contribute to a substantially greater pulmonary risk.

Obesity, a prevalent and serious medical problem throughout the country, directly contributes to the impairment of respiratory function. Over 50 million Americans exceed their ideal weight by 10% or more, and as many as 15 million are morbidly obese, i.e., obese to the extent that health is impaired and life expectancy reduced. In simple obesity, FRC and ERV are decreased. Maximum minute ventilation is also decreased, but tidal volume, vital capacity, forced expiratory volume (FEV), and most other functional components remain within normal limits. As weight increases to 50% above ideal weight, a fall in these other parameters is noted as well. The work of breathing increases dramatically, producing an increase in oxygen consumption and carbon dioxide production. The strapping effect of excess adipose tissue on the chest wall and the restriction of diaphragmatic excursion by the weight of abdominal contents when the obese patient is supine, contribute to the reduction in tidal vol-

Table 2.2.
General Factors Predisposing to Pulmonary Complications

Cigarette smoking	Chronic bronchitis
Asthma	Occupational lung disease
Neuromuscular disease	Coma
Obesity	Tracheal intubation
Nutritional depletion	Hypotension
Acidosis	Hypoxemia
Chronic obstructive	Azotemia
pulmonary disease	

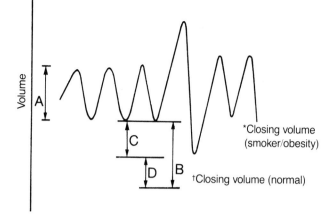

Figure 2.1. Spirometry. **A,** tidal volume; **B,** functional residual capacity; **C,** expiratory reserve volume. **D,** residual volume. *, closing volume (smoker or obesity). +, closing volume (normal).

ume. This results in atelectasis and hypoxemia and contributes to infection. The reduction in ERV is significant, as it may fall below the closing volume of alveoli even during tidal respiration, contributing to further alveolar collapse (Fig. 2.1). Long-standing obesity may result in pulmonary hypertension, due to the increase in pulmonary blood volume and later by hypoxic vasoconstriction. Eventually hypoxemia due to a change in $\dot{V}/\dot{Q}$ relationships and ultimately hypercapnea due to hypoventilation complicate the clinical picture. Even in normal, non-obese patients, ERV, and tidal volume fall postoperatively, as has been discussed. The obese surgical patient, who may have a closing volume that is normally above tidal ventilation, may be further compromised by anesthesia or an abdominal incision.

Age also appears to be a risk factor for pulmonary difficulties. With increasing age there is a progressive decline in static lung volumes, maximum expiratory flow, elastic recoil, and a fall in PaO_2 due to an increase in the alveolar-arterial oxygen gradient. The net effect is a loss of pulmonary reserve. Age itself should not be a contraindication to surgical intervention, but these normal changes with the aging process should be considered. If underlying pulmonary disease is present, spirometry may be used to document the degree of impairment for which aggressive preventive measures may be instituted preoperatively to reduce the risk.

The search for a method to quantify the risks of postoperative pulmonary problems has not met with much success. Spirometry has been able to identify specific abnormalities of the components of respiratory physiology, but the extrapolation to a specific assessment of operative morbidity and mortality from a pulmonary standpoint has not been successful. Maximum breathing capacity (MBC) less than 50% of the predicted value has failed to identify which patients would survive an operative procedure and which would not, even though a mortality rate approaching 50% in patients with an abnormal MBC has been reported. Forced expiratory volume at 0.5 sec ($FEV_{0.5}$) of less than 60% of predicted fares no better as a single predictor.

A combination of a normal MBC and electrocardiogram in one study indicated that if both were normal, the risk of mortality postoperatively was less than 5%. If both were abnormal and age was greater than 40 years, mortality rose to over 70%. Evaluation of other components of pulmonary functions, maximum midexpiratory flow (MMEF), functional ventilatory capacity (FVC), and $FEV_{1.0}$ sec, indicate that if all three components are normal, the risk of pulmonary complications is approximately 3%. With one or more abnormal components, the risk rises to 70%. Some patients with abnormal studies, however, will have no pulmonary complications. Although these may be sensitive indicators, they are not specific. Even attempts to grossly quantitate risk factors into four groups (1, very low risk; 2, low risk; 3, high risk; 4, very high risk) have not been successful. As one might imagine, either end of the spectrum is easily identified. The problem arises in trying to separate the middle two groups. Arterial blood gas analysis has fared no better in specifically sorting out these patients. PaO_2 of less than 50 and/or $PaCO_2$ of greater than 45, while suggesting severe underlying pulmonary disease, cannot stand alone as indicators of operative risk or be used to determine inoperability.

Now that the limitations of pulmonary function studies have been briefly discussed, who is a candidate for them and what do they provide in the way of assessing operative risk? Any patient with significant abnormalities in respiratory function found on routine physical examination (i.e., dyspnea at rest, positive loose-cough test, inability to blow out the match) *may* benefit from preoperative screening if such information would lead to a decision to postpone or even modify a patient's course of therapy. Pulmonary function studies that potentially uncover or quantitate a condition that can be improved in the preoperative period and lessen the risk of postoperative problems are cost effective and justifiable.

Cardiac Evaluation

The preoperative patient with known or suspected heart disease faces additional risk. Because the danger of a postoperative myocardial infarction for patients with a past history of infarction is between 5 and 10%, and the mortality from such infarction is nearly 50%, a detailed history is essential. The incidence of postoperative myocardial infarction is less than 0.5% in patients without clinically evident heart disease.

As previously suggested, it is impossible for our medicine colleagues to clear a patient for surgery from a cardiac or even a general medical standpoint. Like the surgeon, they can only render an opinion based on an estimate of risk. It then becomes dependent on the surgeon to take the necessary steps to minimize the risk. Elective operative procedures immediately after an acute myocardial infarction carry substantial morbidity and mortality. The incidence of an acute cardiac event or cardiac death is approximately 30% within the first three months and reaches a plateau of approximately 5% thereafter. If possible, elective surgery should be postponed for six months after a myocardial infarction.

The patient with unstable angina should avoid surgery, unless it is for coronary artery bypass. Although the patient with stable angina theoretically should be at increased risk, no clear answer pertaining to the extent of increased operative risk is available for this group. In contrast, patients who have undergone coronary artery bypass have a significantly reduced danger of postoperative infarction compared with the angina group. This risk is estimated to be slightly over 1% with a similar mortality. Common sense dictates that patients with any cardiac history be evaluated carefully, the severity of their disease documented, and maximal myocardial performance be achieved before any operative procedure is undertaken. The value of a careful history and physical examination is apparent.

The surgical patient should be questioned carefully concerning the nature, severity, and location of any chest pain. Dates and details about infarctions, documented or suspected, should be noted. A history of dyspnea on exertion may signify cardiac as well as pulmonary pathology. Other potentially significant clues to heart disease include syncope, palpitations, and arrhythmia. A history of rheumatic heart disease generally requires prophylactic antibiotic therapy, even for minor procedures.

Because many diabetics have significant vascular disease, a history of diabetes should increase the index of suspicion of occult cardiac pathology for this group of patients. In individuals with documented diabetes for a period of 5 or 10 years, 60% have vascular problems. After 20 years, nearly all diabetics may be found to manifest some type of vascular abnormality. Additionally, the risk of mortality for the diabetic after a cardiac ischemic event is higher than the nondiabetic. Silent infarctions, ischemic events without symptoms, have historically been reported in the diabetic population. Extensive investigation will often reveal that such episodes probably involved some atypical symptoms, vague pain, breathlessness, syncope, or the onset of mild congestive failure. The diabetic patient therefore should be viewed with suspicion and presumed to have some degree of cardiovascular abnormality, especially those patients with a long-standing history of the disease.

During the physical examination the student should take special note of the patient's overall status. The vital signs themselves can give notable clues to the status of the cardiovascular system, i.e., tachycardia, tachypnea, or postural changes in blood pressure. Jugular venous distension at 30°, slow carotid pulse upstroke, bruits, edema, and a laterally displaced point of maximum cardiac impulse all suggest some type of cardiac disease. Auscultatory findings suggestive of problems include rubs, third heart sounds, and systolic murmurs. For most students, the deciphering of murmurs is perplexing. The patient with hemodynamically significant aortic stenosis usually has a characteristically harsh holosystolic murmur, a slow carotid pulse upstroke, a displaced primary myocardial impulse

(PMI) secondary to left ventricular hypertrophy (LVH, which may also be seen on electrocardiogram), and poststenotic aortic dilation on chest x-ray. Patients with a history of mitral insufficiency have an increased risk of CHF and arrhythmia postoperatively.

Based on history and physical findings, as well as a few simple laboratory studies, efforts have been made to quantify surgical risk. The most commonly used system, the Dripps–American Surgical Association system, has classified patients in four groups, shown in Table 2.3.

This classification may be useful for determining the multipliers for accounting purposes but offers little in determining the specific risk of a cardiac event in the preoperative period or in helping to quantitate the risk of an elective procedure preoperatively.

Goldman and his associates in 1977 published a prospective study that attempted to quantitate the perioperative hazards of myocardial infarction based on history, physical findings, and simple laboratory data. Multiple factors were recorded, including the type of procedures performed and a general assessment of the patient's overall health status. Correlation and regression analysis then identified eight specific elements associated with an increased perioperative risk of infarction. One nonspecific, general category of patients with a greater chance of infarction was also identified. Statistically, each variable was then assigned a point value (Table 2-4).

Poor general health is generally assumed to reflect severe system disease, blood gas signs of respiratory insufficiency ($PaO_2 < 60$ torr or $PaCO_2 > 50$ torr), electrolyte abnormality ($K < 3.0$ mEq/dL or metabolic acidosis, $HCO_3^- < 20$ mEq/dL), acute or chronic renal failure (creatinine > 3.0 mg/dL or BUN > 50 mg/dL), or hepatic dysfunction (abnormal transaminase or stigmata of chronic liver disease). It may be logical to assume that patients with a combination of risk factors (i.e., chronic renal failure *and* metabolic acidosis) should have additive risk (e.g., 3 points + 3 points = 6). Goldman's work does not address this issue in terms of statistical probability. An analysis of these risk factors is shown in Table 2-5. In each case the danger of nonfatal, as well as fatal, postoperative cardiac complications is significantly greater if the risk factor is present.

From these data, a cardiac risk scale can be constructed (Table 2-5). Less than 25 total points implies minimal risk; however, the threat of serious but nonfatal complications increases over sevenfold between class I and class II and over twice that from class II to class III. Any score above 5 multiplies the risk factor of cardiac death by 10, and with over 26 points the danger of a fatal coronary event becomes so prohibitive that elective surgery should not

Table 2.3.
Dripps–American Surgical Association Classification

Class I	healthy patient: limited procedure
Class II	mild-to-moderate systemic disturbance
Class III	severe systemic disturbance
Class IV	life-threatening disturbance

Table 2.4.
An Assessment of Individual Risk Factor [a]

Factor	Life-Threatening/Nonfatal		Cardiac Death		Points	P
	yes	no	yes	no		
1. 3rd heart sound or JVD	14%	3.5%	20%	1.2%	11	<.001
2. MI in past 6 months	14%	3.7%	23%	1.4%	10	<.001
3. Rhythm other than sinus	10%	3.0%	9%	1.0%	7	<.001
4. >5 PVCs/mm	16%	3.3%	14%	1.4%	7	<.001
5. Age >70	6%	3.0%	5%	0.4%	5	.001
6. Emergency procedure	8%	3.0%	5%	1.0%	4	<.001
7. Hemodynamically significant aortic stenosis	4%	4.0%	13%	1.6%	3	.007
8. Aortic, intra-abdominal, intra-thoracic procedure	7%	1.2%	2.5%	1.4%	3	.007
9. Poor general health	7%	2.0%	4.0%	1.0%	3	.027
Total					53	

[a]Adapted from Goldman L, et al: Multifactorial index of cardiac risk factor in noncardiac surgical procedures. *N Engl J Med* 297:845–850, 1977
JVD, jugular venous distension. MI, myocardial infarction. PVC, premature ventricular contractions.

be considered. Patients who fall into class II or class III probably benefit from a period of medical management for several days prior to elective surgery if possible, but data showing a reduction in fatal as well as nonfatal complications are lacking.

Now armed with such scientific ammunition, students still find themselves struggling to ferret out the significance of these findings in a particular patient. For an individual, the risk of cardiac death postoperatively is either 0% or 100%. The patient dies or doesn't. Unfortunately, in Goldman's study only cardiac risk was evaluated, and overall complications and permanent sequelae attendant to these complications were not considered.

The issue concerning the additional risk imposed by a postoperative noncardiac complication as it may relate to additional cardiac stress has also not been addressed. Despite these limitations, the Goldman index is a sensitive indicator of potential risk, although not always specific. Medicine is still an art and relies heavily at times on judgment. Consider the following qualifications of some of Goldman's points.

Age itself may not be as straightforward a risk factor as one would assume at first glance. The student has no doubt encountered septagenarians who could pass for 50-year olds. The converse is also true. The difference between chronological age and physiologic age may be substantial. There is little question that for emergent intrathoracic and intra-abdominal procedures the surgical risk is directly related to age. For nonemergent or minor procedures the relationship is less clear.

The question of hemodynamic significance of an aortic murmur is often difficult for the experienced clinician, much less the student or surgeon. Many older patients have aortic murmurs, and which of these patients deserves special attention preoperatively is confusing. Efforts at cost containment preclude every patient who is found to have a wisp of turbulent flow

on physical examination from having preoperative 2-D ECHO studies or cardiac catheterization. A reliable indicator of hemodynamic significance may be made by a quantitative estimate of the patient's exercise tolerance. A history of dyspnea when climbing a few flights of stairs or other stigmata of aortic valvular disease, such as exertional angina or syncope, suggest the need for careful preoperative evaluation. Loud murmurs, grade III or IV, are significant until proven otherwise.

Any abnormality on a routine electrocardiogram implies increased risk to the adult patient. Rarely, other than an acute myocardial infarction or complete heart block, does the abnormality seen on electrocardiogram require that surgery be postponed or that some presurgical therapy be instituted to modify the aberration in asymptomatic individuals. This includes all types of incomplete heart block and both right and left bundle branch block. In studies in asymptomatic patients, these findings did not correlate with the intra- or perioperative development of complete heart block. The patient with possible cardiac symptoms is another story.

What is not mentioned in Goldman's review may be as important as the risk factors he identified. Preoperative hypertension of mild-to-moderate degrees did not increase the incidence of postoperative infarction, even

Table 2.5.
Cardiac Risk Scale

Class	Points	Potentially Fatal Cardiac Complications[a]	Cardiac Death
I	0–5	0.7%	0.2%
II	6–12	5.0%	2.0%
III	13–25	11.0%	2.0%
IV	>26	22.0%	56%

[a]Postoperative myocardial infarction, pulmonary edema, ventricular tachyarrhythmia.

in those patients taking B-blockers or other antihypertensive medication. Again, only the risk of postoperative infarction was evaluated. The study did not include other less dramatic problems such as electrolyte abnormalities, arrhythmias other than ventricular tachycardia, or hypotension. In general terms, B-blockers should be continued up to the surgical procedure and in the postoperative period as well. Sudden discontinuation of the drugs may precipitate arrhythmias or intraoperative myocardial ischemia in those patients who are taking them for their myocardial preservation effects. Those rebound symptoms, though not as common as originally thought, generally have a peak occurrence at four to seven days after drug discontinuation.

Mild chronic congestive failure was not shown to be associated with an increased occurrence of perioperative infarction. Patients with cardiomegaly on chest x-ray or even those whose clinical course was effectively managed with diuretics or cardiac glycosides do not represent high-risk groups. An abnormal third heart sound or signs of jugular venous distension do indicate decompensation of cardiac function, and these patients are in jeopardy of serious cardiac complications. Digitalis, however, is a drug with a very narrow therapeutic-toxic ratio. Surgical patients frequently are unable to take fluids orally and have multiple tubes removing fluids rich in electrolytes. This predisposes to electrolyte aberrations and further narrows the toxic-therapeutic range.

The patient with a history of rheumatic fever or one who has a prosthetic heart valve requires preoperative antibiotic prophylaxis. The American Heart Association has made the recommendations listed in Table 2-6. In addition to the hemodynamic changes that may attend significant valvular dysfunction, prevention of superimposed endocarditis or seeding of prosthetic valves must be given attention. When in doubt about the history of rheumatic fever, it is better to prevent rather than treat a potential complication. Antibiotic prophylaxis probably should be given to any patient who has had any type of prosthetic device implanted. This includes the patients with prosthetic hip joints, vascular grafts, or other hardware implanted for medical reasons.

While any cardiac abnormality may impose increased risk, the perioperative use of Swan-Ganz catheter monitoring and identification of the high-risk patient may dictate the additional care necessary to assist the patient through an uneventful recovery. Overall risks of fatal and life-threatening cardiac complications have been quantified, but lesser risks have not been as well defined. Careful attention to any abnormality found on preoperative evaluation will help reduce the risk of even minor problems, which can prolong hospital stay or be a source of concern for patients, families, and physicians.

Metabolic Abnormalities

Five abnormal metabolic situations may alter the surgical approach to a particular problem or require extra preoperative preparation. These include diabetes,

Table 2.6.
Endocarditis Prophylaxis in Surgical Patients with a History of Rheumatic Fever or Prosthetic Heart Valves

Rheumatic fever: surgery of upper respiratory tract/dental procedures
  a. Aqueous penicillin G 1 mil units with procaine penicillin 0.6 mil units i.m., 30–60 min preop plus penicillin V 500 mg p.o. g6hx8
or
  b. Penicillin V 2.0 gm p.o. 30–60 min preop with 500 mg p.o. g6hx8
or
  c. Erythromycin 1.0 gm p.o. 60–90 min preop with 500 mg p.o. g6hx8
or
  d. Vancomycin 1 g i.v. over 30 min, 30–60 min preop followed by erythromycin as in c
Prosthetic valves
  e. Penicillin or as in a, plus streptomycin 1 gm i.v. 30 min preop
or
  f. As in d, plus streptomycin as in e
Gastrointestinal, genitourinary, or procedures of instrumentation
  g. Aqueous penicillin G 2.0 mil units i.m. or i.v.
or
  h. Ampicillin 1.0 gm i.m. or i.v.
or
  i. Gentamycin 1.5 mg/kg (max, 80mg) i.m. or i.v.
or
  j. Streptomycin as in e
or
  k. Vancomycin as in d, plus streptomycin as in e

disorders of thyroid function, hepatic dysfunction, adrenal insufficiency, and malnutrition. They are summarized briefly in the following sections.

Diabetes

The diabetic is at increased risk in the perioperative period from a number of perspectives, particularly *1)* metabolic (hyper- or hypoglycemia), *2)* cardiovascular, and *3)* infection. Those requiring insulin for control must have their insulin dose adjusted to compensate for periods when food is not allowed or when the hyperglycemic response to the stress of illness, surgery, or trauma becomes clinically significant. Diabetics previously controlled by diet or oral agents may require insulin in the perioperative period for the reasons mentioned above. Infectious etiologies of surgical disease or infectious problems postoperatively may promote hyperglycemia and even ketoacidosis. Overzealous insulin administration, on the other hand, may lead to hypoglycemia, perhaps the worst management error in the surgical care of the diabetic patient.

Type I diabetics, previously known as juvenile diabetics, are usually insulin deficient, very insulin sensitive, and prone to ketoacidosis. Blood sugar may be quite labile and enormous variations in blood sugar are frequent. The adult onset diabetic, type II, is usually insulin resistant, generally obese, has a variable degree of insulin sensitivity, and is not usually prone to ketoacidosis. It has become common practice to regulate the type I diabetic with intravenous glucose and insulin drips (1–3 units/hr) in the perioperative period when patients can take nothing by mouth. Type II insulin-requiring diabetics are usually managed by giving one-half the usual dose of long-acting insulin on the morning of surgery with a continuous infusion of dextrose and supplemental insulin when needed, based on frequent blood sugar determinations. Finger stick determinations of blood sugar on the ward have replaced the "sliding scale insulin" regime based on the degree of glycosuria. The correlation between blood sugar and urine sugar is not reliable in all cases, especially in older patients.

The cardiac effects of diabetes have been previously discussed. The incidence of vascular abnormalities found on physical examination increases with age and the duration of the diabetes. Males with diabetes may have twice the risk of cardiovascular mortality as their nondiabetic counterparts. Females have as much as four times the risk. Tachycardia for unexplained reasons may be present in the diabetic, thought secondary to autonomic cardiac neuropathy. Often this is associated with orthostatic hypotension without an appropriate increase in pulse. Such findings have been associated with unexplained cardiopulmonary arrest postoperatively.

Gastroparesis, also thought to be due to autonomic neuropathy, may delay gastric emptying and increase the likelihood of aspiration. A splash of fluid heard with the stethoscope over the stomach at a time when the stomach should be empty may require the placement of a nasogastric tube for decompression.

The risk of infection is substantially greater for the diabetic. Hyperglycemia is thought to have an adverse effect on immune function, especially phagocytic activity. The reduced blood flow in those with vascular disease, especially to the extremities, retards wound healing. Because most peripheral vascular disease in the diabetic is small vessel in nature, it is not uncommon to have palpable pulses, even in the face of tissue ischemia. Often the extent of small vessel disease extends deep into the tissue, sparing the skin, much like a cone whose base is directed peripherally and whose apex extends in the central portion of the extremity proximally. Ingrown toenails or minor injuries to the feet in the diabetic are potentially serious problems, frequently leading to amputation or mortality. Therefore even minor procedures on the extremity of the diabetic should be approached with utmost caution.

The surgical diabetic patient should be carefully questioned regarding the duration of the disease, insulin requirements, diet, degree of glucose control, last insulin administration, and peripheral symptoms, i.e, numbness or extremity pain. During the physical examination, special attention should be given to the feet, looking for minor injuries, evidence of poor hygiene, inadequate vascular supply, ulcers, or decreased vibratory sensation. Patients with positive findings should have meticulous care given to foot protection, i.e., daily washing, careful drying, application of softening lotion, protection from minor trauma caused by cradles at the foot of the bed, and avoidance of pressure sores. A careful cardiac history and physical examination should be performed.

The goal of metabolic control in the diabetic patient is a steady state without wide swings in blood glucose concentration. Blood glucose should ideally be kept between 150 and 250 mg/dl. Whatever method of control is chosen, continuous intravenous infusion of glucose and insulin or subcutaneous insulin with glucose infusion, hypoglycemia must be avoided. It is better to keep the diabetic patient a little "too sweet" than to risk the adverse hemodynamic effects of insulin shock.

Abnormalities of Thyroid Function

Signs and symptoms of hyperthyroidism have been described in Chapter 22 and are not to be repeated here. The risk of surgery in the hyperthyroid patient is the risk of thyroid storm. It is often difficult to differentiate the apprehensive preoperative patient from one with signs of hyperthyroidism, as anxiety, nervousness, tachycardia, insomnia, and diaphoresis are nonspecific symptoms. While thyroid storm is most often reported in association with surgery on the thyroid gland itself, it can occur with the induction of anesthesia for procedures outside the neck. The euthyroid state, chemically and clinically, should be achieved before surgery in patients with hyperfunctioning thyroid glands.

In general, hyperthyroid patients are at increased risk for the development of perioperative cardiac arrhythmia. A significant portion will develop atrial fibrillation, which unfortunately is usually resistant to the common cardiac glycosides. Negative nitrogen balance due to a high basal metabolic rate may delay wound healing and alter immune defenses. General muscular weakness may promote pulmonary problems, atelectasis, pneumonia, and difficulty in weaning from the ventilator.

Encounters with patients who are hypothyroid are much less common. Cardiac manifestations of hypothyroidism include reduced contractility and a reduced blood volume, predisposing to hypotension. Respiratory function is altered due to alveolar hypoventilation. Whether the effect is central in origin (i.e., a reduced responsiveness to hypoxia) is unclear. A lower rate of hepatic metabolism reduces drug metabolism and may make the hypothyroid patient very sensitive to narcotics. Pulmonary compliance may be reduced because of secondary obesity.

For a more complete discussion of thyroid disorders, the reader is referred to Chapter 22.

Hepatic Dysfunction

Despite the fact that the liver has an extraordinary amount of reserve and has the ability to regenerate, a significant number of patients (over 15 million individuals) present with evidence of hepatic dysfunction or overt cirrhosis. Usually the etiology is nutritional and secondary to alcohol abuse, but it may also be secondary to an infectious event or idiopathic in nature. General complications and risk of impaired liver function are listed in Table 2-7, and a careful search should be made by the student for these conditions when performing the history and physical examination. Child's criteria have long been used to estimate the risk of nonhepatic surgery in the cirrhotic patient (Table 2-8).

Table 2.7.
Common Problems in the Cirrhotic Patient

Hepatic Dysfunction	H&P Clues	Perioperative Effects/Complications
Drug metabolism	Nonspecific	Sensitivity to narcotics, oversedation, respiratory depression
Protein synthesis	Spider angioma	Abnormalities in coagulation-bleeding
	Petechiae	Reduced factor I, II, V, VII, VIII, IX, X, XI, XIII
	Bruises	Thrombocytopenia
	Changes in sensorium	Exacerbation of encephalopathy, delirium tremens (with ETOH withdrawal), seizures
	Ascites	Fluid retention/respiratory compromise
	Edema	Intraperitoneal sepsis, potential shifts in intravascular volume, potential electrolyte abnormalities
General nutrition	Weight loss (or weight gain with ascites), anemia, muscle wasting, fever, weakness	Vitamin deficiency (A, Bs, D, K): poor wound healing, poor handling of glucose, Wernicke syndrome
	Nausea, anorexia, edema	Magnesium, phosphorous: multiple metabolic abnormalities, arrhythmias Reduced immunocompetence, infection

These criteria only quantitate the degree of hepatic impairment as it relates to increased mortality. Most frequently Child's classification is used with reference to the patient with varices who is a candidate for a portosystemic shunt or a devascularization procedure to combat or prevent the recurrence of gastrointestinal tract hemmorhage. These estimates of mortality are not absolute, and patients may be offered a significant reduction in risk by improving hepatic function preoperatively.

The alcoholic patient must be protected from withdrawal symptoms with use of proper sedatives. The onset of mild withdrawal symptoms can occur anywhere from 1 to 5 days after alcohol is withdrawn. Major symptoms generally peak at about 3 days but have occurred up to 10 days after withdrawal. Valium and Librium are drugs that can prevent major withdrawal symptoms if instituted prophylactically. Untreated delirium tremens carries a postoperative mortality as high as 50% which is reduced to 10% with proper treatment. The use of intravenous ethanol has also been advocated.

Late-stage cirrhotics must have thiamine given parenterally prior to the institution of intravenous glucose. Ataxia, ophthalmoplegia, the severe central nervous system disturbance (Wernicke-Korsakoff syndrome) may follow if such therapy is not instituted. Magnesium and phosphate deficiencies are not uncommon, especially with refeeding, and should be aggressively replaced to prevent abnormalities of glucose metabolism and cardiac arrhythmia.

For more complete discussion of surgical diseases of the liver, the reader is referred to Chapter 23.

Dysfunction of the Adrenal Cortex

The most frequent situation in which a student may be confronted with acute adrenal insufficiency is in the patient on exogenous steroids who develops acute problems secondary to the stress of a surgical procedure, sepsis, or other acute injury. Most often this is a failure to provide adequate supplementation for patients whose adrenal axis has been suppressed. A careful history of steroid use is obviously essential. Prolonged fever and unexplained shock should lead one to suspect the diagnosis. There is little agreement as to the dose and duration of steroid therapy necessary to produce adrenal suppression. Usually, short-term therapy, five days, of less than 40 mg daily produces no suppression. However, suppression has been noted on doses less than 40 mg daily for only three days. It is generally impractical and usually impossible to attempt to wean patients from steroids preoperatively. Exacerbation of the illness for which the drug was prescribed is more than likely. Patients who have been given pharmacologic doses (i.e., 15 mg/day for more than one week) can have suppression of the hypothalmic pituitary axis for up to one year after therapy is withdrawn. Therefore, supplemental steroids should be instituted to cover the stress of surgery in all patients with suspected adrenal suppression. For a more complete discussion of adrenal disorders, the reader is referred to Chapter 21.

Hemostatic Disorders

The majority of bleeding that occurs during and after surgical procedures is mechanical in nature, that is,

Table 2.8.
Child's Classification of Cirrhosis

	Albumin	Bilirubin	Ascites	Encephalopathy	Nutritional State	Mortality
Class A	>3.5	<2.0	Absent	Absent	Good	<10%
Class B	3.0–3.5	2.0–3.0	Minimal	Minimal	Fair	40%
Class C	<3.0	>3.0	Severe	Severe	Poor	>80%

related to transection of vessels and failure to achieve surgical hemostasis. There are patients, however, who may have potential abnormalities of coagulation that predispose them to excessive blood loss. The patient who is taking Coumadin for prophylaxis of an artificial heart valve is a good example. Those with chronic arthritis on large doses of aspirin have platelet dysfunction and increased bleeding tendencies. A careful history of drug use and an understanding of the adverse side effects of common medications, with special attention to potential abnormalities of coagulation, will identify these individuals at increased risk.

The best screening procedure for hemostatic abnormalities is a careful history, substantially better than any laboratory test or combination of tests. It is also more cost-effective. Millions of dollars each year are wasted on needless laboratory determinations of coagulation profiles in healthy patients who are admitted for elective procedures with no history to suggest a coagulation abnormality. The history will identify those patients with excessive bleeding after minor surgical or dental procedures or minor injury. The patient who describes easy bruisability after minor trauma, frequent epistaxis, or a history of chronic excessive alcohol use has a coagulopathy based on a reduced production of coagulation factors. Only individuals whose history suggests the potential for excess bleeding should have preoperative laboratory screening. A coagulopathy discovered intra- or postoperatively is a failure to take an adequate history, not a failure to order laboratory tests. Findings on physical examination that suggest bleeding disorders include multiple petechiae, joint deformity, generalized lymphadenopathy, hepatosplenomegaly, and severe malnutrition. These findings should confirm the suspicions identified in the patient's history. Specific questions must be asked of the patient, and the student should not rely on the patient volunteering the information. For a more complete discussion of bleeding disorders, the reader is referred to Chapter 8.

Nutritional Status

Poor nutritional status predisposes to operative complications related to wound healing, respiratory insufficiency, and reduced immunocompetence leading to infection. Mortality is substantially higher in patients with poor nutritional status. In some studies as many as 50% of patients admitted to hospitals in the United States could be shown to have some element of malnutrition. Until recent years little attention was given to nutritional assessment, and many hospitalized patients with illnesses longer than 20–30 days either starved to death or died of septic complications related to malnutrition. The ability to support patients enterally and parenterally with adequate calories and protein has significantly reduced morbidity and mortality. Elements in the history that suggest poor nutritional status include anorexia, weight loss, chronic vomiting and diarrhea, and chronic illness. Chronic renal failure is frequently associated with malnutrition, as is chronic hepatic dysfunction.

Findings on physical examination of muscle wasting in the temporalis muscle or over the thenar or hypothenar eminence, peripheral edema, or neuropathy suggest possible protein-calorie malnutrition. Glossitis, loss of rugae on the tongue, or smoothing of the edges of the tongue alone suggest vitamin B deficiency. Cheilosis or scaling and cracking of the vermilion border of the lips or corners of the mouth likewise suggest vitamin B–complex deficiency.

Several visceral protein markers, albumin, prealbumin, transferrin, retinal binding protein, and carnitine have been used to estimate nutritional deficiency. Delayed hypersensitivity to recall antigens and total lymphocyte count are useful in some cases to quantitate immune function. Anthropomorphic measurements to assess body reserves (i.e., tricep skin-fold thickness for body fat) or attempts to estimate bodycell mass (e.g., midarm muscle circumference or the creatinine-height index) are advocated by some. None of these simply or in combination have proven to be more useful than careful history.

Attempts have also been made to quantitate the risk of surgical procedures based on nutritional parameters alone. The prognostic nutritional index, Table 2-9, attempts to define such risk. In an effort to likewise define mortality, the Hospital Prognostic Index has also been developed (Table 2-9). More important perhaps than the specific identification of a statistical probability of death or of developing a complication, these methods may help identify those patients who would benefit from preoperative nutritional support in one form or another. Morbidity and mortality can be reduced in nutritionally depleted patients, and it is not necessary to wait until all parameters return to normal. Such is not practical, as it may require many weeks in some cases, and surgical intervention cannot be postponed for that period of time. For a more complete discussion of the evaluation and treatment of nutritional problems, the reader is referred to Chapter 7.

Chronic Renal Disease

In the United States alone, over 45,000 patients with end-stage renal disease (ESRD) are maintained on dialysis. An even greater number of individuals can be identified who have renal function that is significantly below normal. The metabolic and nutritional aberrations that accompany ESRD frequently require special preparation of the patient for an elective surgical procedure. Most procedures can be performed in patients with chronic renal failure (CRF) with an acceptably low complication rate, provided meticulous attention to perioperative care is given. Most surgical diseases occur with at least the same frequency in this population as in the normal, and no patient should be denied a necessary surgical procedure based on a history of renal disease alone.

The student who evaluates the patient with CRF must be aware of the changes that occur in these patients as the sequelae of their renal disease. The ability to handle water and sodium and maintain homeostasis is impaired. Extracellular volume expansion usually does not occur until renal function reaches less than

Table 2.9.
Predictors of Morbidity and Mortality on Nutritional Parameters

(PNI)	(HPI)
PNI = 158% − 16.6(ALB) − 0.78TSF − 0.2(TFN) − 5.8(DH)	HPI = 0.91(ALB) − 1.0(DH) − 1.44 (sepsis) + 0.98(Dx) − 1.09
DH > 5 mm = 2	DH >/.5 mm = 1
	anergy = 2
DH 1–5 mm = 1	Sepsis = 2; no sepsis = 1
anergy − 0	
	Dx (cancer) = 1; no cancer = 2
	HPI = −3 = 5%
	HPI = −2 = 10%
	HPI = −1 = 20%
	HPI = 0 = 50%
	HPI = +1 = 74%
	HPI = +2 = 88%

PNI, prognostic nutritional index, risk of complication. HPI, hospital prognostic index, probability of survival. ALB, albumin (g/dL). TSF, tricep skin-fold thickness (mm). TFN, transferrin. DH, delayed hypersensitivity.

10% of normal. Other disease states that complicate sodium excretion and that are, unfortunately, frequently found in these patients (congestive heart failure or the nephrotic syndrome) may contribute to volume overload with lesser degrees of renal insufficiency. Nonetheless, the ability to handle large volumes of intravenous fluids and sodium is impaired and should be carefully monitored. Chronic volume depletion is perhaps as frequently encountered in these patients as is volume overload and can be reversed, if present, in the same fashion as in those individuals with normal renal function. Achieving appropriate fluid balance in the perioperative period may require more invasive monitoring techniques (i.e., central venous pressure monitoring or right heart catheterization) particularly in those patients who may be kept NPO or who have additional losses of fluid and electrolytes from fistulae or nasogastric tubes.

Impaired ability to excrete potassium is also present and is secondary to altered acid-base equilibrium. Major problems with hyperkalemia do not occur until the patients reach ESRD, but patients with impaired renal function do not tolerate sudden changes in potassium. The surgeon's and anesthesiologist's primary concern is the development of hyperkalemia intraoperatively and immediately postoperatively. For patients on dialysis, this risk is directly proportional to the serum potassium level *before* the last dialysis. Potassium levels should be below 5 mEq/liter before surgery, and this may require the use of ion-exchange resins.

Chronic renal failure is usually accompanied by a chronic metabolic acidosis due to the impaired ability of the kidneys to excrete acid end products of metabolism, including sulfates, phosphates, and lactate. With milder degrees of renal compromise, respiratory compensation is able to maintain the serum pH at an acceptable level slightly below normal. Serum bicarbonate should be greater than 18 mEq/liter, and this may re-

quire exogenous bicarbonate administration or dialysis against a bicarbonate bath. Postoperatively the acid load may rise substantially due to the release of hydrogen ions from damaged cells. Hyperventilation may compensate for this phenomenon, but if PCO_2 rises even slightly, a profound exacerbation of the acidosis may occur. It is therefore advisable to consider the CRF patient's ability to ventilate, and preoperative blood gases are indicated. Because of the pulmonary changes that occur postoperatively, aggressive pulmonary toilet directed at preventing hypoventilation, atelectasis, pneumonitis, and oversedation is mandatory.

Other electrolyte abnormalities are often encountered in patients with chronic renal failure; hypocalcemia is the rule, secondary to hyperphosphatemia, and hypermagnesemia is not unusual, so magnesium-containing antacids should be avoided. Oral phosphate binders and dietary restriction of phosphates may be required.

Most patients with long-standing CRF are malnourished. Anorexia secondary to azotemia, as well as the inability to handle the accumulation of nitrogenous end products, promote the depletion of both skeletal muscle and visceral protein stores. Malabsorption syndromes are common, as are overt vitamin deficiencies. Patients who receive chronic peritoneal dialysis may lose as much as 6–8 g of protein per day and complicate the situation. A careful dietary history and a history of weight loss should be sought and consideration given to early nutritional support.

A number of other aberrations are usually present in the patient with CRF. A normochromic, normocytic anemia is usually well tolerated, but the reduced oxygen-carrying capacity may have a profound effect in the surgical patient. Chronic dialysis is estimated to remove as much as 3 liters of blood per year, and the reduced production of erythropoietin by the kidney hampers replacement. Red blood cell life span is also reduced in the uremic state. Deficient immune responses are also present in this population and theoretically enhance the potential for infectious complications. Because of multiple transfusions, many of these individuals are carriers of hepatitis B. Chronic coagulopathy due to heparinization during dialysis, or uremia itself, may exaggerate blood loss during surgery or immediately after.

With the knowledge of the potential problems the renal failure patient may face, a careful preoperative evaluation and preparation of the patient will, in most instances, minimize operative risks. Careful attention to volume status may necessitate invasive hemodynamic monitoring. Daily weights and accurate intake and output records are mandatory. Baseline renal function studies should be obtained preoperatively, including determinations of BUN and creatinine, as well as an evaluation of glomerular filtration. Exacerbation of renal failure should be prevented if hypotension is avoided, and proper dosing of potentially nephrotoxic drugs is considered. A coagulation profile may be helpful to identify intrinsic deficiencies, and time should be allowed for the effects of the heparin used during dialysis to clear prior to the operative procedure itself.

Such practices will reduce the risk of excessive blood loss. The presence of renal failure may require major modifications in the anesthetic techniques employed, and the anesthesiologist should become a part of the preoperative evaluation. Antibiotic prophylaxis may be instituted safely if attention to proper dosing is given. Postoperatively, aggressive pulmonary physiotherapy, attention to volume and electrolyte status, and nutritional support will substantially reduce many metabolic sequelae.

Despite the formidable spectrum of potential problems the surgical patient with CRF faces, elective surgery can be performed safely with a modicum of risk. Modification in the timing and type of dialysis may be necessary, and close consultation with the nephrologist is advisable.

Summary

The intent of this chapter was not to provide an in-depth analysis of the diagnosis of surgical disease, but to give the student who is new to the surgical ward an approach to the assessment of surgical risk so that he or she may begin to develop the judgment necessary for clinical practice. Clinical encounters are opportunities to practice these assessment skills, question and review the responses to therapy, and help the surgical team plan appropriately to make the proposed surgical procedure as safe and effective as possible.

SUGGESTED READINGS

Alberti KGMM, Thomas DJV: The management of diabetes during surgery. *Br J Anaesth* 51:693, 1979.
Alder AG: *Medical Evaluation of the Surgical Patient.* Philadelphia, WB Saunders, 1985.
Bartless RH, Gozzariga AB, Geraghty TR: Respiratory maneuvers to prevent postoperative pulmonary complications. *JAMA* 224:1017–1021, 1973.
Byyny RL: Preventing adrenal insufficiency during surgery. *Post Grad Med* 67:219, 1980.
Cerra FB: *Pocket Manuel of Surgical Nutrition.* St. Louis, CV Mosby, 1984.
Conrad SA, Kinasewitz GT, George RB (eds): *Pulmonary Function Testing; Principles and Practice.* New York, Churchill Livingstone, 1984.
Goldman L: Cardiac risk and complications of non-cardiac surgery. *Ann Intern Med* 98:504–513, 1983.
Goldman L, Caldera DL, Nussbaum SR, et al: Multifactorial index of cardiac risk in non-cardiac surgical procedures. *N Engl J Med* 297:845–850, 1977.
Gower, WE, Kerstein H: Prevention of alcohol withdrawal symptoms in surgical patients. *Surg Gynecol Obstet* 151:382, 1980.
Hoffenberg R: Thyroid emergencies. *Clin Edocrinol Metab* 9:503, 1980.
Plumpton FS, Besser GM, Cole PV: Corticosteroid treatment and surgery: the management of steroid cover. *Anesthesiology* 24:13, 1969.
Stone HH: Preoperative and postoperative care. *Surg Clin N Am* 47:409, 1977.
Tisi GM: Preoperative evaluation of pulmonary function. *Am Rev Respir Dis* 119:293–310, 1979.
Watts LF, Miller J, Davidson MD, et al: Perioperative management of diabetes mellitus. *Anesthesiology* 55:104, 1981.

Skills

1. Perform a complete history and physical examination, preferably under the supervision of an attending physician, of a preoperative elective patient, and a patient with a surgical emergency.

2. Present the patient to the surgical team on rounds.

3. Discuss the specific methods of determining surgical risks.

Study Questions

1. A 56-year-old male presents for elective surgery for chronic peptic ulcer disease. He has a history of vague anterior chest pain with exertion.
   a. What additional elements of history may be important for your assessment?
   b. What should you look for on physical examination?
   c. What laboratory or special diagnostic procedures would be helpful in determining operative risks?

2. A 60-year-old insulin-dependent diabetic is admitted because of acute cholecystitis and needs a cholecystectomy within the week.
   a. Describe how you would evaluate the patient's operative risk.
   b. Suppose the patient reported having a mild myocardial infarction 4 months ago (6 months ago), developed symptoms of acute cholecystitis 4 days after coronary artery bypass grafting.

3. Discuss the preoperative evaluation and care of a patient with chronic obstructive pulmonary disease admitted for an elective hernia repair.

4. A 28-year-old football player is admitted for removal of a right-sided branchial cleft cyst. Describe his preoperative evaluation and care.

5. A 38-year-old female is admitted for a bariatric surgical procedure. She weighs 130 kg, takes Biakenese, and smokes one pack of cigarettes per day. What should be done to evaluate this patient preoperatively?

6. A 48-year-old male develops an obstructing duodenal ulcer and requires an operation. He has chronic renal failure and is maintained on hemodialysis. Describe the preoperative evaluation and preparation of this individual for his surgical procedure. Describe the evaluation and preparation
   a. for the same patient who is to have a renal transplant;
   b. for the same patient who is to have a thoracotomy for removal of a biopsy-proven malignant lesion in the right upper lobe.

3

Surgical Record Keeping

Richard M. Bell, M.D.
Paddy M. Bell, C.S.T.

ASSUMPTIONS

The student is allowed to make entries in the patient's hospital record or another mechanism is available for students to document a patient's progress.

OBJECTIVES

1. Demonstrate an understanding of the elements of the surgical admission order by writing complete, concise, and clear orders.
2. Demonstrate an understanding of the optimal preoperative evaluation of a patient by writing a preoperative assessment note.
3. Demonstrate an understanding of a surgical procedure by recording the relevant information in a brief operative note and discuss its importance.

Admission Orders

The Medical Record

The medical record should be a concise and explicit document that chronologically outlines the patient's course of treatment. Although records remain the property of the physician, clinic, or institution in which the patient received his or her care, the patient has the legal right to the information contained in these records, and such information may not be denied the patient. Most states have initiated legislation that allows patients access to their records and permission to obtain copies of them. Careful thought must be given to the information placed in the record, and this information must be relevant to the course of treatment or diagnostic workup. The medical record should not be used to relay messages among consulting services or as a forum for trading derogatory expressions. Such action is unprofessional. It does not enhance patient care in any fashion and opens physicians, house staff, and students to legal inquiry or litigation. Before a progress note is written, the physician should ask himself or herself the following questions.

1. Does the information pertain to patient care?

2. Is the information of value in documenting the treatment course?
3. What details will be important for future care of the patient or valuable for future review?
4. Is the information accurate?
5. If suspicions or theories regarding the diagnosis, treatment, or the possible development of complications are recorded, are they clearly identified as suspicions, theories, or possibilities?
6. Does the note serve the best interests of the patient, the physician, and the health care team?

Consideration of each of these points will illustrate how potential problems can be avoided.

1. *Does the information pertain to patient care?* The following note was written by a surgical house officer when asked by a medical service to consult on an acute gastrointestinal bleeder:

> has obviously been mismanaged! Surgical consultation before transfusing twelve units of whole blood would have allowed earlier intervention, reducing operative risks.

Although this is an extreme example, it is unfortunately a true one. Such a note adds nothing to the care of the patient.

2. *Is the information of value in documenting the treatment course?* There is little value in repeating what has previously been documented. In teaching institutions it is common to see history and physical examination or progress notes recorded by the student, the acting intern, the junior resident, and the chief resident. The delivery of care in an educational environment is by necessity repetitive; this repetitiveness, which is essential for the educational activities of the institution, clutters the record and makes it cumbersome. Some facilities have a special area of the chart for student notes; others delete student notes when the records are shelved. Although it is important that the student gain experience in writing progress notes, it serves no purpose to rewrite what has been written previously.

3. *What details will be important for future care of the patient?* Operative notes are perhaps the best illustration of the importance of the note in identifying potential needs for future care. Recording the findings at

surgery is more important than noting the type of suture that was used to close a perforated duodenal ulcer or to ligate a vessel. Consider the 38-year-old female who presents to the gynecologist with pelvic pain six weeks after an elective cholecystectomy. Information concerning palpation of the uterus and ovaries at the time of surgery is more helpful than the fact that 3-0 silk suture was used to tie the cystic artery. Consider the house officer who is asked to see a patient six hours after a subtotal gastrectomy for fever and oliguria. Information concerning blood loss, blood and fluid replacement, and operative time are more relevant than the method of skin closure. The thought process used in unraveling a patient's illness or selecting diagnostic studies is often more important than minor technical details.

4. *Is the information accurate?* Unfortunately, discrepancies in the records are frequently encountered. Verbal reports of diagnostic studies written into progress notes that do not agree with formal reports once typed, signed, and filed, cause confusion. Erroneous information can lead to disastrous results.

5. *Are suspicions and theories clearly defined as such?* A note written by an inexperienced member of the medical team that confuses suspicions with documented and confirmed medical/surgical problems is a potential legal liability. This leads to distortion of the facts in the record and misconceptions on the part of others who may be peripherally involved with the patient or the patient's care. Inaccuracy is a powerful opponent of quality patient care at all levels.

6. *Does the note serve the best interests of the patient, the physician, and the health care team?* The record is kept on behalf of the patient and to document the events, timing, and thinking that relate to the care given during the period of hospitalization. The record is a confidential document and cannot be revealed to anyone who is not directly involved with the care of the patient

without the patient's (or a responsible agent's) written consent. Without this consent the individual who discloses such information breaches the ethical contract between patient and physician and can be held legally accountable for such actions.

The medical record can be both the physician's and the patient's best ally or worst enemy. Documentation of findings, results, and what has been explained to the patient, particularly in terms of risks, benefits, anticipated results, and therapeutic alternatives, can protect both the patient and physician.

The medical record resembles a small novel, in that it details a patient's illness and progress, but it should be nonfiction. As health care has increasingly become a team effort, with evaluation and therapy directed by many members, the chart has grown from a simple paperback to an epic trilogy in many respects. Most hospitals adopt their own methods of recording and retaining information, but Table 3-1 depicts the general organization with respect to individual chapters.

The Order Sheet

The physician's order sheet is one of the most crucial aspects of the patient's medical record. Its purpose is to provide detailed guidelines for members of the health care team who will provide clinical and diagnostic services for the patient. Orders, therefore, are to be *followed* and *not interpreted.* Unfortunately, too often the latter is the case, because of the hasty scribblings of physicians that may be unclear, illegible, or inaccurate. Orders should be written with sufficient detail to eliminate possible misunderstandings. The student physician should remember that from the time of admission to the hospital every aspect of the patient's life (e.g., diet, level of activity, access to the bathroom, and even what the patient is to breathe) is the responsibility of the physician. Errors of omission could result in assumptions by nursing personnel as to what the physician wants or what is appropriate.

Generally the orders should include those elements listed in Table 3-2. Content and format may vary among institutions, but the principles are the same. Usually the first orders written concern general nursing care. Identification of the physician or team responsible for the patient is important so that the staff knows who to contact if problems or questions arise. Listing the working diagnosis or reason for admission gives the staff a general idea of what the problems may be and sets the tone for the delivery of services. The frequency of vital signs and which are to be recorded is next. Any special nursing evaluations (e.g., neurologic function) should also be indicated. If the physician wishes to be notified of any of these assessments (e.g., temperature > 102°), the staff should be so informed.

Diet specifications or NPO orders for the patient should be indicated. Special diets are required by patients such as diabetics or those undergoing special diagnostic procedures. Too frequently hospitalization may be prolonged or expensive procedures may need to be repeated because attention to the details of pre-

Table 3.1.
Organization of Information for Medical Records

Administrative information	*Ancillary personnel notes*
Name	Physical therapy, respiratory
Address,	therapy, dietary, social ser-
Insurance information	vices, etc.
Emergency notification informa-	*Physicians orders*
tion	*Laboratory, pathology, blood*
Consent for general treatment	*bank reports*
(Invasive procedures require	*Radiology reports*
specific consent by the patient	Operative record
or responsible agent)	Operative consent form
Medical summary	Anesthesia record
Discharge summary	Operative report
History and physical examina-	Postoperative, recovery room
tion	record
Physician's progress notes	*Consultation reports*
Nursing notes	(frequently found in progress
Vital signs	notes)
Intake/output sheets	*Miscellaneous*
Written nursing assessments/	
nursing observations	

Table 3.2.
General Considerations for Writing Orders

1. Physician/team responsible
2. Diagnosis/condition
3. Immediate plans
4. Vital signs/special checks/notification parameters
5. Diet
6. Level of activity
7. Special nursing care instructions
   a. Positioning
   b. Wound care
   c. Tubes/drains: management and care
8. Intake/output: frequency
9. Intravenous fluids
10. Medications: drug, dose, route, frequency
    a. Routine
    b. Special
11. Laboratory orders
12. Special procedures/x-ray
13. Miscellaneous

scribing the appropriate diet were overlooked. The level of patient activity must be specified for obvious reasons. Such orders are generally considered routine, and some hospitals may have standard protocols for many of them. Prudent physicians, however, will specifically write their own routine in sufficient detail to ensure that their plans are carefully followed.

Those nursing care functions that are not usually considered routine need to be identified. These include special positioning, turning, pulmonary exercises, and care of wounds or drainage tubes. Foley catheters are usually placed to gravity drainage, nasogastric tubes to some type of suction apparatus, and wound drains to either suction or dependent drainage. The staff should be informed specifically as to management of these drains or tubes. Daily care of the incision site should be clearly noted. Retrograde infection from incision sites, especially with urinary catheters and wound drains, is a major contributor to morbidity. Patient positioning becomes extremely important in preventing pulmonary problems or preventing aspiration of gastric contents in an individual receiving enteral tube feedings. Other nursing instructions include the periodic assessment of glycosuria in the diabetic, the recording of fluid intake or output from urinary catheters and drains, and the specific instructions for tube care, stripping, irrigation, or notification of the physician in the event of some occurrence (e.g., urine output < 30 ml/hr or chest tube drainage > 100 ml/hr).

The type and rate of intravenous fluid administration should be specified. When multiple intravenous sites are being used, it is frequently helpful to specify which fluids are to be infused at which sites. This may avoid the infusion of incompatible drugs or solutions through the same catheters. Noting total fluid intake per hour is also helpful for the nursing staff.

The medication section of the physician's orders is perhaps the most common source of errors. Meticulous attention to detail is mandatory to prevent potentially fatal medication errors. The notation sequence should

be type of drug, dosage, route of administration, and frequency. These orders should be absolutely clear and legible. If the spelling of a drug is uncertain, a reference should be consulted. Only standard abbreviations should be utilized. It may be advantageous to write medications in a separate section of the order sheet so they are not mixed in with other nonmedication orders. This helps avoid confusion and oversights. Routine medications such as analgesics, laxatives, and sleeping pills should be written first, followed by those medications that are special for an individual patient. It is good practice to review the medication lists on a daily basis. Changes in drugs, dosage, or frequency can be confusing for both the pharmacy and the nursing staff. If drugs are changed, it is best to write an order to stop the original drug, then order the new one. In most institutions parenteral nutritional products are prepared in the pharmacy, therefore total parenteral nutrition (TPN) orders should be placed with the medications.

The prudent physician will specify the laboratory studies and special diagnostic procedures that are desired. Special procedures, such as x-rays, require some additional thought. Request slips for these studies should specifically state the presumptive diagnosis and the reason for the test. Personal consultation with the radiologist or technician will avoid confusion and prevent delays or unnecessary repetition of procedures. If those performing the tests are aware of what the physician is looking for, the results are nearly always more productive. Some procedures require special preparation of the patient, so be certain these instructions are included in the orders. "Routine" or "daily" laboratory orders should be avoided. Although these may simplify order writing for the physician, they are an expensive practice and usually result in needless blood work or radiation exposure. Order the tests that are needed. If the results of a test will make no therapeutic difference or change the course of treatment, there is little to be gained by ordering it. Study protocols may be an exception to this rule. Laboratory and diagnostic studies should be used to confirm clinical suspicions and not as a shotgun approach to ferret out a diagnosis.

The miscellaneous category in Table 3.2 is for other orders that may be necessary, including requests for consultation, obtaining procedural permits, obtaining old records, or entering a patient into a special study or protocol.

The orders are only as complete as you make them. Clarity and legibility will make the delivery of services efficient and appropriate.

Preoperative Evaluation

A brief preoperative note to summarize the workup, proposed surgery, and pertinent physical and laboratory findings is usually written the day before surgery. Such notes also serve as a check list to ensure that the important aspects of preoperative preparation have been completed. An example is shown in Table 3-3.

Table 3.3.
Sample Preoperative Note

1. Diagnosis:	Cholelithiasis
2. Proposed surgery:	Cholecystectomy with operative cholangiogram
3. History and physical:	Completed (dictated)
	Grade II/VI systolic murmur at apex
	Hypertension (controlled)
4. Labs:	CBC: $\dfrac{14.5}{41.5\%}$ 7,500
	Electrolytes: 140 | 4.2 BUN 10
	26 | 101 Glu 105
	CXR: NAD
	ECG: NSR-normal
	Present meds: HCTZ 50 mg qd
	Blood: type and hold (specimen in blood bank)
5. Operative permit:	Signed and on chart; risks, rationale, benefits and alternatives have been explained in detail; patient understands and agrees to proceed with the surgical plans.
6. Miscellaneous information	
	Signature _____

Preoperative notes assist the anesthesiologist in his or her evaluation of the patient and aid any others who need to know about the patient. Any information that may be pertinent to the efficiency or safety of the proposed procedure should be listed. In general, the note is only beneficial when it reflects the thought that goes into the preoperative evaluation and plans.

Operative Permit

An operative permit, sometimes called a signed surgical consent, is required in most hospitals before the proposed operation can take place. Regardless of which member of the health care team obtains the permit, it is the surgeon's responsibility to ensure that the patient or the patient's legal guardian is adequately informed about the proposed surgery, the potential complications, anticipated outcome, and alternatives. Although a signed operative permit implies that such conditions have been met, it in no way is legal protection for the surgeon, the surgical team, or the hospital. The degree to which a physician must ensure that informed consent has been given varies greatly across the country. In general, patients should be given enough information to make an intelligent decision of their own free will regarding the proposed surgery, based on potential complications, outcome, and alternatives. While it is not practical to discuss in detail every remotely possible risk with the patient or the patient's representative, sufficient information about the usual or more common contingencies should be provided. It is good practice to record in the medical record the details of what the patient was told and that

the patient indicated his or her understanding of those facts. It is also prudent to have this note witnessed by a person other than a member of the operative team. Failure to provide full disclosure has led to successful negligence suits. Following such protocol is more than defensive medicine, as it helps ensure that the patient is aware of what is about to take place.

If competent, the patient is the only one who need give consent. It is, however, appropriate that family members be a part of the decision-making process. Consent of a spouse is not necessary. Consent of both parents in the case of a minor is usually requested and should follow the guidelines discussed above. In the emergency situation the surgeon is often forced to do what is necessary to save a life or prevent grave harm. A detailed note describing the situation should be recorded as soon as practical, listing the reasons for emergency intervention and why informed consent could not be obtained.

Operative and Postoperative Records

The operative note is a brief handwritten account of the surgical procedure. A detailed note is usually dictated by the surgeon but, because of delays in transcription or dictation, is not immediately available in the record. The brief operative note is valuable. Important components are listed in Table 3-4.

The surgical record form is filled out by the circulating nurse while the patient is in the operating room. The following information is included: name, date, surgeon and assistants, anesthesiologists, type of anesthesia, preoperative diagnosis, postoperative diagnosis, procedure, surgical technologist, circulating nurse, time of procedure (beginning and end), intravenous fluids and drugs administered, sponge and needle count data, and supplies used. Other special records include reports for frozen section, specimen, artificial implanted devices, transplantation, sterilization, amputation, death, and incident reports (unusual occurrence).

The anesthesia sheet is a record of the patient's condition throughout the operation. Vital signs are recorded periodically on the graph on the sheet. Type of anesthesia, means of administration, drugs administered, intravenous fluids or blood given, and other per-

Table 3.4.
Operative Note

1. Procedure:	
2. Findings:	
3. Surgeons:	Attending surgeon:
4. Estimated blood loss:	
5. Crystalloid replaced:	Blood products:
6. Anesthesia:	
7. Complications:	
8. Tubes/drains:	
9. Disposition:	
	Signature:

tinent data relating to the physiologic function are recorded.

Progress Notes and Discharge Notes

Progress notes record the clinical course of the patient. Frequently it is helpful to first note the hospital day number, the postoperative day, or days after injury. The details of this note have been described. Listing by problem number, using the SOAP format (Subjective, Objective, Assessment, and Plans), or arranging the notes by organ system can improve organization. The format used varies among hospitals and even services within the hospital. All notes should be dated, timed, and signed.

The discharge note should contain the elements listed in Table 3-5. A formal dictated summary is required by most hospitals, but the handwritten note is useful until the transcribed summary is appended to the chart. Items 1–3 are self-explanatory. Item 4, the hospital course, is a very brief account of what transpired during the admission. Item 5 indicates where the patient went or was intended to go after discharge. Item 6 is an important but frequently overlooked addition to the note. In many instances home care instructions contribute substantially to the patient's recovery and can have significant legal implications. Not only should information disclosed to the patient be documented, but the physician should make every effort to ensure that the patient *understands* what he or she is to do, or not do, after discharge. A list of medications the patient is instructed to take, as well as the

Table 3.5.
Discharge Note

1. Admission diagnosis: Date:
2. Discharge diagnosis: Date:
3. Operative procedure:
4. Hospitalization course:
5. Disposition:
6. Home care instructions:
   a. Activity
   b. Diet
   c. Restrictions
   d. Wound care
   e. Other
7. Discharge medications:
8. Follow-up instructions:
9. Miscellaneous:

dosage and frequency, should be included. This is followed by noting when the patient is to return for follow-up examination. It is more effective to give the patient a specific date and time for a follow-up visit than to simply indicate "return in two or three weeks." Compliance with follow-up appointments under these circumstances is much greater.

In summary, the medical record should be accurate and informative. If physicians think carefully about what information would be helpful if the details of this illness were to be reviewed by themselves or someone else, the value of the medical record for subsequent patient care, research, or medicolegal opinion will be greatly enhanced.

Skills

1. Demonstrate your understanding of appropriate medical record keeping by writing admission orders, a preoperative note, an abbreviated operative note and progress notes.

Study Questions

1. Write the admission orders for a 56-year-old diabetic female on insulin (20 units NPH/day) who is to be admitted for an elective cholecystectomy in the morning.

2. Prepare a preoperative note on one of your patients.

3. Discuss the content of an operative note for the patient in question.

4. Describe how you would write a daily progress note on a patient with multiple organ failure who is in the intensive care unit.

5. You are asked to see a patient who is four hours postoperative following a cholecystectomy, because of mild hypotension and decreased urinary output. What information in the preoperative and operative notes would be most beneficial?

4

The OR—Home of the Surgeon

Richard M. Bell, M.D.
Paddy M. Bell, C.S.T.

ASSUMPTIONS

The student is allowed access to the operative theatre and is allowed to participate in operative procedures.

> ### OBJECTIVES
> 1. Discuss operating room protocol and the rationale behind the rules of conduct and attire.
> 2. Demonstrate the proper technique for surgical scrubbing and assisted and unassisted gowning and gloving.
> 3. Demonstrate knowledge of aseptic technique and discuss the microbiological principles involved.
> 4. Name the three sterilization methods.
> 5. Name at least nine basic principles regarding sterile technique.
> 6. Identify areas that are considered part of the sterile operative field.
> 7. Outline and discuss the responsibilities of an assistant in the operating room environment.
> 8. Define the classification of operative procedures with reference to their potential for infectious complications. Discuss the importance of this classification system.

The Operating Room

The surgical theater is at best an uncomfortable place for the novice. The intensity of the environment and the regulations that govern maintenance of sterile technique add to the awkwardness and anxiety experienced by the student who enters the operating room suite for the first time. Fortunately, the code of conduct is straightforward, serves the purpose of protecting the patient, and is easily learned. The operating room is also the arena where the student can actually see and touch the pathology and thus is one of the best educational activities in which the surgical clerk can participate. Surgeons use the opportunity to demonstrate precisely how surgical therapy affects disease process, as well as to demonstrate living human anatomy and to discuss normal and pathologic physiology.

Operating Room Attire

Every member of the health care team must understand the strict protocol that is mandatory in the operating room and adhere to the prescribed rules of conduct, attie, and function. Careful attention must be given to the construction and maintenance of a therapeutic environment for the surgical patient, and every possible measure must be utilized to prevent complications.

Knowledge of the surgical environment and the meticulous practice of asepsis and sterile technique is required. This knowledge ensures that operative procedures will be performed with maximal protection for the patient and that the risk of contamination will be kept to an absolute minimum. Infectious complications increase hospital stay, patient discomfort, and costs, as well as the risk of death and disfigurement. Operating suites are designed to be functional, but it is the responsibility of the personnel to safeguard the integrity of this environment. High standards of discipline must be maintained, and students should consider their participation in the care of the surgical patient and admission to the surgical suite a privilege.

Proper design of facilities and regulations for proper attire and conduct in the surgical suite are important measures in preventing transportation of microorganisms into the operating room. Street clothes should never be worn within restricted areas of the surgical suite, and operating attire should not be worn outside of the operating area. This minimizes the transportation of virulent hospital pathogens directly into the surgical arena. All persons who enter restricted areas should be required to wear clean surgical apparel, including hats, scrub clothes, shoe covers, and face masks. Each item of surgical garb is a specific means of protecting the patient from contamination from the hair, fomites, and microorganisms in the air.

The hat or hood should cover and contain all hair. It should fit snugly, with edges secured by elastic or drawstrings. For those with long hair, hoods that tie under the chin are available.

Scrub clothes are made of a closely woven fabric that is flame-resistant, lint-free, cool, and comfortable. A large variety of scrub suits and dresses are available. All must fit the body closely, and shirts and drawstrings should be tucked inside the pants.

Shoe covers are worn by all persons entering the restricted areas of the surgical suite. To prevent cross-contamination from other areas of the hospital, shoe covers should be changed between operative procedures and never worn outside the operating area.

High-filtration efficiency disposable masks should be worn at all times in the operating room. The mask must cover the mouth and nose entirely and be tied securely. To prevent cross-infection, masks should be handled only by the strings, never lowered to hang loosely around the neck, changed frequently, and promptly discarded after use.

Sterile gowns and gloves are added to the basic attire for scrubbed team members to permit the construction of the sterile field and participation in the operative procedure.

Both reusable and disposable gowns of water-repellent material or densely woven cotton are in use. Although the entire gown is sterilized, neither the back nor any area below the waist or above the chest is considered sterile once the gown is donned. The cuffs are stockinette to tightly fit the wrist. The sterile glove covers the wrist of the gown. Gloves are worn to permit the wearer to handle sterile supplies or tissue of the operative wound.

Operating Room Personnel

The operating room team is divided according to the function of its members: scrubbed sterile personnel or unscrubbed unsterile personnel. The scrubbed sterile team is composed of the operating surgeon, the surgical assistants, and the scrub nurse or operating room technician. These persons scrub their hands and arms, wear sterile gowns and gloves, and enter the sterile area that immediately surrounds and is especially prepared for the patient. To establish the sterile field, all instruments and items needed for the operation are sterilized. The instrument tables and stands are covered with sterile sheets, and the operative site is prepared and also draped. Thereafter, the sterile team members function within this limited area and handle only sterile items.

The unscrubbed unsterile team members include the anesthesiologist, the circulating nurse, and others such as x-ray technicians or biomedical engineers. Although these persons do not enter the sterile field, they must assume responsibility for maintaining the integrity of the sterile environment during the operation. They handle supplies and equipment not considered sterile and keep the sterile team supplied. They give direct patient care and handle other special requirements necessary during the surgery, such as obtaining medications and blood products or managing special equipment.

The operating surgeon is responsible for the preoperative diagnosis and care of the patient, the selection and performance of the surgical procedure, and the postoperative management and care. The surgeon assumes full responsibility for the medical acts of judgment and the management of the surgical patient. Under the operating surgeon's direction, one or two assistants are available to provide exposure of the operative site and assist with the surgical procedure. Other assistants may include medical students, nurses, and technicians. The scrub nurse is the member of the sterile team who may be a registered nurse, practical nurse, or operating room technician. He or she is responsible for preparing and arranging instruments and supplies and assisting the surgeon during the operative procedure. The scrub nurse maintains the integrity, safety, and efficiency of the sterile field throughout the operation.

The anesthesiologist is responsible for inducing anesthesia, maintaining anesthesia at the required levels, and managing reactions to anesthesia for the surgical patient. The circulating nurse manages activities of the operating room outside the sterile field and provides nursing care required for each patient. The circulating nurse is not scrubbed but is free to move about to assist others with supplies and equipment. This nurse maintains documentation during the procedure, completing information for the chart and surgical records.

Of utmost importance in the operating room is the team concept and the acceptance of each person as a vital contributor in the cooperative effort. All personnel must conform to accepted standards of conduct, honesty, consideration, and observation of policies and regulations at all times, with optimum patient care the primary objective.

Scrubbing

Skin sterilization is not possible; however, every effort is made to reduce the bacterial count of the skin to minimize the possibility of microbial contamination. This is accomplished through the surgical scrub, a process of mechanical scrubbing with a chemical antiseptic solution. Scrubbing procedures should be standardized and followed by all without exception. General preparations for the surgical scrub include the following: short, unpolished fingernails; removal of all hand jewelry; cleaning under the nail of each finger; and short prescrub of hands and arms. The length of procedure of the surgical scrub varies from one institution to another, but the recommended methods are applications of the principles of aseptic technique. These may be either *time method* or *counted-stroke method*.

Time Method

Fingernails, fingers, hands, and arms are scrubbed by allotting a prescribed amount of time to each anatomical area or each step of the procedure. Recommendations are for either a 5-minute total scrub or a 10-minute total scrub. This depends on the antimicrobial agent used and the frequency of scrubs. Many hospitals require a 10-minute scrub for the initial scrub of the day and subsequent scrubs of 5 minutes.

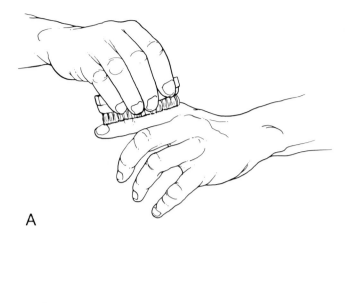

A

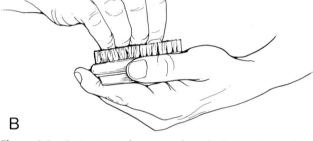

B

Figure 4.1. **A**, Anatomical pattern of scrub; four surfaces of each finger. **B**, bristle brush used to scrub fingernails.

Counted-Stroke Method

A prescribed number of brush strokes is used for each surface of the fingers, hands, and arms. The recommendation is for a repeat pattern of 50 strokes for nails, 40 strokes of each side for each finger, 10 strokes for the back and the palm of the hand, and 40 strokes for each third of the arm to the elbow.

Both methods follow an anatomical pattern of scrub: fingernails, four surfaces of each finger, the dorsal surface of the hand, the palmar surface of the hand, over the wrists and up the arm, ending 2 inches above the elbow (Fig. 4.1). Because the hands are in most direct contact with the sterile field, all steps of the scrub procedure begin with the hands and end at the elbows. After the scrub, hands and forearms must be held higher than the elbows so that contaminated water can roll off at the elbow and not run down the arms to contaminate the hands (Fig. 4.2). Hands and arms are also held away from the body.

To dry the hands, grasp a folded sterile towel with one hand and permit it to unfold, making sure it does not touch any sterile object. Dry one arm by holding the towel in the opposite hand: begin at the fingers and hand, rotate the arm, and draw the towel up to the elbow. Be sure the used portion is never brought back

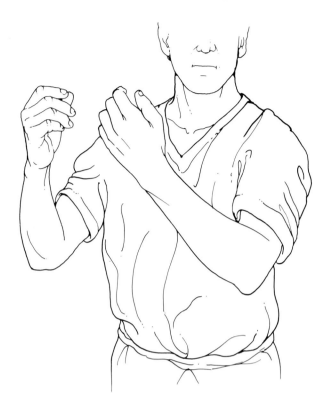

Figure 4.2. Hold hands and forearms away from the body and higher than the elbows.

into the dry area. Carefully reverse the towel and dry the opposite hand and arm on the unused end of the towel. Discard the towel in the appropriate container.

Gowning and Gloving

If you are gowning unassisted, pick up the gown, being careful to touch only the inner surface. Hold the inside of the neckband and let the gown unfold, keeping the inside of the gown toward you. With your hands at shoulder level, insert your arms into the sleeves, keeping your arms extended. The circulating nurse will assist by pulling the gown over the shoulders and tying it in the back.

If a closed-gloving technique is to be used, advance hands only to the edge of the cuff and not through (Fig. 4.3A). With this method the gloves are handled through the fabric of the gown sleeves and the hands are pushed through the cuff openings as the gloves are pulled on. This is done by placing the glove palm down onto the pronated forearm of the matching hand, with the fingers of the glove pointing toward the elbow and the glove cuff on the gown wristlet (Fig. 4.3B). Hold the glove cuff securely by the hand on which it is to be placed and use the other hand to stretch the cuff over the sleeve opening to cover the gown wristlet (Fig. 4.3C). Draw the cuff back onto the wrist and adjust the fingers (Fig. 4.3D). The gloved hand is then used to position the other glove on the opposite sleeve in the same fashion (Fig. 4.3E).

If open-gloving technique is used, advance hands completely through the cuffs of the gown (Fig. 4.4).

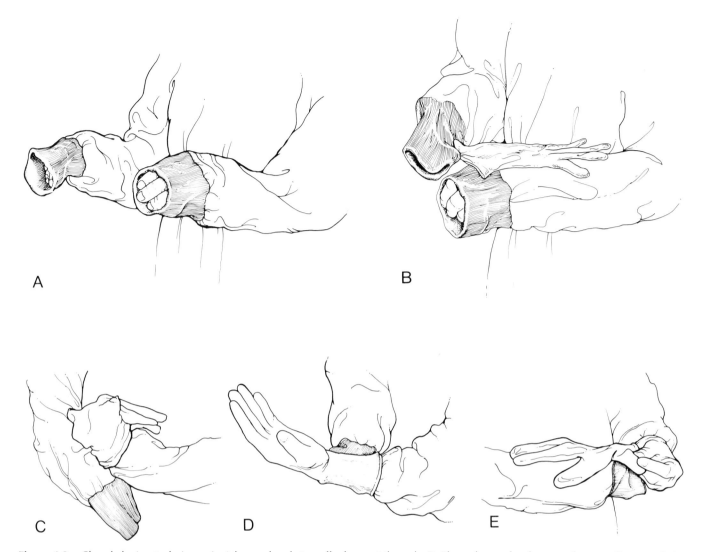

Figure 4.3. Closed-gloving technique. **A**, Advance hands to cuff edge, not through. **B**, Place glove palm down on forearm, fingers pointing toward the elbow. **C**, Use other hand through gown fabric to stretch glove over gown wristlet. **D**, Draw cuff back onto wrist. **E**, Use gloved hand to pull on remaining glove in same fashion.

Take the left glove by placing the fingers of the right hand on the folded-back cuff, touching only the inner surface of the glove. Insert the left hand into the glove, but do not turn up the cuff. Now take the second glove from the package by slipping the gloved left fingers under the inverted cuff, and pull the glove onto the right hand. The cuffs are now pulled over the gown wristlet by slightly rotating the arm.

If the scrub nurse helps you gown and glove, she or he will hold the gown open with the inner side toward you. Insert your arms, and the circulating nurse will reach inside the gown to grasp the sleeve seam, pull the gown on, and tie the back closure. When the gown is on, the scrub nurse will hold the gloves open with the palm toward you, allowing you to slip your hands into the gloves.

When gloved, untie the exterior gown ties in the front of the gown and hand the tie attached to the back of the gown to another gowned and gloved person. Hold the other tie securely and turn in the opposite direction, so the back panel of the gown is closed. Retrieve the tie and tie securely at the side.

If a glove becomes contaminated, it must be changed immediately. Extend your hand to the circulating nurse, who can then grasp the outside of the glove cuff and pull it off inside out. Do not attempt to remove the glove yourself, as you will likely contaminate the other hand. It is also important to not allow the sleeve wristlet to be pulled down over the hand when the glove is removed, as contamination of the new glove by the gown sleeve would occur. It is preferable for another sterile team member to assist with the regloving; however, if this is not possible, step aside and utilize the open-gloving technique to apply the new glove.

To remove the gown and gloves properly, first remove the gown by pulling it down from the shoulders and turning the sleeves inside out as the arms are pulled from the sleeves. Remove the gloves, turning them inside out and protecting hands by not touching the outer soiled part of the gloves (Fig. 4.5). As a mat-

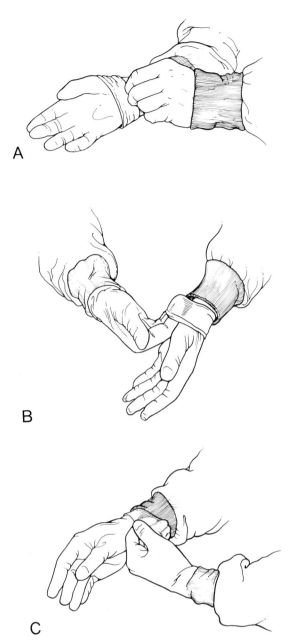

Figure 4.4. Open-gloving technique. **A,** Left *ungloved* hand pulls on right glove, touching only the inner surface of the glove. **B,** Insert gloved fingers of right hand under the inserted cuff and pull onto left hand. **C,** Pull glove cuffs over gown wristlets.

ter of courtesy as well as containment of contaminants, discard the gown and gloves in receptacles provided. Do not throw soiled apparel on floor or furniture.

Some procedures have an added infection risk and may be labeled ''dirty,'' ''contaminated,'' or ''septic.'' Special protocol may be dictated to confine organisms and prevent their transmission. Examples of such cases might be *1)* intra-abdominal sepsis, *2)* empyema, *3)* gross fecal contamination, or *4)* perirectal abscess. Personnel will be required to remove gown, gloves, footcovers, hat, and mask prior to leaving the operating room. Additional aspects of protocol may differ in each institution, and the surgical staff should advise the student as to specific protocol in such cases.

Principles of Asepsis and Sterile Technique

A simple definition of asepsis is the absence of any infectious agents. However, asepsis it also used as a broad term to describe a wide variety of procedures that reduce the incidence of infection in patients and personnel. Such practices include sterilization of goods and supplies, disinfection of the hospital environment, antisepsis of animate objects, and environmental control of the operating room.

Sterilization is the process that kills all forms of living matter (including bacteria, virus, yeast, mold) with the use of special equipment employing moist heat, dry heat, or ethylene oxide gas.

Moist heat destroys all forms of microbial life, including spores, through denaturation and coagulation of intracellular protein. The essential factors are temperature, time, and pressure. A temperature of 250°F, a time exposure of 15–30 minutes, and a pressure of 15–17 pounds per square inch are required to kill microorganisms. Other variables are the size, contents, and packaging methods of the materials to be sterilized. The type of moist heat sterilizer commonly used in the operating room is a high-speed instrument sterilizer (autoclave), often called a flash sterilizer, which is designed to function rapidly at a high temperature and increased pressure. The requirements for unwrapped instruments are 270°F, 27 pounds of pressure, and minimum exposure time of 3 minutes.

The use of dry heat sterilization is limited to articles that cannot stand the corrosive action of steam or products that cannot be penetrated by steam or gas. Examples of such items are petroleum products, powders, glassware, and delicate instruments. In the absence of moisture, higher temperatures and longer exposure times are required: 340°F for 1 hour, 280°F for 3 hours, 250°F for 6 hours.

Ethylene oxide gas sterilization is a process that kills bacteria by reacting with the chemical components of the protein of the cell. It is particularly useful for non-heat-stable items or moisture-sensitive items such as lensed instruments, air-powered instruments, glassware, and paper or rubber products. This form of sterilization is dependent on gas concentration, temperature, humidity, and exposure time.

Assurance that sterilization conditions were achieved can be obtained only through a biological control test. Process monitors, such as heat-sensitive tape, indicate that materials were exposed to sterilization conditions; however, they do *not* assure sterility. Packaged items are also marked with a sterilization date. The time a sterile package may be kept in storage without compromising the sterility is the shelf life. The shelf life is dependent on conditions of storage, packaging materials, seal of package, and integrity of package. Any package that is outdated, exposed to moisture, dropped on the floor, or receives a tear or puncture is considered contaminated.

Disinfection of the hospital environment is achieved through the use of chemical agents to destroy pathogenic bacteria on inanimate surfaces. The operating

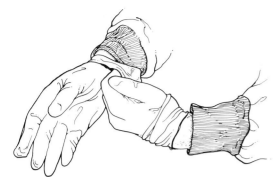

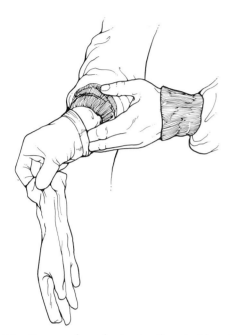

Figure 4.5. Remove gloves by turning them inside out, being careful to not touch the soiled part with hands.

depends on strict adherence of all personnel to sterile technique. The following basic principles regarding sterile technique must be conscientiously practiced.

1. Only sterile items are used within a sterile field. The sterility of those items must be provided by proper packaging, sterilization, and handling.
2. Parts of a gown considered sterile are the sleeves and the front from the waist to the shoulder level.
3. Tables are sterile only at table level (top); the edges and sides below table level are unsterile.
4. The edges of anything that encloses sterile contents are considered unsterile.
5. Persons who are sterile touch only sterile items; persons who are not sterile touch only unsterile items.
6. Sterile persons keep within the sterile area; unsterile persons avoid the sterile area.
7. Sterile persons avoid learning over an unsterile area; unsterile persons avoid reaching over a sterile area.
8. Sterile persons keep contact (sitting, leaning) with an unsterile area to a minimum.
9. A sterile field is created as close as possible to the time of use.
10. Sterile areas are continuously kept in view.
11. Destruction of the integrity of microbial barriers results in contamination.
12. Microorganisms must be kept to a minimum.

Careful attention to these sound principles of sterile technique is mandatory for the safety of the patient. Once the principles are understood, the need for their application becomes obvious.

The Sterile Field

The sterile field is the area of the operating room that immediately surrounds and is especially prepared for the patient. It is the area around the site of incision and the area that has been prepared for holding sterile supplies and equipment. All items needed for the operation are sterilized and used within the restricted area to prevent the transportation of microorganisms into the open wound. The sterile field is created by the placement of sterile sheets and towels in a specific position to maintain the sterility of surfaces where the operation will be performed. The patient and operating table are covered with drapes so the site of incision is exposed yet isolated (Fig.4.6). Objects that are draped include instrument tables, basins, the Mayo stand, and trays. The sterile team members function within this limited area and handle only sterile items. All members of the operating team must constantly safeguard the sterility of the operative field.

Skin Preparation

Prior to the placement of the drapes, skin preparation at the site of incision is performed. A wide area of

room and all the furniture (e.g., the operating table, instrument tables, lights) are cleaned after each operation with chemical disinfectants.

Antisepsis refers to the use of chemical agents on animate surfaces to destroy bacteria. Personnel perform the surgical scrub on hands and arms before the operative procedure with antiseptic soaps, and careful attention is given to preoperative preparation of the patient's skin to construct an area with reduced bacteria.

Environmental control of the surgical suite is essential to keep contamination to a minimum and provide maximum protection for the patient. These factors include greater room air pressure than in the hallway, which forces airflow out of the surgical area; restricted traffic; controlled room temperature of 68°–72°F; controlled humidity of 50%; and air change rate of 18–25 times per hour.

A variety of measures and controls are employed to maintain an environment that is as sterile and free of bacteria as possible. The integrity of this environment

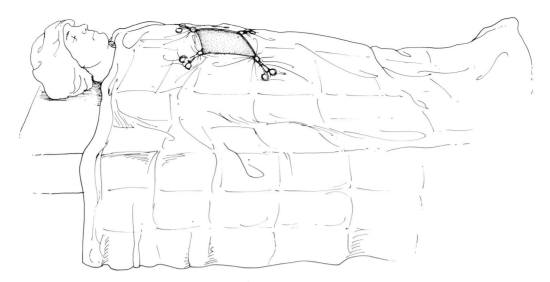

Figure 4.6. Incision site is exposed, yet isolated.

skin around the operative incision must be meticulously prepared by shaving and scrubbing. Shaving, if required, should be performed just prior to the procedure and ideally outside the operative theater. The skin preparation cleanses the operative site of transient and resident microorganisms, dirt, and skin oil so that the danger of infection is minimized.

Skin preparation is usually carried out from a separate table called a "prep" table. Commercially made disposable trays are available that contain towels, gauze sponges, antiseptic soap, and disposable razors. After the positioning of the patient on the operating table, one member of the surgical team prepares the patient's skin with antiseptic. Sterile gloves are worn, and gauze sponges or a sponge forceps to hold the gauze are used. The incision line is scrubbed first and the antiseptic is applied to an increasingly larger area, working outward toward the periphery of the field (Fig. 4.7). Theoretically, the incision line should be the cleanest, and, as one moves away from this site, the number of organisms increases. Once the lateral limits of the operative field are reached, the sponge is discarded and a new one is used to repeat the process. The sponge is never brought from the outside of the field to repeat the scrub of the central incision area. Areas likely to contain large numbers of bacteria, such as the perineum, groin, or axillae, are washed last before discarding the sponge. Cleansing should be done vigorously, employing both chemical and mechanical action. Particular attention to difficult areas such as the umbilicus must be given. Cotton-tipped applicators may be used in this area. Towels should be used to absorb excess solution and prevent the solution from pooling under the patient. The procedure for applying antiseptic solution on various parts of the body may vary, depending on the site and the surgeon preference. Painting of the operative area follows the same principles as the scrub, i.e., central toward the periphery. After the skin has been prepared, the patient is ready for draping.

Draping involves covering the patient and surrounding areas with a sterile barrier to construct a sterile area. Drapes must be fluid-resistant, antistatic, abrasive-free, lint-free, and drapable (to fit contours). Varieties include textile, plastic, and nonwoven disposable (paper). Textile drapes are usually tightly woven muslin of double thickness, preferably blue, green, or grey, as color reduces glare and eye fatigue. The drape is folded before sterilization in such a way for easy and safe handling. Styles of drapes include the following:

- Towels: used to outline the operative site; the folded edge is placed toward the incision and secured with towel clips.
- Stockinette: seamless tubing of stretchable material that contours to fit snugly to the skin; may be used for extremities.
- Fenestrated sheets: usually 108 × 72 inches with longitudinal or transverse fenestration that exposes the operative site.
- Split sheet: longitudinal cut from one end up the middle usually one-third the length, forming two free ends; may be used to drape an extremity or the head.
- Single sheet: 108 × 72 inches for draping nonspecific areas.
- Plastic incise drape: transparent self-adhering drape can be applied after the fabric drape, alleviating need for towel clips; facilitates draping of irregular body surfaces.

The following are standard basic draping principles:

1. Place drapes on a dry area.
2. Handle drapes as little as possible; avoid shaking drapes (air currents carry contaminants).
3. Make a cuff over the gloved hand to protect hand from contacting an unsterile area.
4. Never reach across the table to drape the opposite side; go around the table.
5. Hold the drape high enough to avoid touching nonsterile areas.

6. Once the drape is placed, do not adjust; if incorrectly placed, discard it.
7. Unfold toward the feet first.
8. Place the folded edge toward the incision (this provides a smooth outline of the field and prevents instruments or sponges from falling between layers).
9. Any part of the drape below waist level or table level is considered contaminated and not to be handled.
10. Towel clips fastened through the drapes have contaminated points; remove only if necessary and discard.
11. If a hole is found after a drape is placed, cover that area with another barrier.

Draping procedures may vary from one hospital to another; however, standardized methods of application should be followed.

Functioning as an Assistant in the Operating Room Environment

Frequently the student is asked to function as an assistant during an operative procedure. This can produce a spectrum of emotional responses, varying from elation to fear and trepidation. More commonly, undergraduates are asked to hold retractors or provide other measures to gain exposure for the operating surgeon. Occasionally the student is excluded from the field of view, asked to contort into uncomfortable positions while pulling on a retractor that he or she cannot see, with strength that has long been spent, and while feeling ill, exhausted, or worried and anticipating a barrage of questions concerning regional anatomy, physiology, or surgical technique. Almost every

surgical clerkship has been "branded" at one time or another by an anecdotal account of physical, mental, and emotional horror experienced in the operating room, but this is rarely the situation. Most surgeons respond positively to students who demonstrate an interest and some evidence of independent study about the patient or the operation. The elective nature of most surgical procedures allows sufficient time for the student to become familiar with the basic operative steps.

The following checklist may help the student prepare for the role as an assistant or an observer in the operating room. The better prepared the student, the more likely that the experience will be educational and the greater will be the student contribution to what is taking place.

- What procedure is to be done?
- What is the regional anatomy?
- What is the normal physiology and the pathophysiology of the organ?
- What are the surgical and nonsurgical options?
- What is the effect of the procedure on the pathophysiology?
- What are the potential complications?

In most clinical circumstances the operative plan is usually very clear (e.g., cholecystectomy for cholelithiasis) and has been discussed on rounds. If it has not been discussed, ask! A review of the regional anatomy is always beneficial. The blood supply to the organ(s) involved, the lymphatic drainage, and the proximity to other vital structures (e.g., relationship of common bile duct to the portal vein or hepatic artery) become important. A surgical atlas may be the best reference to refresh the memory on anatomical detail, as these texts approach the subject from a surgeon's perspective rather than that of an anatomical dissector.

Most surgeons assume that students are able to de-

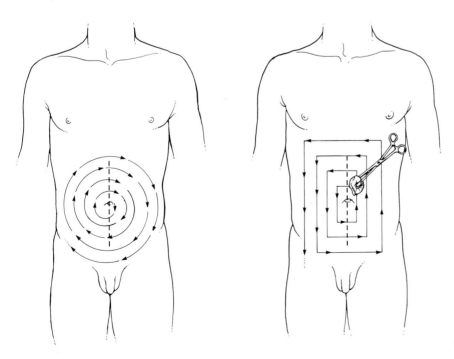

Figure 4.7. Preparation of the operative site. Movement from the center toward the periphery.

scribe the normal physiology of the organ or organ systems involved. If this is not fresh in your mind, a review is in order. An understanding of the abnormal or pathophysiologic process is the goal of most undergraduate clerkships. For many disease processes, a clear description can be found, and for others there may be several theories. Even when there are several theories, students should be able to provide some intelligent explanations if asked.

There is frequently more than one surgical approach to a problem and nonsurgical alternatives as well. Surgery for peptic ulcer disease and the approach to the solitary thyroid nodules are excellent examples. Knowledge of how the surgical procedure reverses or changes the pathophysiologic process involved enhances the student's concept of what is happening in the operating room.

Every surgical procedure carries with it the risk of complication. Some complications are related specifically to the technical aspects of the procedure itself, such as anastomotic leak or stenosis, pseudoaneurysm, and common duct stricture. Others may relate to the physiologic or anatomic alterations imposed by surgery, such as marginal ulcers at the site of gastrojejunostomy, dumping syndrome, or afferent loop syndrome. Many surgical atlases list the common complications that are specific to the procedure. The risks of the anesthetic, pulmonary compromise, atelectasis, thrombophlebitis, and wound infection are complications commonly shared by multiple procedures and should not be forgotten.

Functioning as a good assistant can be as demanding as serving as the primary surgeon. Being a good assistant is a learned behavior and requires experience. A proficient assistant can often make a mediocre surgeon appear expert. This requires a knowledge of what is to be done. The assistant should anticipate the steps in the procedure and help rather than compete with the operating surgeon. Keeping the field dry, anticipating the cutting of suture, and providing adequate exposure are within the capabilities of even the novice in the operating room. Most surgeons recognize that the undergraduate student is in unfamiliar territory, and instruction on how to help is usually provided by the senior members of the team. The assistant must pay attention to the procedure itself and avoid needless distractions.

Conversation should be limited and pertain to the case. This is especially important if the procedure is being done under local or spinal anesthesia while the patient remains awake. Needless chatter, jocular remarks, or the inadvertent "oops" does not promote confidence in the patient's mind and is not professional. Care must be taken not to inadvertently lean on the patient while standing at the operative table, as nerve damage or the inability to ventilate could result.

The surgical technician will pass the requested instruments; attempts by the student to retrieve or replace instruments on the Mayo stand disrupt the organization and flow of the operation. Many surgical technicians consider the Mayo hallowed ground, and

trespassers are frequently harshly chastized. This is for good reason, as the ability to provide requested instruments, ties, or suture quickly is hampered by extra hands or disorganized instruments. The operative field should be kept as tidy as possible. Sponges used during the procedure should be dropped into the container provided. This helps to contain contamination, simplify accounting of sponges, and aids in providing a rough estimate of blood loss. Searching for a misplaced sponge tries everyone's patience! Members of the surgical team should remain in the room until the patient leaves or permission to leave has been given by the surgeon. The student should remain available to assist with completion of dressing application, transferring of the patient to the stretcher, or other incidental tasks as required.

In addition to serving as an assistant during the technical aspect of the procedure, the medical student should be prepared to assist with the transfer of the patient to the operating table, positioning of the patient, skin preparation for the patient, and other miscellaneous procedures. A familiarity with basic equipment and supplies is most helpful.

Proper positioning of the patient for the operation is determined by the surgeon. The following principles should be considered:

- Proper maintenance of respiratory function
- Unimpaired circulation
- Protection of muscles and nerves from pressure
- Accessibility and exposure of the operative field
- Uninterrupted administration of anesthetic agents
- Accessibility for administration of intravenous fluids
- Comfort and safety of the patient

Important safety measures that must be observed during transfer or positioning of a patient include the following:

- Table securely locked in position
- Protection of patient's head during movement by the anesthesiologist
- Uninterrupted flow of intravenous fluids
- Care to not hyperextend arms
- Slow and gentle movement to avoid circulatory or respiratory compromise
- Prevention of pressure on nerves (make certain legs are not crossed with patient in supine position; place pillows or rolls under chest if patient is prone)
- Unobstructed tubings

Operating tables are divided into three or more hinged sections that can be flexed or extended so the desired position can be obtained. This procedure is often called "breaking" the table, and the joints of the table are referred to as "breaks." The operative table can be placed in a number of positions, including head up (reverse Trendelenburg), head down (Trendelenburg), rotated laterally, flexed, raised, or lowered. Special equipment and table attachments may be used to stabilize the patient on the table. Examples of such accessories are safety belts, arm straps, arm boards, braces, supports, stirrups, and bandage rolls. Although the circulating nurse assumes the major responsibility in the actual positioning of the patient, the safety of the patient during the operative experience is a responsibility shared by every member of the surgical team.

Classification of Operative Wounds

Operative wounds may be specifically classified according to the risk of contamination or infection as clean, clean-contaminated, and contaminated or dirty. This classification allows a prediction of subsequent wound infection risk and helps to allow comparisons of one surgical team's technique with another. Clean wounds are those in which the gastrointestinal, respiratory, or urinary tract is not entered. Inflammation is not present, and no break in technique occurs. The risk of infection is negligible. Clean-contaminated wounds include those in which the gastrointestinal, respiratory, or urinary tract is entered without significant spillage, or a break in operative technique occurs. The risk of infection is minimal. Contaminated wounds involve gross spillage of gastrointestinal or urinary tract contents, or acute inflammation is encountered. A major break in operative technique occurs. Fresh traumatic wounds are also included in this category because of potential contamination. The risk of infection may approach 5%. The wound is considered dirty if pus or a perforated viscus is encountered. Old traumatic wounds with necrotic tissue, foreign body excision, or cases with gross fecal contamination present are also considered dirty. The infection rate is quite high if these are closed primarily, and therefore they are often managed by leaving them open.

The prevention of wound infection in the surgical patient requires the following:

- Control of endogenous infection
- Strict sterile technique
- Careful operative technique and wound closure
- Reduction of exogenous or environmental sources of contamination
- Thorough, prompt cleansing and debridement of traumatic wounds
- Prevention of intraoperative wound contamination
- Prophylactic antibiotics in selected patients
- Sterile technique for dressing changes
- Documentation of wound infection statistics

Wound infections are associated with prolonged hospitalization, significant patient discomfort, incisional hernia formation, and frequently with unfavorable cosmetic result. Through adherence to these principles the morbidity associated with wound infections can be minimized.

SUGGESTED READING

Atkinson LJ, Kohn ML: *Berry and Kohn's Introduction to Operating Room Technique.* New York, McGraw-Hill, 1978.

Skills

1. Perform a preoperative surgical prep on a patient having an abdominal or thoracic procedure.

2. Demonstrate a surgical scrub and sterile gowning and gloving.

3. Assist with an operative procedure.

Study Questions

1. Describe what is considered "sterile" in the operating room.

2. Discuss the role of the student in an operative procedure and how the student should prepare to participate in an operative procedure.

3. Prepare a list of questions a surgeon might ask a student during
   a. an elective cholecystectomy
   b. an inguinal herniorrhaphy
   c. a thyroidectomy for malignancy
   d. an elective abdominal aortic aneurysmectomy
   e. an emergency celiotomy for a perforated ulcer

4. Describe the procedure for the surgical preparation of a patient who is to undergo a modified radical mastectomy.

5

Surgical Procedures for Medical Students

Richard M. Bell, M.D.
Paddy M. Bell, C.S.T.

ASSUMPTIONS

Students are allowed to perform basic invasive procedures commonly utilized in patient care.

OBJECTIVES

1. Discuss the purpose of a nasograstic tube and list the risks, indications, and contraindications for insertion and removal.
2. Given an actual patient, demonstrate the ability to intubate the stomach with a nasogastric tube, including proper positioning and secure taping.
3. Demonstrate proper care of a nasogastric tube: describe the care of other gastrointestinal tubes, including gastrostomy tubes, T-tubes and jejunostomy tubes.
4. List the indications, contraindications, and possible complications of passage of a urethral catheter.
5. Demonstrate the ability to insert a urethral catheter and provide daily catheter care and maintenance necessary for preventing stricture formation and retrograde infection.
6. Demonstrate proper technique for sampling urine (i.e. through a catheter or a spontaneously voided specimen).
7. Describe the indications for drain placement, advancement, and removal as well as possible complications associated with their use.
8. Appropriately advance and remove surgical drains, including Penrose drains, Hemovac sumps, nasogastric tubes and urethral catheters.
9. List the indications, contraindications and complications associated with the insertion of central venous catheters, Swan-Ganz catheters and arterial catheters and participate in their placement.
10. Demonstrate the ability to insert intravenous catheters for the delivery of intravenous fluids or medications.
11. Demonstrate the routine maintenance of central venous catheters, including care and management of the tubing and solution containers.
12. Perform venipuncture for blood sampling.
13. Demonstrate the ability to sample arterial blood by performing arterial puncture.
14. Describe, identify and manage complications secondary to venipuncture or arterial puncture.

Surgical Tubes and Drains

The proliferation of ancillary medical services has reduced the necessity for the physician or student physician to perform the majority of routine ward or laboratory procedures. Nursing services may place most of the nasogastric tubes and Foley catheters and initiate intravenous therapy. Respiratory therapists may sample arterial blood, and physician assistants may assume additional responsibilities, relieving the physician of many day-to-day chores. Nevertheless, the physician must be proficient in the skills to offer assistance when necessary and to perform them when ancillary help is not available. More importantly, it is imperative that the physician know the indications and contraindications for these procedures, as well as how to manage catheters, tubes, and drains. This chapter, which is not a complete listing of all psychomotor skills the student must master, includes those more frequently performed on the wards. The student is referred to the videotape collection that accompanies the rest of this educational package for demonstrations of these various skills.

Nasogastric Intubation

As the term *nasogastric* implies, a tube is passed from the nose into the stomach. Indications for such a procedure are listed in Table 5.1.

Gastric decompression is perhaps the most common indication encountered on a surgical service. Postoperatively, many surgical patients manifest an ileus, and the tube is placed to remove gastric secretions. Because the stomach may produce 800–1200 cc of acid-rich se-

Table 5.1.
Indications for Nasogastric Intubation

Gastric decompression
Sampling gastric content for analysis
Gavage (feeding)
Lavage (irrigation or dilution of gastric content)

Table 5.2.
Equipment Required for Nasogastric Intubation

Tube
Anesthetic spray or gel
Lubricating gel
Bulb syringe or Asepto
Tape
Stethoscope
Suction apparatus (optional)
Water cup and straw
Water for irrigation
Ice to stiffen the tube
Emesis basin

cretions per day, gastric distension may result in esophageal reflux, vomiting, and even aspiration in the absence of normal gastrointestinal motility. With mechanical small bowel obstruction the situation is compounded. Reflux of small bowel contents into the stomach produces further distension, usually resulting in the vomiting of feculent material, classically associated with mechanical small bowel obstruction. Nasogastric tubes are also used therapeutically to prevent antral distension in treating acute inflammatory diseases of the pancreas and biliary tract. Because antral distension produces the most powerful physiologic stimulus to acid secretion via the release of gastrin, nasogastric tubes are often utilized to reduce this stimulus by decompressing the stomach. Acid in the duodenum is the initiator of most secretory mechanisms in gastrointestinal physiology, and the prevention of antral distension helps minimize gastrointestinal function by this mechanism. It is a common misconception that the use of a nasogastric tube will prevent the aspiration of gastric contents; although the risks may be minimized, the presence of a tube in the stomach is no guarantee that aspiration will not occur.

Some tubes are placed for diagnostic reasons, to help identify the site of gastrointestinal blood loss or to collect gastric samples for acid analysis. Although it is usually not possible to aspirate blood from beyond the ligament of Treitz, this can provide preliminary information as to the general area of bleeding. Nasogastric and nasoenteric tubes are frequently utilized for gavage or feedings in those patients who cannot or will not eat sufficiently. Lavage, or washing of the stomach, to remove blood or ingested material is also a frequent indication.

Generally there are few contraindications to the passage of a nasogastric tube. Obstruction of the nasal passages secondary to old or acute trauma and suspected basilar skull fracture are absolute contraindications. In these situations the tube may be placed through the mouth. Maxillofacial fractures are relative contraindications, and it is advisable to use the oral route in these cases as well. The passage of a tube into the stomach through or close to a fresh anastomosis should be done only by a very experienced individual and usually with the aid of fluoroscopy.

Before attempting to pass the tube, tell the patient what to expect and why the tube is necessary. Make the patient as comfortable as possible to alleviate any anxiety. Sump tubes are usually used for routine gastric intubation, and most adults will tolerate a 16–18 French tube. Although silicone tubes are softer and better tolerated by patients, they may be more difficult to pass. As with all procedures, assemble all the equipment you may need before you begin. Table 5.2 lists most of the usual requirements.

Have the patient who is awake in the sitting position. If the patient is not awake, be prepared to remove vomitus by suctioning or turning the head. Examine the nasal passage and choose the side that does not appear to be obstructed. Spraying the posterior pharynx and nasal passage with a topical anesthetic spray or gel may so reduce the discomfort of insertion. While the anesthetic is taking effect, tell the patient that pressure and some discomfort will be felt as the tube passes through the nose. When the patient feels the tube in the back of the throat, ask him or her to swallow. Provide water and straw for sipping.

Lubricate the tip of the tube to make passage through the nose easier. The distance to the stomach can be estimated from the tip of the nose posteriorly to curve just in front of the aural tragus and end in the midepigastrum. Direct the tip of the tube directly posterior toward the base of the neck. Most beginners attempt to direct the tube superiorly, encountering resistance (Fig. 5.1). Once the tube is in the hypopharynx, ask the patient to swallow. This elevates the larynx and tucks it under the base of the tongue and helps to prevent inadvertent tracheal intubation. Gentle but firm pressure usually results in the passage of the tube past the glottis and into the proximal esophagus. Repeated swallowing aids the passage of the tube into the stomach.

Frequently patients gag when the tube passes the hypopharynx, and occasionally they vomit. Mentioning this to them virtually ensures its occurrence. If gagging prevents the passage of the tube, it may be prudent to repeat the application of the topical anesthetic and try again. Fortunately the gagging is usually transient, and once the tube enters the esophagus it ceases. Pass the tube to the predetermined mark (obtained by measurement as directed previously). Once it is felt that the tube has been passed an appropriate distance, the Asepto or bulb syringe is used to aspirate gastric contents. Fifty to 100 cc of air may be insufflated while auscultating over the upper abdomen for gurgling sounds. Once it is determined that the tube is appropriately positioned, anchor the tube to the nose with tape. Be careful not to pull the tube into the corner of the nasal alae, as this may result in ischemic necrosis of the skin and nasal alar cartilage. Patients

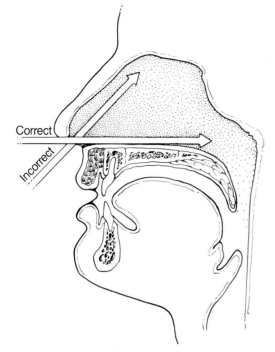

Figure 5.1. Correct insertion of nasogastric tube.

are most unappreciative of being marked with a permanent crescent-shaped divit on one side of their nose. Connect the tube to the appropriate suction device.

Although the procedure sounds relatively simple, a few misadventures may occur. If the tube will not pass through the nasopharynx on one side, try the other. If gagging and/or vomiting become a problem, it may be expeditious to allow the patient to regain composure and try again later. Tracheal intubation is usually manifested by a paroxysm of coughing, inability to speak, and a look of impending doom on the face of the patient. Simply remove the tube, wait a while, and repeat the attempt.

Rarely, epistaxis may occur. Although this usually resolves spontaneously, ephedrine nasal drops may help. Injury to the mucosa of the posterior pharynx and submucosal tube placement have virtually been obviated with the softer tubes and gentle manipulation while placing them. Esophageal perforation can occur but can be avoided by gentleness and stopping if resistance to passage is met. Occasionally the tube may curl in the hypopharynx and extrude through the mouth. If this occurs, remove the tube and make another attempt. If problems are encountered, ask for help from someone with more experience.

Nasogastric tubes are very uncomfortable and a source of extreme agitation for many patients. Unfortunately there is very little that can be done to completely alleviate the problem. Analgesic throat lozenges or sprays may help some. A mixture of 1% Xylocaine® and Neo-Synephrine® used as nasal drops may afford some relief. Occasionally, patients may complain of ipsilateral otalgia, which is secondary to an obstructive serous otitis from blockage of the tympanopharyngeal orifice. Removal of the tube or moving it to the other nostril nearly always relieves the complaint. Decongestants or nasal sprays may offer additional relief. Re-

Table 5.3
Bladder Catheterization

Indications
1. Provide for accurate assessment of urinary output
2. Decompress the bladder
3. Relieve obstruction
4. Diagnosis
4. Therapy

Contraindications
1. Suspected urethral disruption
2. Difficulty encountered in attempting to pass the catheter

moval of the tube is quite simple and, as a rule, is accompanied by profuse expressions of gratitude by the patient. Disconnect the suction to avoid mucosal biopsy and gently remove the tube from the nose. A tissue for the patient to wipe both nose and eyes is nearly always appreciated.

Urethral Catheterization

The indications for bladder catheterization are listed in Table 5-3. On a general surgical service, the Foley catheter is frequently placed for a determination of hourly urine output, as an indication of adequate assessment of intravascular volume replacement. Because urinary output is a simple indicator of effective renal perfusion, catheters are often inserted for this purpose.

Prior to abdominal procedures, a catheter is placed to decompress the bladder. This is done to ''shrink'' the organ from the proximity of the incision and thus minimize the risk of inadvertent cystotomy when opening the abdominal cavity. The same principle is employed prior to performing diagnostic peritoneal lavage (see Chapter 13), as inadvertent lavage of the bladder rarely provides useful information.

Catheters are also placed to relieve obstruction, as in the case of benign prostatic hypertrophy. The majority of catheterizations are employed for diagnosis, to obtain uncontaminated urine for analysis or culture, cystograms, cystometrograms, reflux studies, or to determine the volume of residual urine.

Additionally, they are used therapeutically in patients who are unable to void spontaneously secondary to neurologic injury or disease, to treat bladder inju-

Table 5.4.
Equipment for Bladder Catheterization

Sterile drapes
Sterile gloves
Collection bag and drainage system (if retention catheter used)
Sterile water-soluble lubricant
Sterile cotton or gauze sponges
Sterile sample container
Prep solution
Forceps
Syringe and sterile water (for balloon inflation)
Tape
Catheter
    14 French for female
    16 or 18 French for male

ries, or even to provide hemostasis by tamponade, such as after prostatectomy.

An obvious contraindication to transurethral bladder catheterization is the suspicion of urethral injury, usually associated with pelvic fracture. (see Chapter 13). A relative contraindication for students, who are usually novices in the procedure, is a patient with a known history of stricture and obstruction, or resistance while attempting to pass the catheter. Such situations are best handled with assistance from a member of the resident staff or by obtaining a urology consultation.

Most hospitals provide a packaged kit that contains all the needed equipment, as listed in Table 5.4. The equipment is opened sterilely and placed where it is easily accessible. Unless there is some urgency, a few minutes taken to explain the procedure to the patient will help allay anxiety and make the insertion of the catheter less traumatic. Males should be told that they will feel pressure and some discomfort as the catheter enters the bladder and that relaxation helps minimize the discomfort. Patients should also be advised of the sensation of the need to void after insertion.

The patient's perineum is exposed and draped. This is usually not difficult for catheterization of males but may be a problem in females. An assistant may be necessary to spread the labia or hold the thighs apart so that the urethral meatus can be clearly seen. Make sure the lighting is adequate and properly adjusted.

Before starting, fill the syringe with the correct amount of sterile water, attach it to the catheter, and inflate the balloon to test for its integrity. The sterile lubricant is then opened and applied to the catheter tip. Prep solution is opened and the cotton swabs saturated.

Sterile gloves are worn. One hand grasps the shaft of the penis and holds it straight or spreads the labia so the meatus can be seen (Fig. 5.2) This hand is considered contaminated and should not touch any of the sterile equipment or the catheter. The sterile hand uses the forceps to hold the prep swabs. The foreskin is retracted to expose the glans, and the glans is washed with the prep solution. In the female, the urethral meatus is wiped with prep solution toward the vagina. In some situations it is almost impossible to perform the procedures under sterile conditions; however, every effort should be made to maintain aseptic technique to decrease the incidence of urinary tract infection.

The penis is held erect, thus providing the straightest path via the urethra to the bladder. It is helpful to have the catheter well lubricated, especially in the male. The tip is inserted into the urethral meatus and advanced with steady and firm pressure. In the male the catheter tip will induce spasm of the external urethral sphincter, occasionally creating resistance. Steady firm pressure will result in fatigue of the sphincter mechanism and the catheter will usually pass. When the tip is in the bladder, urine will flow into the collection system. The catheter is advanced another 2–3 cm to ensure that the balloon will not be inflated in the urethra. If the balloon does not inflate easily, advance the catheter further and try again. Do not forcefully expand the

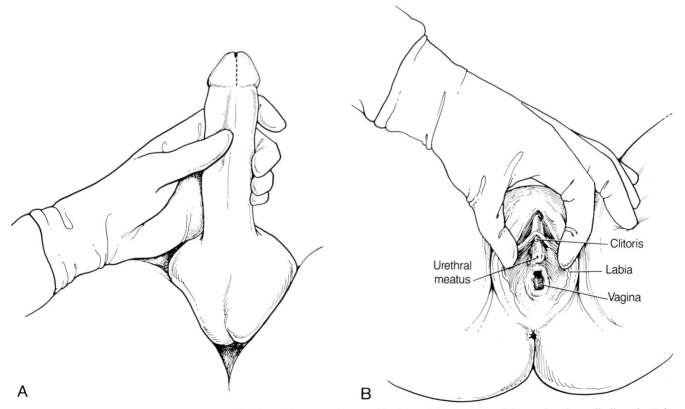

A   B

Figure 5.2. Foley catheter insertion. **A,** Penis is held straight upward to provide the straightest course of the urethra that will allow the Foley access to the urinary bladder. **B,** Anatomical relationship of the female urethra. With the hips abducted, a gloved hand spreads the labia to expose the uretha. The other hand prepares the area and inserts the lubricated catheter.

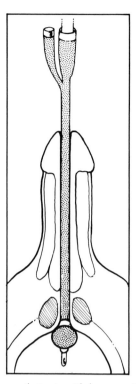

Figure 5.3. The Foley catheter is withdrawn until the balloon seats itself against the outflow tract. The catheter may be taped to the lower abdomen in males or the leg in females.

balloon. If you are uncertain, it is better to try insertion again or ask for help rather than risk urethral injury.

Complications encountered during catheterization include possible bacteremia, urethral disruption or tear, and creation of a false passage. These are minimized by following the procedure outlined above.

Once the balloon is inflated, withdraw the catheter until the balloon rests against the urethral orifice inside the bladder (Fig. 5.3). In the female the catheter may be taped to the inner thigh. In the male it is better to tape the catheter to the right or left side of the lower abdomen. This forces the urethra to take a gently curved path, reducing the effect of kinking and pressure necrosis imposed by the catheter. The latter may result in stricture formation. The foreskin must be replaced over the glans to prevent phimosis.

Secondary bladder colonization is usually produced by retrograde migration of bacteria around the meatus. Once the catheter has been placed, the barrier to bacteria has been lost. Because of the relatively short urethra in the female and the proximity to the vagina, secondary infection is common. For these reasons, catheter care is vital to reducing infectious complications. The meatus and catheter should be cleansed of debris and encrustations at least daily, more often if necessary. An antimicrobial agent, such as Betadine ointment, is applied around the urethral meatus and the catheter is retaped into the appropriate position. The collection system should remain closed, thus reducing the likelihood of contamination.

Catheters are removed when they have accomplished the purpose for which they were inserted. Removal of the catheter is quite simple. A syringe is used to remove

the water in the balloon. The same volume should be removed as was inserted to assure complete decompression of the balloon. The catheter is withdrawn using gentle traction. Culturing catheter tips rarely provides clinically useful information, as contaminants from around the meatus are usually cultured. If culture information is necessary, a midstream collection of the first voiding after removal is more appropriate.

Wound Drains

Drains are utilized to provide for the egress of air or liquid accumulations in spaces or potential spaces after surgical procedures. Most frequently they are used to evacuate serum, blood, lymph, gastrointestinal tract secretions, pus, or necrotic debris from areas that do not lend themselves to repeated exposure or packing. (Table 5-5). Persistence of such collections may promote infectious complications or hinder the resolution of an existing infectious process. Drains are usually placed at the time a surgical procedure is performed, and, for the most part, the medical student is concerned about their care and removal.

Drains come in a variety of sizes and shapes, depending on the purpose for which they are used. They function by gravitational flow (e.g., T tube in bile duct), suction (e.g., sumps or closed suction drains), or capillary action (e.g., Penrose or wick drains).

The simplest drains are those that act as wicks or promote drainage by capillary action. The Penrose drain is a soft, collapsible Latex cylinder, frequently placed into an abscess cavity to allow purulent material to escape to the outside. Historically, Penrose drains were placed near pyloroplasties or near the duodenal stump to indicate early breakdown and leak of intestinal content. These are rarely used today. A gauze roll placed inside the Penrose drain promotes drainage utilizing a wicking action.

Constant gravity drains are usually placed in cavities, conduits, or structures that secrete fluids or drain organs. A T tube in the common bile duct, a nephrostomy tube, or a cholecystostomy tube are examples. Fluid is removed with the help of gravity and the secretory pressure of the organ producing the fluid. Many such drains are simply vents to allow excess pressure from secretions to escape, thus preventing overdistension of the cavity or conduit and disruption or breakdown until normal internal drainage can be reestablished.

Closed suction drains are usually rubber or silicone tubes with numerous holes that allow secretions to be evacuated from the area by a suction device. Wall suc-

Table 5.5.
Purpose of Drains

1. Evacuation of air or secretions
2. Prevention of collections that would elevate skin flaps and retard viability
3. Minimizing dead space
4. Decompression (e.g., T tube in common duct)
5. Stents

tion or a collapsible receptacle provides the vacuum into which secretions are collected. Sumps are simply modifications of such systems, but an additional tube, usually within the drainage tube itself, permits a steady flow of air from outside through the drainage catheter to help ensure patency. Frequently this air passes through a small filter to remove particulate matter.

The selection of the system to use is dictated by the nature of the materials to be evacuated, the area needing drainage, and, perhaps most importantly, by inherent bias and personal preference of the surgeon. Most drains are anchored to the skin by tape or sutures to avoid inadvertent removal. In some circumstances, premature removal can have disastrous consequences, producing excessive morbidity and even mortality. Drains should always be handled with care, and every effort made to protect them. The insertion sites should be inspected daily and the sutures securing them cleaned. An antimicrobial ointment can be used sparingly around the anchoring sutures to reduce bacterial colonization.

Drains are two-way streets. Retrograde infection from the skin to the inside is a real and clinically significant problem. Sterile gloved hands, attention to aseptic technique, and attentive dressing of the drain site can help reduce these problems. Drains should never be advanced or removed unless hands are properly gloved.

Drains are removed or advanced when they have fulfilled the purpose for which they were placed or have become nonfunctional. Closed suction systems and gravity drains are usually removed all at once, while the others are gradually advanced to allow closure of the drainage tract from inside to outside. This prevents the skin from sealing prematurely and helps to avoid tract infections. Because the tract communicates with the skin and the integument has been broken, the tract is contaminated by microorganisms and infection may result if the tract itself is not allowed to drain. Once the drains are removed, the skin site is allowed to heal by secondary intention. When advancing drains, reanchor the drain after advancement to prevent migration back inside the body cavity.

Vascular Catheterization

Intravenous therapy is such a common practice in medicine that every student *must* be comfortable with the procedure. Unfortunately, in many medical centers, nurses or intravenous teams have reduced the opportunities for the student to place venous catheters and thus become truly proficient in this skill. Nonetheless, future physicians must be able to gain access to the venous circulation for fluid therapy, the delivery of medications, and blood sampling. Often you will be called on when the intravenous technician fails to gain access.

The ability to deliver intravenous fluids to a patient is a relatively new technique. Early in the twentieth century, because of a lack of prepackaged fluids, sterile tubing, and plastic catheters, fluids were administered in limited quantities by a technique known a clysis. Large-bore steel needles were used to infiltrate fluids into subcutaneous tissue of the flank, thigh, or abdomen with hopeful absorption into the circulation. With the development of plastic catheters, the intravenous installation of electrolyte solutions has become a safe and efficient method of correcting metabolic or electrolyte abnormalities.

Several types of catheters are available, depending on the infusion requirements and size of the vein. These are available in prepackaged, presterilized kits. Small veins usually require small catheters (18- or 20-gauge), whereas large veins can accept catheters (sizes 12–18). The smaller the number, the larger the catheter. For surgical patients who may require the administration of large volumes of fluid or the transfusion of whole blood or blood products, a 16-gauge catheter or larger is preferred.

Insertion sites are numerous, and the student should choose a location with a large vein that minimizes patient discomfort and one that avoids motion around a joint. The antecubital fossa usually contains large veins that can be easily cannulated, but the problems of motion at the elbow frequently reduce the longevity of catheters inserted in this area. It is also very uncomfortable for patients to have their arms immobilized by restriction of elbow motion. The dorsum of the hand is a better choice, although the large veins of the forearm are most preferred. Intravenous catheters in the lower extremity of the adult patient should be avoided if at all possible, except in emergent situations. The development of phlebitis associated with the lower extremity cannulation can be a significant clinical problem.

If possible, inform the patient about what you are to do and the necessity of the procedure. Make the patient as comfortable as possible, keeping the extremity selected in a dependent position to promote venous filling. Use towels to protect the bed linens and patient's clothing from inadvertent soilage by blood or other solutions. (This will win points from the nursing staff.) Apply a tourniquet above the chosen site. Rubber tubing, a Penrose drain, or a more sophisticated constricting device (often available from drug companies) may be used. The tourniquet need only be tight enough to constrict venous return, not to disrupt total circulation to the extremity. Have all the equipment ready and easily accessible, especially the fluids to be infused.

Prepare the site adequately with alcohol or other antiseptic solution. Often it is advisable to shave the area to decrease the discomfort of tape and dressing removal. The apex of the junction of two veins is a convenient spot to perform the vein puncture. The

Table 5.6.
Equipment for Intravenous Cannulation

1. Catheter of appropriate size
2. Alcohol swabs for skin prep
3. Tourniquet
4. Tape
5. Fluids/administration set
6. Antibiotic ointment
7. Band-Aid
8. Additional catheter
9. Local anesthesia (if required)

prepped site is punctured near the vein and the catheter is inserted until blood return is visible at the hub of the set, or the skin may be punctured adjacent to a vein, and the vein entered at the side. Direct skin puncture over a large vein, if one is so fortunate, is also acceptable. The catheter is inserted, and once blood return is noted into the hub, the outer plastic sheath is advanced into the vein, the needle withdrawn, and the tourniquet released. The solution and tubing prepared prior to venipuncture are now connected. Tape is used to secure the catheter to the skin. There are many ways to accomplish this, and students will develop their own preferences. Antiseptic ointment is applied to the puncture site and covered with a sterile dressing, e.g., Band-aid. The infusion rate is then adjusted as necessary. Carefully inspect the vein proximal to the cannula to ensure that inadvertent infiltration of intravenous fluids is not taking place. Patients may notice a cool sensation up the arm but should feel no pain as the fluids infuse. If burning or stinging is noticed, infiltration is suspected, and the infusion should be stopped. If a joint needs to be immobilized, an arm or wrist board may be taped into place to prevent flexion or extension. Be sure that a loop of the extension set is taped to the extremity. This may prevent the inadvertent loss of the intravenous line if the tubing is caught on some object, the bed, or the patient.

Arterial Catheterization

Continuous blood pressure monitoring and the frequent determination of arterial blood gases in the intensive care unit has led to the placement of intra-arterial catheters for monitoring and repeated sampling. The insertion of an arterial catheter requires more skill and patience than venous catheterization. The necessary equipment is listed in Table 5.7. Patients with arterial lines must be under constant observation, as inadvertent disconnection of the system can have fatal consequences.

The radial artery is frequently selected as the site for cannulation, although others (e.g., brachial, dorsalis pedis, or posterior tibial) are sometimes chosen. It is wise to avoid the lower extremity, especially in older patients whose distal circulation may be impaired. Brachial and femoral arteries should be reserved for only the most extreme circumstances where information gained would outweigh the attendant risks of arterial injury.

Before insertion of the catheter, it is imperative to determine that the patient has sufficient collateral circulation. Both dorsalis pedis and posterior tibial pulses must be palpable in the foot. In the hand, the Allen test ensures sufficient collateral circulation. The patient is asked to make a fist while digital compression occludes both radial and ulnar arteries. The patient opens and closes the fist to empty the hand of blood. With the palm open, the pressure on the ulnar artery is released while maintaining occlusion of the radial artery. The hand should show a blush as reperfusion of the digits and palm occurs from flow through a patent ulnar vessel. If reperfusion does not occur, if it is delayed beyond two seconds, or if the entire hand is not reperfused, then it is unwise to utilize that radial artery, as

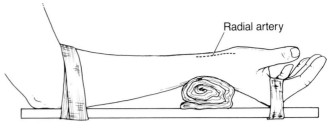

Figure 5.4. A roll of gauze may be placed under the dorsum of the wrist to provide a degree of hyperextension with the hand and forearm taped to the intravenous board as shown. This provides easier access to the radial artery.

the blood supply from the ulnar artery is not adequate to perfuse the hand. If there is any question concerning the adequacy of the collateral circulation, another site should be chosen.

Positioning the patient's wrist in slight hyperextension with a small roll of gauze or washcloth helps expose the radial artery (Fig. 5.4). All fluid lines and monitoring equipment are made ready before insertion of the catheter. The skin is prepared and draped using sterile technique and anesthetized with a local agent. A small amount of local anesthetic is infiltrated *around* the artery to help reduce spasm. It is important not to inject the artery itself, to distort the anatomy with excessive local anesthesia, or to obliterate the palpable pulse. One finger palpates the pulse to serve as a guide to direct the catheter. Once the artery is punctured, arterialized blood should be visible in the hub of the cannula. The plastic sheath is then slowly directed over the needle and the needle withdrawn. Proximal pressure on the artery will reduce the loss of blood through the catheter while the monitoring line is connected. After connection to the monitoring system, an arterial pressure tracing should be visible on the screen, or the digital readout of the monitor should show arterial pressure. The system is flushed with heparinized saline to clear the catheter and lines of blood. If the system is functional, the catheter is sutured to the skin, the insertion site is cleaned, and antibiotic ointment is applied. A sterile dressing is placed over the puncture site, and the tubing is taped securely to prevent disconnection. Once the procedure has been completed, recheck the hand by compressing the fingernails or palm, and watch for the blush, indicating adequate blood flow. If there are any questions or problems, ask for help from someone with more experience.

Occasionally complications can occur, but if meticulous technique is followed, these can be kept to a minimum. Ischemia in the extremity should never occur if an adequate evaluation of collateral blood flow was made before the procedure. Hematoma formation at the puncture site, thrombosis of the artery or the catheter, or distal microemboli from the tip of the catheter are other potential problems. Bleeding and septic complications should not occur with adequate care and protection of the system.

To remove the catheter, remove the sutures and tape that have fixed the system to the patient. Smoothly withdraw the catheter from the artery and apply digital pressure over the puncture site for 10 minutes or until bleeding ceases. A dressing is then applied.

Table 5.7.
Equipment for Placement of Intra-arterial Catheters

Plastic catheter (size 18–22)
Skin prep solution
Local anesthetic
Suture
Heparinized saline
Pressure tubing
Pressure bag
Monitoring equipment and transducers
Antibiotic ointment, dressings

Blood Sampling

Although most phlebotomy is performed by ancillary services, blood sampling is another skill that all physicians must acquire. Sites for venipuncture are numerous and, at some time, almost every accessible vein has been utilized. The arms are preferred, as these large superficial veins present good targets. The patient should be made as comfortable as possible, preferably in a sitting or reclining position. The site is prepared with antiseptic solution and the tourniquet applied above the puncture site. Remember that it is necessary only to restrict venous return. An appropriate gauge needle (18- or 20-gauge), and a syringe adequate to hold the amount of blood required are chosen. Preliminary thought here will prevent the need for a second phlebotomy due to an inadequate volume of blood being withdrawn on the first stick.

The vein is punctured with the bevel of the needle up. Gentle traction is applied to the plunger of the syringe as the needle and syringe are steadied against the patient's arm. Once sampling has been completed, the tourniquet is released, and the needle is withdrawn. This helps reduce bleeding and hematoma formation at the puncture site. A dry piece of gauze is used to hold pressure over the puncture site until hemostasis is secure.

The vacutainer system, used in many hospitals and laboratories, allows the direct filling of collection tubes. The technique of venipuncture is the same. Initial consideration and procurement of the specific containers required for each type of test can eliminate the frustration of having to repeat the procedure because the samples clotted in the syringe or the wrong tubes were used. Some samples require anticoagulation or special preservatives. If there is any question, consult the laboratory or the laboratory reference manual to be sure before proceeding. Plan carefully so that needless repeat phlebotomies are not done. Furthermore, frequent venous sampling can actually deplete the blood volume of small children.

Arterial sampling is slightly more difficult. The brachial, radial, and femoral arteries are common sites. For arterial blood gas analysis, the syringe must be heparinized. If the collection system being used does not have a "heparin button" in the pre-packaged set, then the student must heparinize the syringe. A small amount of heparin solution is drawn into the syringe from the vial (1–1½ ml of 1000 U/ml is sufficient), and the solution is allowed to coat the inside of the syringe. The excess is then expelled. Even small amounts of heparin in the syringe may make the results inaccurate.

The skin is prepared in the usual fashion. The pulse may be palpated with the index finger or the artery may actually be positioned between the index and long finger to provide a target. The needle and syringe may be held much like a dart and, by feeling the pulse, the artery can be punctured. If a glass syringe is used, the successful arterial puncture will be heralded by the flow of blood into the syringe due to arterial pressure. Plastic syringes with rubber plungers usually require manual withdrawal of the sample. In this case, the syringe must be steadied while the plunger is withdrawn. Blood gas analysis rarely requires more than 1 or 2 ml. The needle is withdrawn and firm pressure is held over the puncture site to prevent hematoma formation. All air should be removed from the syringe to prevent gas exchange with the blood, and the syringe should be capped. Samples for gas analysis should be run immediately or iced for no more than 15 minutes.

The complications that can occur from arterial puncture are obvious. Hematoma formation and thrombosis of the artery are the most frequent, especially with repeated sampling from the same site.

Tying Surgical Knots

Two-Handed Tie

Tying suture properly requires practice. It is helpful to ask the operating room technician for the leftover surgical ties to take home and perfect this skill. "Knot boards" are often available for use around the hospital.

The ends of the suture are held, one in each hand. The thumb of the left hand catches the right hand strand near the base of the thumb and loops the left-handed strand at the base of the nail (Fig. 5.5A and 5.5B). The right-handed strand is pinched between thumb and index finger of the left hand and is pushed through the loop created, as shown in Figure 5.5C. In this step the index finger can "follow" the thumb through the loop. The right hand releases the end of the suture and the left thumb and index finger pull the end through to complete the first half hitch (Fig. 5.5D). The half hitch just formed is tightened just enough to approximate the edges of the tissue. Notice that the hands are crossed to seat the knot flat. If this is not done, a slipknot is formed and tension can be lost. Some prefer to loop the right-handed strand twice (Fig. 5.5B–D) to form the surgeon's knot. This is necessary only in rare circumstances. The hands are uncrossed after securing the first half hitch, the left thumb catches the left strand just as in the first step, but the right-handed strand is above, not below, the left strand (Fig. 5.5G). This forms a loop through which the left index finger can be passed. The left strand is now pinched between the left index finger and the left thumb, and the thumb "follows" the index finger (with the suture) back through the loop (Fig. 5.5H). The right hand releases the strand temporarily and then pulls the end through, completing the second half hitch. The half hitch is seated squarely on the first, forming the knot

(Fig. 5.5I). If additional half hitches are necessary, the steps are repeated. This is often necessary for nylon suture, which unties itself quite easily, or to add some insurance that the knot will not come undone.

Instrument Tie

After the suture has been placed, grasp the long end in the left hand, point the needle holder held in the right hand toward the fingers of the left hand, and wrap the long end around the instrument in a clock-wise manner. Now grab the short end of the suture with the needle holder and pull the short end through the loops (Fig. 5.6A). The first half hitch can now be seated across the edges of the tissue (Fig. 5.6B). If a surgeon's knot is desired, simply loop the long end around the instrument twice before grasping the short end. Remember when wrapping to point the instrument toward the fingers of the left hand. The second half hitch is made by repeating the step, but wrapping counterclockwise, then grasping the short end with the

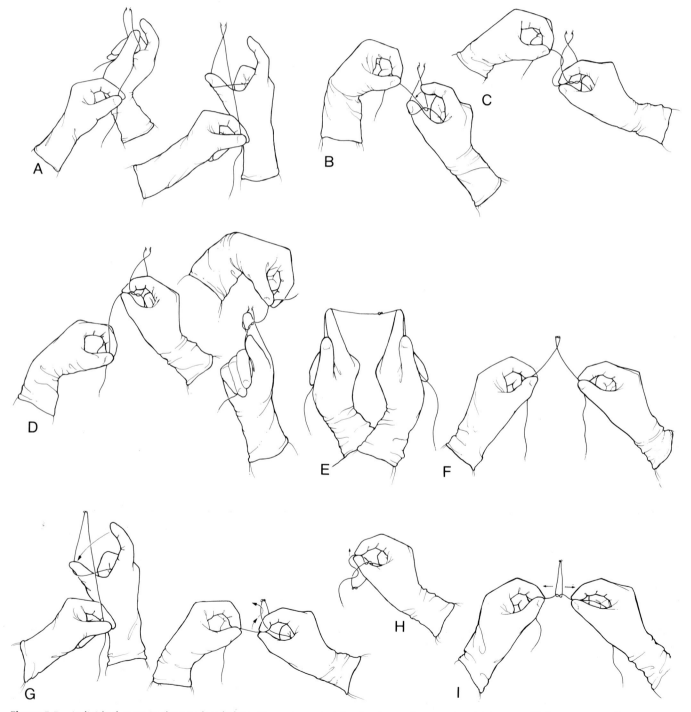

Figure 5.5. Individual steps in the two-handed tie. Competence in tying knots requires practice. Make use of leftover suture after a surgical procedure.

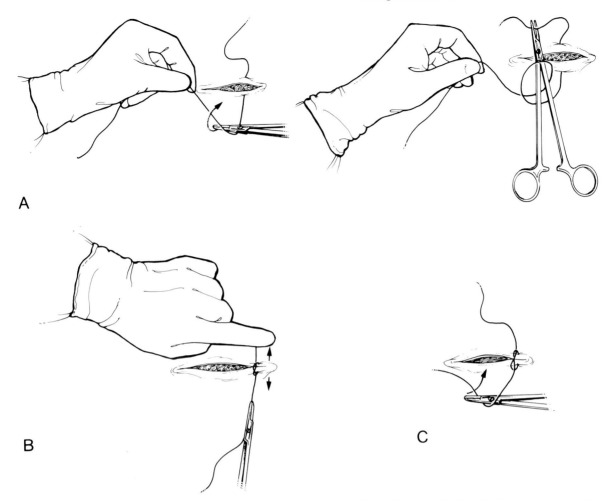

A

B

C

Figure 5.6. Instrument tie. Notice how the tip of the instrument points toward the fingers of the hand holding the suture. (See text for description.)

instrument (Fig. 5.6C). The second half hitch is now tightened on the first. Be sure the knots are seated flat across the tissue edges to prevent placing slipknots. The procedure is repeated as often as needed, wrapping first in one direction and then the other.

SUGGESTED READINGS

Nealon TF: *Fundamental Skills In Surgery.* Philadelphia, WB Saunders, 1971.
Peacock EE, Van Winkle W Jr: *Surgery and Biology of Wound.Repair,* ed 2. Philadelphia, WB Saunders, 1976.

Skills _____

1. Insert under supervision a nasogastric tube, a foley catheter, and an intravenous cannulae for fluid administration.

2. Perform phlebotomy and arterial blood sampling.

3. Demonstrate simple suturing of a wound and knot tying techniques.

Study Questions _____

1. Describe the process of positioning a
   a. nasogastric tube
   b. Foley catheter

2. Discuss the complications and contraindictions to the placement of a nasogastric tube, Foley catheter, and the alternatives available.

3. Demonstrate an instrument tie and a two-handed tie of suture.

4. Demonstrate your ability to perform venipuncture for blood sampling, arterial puncture, and the placement of an intravenous cannula for the infusion of intravenous fluids.

6 Fluid and Electrolyte Balance

Arthur Naitove, M.D.
Douglas B. Evans, M.D.
Janet K. Ihde, M.D.

ASSUMPTIONS

The student understands the distribution of fluids and electrolytes in the body compartments.

The student understands the role of the kidney in regulating fluid electrolyte, and acid-base balance.

The student understands the role of the lung in regulating acid-base balance.

OBJECTIVES

1. Complete the following table of normal values:

	Na	K	HCO$_3$	Cl
Serum				
Gastric aspirate				
Bile				
Ileostomy aspirate				
Perspiration				

2. Describe the extracellular, intracellular, and intravascular volumes in a 70-kg man.
3. List at least four endogenous factors that affect renal control of sodium and water excretion.
4. List at least six physical findings or symptoms of dehydration.
5. List and describe the objective ways of measuring fluid balance.
6. Describe the 24 hr. sensible and insensible fluid and electrolyte losses in the routine post-op patient.

7. List the composition of electrolytes in the following solutions:

	Gluc	Na	K	Cl	HCO$_3$	Ca
Normal Saline (.9%)						
Ringers lactate						
5% dextrose in water						
5% dextrose in Ringers lactate						

8. Given a patient with the condition in the left columns, list representative values and pH for the serum electrolytes observed.

	Na	K	HCO$_3$	Cl	pH
Excessive gastric losses					
High volume pancreatic fistula					
Small intestinal fistula					
Biliary fistula					

Diarrhea

_____

Closed
head
injury

_____

9. List representative values that might be obtained
   in patients with the conditions listed in the left
   column.

SERUM

	Na	K	HCO$_3$	Cl	Osmolality
ATN					
Dehydration					
Inappropriate ADH secretion					
Diabetes insipidus					
Congestive heart failure					

URINE

	Na	K	HCO$_3$	Cl	Osmolality
ATN					
Dehydration					
Inappropriate ADH secretion					
Diabetes insipidus					
Congestive heart failure					

10. Describe the possible causes (differential diag-
    nosis), appropriate laboratory studies needed, and
    treatment of the following conditions:
    A. Hypernatremia
    B. Hyponatremia

C. Hyperkalemia
D. Hypokalemia
E. Hyperchloremia
F. Hypochloremia

11. List the physiological limits of normal blood
    gases.
12. List representative values that might be obtained
    in patients with the conditions listed in the left
    column:

ARTERIAL BLOOD

	pH	PO2	PCO2	HCO3	Base Excess
Acute metabolic acidosis					
Acute respiratory acidosis					
Chronic respiratory acidosis					
Acute respiratory alkalosis					
Compensated metabolic acidosis					

15. List the differential diagnosis and describe the
    treatment of metabolic acidosis, metabolic alka-
    losis, acute hypoxia, and acute respiratory aci-
    dosis.

Fluids and Electrolytes

The recognition and management of fluid, electrolyte, and related acid-base problems are common challenges on a surgical service. The nature of the diseases
and trauma being treated, as well as the physiologic
stresses of the operations performed, contributes to
these circumstances. This chapter attempts to provide
students with a working base of information to enable
them to be aware of the daily fluid and electrolyte
needs of surgical patients and the factors that can modify them, to better understand and recognize imbalances that can be encountered, and to formulate
effective therapeutic plans for preventing the occurrence of imbalances or correcting them when they oc-

cur. Before dealing with specific clinical problems, we start with a simple overview of basic concepts pertaining to fluid, electrolyte, and acid-base balance that must be kept in mind and utilized to achieve the stated goals. This chapter is intended to be an introduction to the subject material covered; students should seek more complete and comprehensive information from the many available texts and articles in the literature, some of which are listed at the end of this chapter.

Overview

Anatomy and Composition of Fluid Compartments

Total body water (TBW) in the adult can represent 45–70% of body weight, the value varying as a function of age, sex, and lean body mass. At the extremes, it is lowest in the aged and obese and highest in the very lean and young. TBW is estimated as 60% of body weight in the idealized 70-kg adult male and 50–55% in his female counterpart. Functionally TBW is partitioned into two main compartments. The intracellular space represents two-thirds of the total, and the extracellular space one-third, amounting to 40% and 20% of body weight, respectively, in the average adult male (Fig. 6.1). The extracellular compartment is further divided into the larger interstitial space (16%) and the smaller intravascular plasma fluid space (4%).

The electrolyte composition of the two subdivisions of the extracellular fluid space are similar. As present in plasma (Table 6.1), sodium is the chief extracellular cation, with small amounts of potassium, calcium, and magnesium also present. The corresponding anions are chloride, bicarbonate, and smaller amounts of proteins, phosphates, sulfates, and organic acids. The ionic composition of the interstitial fluid differs only with respect to its lower concentration of protein, and the related minor changes in chloride and bicarbonate levels as determined by the Gibbs-Donnan equilibrium. In contrast, in the intracellular compartment the cations potassium and magnesium and the anions phosphates, sulfates, and proteins are the dominant ionic species.

Table 6.1.
Normal Plasma Values

	Concentration, mEq/liter
Cations	
Sodium	135–145
Potassium	3.5–5.0
Calcium	4.0–5.5
Magnesium	1.5–2.5
Anions	
Chloride	95–105
Carbon Dioxide content	24–30
Phosphate	2.5–4.5
Sulfate	1.0
Organic acids	2.0
Protein	1.6

The striking differences in the intracellular and extracellular electrolyte composition are maintained by the selective permeabilities of cellular membranes. Free diffusion of proteins, chloride, and multivalent ions is limited and active metabolic "pumps" in the cell wall promote the movement of sodium out of the cell and the passage of potassium into it.

Movement of water from one compartment to another is passive, determined by the action of physical forces exerted across the intervening membranes. The capillary membrane separating the interstitial and intravascular spaces under most circumstances is freely permeable to water, electrolytes, and solutes but not to proteins. Consequently the net flow of water between these two spaces is a function of the balance between fluid pressures generated on either side of the membrane and the effective colloid oncotic pressures generated by the higher concentrations of nondiffusible protein in the plasma. The exchange of water between the intracellular and extracellular interstitial compartments, on the other hand, is totally determined by osmotic gradients across the cell membranes. Normally there is no gradient and no significant net water flow in either direction, as the osmolarity or number of osmotically active particles per liter of solution on either side of the membrane is the same. Under usual circumstances this measures approximately 290 mOsm/liter. When extracellular fluid becomes hyposmolar (or hypotonic) relative to normal values, water will flow into the cells where the osmolarity is higher. A new equilibrium will be reached with the osmolarity of both compartments less than the normal 290 mOsm/liter. Similarly, hyperosmolarity (or hypertonicity) will develop in both compartments should extracellular osmolarity be raised. Osmotic equilibrium is reached by an egress of water from the cell into the extracellular space. Isotonic fluid expansion or contraction of the extracellular space, in contrast, having no effects on osmolarity, will not include such movements of water between the cells and interstitial fluid.

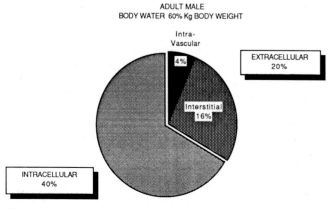

ADULT MALE
BODY WATER 60% Kg BODY WEIGHT

Intra-Vascular
4%

EXTRACELLULAR
20%

Interstitial
16%

INTRACELLULAR
40%

Figure 6.1.

Regulation of Sodium, Water, and Osmolarity

Total body sodium is estimated to be 40 mEq/kg (2800 mEq in a 70-kg man). One-third is fixed in bone, and the other two-thirds, most of which is extracellular, is the exchangeable fraction. Sodium and its related anions represent 97% of the osmotically active particles normally present in the extracellular fluid compartments. In practice, extracellular osmolarity can be estimated by the formula

$$\text{extracellular osmolarity} = 2 \times [Na]_s + 10^1 \qquad (1)$$

where $[Na]_s$ is serum sodium concentration and 10^1 is the osmolar contribution of other solutes, including blood glucose (mg/dl/18) and BUN (mg/dl/2.8).

If the value approximates 290 ± 10 mOsm/liter it can be reasonably assumed that extracellular osmolarity is within normal limits. The central role of sodium in the determination of the extracellular as well as the intracellular osmolarity is evident; factors that alter sodium concentration, whether by manipulation of the ion or the water in which it is dissolved, must be understood.

Renal Mechanisms to Control Fluid and Electrolytes. Under usual circumstances regulation of salt and water balance is primarily done by the kidney. Assuming normal renal perfusion and membrane function, sodium and water are both filtered at the glomerulus. In the proximal tubules large amounts of each are recovered. Ultimately, however, determination of renal conservation or excretion of sodium and/or water depends on selective processes occurring at more distal tubular sites.

Sodium reabsorption in exchange for potassium and hydrogen ion secretion in the distal tubules is a direct effect of the adrenal cortical hormone, aldosterone. This action can help to maintain both extracellular volumes and osmolarity. Extracellular volume reduction, particularly in the intravascular space, is a potent stimulus for aldosterone release. This response is triggered by a decrease in renal perfusion, which promotes the juxtaglomerular apparatus to secrete renin, which in turn promotes the secretion of angiotensin I and its conversion to angiotensin II, which is a potent stimulator of aldosterone secretion. Volume receptors in the right atrium are present also, which when activated will cause aldosterone secretion. The juxtaglomerular apparatus and its renin-angiotensin mediated aldosterone secretion is also activated by low extracellular fluid sodium concentrations. In addition, aldosterone secretion can be stimulated by an increase in serum potassium levels and the action of ACTH. Aldosterone is suppressed by extracellular volume expansion and increased sodium and decreased potassium concentrations.

Antidiuretic hormone (ADH) released from the posterior pituitary has a potent direct effect on the kidney to increase tubular reabsorption of water. This effect and its modulation are important in the regulation of fluid volumes and osmolarity in the body. Intracranial osmoreceptors serve as the sensors initiating events promoting ADH secretion when plasma osmolarity increases and, conversely, inhibiting ADH secretion when plasma osmolarity decreases. Importantly, ADH production and release also are dependent upon volume receptor activity in the right and left atria. Decreased extracellular volume sensed in the right atrium leads to ADH secretion. Increased volume sensed in the left atrium leads to inhibition of ADH release. Volume dependent responses can and usually do override the influences of the osmoreceptor controlling system when the two are in conflict.

Potassium Metabolism

Total body stores in the normal adult are of the order of 3500 mEq (50–55 mEq/kg), approximately 98% of which is located intracellularly at a concentration of 150 mEq/liter of cell water. In the extracellular fluid compartment, a total of 70 mEq (including plasma) is present at a concentration of 3.5–5.0 mEq/liter. Normal daily intake of potassium averages 100 mEq, 95% of which is excreted in the urine and 5% of which is lost in feces and sweat. In the kidney most of the filtered potassium is reabsorbed in the proximal tubular system. Nevertheless, selective secretion or absorption in the distal tubule determines net renal excretion or conservation. Potassium excretion is directly related to circulating levels of aldosterone, cellular and extracellular potassium content, and tubular urine flow rates. Acid-base disturbances also exert significant influence. Alkalosis enhances excretion by promoting distal tubular secretion of potassium in exchange for the reabsorption of sodium and hydrogen. Conversely, acidosis prompts renal conservation of potassium in proportion to the urinary excretion of the other cations.

Acid-Base Balance

Acid-base balance is in effect the management of large amounts of hydrogen ion produced endogenously each day. There is a 40–60mM load of fixed nonvolatile organic acids (i.e., sulfuric, phosphoric, and lactic acid), some of which are ingested and some of which are produced by metabolic activity; and there is the 13,000–20,000 mM of carbon dioxide comprising the volatile acid load. Normally the free hydrogen ion concentration of extracellular body fluids, measured as pH, is maintained at 7.40 ± 0.05. This is accomplished by the combined action of three mechanisms: (1) buffering systems present in body fluids that immediately offset changes in hydrogen ion concentrations; (2) pulmonary ventilation changes that can promptly adjust the excretion of carbon dioxide; and (3) renal tubular function, which over time can contribute by modulating the urinary excretion or conservation of acid or base.

The bicarbonate/carbonic acid buffer system in extracellular fluid is one of the most important. Its relationship to pH is described by the Henderson-Hasselbalch equation and its modifications:

$$pH = pK^a + \log \frac{[HCO_3^-]}{[H_2CO_3]} \qquad (2a)$$

$$pH = 6.1 + \log \frac{[HCO_3^-]}{0.03 \times PCO_2} \quad (2b)$$

$$7.4 = 6.1 + \log \frac{24 \text{ mEq/liter}}{1.20 \text{ mEq/liter}} \quad (2c)$$

where $PaCO_2 = 40$ mm Hg.

The value for $[H_2CO_3]$ can be determined as the arithmetical product of a proportionality constant and the $PaCO_2$. In clinical practice, direct measurements of arterial pH and $PaCO_2$ are readily available and $[HCO_3^-]$ can be calculated or derived from a nomogram. The pH is determined by the ration $[HCO_3^-]/[H_2CO_3]$, which normally is approximately 20:1. A change in either the numerator or denominator can alter the ratio and the resulting pH value. As well, a change of either $[HCO_3^-]$ or $PaCO_2$ can be compensated for by a corresponding change in the same direction of the other, restoring the ration to 20:1 and the pH to 7.40. Thus pulmonary regulation of $PaCO_2$ and renal tubular regulation of plasma HCO_3^- can be appreciated as important determinants of extracellular pH.

As effective as the HCO_3^-/H_2CO_3 buffer system is, and as available as its substrates are from metabolic sources, it, in combination with all other extracellular buffers, cannot maintain arterial pH at normal levels in the face of all challenges. A major role is played by intracellular buffer systems. It is estimated that as much as 50% of fixed acid loads and 95% of hydrogen ion changes resulting from excessive retention or excretion of carbon dioxide are buffered in the cells. These movements of hydrogen into and out of the cell involve cationic exchanges that induce reciprocal shifts of potassium. Thus acidosis induces movement of potassium out of the cell, which raises its extracellular fluid concentration, and alkalosis causes the opposite movement into the cell, which decreases its extracellular concentration. The impact such acid-base-related exchanges can have on serum potassium concentrations must be remembered. The usual assumption of a direct relationship between serum levels and total body stores is no longer valid. Serum potassium concentration changes induced by acid-base alterations can have significant clinical implications, particularly with regard to myocardial irritability and function.

Disorders of Volume

Volume Depletion

Combined losses of fluid and electrolyte are frequently encountered in surgical patients. Among the most common are gastrointestinal fluid losses due to vomiting, nasogastric suction, diarrhea, and external drainage from enteric, biliary, or pancreatic fistulas. Such losses for the most part (Table 6.2) result in isotonic depletion of extracellular fluid volume, which in the absence of osmolar alterations are not shared with the intracellular fluid compartment. Isotonic depletion is also true of "third-space" losses of body fluids that

Table 6.2.
Approximate Electrolyte Composition of Gastrointestinal Contents

mEq/liter	[Na$^+$]	[K$^+$]	[Cl$^-$]	[HCO$_3^-$]
Gastric				
pH > 3.0	100	10	100	[a]
pH 1.0–2.0	25	15	140	[a]
Bile	140	5	60–120[b]	30–50[b]
Pancreatic	140	5	60–90[b]	90–115[b]
Small bowel[c]				
proximal	140	5	130	30
Distal or ileostomy	90	10	90	40
Diarrhea[d]	25–130	10–60	20–90	20–50

[a]Not measureable.
[b]At higher flow rates [HCO$_3^-$] increases and [Cl$^-$] decreases.
[c]Differences reflect increased absorption of Na$^+$ and Cl$^-$ and secretion of K$^+$ and HCO$_3^-$ in the progression from proximal to distal in the gut.
[d]Differences reflect whether diarrheal stool content is predominantly derived from the small bowel where [Na$^+$] and [Cl$^-$] are higher and [K$^+$] and [HCO$_3^-$] are lower, or from the colon where the other extremes of the ranges shown prevail.

are sequestered in injured tissue after trauma or surgery, and can be particularly significant in burns, crush injuries, long bone fractures, peritonitis, acute hemorrhagic pancreatitis, intestinal obstruction, pleural effusions, and large areas of soft tissue infection. Excessive urinary loss of water and electrolytes also can lead to volume depletion, as can be seen with diuretic therapy, high-output renal failure, and osmotic diuresis associated with nonelectrolyte hyperosmolar solute loading (e.g., glucose, mannitol, angiographic contrast media). Finally, there are volume depletions that involve losses of water in excess of solute. These include excessive renal free water excretion associated with primary deficiencies of ADH or nephrogenic causes of diabetes insipidus, increased evaporative losses from burned surfaces, and increased sweating and evaporative losses from the skin and respiratory tract in febrile patients. These hypotonic losses, however, create a hypernatremic hyperosmolar state in the extracellular compartment that will draw volumes from the cell fluids. This repletion of the extracellular space can blunt the clinical picture of volume depletion, which for the most part reflects extracellular deficits.

Extracellular volume depletion involves equivalent reductions of interstitial and plasma fluid volumes. The clinical consequences, therefore, can be viewed as twofold; consequences related to interstitial fluid deficits that can be appreciated by signs of decreased tissue turgor and volume, and consequences related to intravascular plasma volume deficits with signs of restricted tissue perfusion similar to those seen with whole blood loss. As outlined in Table 6.3, the clinical findings of extracellular volume depletion are directly related to the magnitude of the deficit involved. Weight loss can be a valuable indicator when previous values are known and the fluid losses are external. This is not true, however, if the depletion is due to internal third-

Table 6.3
Signs of Extracellular Fluid Volume Depletion

10% ECF reduction (~1.5 liters[a])-threshhold changes that can be overlooked.
    2% weight loss
    Thirst, mild reduction of urinary output.
    Laboratory: slight elevations of hematocrit[b] and urine sp gr.
20% ECF reduction (3 liters[a]): findings are always evident
    4% weight loss
    Apathy, drowsiness
    Decreased skin turgor, dry mucous membrane, longitudinal furrowing of the tongue
    Tachycardia, orthostatic hypotension
    Oliguria moderate with urine output <30 ml/hr

    Laboratory
      Hematocrit: elevated[2] (as will be RBC, Hgb, WBC)
      Urine: Sp Gr 1.020 or higher, osmolarity >500
                    mOsm/liter [Na$^+$] 10–15 mEq/liter or lower
      BUN/Cr: Both values modestly elevated with BUN/Cr
                    ratio > normal 10:1 (as high as 25:1)
30% ECF reduction (~4 liters[a]): findings are extreme
    6% weight loss
    Stupor or coma
    Skin cool, pale, cyanotic with poor turgor
    Eyes sunken
    Pulse rapid weak and thready, hypotension
    Oliguria pronounced with urine output <10–15 ml/hr
Laboratory:
Hematocrit: further elevated[b]
Urine: findings as above, excepting changes indicative of acute tubular necrosis (e.g., [Na$^+$] >20 mEq/liter, BUN/Cr ratio falling towards
    normal of 10:1, sp gr, and osmolarity decreasing below 1.020 and 500 mOsm, respectively)

[a]Calculated for 70-kg man.
[b]Rule of thumb—1% hematocrit rise for each 500-ml ECF deficit if RBC loss is nil.

space fluid sequestration in tissue spaces. In such circumstances, one becomes more dependent on hemodynamic parameters, elevated hematocrit, oliguria, and urinary concentration studies as guidelines. As renal perfusion becomes more restricted and levels of BUN and serum creatinine rise, one has to be sure that these are manifestations of prerenal azotemia and not renal failure secondary to acute tubular necrosis. Urine sodium concentrations of 10–15 mEq/liter or less and BUN creatinine ratios >20:1 are characteristic of prerenal azotemia. With renal tubular damage, on the other hand, renal tubular reabsorption of sodium and urea are impaired, urinary sodium concentration rises above 20 mEq/liter, and the ratio of BUN/creatinine falls toward a more normal value of 10:1.

Treatment of Volume Depletion. Successful treatment of any fluid or electrolyte disturbance depends on an understanding and correction of the underlying cause(s). Appropriate repair of volume depletion is determined by the composition as well as the amount of fluid administered (Tables 6.4 and 6.5). Information gathered by history, physical examination, and direct clinical observations of the losses involved, as well as measurements of serum electrolytes and arterial blood pH and PaCO$_2$ can be critical in determining the nature of the fluid therapy to employ. Treatment of isotonic extracellular volume deficits due to intestinal, biliary, pancreatic, or third-space fluid losses by intravenous infusions of Ringer's lactate or normal saline with potassium supplements is usually appropriate. On the other hand, lactate-containing solutions should not be used as replacement for acidic stomach contents lost by nasogastric suction or vomiting. In vivo conversion of the lactate to bicarbonate would make such solutions inappropriate in the treatment of fluid losses associated with metabolic, hypochloremic alkalosis. Comparably, glucose-containing solutions should not be used in repairing volume deficits secondary to osmotic diuresis induced by hyperglycemia. Therapeutic needs would be better served by infusion of glucose-free saline solution to restore volume and parenteral administration of insulin to reduce blood sugar levels.

As a rule, the rate of volume correction should be commensurate with the need and the ability of the patient to accept the fluid loads being delivered. When the deficits are moderate, complete replacement should be temperately carried out over at least a 24-hr period. If deficits are large and the consequences severe, the needs become more urgent. The therapeutic approach in such cases is to correct hemodynamic and perfusion inadequacies as rapidly and safely as possible and then to complete volume restoration at a much slower rate over the next 18–24 hr. The initial phase of treatment may require rapid infusion of up to one or more liters over 15–30 min to achieve hemodynamic stability. In this situation central venous or pulmonary arterial catheter pressure monitoring should be considered in

Table 6.4
Commonly Used Intravenous Solutions

	Glucose	Na$^+$	K$^+$	Cl$^-$	Lactate[a]	Ca^{++}
	g/liter	mEq/liter	mEq/liter	mEq/liter	mEq/liter	mEq/liter
5% Dextrose/water	50					
10% Dextrose/water	100					
"Normal" saline[b]		154		154		
5% D/saline[b]	50	154		154		
5% Dextrose/½ normal saline[c]	50	77		77		
3% NaCl		513		513		
Ringer's Lactate		130	4.0	109	28	3.0
5% Dextrose/Ringer's lactate	50	130	4.0	109	28	3.0

[a]Converted to HCO$_3^-$.
[b]0.9% NaCl.
[c]0.45% NaCl.

the management of high-risk patients whose cardiovascular status may be compromised by such therapeutic manipulations. This may become an absolute necessity in patients requiring emergency surgery and for whom the time course for volume correction is compressed even further. In general, it is also wise to avoid using glucose-containing solutions when rapidly repleting a volume deficit, thereby minimizing the risk of further fluid losses in response to a hyperglycemic-related osmotic diuresis.

Monitors of Fluid Repletion. Although hemodynamic data, measurements of weight change, and records of fluid intake and output can provide important information, urine flows and concentrations remain excellent guides to fluid needs and the adequacy of the replacement being given. Barring high-output renal failure, osmotic consequences of glycosuria, and the use of diuretics, urinary outputs of normally concentrated urine (sp gr ~ 1.015–1.020) at rates in excess of 40 ml/hr indicates adequate repletion of the extracellular fluid compartments. Similarly, in the absence of continuing whole blood loss, the lowering of hematocrit and hemoglobin values to normal levels also signifies extracellular volume correction. Reductions of BUN and serum creatinine to more normal values would be consistent with restoration of adequate renal perfusion as a result of extracellular volume repletion.

Volume Excess

Volume expansion can be the result of excessive fluid administration, abnormal fluid retention, or a combination of both factors. Excessive intravenous fluid therapy with balanced salt solutions is a common iatrogenic cause of isotonic fluid overload. This produces an extracellular expansion, which, in the absence of attendant osmolar changes, is not shared intracellularly. As such, isotonic extracellular expansion becomes manifest both as intravascular overload and excess interstitial fluid. These consequences are more apt to occur in the period immediately after surgery or trauma when maximal hormonal responses to stress are operating to

diminish sodium and water excretion by the kidney. The risk of fluid overload is even greater in the elderly and patients in whom underlying cardiac, renal, or hepatic disorders can contribute to fluid accumulation. Congestive heart failure, oliguric renal failure, and hypoalbuminemia secondary to hepatocellular dysfunction stand by themselves as recognized causes of extracellular fluid volume expansion.

Hypotonic as well as hypertonic fluid overloading also can occur. Inappropriate administration of salt-poor solutions as replacement for isotonic gastrointestinal or third-space fluid losses is a common cause of hyponatremic hypotonic volume expansion. Enhanced secretion of ADH in surgically stressful situations and inappropriate ADH activity associated with intracranial disorders or ectopic production by malignancies also are causes of selective restriction of water excretion that can lead to hypotonic fluid expansion. On the other

Table 6.5.
Concentrated Electrolyte and Glucose Solutions for Addition to Intravenous Fluids[a, b]

	Cation (mEq)	Anion (mEq)
Ammonium chloride	5.0	5.0
Calcium chloride	1.4	1.4
Calcium gluconate	0.5	0.5
Magnesium sulfate	4.1	4.1
Potassium acetate	2.0	2.0
Potassium chloride	2.0	2.0
Potassium phosphate	4.4	3.0 mM[c]
Sodium bicarbonate	1.0	1.0
Sodium Chloride	2.5	2.5
Sodium Lactate	5.0	5.0
Dextrose 50%	<0.5 gm>	

[a]Available in various concentrations. Check your hospital formulary.
[b]Incomplete list. All solutions are available in various concentrations. Other solutions are available, including trace metals for use in preparing parenteral nutrition solutions. Check your hospital formulary.
[c]Phosphate expressed in millimolar concentrations, as pH dependent multivalences preclude milliequivalent designation.

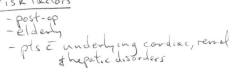

IV fluid overload risk factors
- post-op
- elderly
- pts c̄ underlying cardiac, renal & hepatic disorders

hand, administration of sodium loads that are not balanced by appropriate water intake result in hypernatremic hypertonic extracellular volume expansion. In such instances, water moving out of the cells in response to increased extracellular osmolar concentrations also contributes to intravascular and interstitial fluid overload. The resulting hypervolemic state can become even more pronounced when renal tubular excretion of salt and/or water is compromised. Hypertonic extracellular volume expansion also can be induced by the rapid infusion of nonelectrolyte osmotically active solutes (e.g., glucose, mannitol). Such a circumstance, however, is accompanied by hyponatremia, not hypernatremia. Plasma sodium concentration falls as a consequence of dilution by the solution that is being infused and the sodium-free water drawn from the cells into the extracellular space in response to the osmolar gradient created by the infused nonelectrolyte solute load.

The clinical picture of extracellular volume excess can vary, depending on the cause, nature, and severity of the challenges. Thus the signs can range widely. At the lower end of the scale are simple weight gain, small decreases of hemoglobin and hematocrit levels signifying hemodilution, modest elevations of peripheral and central venous pressures, and the appearance of dependent sacral or lower extremity edema. At the other end there are extreme consequences of vascular and interstitial fluid overload with frank congestive heart failure, as evidenced by pulmonary edema, pleural effusion, anasarca, and hepatomegaly.

Treatment of Volume Excess. Treatment is adjusted according to the severity of the extracellular fluid excesses and the related clinical findings. Lesser problems are treated by fluid and or salt restriction. As the

Table 6.6.
Causes of Hyponatremia

Dilution
  Accumulation of excess water
    Ingestion or infusion of excess free water.
    Hypotonic fluid replacement of isotonic gastrointestinal and "third space" fluid losses.
    Enhanced metabolic production of free water occurring with surgical stress and caloric deprivation.
  Retention of excess water secondary to enhanced ADH activity
    Physiologic response to surgical stress and/or hypovolemia
    Syndrome of inappropriate ADH (SIADH)
    Advanced cardiac, renal, and hepatic disease
Excessive Renal Loss of Sodium
  Salt wasting nephropathy
  Metabolic alkalosis
  Ketoacidosis
  Diuretics
  Adrenal insufficiency
Artifactual
  Hyperlipidemia
  Hyperproteinemia

magnitude of the problems increases, diuresis with furosemide administered in parenteral doses of 10–50 mg frequently becomes necessary. Potassium losses associated with the induced diuresis should be monitored and replaced by appropriate supplements. Cardiotonic drugs, oxygen therapy, and artificial ventilation may also be needed in the management of cardiac failure and respiratory insufficiency. The particular issues of therapeutic management of related hyponatremic and hypernatremic states are discussed in the next section.

Disorders of Electrolyte Concentrations

Sodium

The sodium ion is the principle solute determining osmolarity in the extracellular fluid compartments. Related increases or decreases of extracellular sodium concentration and tonicity are associated with movements of water across cell membranes, the direction of which depends on the osmotic gradient created by the extracellular alterations. The resultant cell volume changes are responsible for the adverse symptomatic consequences associated with low (hyponatremia) or high (hypernatremia) extracellular sodium concentrations.

Hyponatremia. Hyponatremia is defined as a low serum sodium concentration, which when clinically significant usually is below 130 mEq/liter. The causes of hyponatremia are outlined in Table 6.6. Hyponatremia can be the consequence of dilution related to the accumulation and retention of water in excess of salt, primary losses of sodium in excess of water, or a combination of both. In the surgical patient, dilutional hyponatremia commonly is caused by the infusion or ingestion of too much water, or the use of hypotonic fluids to replace isotonic gastrointestinal or third-space fluid losses. Accumulations of sodium-free water also can be generated metabolically by the catabolic breakdown of body tissues, as occurs with surgical stress and caloric deprivation (approximately 1 liter of water per kilogram of body fat or muscle). Perioperatively or post-traumatically, the usual compensatory mechanisms leading to renal excretion of excess water and correction of the hypotonic state may not be operative. In these circumstances, secretion of high circulating levels of ADH induced by a number of stress-related stimuli is not subject to hyposmolar inhibition, and hypotonic fluid retention persists. Similarly, hyponatremia secondary to unremitting ADH-induced accumulation of water in excess of salt is characteristic in patients with advanced diseases of the heart, kidney, or liver. Finally, there is the classical picture of dilutional hyponatremia associated with the syndrome of inappropriate ADH secretion or activity (SIADH). Clinically SIADH can be seen with tumors of the lung, pancreas, and duodenum; intracranial disease, trauma, and surgery; and the use of any of a number of medications.

In many instances, dilutional hyponatremia occurs as a concomitant of extracellular and total body water volume expansion. However, this need not be so, nor is it universally true that serum sodium concentrations necessarily reflect the true state of body sodium content or even osmolarity. Dilutional hyponatremia can occur as well with volume depletion (e.g., inadequate volume replacement of isotonic fluid losses with hypotonic fluid). Despite normal or low serum sodium levels, total body sodium frequently is increased in patients with chronic cardiac, hepatic and renal disease. In some circumstances, as with severe hyperlipidemia or hyperproteinemia, low serum sodium values can be an artifact of measurement. The osmotically active sodium ions in serum are in solution in the aqueous phase. Excess lipid or protein in serum displaces water and its sodium content in a given standard volume of serum taken for measurement. Consequently the measured serum sodium concentration in the sample can be low, even though the concentration in serum water remains unchanged. Presently this is the most apt to occur in surgical patients being given a course of total parenteral nutrition, in whom serum sodium determinations are made within 6–8 hr of an infusion of intravenous lipids. Lastly, as has already been discussed, hyperglycemia can cause hyponatremia associated with a hypertonic rather than a hypotonic volume expansion (see ''Disorders of Volume'').

Primary extracellular sodium losses leading to hyponatremia are most often due to decreased renal tubular reabsorption of salt, as seen with sodium-wasting nephropathies, renal tubular acidosis, metabolic alkalosis, diabetic ketoacidosis, diuretics, and adrenal insufficiency. Gastrointestinal losses of sodium-containing fluids also can contribute, as can intracellular shifts of sodium in patients with chronic debilitating and energy-depleting disorders that alter cell membrane integrity and function. In many of the instances in which loss of extracellular salt content is a primary factor, volume depletion also occurs.

Symptoms and signs of central nervous system dysfunction are the primary clinical manifestations of hyponatremia. Due to the enhanced intracellular fluxes of water occurring when serum sodium concentration and extracellular osmolarity decrease, cerebrospinal fluid pressures rise as cell volumes in the brain and spinal cord expand and neurologic disturbances result. The severity of the disturbances produced is directly related to both the degree of hyponatremia and its rate of development. Serum sodium levels no lower than 130 mEq/liter are rarely symptomatic. Below this value and down to 120 mEq/liter, findings of weakness, fatigue, hyperactive deep tendon reflexes, and muscle twitches may become evident. This is particularly true when serum sodium concentrations decrease relatively rapidly (equal to or faster than 10–15 mEq/liter in <24–48 hr); whereas at slower rates of change, a number of patients exhibit no abnormalities. However, as hyponatremia becomes more severe, with serum levels falling below 120 mEq/liter and progressing toward 110 mEq/liter or less, convulsions, coma, areflexia, and even death will occur unless therapy is promptly instituted.

Treatment of Hyponatremia. The treatment of a low serum sodium value is determined by its cause, severity, and whether there is an accompanying volume excess or deficit. In most instances of dilutional hyponatremia that is iatrogenically induced in the perioperative period, the associated asymptomatic decrease of serum sodium and modest extracellular volume expansion are readily treated by simple restriction of fluid intake. This approach also suffices to correct hyponatremia secondary to SIADH, although the daily fluid intake may have to be limited to 500 ml or less. Similarly, fluid restriction is employed in the management of hyponatremia secondary to water retention, as occurs in advanced cardiac, renal, or liver disease. However, with these disorders, limitation of salt intake as well as other therapeutic measures directed at the underlying disturbances also must be employed to restore fluid and electrolyte balance.

In contrast, hyponatremia associated with volume contraction, as seen with inadequate replacement of isotonic fluid losses or renal salt-wasting syndromes, is treated with combined salt and volume repletion. Most often this entails the use of intravenous normal saline or a balanced Ringer's lactate solution, given in an amount to raise the serum concentration to about 130 mEq/liter, at a rate appropriate to the need for repairing the volume deficit. Care should be exercised to avoid causing a volume overload by too rapid infusions. The restoration of the serum sodium toward normal should also be gradual. This helps to avoid rapid changes of extracellular osmolarity that can cause related rapid shifts of intracellular water and resultant undesirable neurologic consequences. For the same reasons, a slow-paced approach to correction of low serum sodium values becomes even more important on the rare occasions that hypertonic 3% saline solutions are brought into use in the treatment of hyponatremia. This is indicated only when hyponatremia is severe enough to induce clinically manifest life-threatening neurologic disturbances. Proper use of hypertonic saline first requires an estimate of the amount of sodium ion needed to completely correct the serum concentration deficit. As shown in Equation 3, this involves multiplying the milliequivalents per liter decrease in serum sodium concentration by the liters of total body water, calculated as a percent of total body weight (calculated here for a 70-kg male).

$$\text{mEq Na}^+ \text{ needed} = (140 - \text{serum Na}^+) \times (0.6 \times \text{kg wt}) \quad (3)$$

No more than one-half of the total amount calculated should be given in the first 12–18 hr. The goal is to bring sodium concentrations up to levels that are no longer symptomatic. Over the next 24–48 hr further correction can be carried out, using normal saline in the amounts dictated by the clinical picture and the laboratory findings.

Table 6.7
Causes of Hypernatremia

Decreased Body Water
  Excessive loss of water
    Skin: Hypotonic sweat and insensible water loss, both of which
      are enhanced in the presence of hyperpyrexia. Increased
      evaporative loss from altered skin surfaces (e.g., burns).
    Lungs: Insensible losses enhanced in presence of hyperpyrexia,
      particularly with tracheostomy and unhumidified inspired
      air source.
    Renal: Osmotic diuresis. High output renal failure with inability
      to excrete concentrated urine. Diabetes insipidus, whether
      hypothalamic or nephrogenic. (lack of ADH)
  Limited water intake
    Comatose and disoriented patients who cannot drink.
    Gastrointestinal disorders preventing oral intake of fluids.
    Hypothalamic tumor or disorder with decreased thirst.
Increased Body Sodium Content
  Excessive intake of salt
    Iatrogenic administration of excess salt (e.g., overzealous treat-
      ment with intravenous hypertonic salt solutions).
  Decreased sodium excretion
    Hyperaldosteronism, whether iatrogenic, primary, or secondary
      in origin.
    Cushing's disease or syndrome.

Hypernatremia Hypernatremia is defined as an elevated serum sodium concentration, which when clinically significant is in excess of 150 mEq/liter. Less frequent in occurrence than hyponatremia, it can be just as lethal if allowed to persist and progress unchecked. Hypernatremia can be the result of a decrease in body water content secondary either to excessive losses or limited intake of water, or an increased body sodium content due to an excessive intake or a decreased excretion of this cation. The various circumstances leading to hypernatremia and the particular disorders relating to them are listed in Table 6.7.

The pathophysiologic consequences of hypernatremia reflect both extracellular volume losses that can occur and intracellular dehydration when water is drawn from the cells in response to extracellular hyperosmolarity. As with hyponatremia, the severity of the clinical manifestations is directly related to the degree of hypernatremia and the rapidity with which it develops. Serum sodium concentrations in excess of 160 mEq/liter are cause for concern. The constellation of symptoms and signs include restlessness, weakness, decreased salivation and lacrimation, dry mucous membranes, dry flushed skin, decreased tissue turgor, oliguria (except when renal water losses are responsible), hyperpyrexia, tachycardia, hypotension, and ultimately delirium, coma, convulsions, and death. In patients dying of hypernatremia, intracranial hemorrhage is a common finding at postmortem examination. The genesis of this complication is not clear, but it is believed that cell shrinkage with associated decreases in brain volume and intracranial pressure can contribute to the tearing or disruption of intracranial blood vessels.

Treatment of Hypernatremia. The treatment of hypernatremia is correction of the pure water deficit that exists. This deficit can be estimated in a number of ways, but the simplest accurate general rule is the following: *For every liter of water deficit, the serum sodium concentration will rise 3 mEq above normal (140 mEq/liter).* When the deficits are modest and the underlying condition can be controlled, simple oral ingestion of water or intravenous administration of 5% dextrose in water can reduce sodium concentrations to normal. When the hypernatremic state is more prolonged and severe (i.e., serum sodium levels >160 mEq/liter), the correction process becomes more complicated. The nature of fluid given may have to change as different needs become apparent. If contraction of the extracellular space, hypotension, and symptoms and signs of poor tissue perfusion are present, infusions of normal saline until hemodynamic stability is restored can be appropriate. Similarly, one can find circumstances in which the administration of half-strength saline might also be used to replace water deficits that are associated with hypotonic salt losses. It is important that the repair of a significant water deficit be at a controlled slow pace. If fluid replacement is too rapid, intracellular swelling can occur and the treatment can become as hazardous as the hypernatremic state being treated. This is particularly true of neurologic sequelae. Brain cells accommodate to slowly developing extracellular hypertonicity by accumulating extra intracellular solute. A sudden decrease in extracellular osmolarity without time for elimination of these extra intracellular milliosmoles leads to rapid swelling of brain cells, which in turn can cause serious neurologic dysfunction. Thus the correction should be phased, with no more than half of the calculated fluid deficit being made up in the first 12 hr and the remainder over the next 24–48 hr. It has been suggested that the fall of serum sodium concentration should not exceed 15 mEq/liter in any 6-hour period. An essential part of the treatment of hypernatremia is correction or treatment of the underlying cause whenever possible.

Potassium

Disturbances of potassium balance are common in surgical patients. Their importance relates to the significant role the potassium ion plays in cellular metabolism and the excitation of muscle and nerve.

Hypokalemia. Hypokalemia is defined as a serum potassium concentration of <3.5 mEq/liter, although it rarely becomes clinically significant until levels fall between 2.5 and 3.0 mEq/liter. Causes of hypokalemia in the surgical patient are outlined in Table 6.8. The causes are multifactorial, involving increased gastrointestinal and/or renal losses, movement of potassium from extracellular fluids into the cells, and negative potassium balance resulting from inadequate intake or replacement of losses.

Disorders of the gastrointestinal tract can be major contributors to hypokalemia (see Table 6.2 for a comparison of electrolyte losses from various sites). Large fluid volume losses from any level of the gastrointestinal system, biliary tract, or pancreas will lead to potassium depletion. With diarrhea, this is particularly true when losses are due to disorders of the colon and rectum, where the concentrations of potassium in the intraluminal intestinal contents are the highest.

Table 6.8
Causes of Hypokalemia

Gastrointestinal Losses	
Gastric	Vomiting or nasogastric aspiration of acid secretory contents.
Diarrhea	Infectious diarrheas, particularly when colonic fluid losses are major.
	Pseudomembranous enterocolitis (C. difficile).
	Villous adenoma of the rectum or sigmoid.
	Rare watery-diarrhea syndrome associated with pancreatic islet tumor secretion of vasoactive intestinal peptide (vipoma).
Fistulas	External high output losses of duodenum and small bowel contents, bile, and pancreatic juice.
Obstruction	Potassium containing "third space" fluid losses into intestinal lumen and wall (particularly small bowel).
Renal Losses	
Alkalosis	Metabolic or respiratory.
Diuresis	Secondary to diuretic agents or osmotic and volume loading.
Hypochloremia	Most common in association with losses of gastric acid secretory contents.
Hypomagnesemia	Inadequate gastrointestinal uptake (e.g., inflammatory bowel disease, prolonged diarrhea or ileus, and specific malabsorptive disorders.)
Mineralocorticoid	Enhanced aldosterone activity triggered as a physiologic response to hypovolemia or sodium depletion.
	Hyperaldosteronism, primary or due to hypersecretion of renin.
Glucocorticoid	Enhanced activity due to glucocorticosteroid therapy.
	Cushing's disease or syndrome.
Nephropathy	Intrinsic salt-wasting renal disease.
Medications	Sodium binding nonreabsorbable anions (e.g., carbenicillin)
Intracellular Shifts	
Alkalosis	Potassium exchange for hydrogen ion.
TPN	Rebuilding of cell mass and maintenance of metabolism during course of total parenteral nutrition involves increased intracellular needs for potassium.
Insulin	Insulin enhances associated movements of glucose and potassium into cells.
Inadequate Intake	
Dietary	Inadequacies of diet, per se, very uncommon.
Therapeutic	Failure to provide adequate amounts of potassium in maintaining or treating perioperative or posttraumatic surgical patients is far more common.

Vomiting or nasogastric aspiration of the acid secretory contents of the stomach with potassium concentrations well above that of serum also can account for significant potassium losses. However, a number of other factors contribute to the hypokalemia commonly occurring in such circumstances. External losses of gastric acid contents containing significant amounts of hydrogen and chloride ions as well as potassium, in association with an extracellular accumulation of bicarbonate, lead to the development of metabolic, hypochloremic, hypokalemic alkalosis. The increase in extracellular pH causes intracellular movement of potassium ions, which further aggravates the hypokalemic state. As a general rule, *an increase of 0.1 pH unit results in a 0.4–0.5 mEq decrease in serum potassium concentration.*

With alkalosis there is also renal compensation in the form of distal tubular hydrogen ion reabsorption at the expense of potassium excretion. Similarly, the delivery of greater amounts of sodium ion to be reabsorbed in the distal tubular system, secondary to the high-bicarbonate and low-chloride concentrations in tubular fluid, leads to additional loss of potassium in the urine. Finally, extracellular volume depletion associated with the gastric fluid losses can stimulate aldosterone activity, introducing still another factor that will increase renal excretion of potassium. Ultimately all of these influences interact to produce a marked potassium depletion, both intra- and extracellularly. At this point, dictated by the need to conserve potassium, renal tubular hydrogen ion excretion increases, urinary pH becomes acidic, and external losses of potassium are reduced. This "paradoxical aciduria" occurs despite the severity of the alkalosis still present. When evident, this aciduria is an indication of profound total body depletion of potassium that urgently needs restoration.

In patients who are persistently hypokalemic, in the absence of any obvious gastrointestinal disorders or reasons for increased intracellular movement of potassium (e.g., total parenteral nutrition, insulin), disorders of renal origin or the effects of diuretic agents should be considered (Table 6.7). Another important but often overlooked cause of hypokalemia in surgical patients is hypomagnesemia, which (for reasons that are not entirely clear) acts to decrease distal renal tubular reabsorption of potassium. If the magnesium deficiency is not repaired, it is extremely difficult to correct the hypokalemia.

The clinical manifestation of hypokalemia reflects the role of potassium in muscle and nerve function. In general, their severity is proportional to the degree of decrease in serum levels and the rate at which they develop. Additionally, adverse consequences of hypokalemia can be exaggerated by alkalosis, hypocalcemia, and in the case of cardiac effects, digoxin therapy. Skeletal muscle weakness may be noted with serum potassium of 2.5 mEq/liter or less and can progress to hyporeflexia, paraesthesias, and paralysis as serum concentrations fall even lower. Nausea and vomiting due to paralytic ileus and attendant abdominal distension can at times be attributed to low serum potassium levels. Also, increased renal tubular production of ammonia induced by hypokalemia can have a significant impact on serum ammonia levels and the clinical course of patients with hepatic encephalopathy. However, cardiac abnormalities are the most important and worrisome consequences of hypokalemia. Rarely appearing at serum levels >3.0 mEq/liter in the absence of digoxin therapy, electrocardiographic changes signifying decreasing serum potassium concentrations include low voltage, flattening of the T waves with prominant U waves, prolongation of the P-R interval, and finally (when values fall to 2 mEq/liter or less) widening of the QRS complex.

Treatment of Hypokalemia   Treatment of hypokalemia involves the replacement of potassium losses and the correction of the underlying condition(s) responsible for them. When possible, oral supplements of potassium salts are used in doses of 40–60 mEq. If intravenous replacement is required, the rate of administration usually is limited to 10 mEq/hr, the dose being repeated as necessary to raise serum levels to a satisfactory level. Even at this rate it is advisable to use electrocardiographic monitoring for evidence of hyperkalemia during the infusion. If higher dose rates are used (e.g., 20 mEq/hr), such monitoring becomes mandatory. When giving intravenous potassium supplements, it is wise to avoid using glucose-containing solutions as the diluent. Intravenous dextrose can increase endogenous insulin levels, which in turn can induce movement of potassium with dextrose into the cells. Initially this can cause serum levels to fall even further and, in the long run, can impair efforts to overcome the hypokalemic state.

Hyperkalemia.   Hyperkalemia is defined as a serum potassium concentration >5.5 mEq/liter, although usually not clinically significant until values rise to >6.0 mEq/liter. As with hypokalemia, the etiology is multifactorial (Table 6.9). Increased potassium levels can be the result of exogenous loading due to excessive dietary intake or parenterally introduced potassium loads (e.g., multiple transfusions of stored banked blood and high-dose penicillin therapy). Endogenous loading occurs whenever large amounts of cellular potassium are released into the extracellular fluid space (e.g., crush injuries, intravascular hemolysis, lysis and absorption of large hematomas, catabolism of fat and muscle tissue due to stress or starvation, and rapid rewarming of the severely hypothermic patient). Decreased urinary excretion of potassium is another important cause of hyperkalemia, most often as the consequence of intrinsic renal disease. Adrenal insufficiency and impaired aldosterone activity also reduce excretion by the kidneys. Extracellular shifts of intracellular potassium, as seen with acute acidosis, represent another manner in which serum levels can be elevated. This phenomenon is not a feature of chronic acidotic states. Increased serum concentrations also can be caused by insulin deficiency, which reduces intracellular deposition of potassium, and the use of digitalis and related cardiotonic agents that encourage the exit of potassium from cells. Finally, an elevated serum potassium level can be an artifact of blood sampling. Falsely high values are obtained when there is hemolysis of the sample drawn or when the sample is taken from a vein into which a potassium-containing solution is being infused.

As is true of hypokalemia, with hyperkalemia muscle weakness may occur, but the most significant complication is cardiotoxicity. The absolute serum values at which it occurs can vary. The appearance of adverse cardiac effects are accelerated by acute acidosis, hypocalcemia, hyponatremia, and rapid increase of serum potassium concentration. In the absence of such factors, peaked T waves, best appreciated in the precordial leads, appear at serum concentrations of 6.0–7.0 mEq/liter. At serum values of 7.0–8.0 mEq/liter, electrocardiographic changes include diminished P waves, increased P-R intervals and heart block, decreased Q-T intervals, widening of the QRS complexes, and, depressed S-T segments. Elevations >8.0 mEq/liter, with loss of T waves and diastolic asystole, can be lethal.

Treatment of Hyperkalemia   The primary goal for treatment of hyperkalemia is to reduce serum potassium concentrations to levels that are not life threatening. A variety of therapeutic measures are used. The most simple are restrictions of potassium intake and the administration of a potassium-depleting diuretic agent. Next in the progression of treatment is the use of sodium polystyrene sulfonate (Kayexalate®), a cation-exchange resin. Each gram of the resin can bind approximately 1 mEq of potassium. Orally, doses of 25 gm suspended in 50 ml of a 20% sorbitol solution are given every 4–6 hr. Rectally, 50 gm in 200 ml of a 20% sorbitol solution are given every 4 hr. The above measures usually will be all that are needed for modest elevations of potassium up to 6.5 mEq/liter. With

Table 6.9
Causes of Hyperkalemia

Increased Potassium Load
  Exogenous
    Excessive dietary intake, per se, very uncommon
    Transfusions of bank blood or packed RBCs
    High dose potassium penicillin therapy
  Endogenous
    Extensive tissue trauma and rhabdomyolysis (crush injuries).
    Hemolysis
    Catabolic breakdown of tissue with trauma, starvation, etc.
    Cellular breakdown with rapid rewarming in severely hypothermic patients.
Decreased Potassium Excretion
  Renal failure
  Adrenal insufficiency and impaired aldosterone activity
Extracellular Shifts
  Acute acidosis, metabolic or respiratory
  Insulin deficiency
  Digitalis and related cardiotonic drugs
Pseudohyperkalemia
  Blood sample hemolysis
  Blood sample contaminated by infused potassium solution

greater increases to levels up to 7.5 mEq/liter, 10 units of insulin given subcutaneously, in conjunction with an intravenous infusion of 25 gm of glucose over a 5-minute period, can be added to the regimen. This may reduce serum levels by as much as 1 mEq/liter by driving potassium into the cells. Metabolic alkalosis induced by the infusion of 45 mEq of sodium bicarbonate over 5 min also may effect a decrease in serum potassium concentrations lasting up to 2 hr. Finally, if potassium levels rise even higher to levels >7.5 mEq/liter, 10 ml of a 10% calcium gluconate solution infused slowly over 5 min can help to reduce the electrical excitability of heart muscle and minimize the lethal potential of this degree of hyperkalemia. The hazards of calcium infusion mandate that it should only be used when hyperkalemia is very severe and the risks are justified. It is always advisable to employ electrocardiographic monitoring when dealing with hyperkalemic states; such a precaution is absolutely necessary when infusing calcium. In addition to all of the above, dialysis (renal or peritoneal) is an option to be exercised in the treatment of hyperkalemia, particularly in cases of renal failure.

Calcium

Although most of the body calcium is in bone, the small amount in extracellular fluid is important. This is true of the physiologically active and hormonally regulated ionized fraction that accounts for approximately 50% of the extracellular content. The remainder is inactive, with 40% bound to plasma protein and 10% complexed with bicarbonate, citrate, and phosphate. Normal dietary intake is 1 gm or more, two-thirds of which is excreted in stool and one-third is absorbed in the small bowel, where vitamin D plays a regulatory role. Intake is balanced by renal excretion, largely determined by the fate of the 10% of filtered calcium reaching the distal tubular collecting system. There a variety of influences on urinary calcium excretion occur (e.g., parathyroid hormone and metabolic alkalosis increase tubular reabsorption, and hypophosphatemia and metabolic acidosis decreases it). Severe abnormalities of calcium metabolism are uncommon in the surgical patient, but as described next, symptomatic alterations of serum calcium concentrations are seen. For a more complete review of calcium metabolism, its hormonal regulation, and disorders, the reader is referred to the section of parathyroid disease in Chapter 22.

Hypocalcemia. Hypocalcemia occurs when serum calcium levels fall below 4 mEq/liter (8 mg/dl). Common causes in surgical patients are as follows. Hypocalcemia associated with surgically induced hypoparathyroidism can be present transiently after removal of a parathyroid adenoma in a hyperparathyroid patient or be a more permanent problem as the result of inadvertent removal or damage of parathyroid tissue during thyroid gland surgery. Hypocalcemia is also a feature of acute pancreatitis due to calcium binding in saponified tissue, parathyroid hormone dysfunction,

and decreased protein-bound fraction secondary to hypoalbuminemia. Low serum calcium levels also are seen with severe soft tissue infections such as necrotizing fasciitis. As well, inadequate intestinal absorption related to inflammatory bowel diseases, pancreatic exocrine dysfunction, or mucosal malabsorptive syndromes can cause hypocalcemia. Excessive fluid losses from pancreatic and intestinal fistulas or chronic diarrhea also seriously deplete the extracellular calcium pool. Similarly, impaired tubular reabsorption and increased urinary losses of calcium associated with renal insufficiency can lead to extracellular calcium depletion. Finally, low calcium serum levels may be related to severe magnesium depletion.

The clinical manifestations of hypocalcemia reflect the importance of the role of this ion in neuromuscular excitability. Symptomatically this includes circumoral paraesthesias, numbness and tingling of the tips of fingers, and muscle cramps. The signs are hyperactive deep tendon reflexes, a positive Chvostek sign, tetany with carpopedal spasm, and convulsions when hypocalcemia is very severe. Electrocardiographically, prolongation of the Q-T interval is the most typical finding. It should be remembered, however, that there are circumstances in which measured serum calcium levels do not correlate well with the appearance of the signs and symptoms described. Hypocalcemia in association with hypoproteinemia is due to the decrease in bound calcium, not the biologically active ionized fraction. Thus no symptoms become evident when decreased total serum levels are the consequence of low serum protein concentrations. In acidosis the ionized fraction of extracellular calcium increases at the expense of the bound portion. Thus it is possible that the concentration of ionized calcium can be adequate to prevent symptoms, even though the total calcium level in serum is lower than normal. A pH-dependent change in the ionized fraction occurs with alkalosis, as well. As the pH rises the ionized fraction grows smaller as more calcium becomes bound. Thus severe alkalosis can be associated with symptoms and signs of hypocalcemia when measured levels of total serum calcium are normal.

Treatment of Hypocalcemia Treatment of hypocalcemia is aimed at correcting the calcium deficit, the underlying cause(s), and any associated condition that aggravates the severity of the clinical manifestations (e.g., alkalosis). Replacement can be accomplished by the intravenous administration of calcium gluconate or calcium chloride when the symptoms and signs are pronounced and the need is urgent. Oral ingestion of calcium lactate, with or without accompanying vitamin D supplements, is more often used in the long-term treatment of hypocalcemia associated with chronic disorders. In general, the use of intravenous calcium supplements during transfusions of blood or packed red blood cells is unnecessary. Most evidence suggests that at moderate rates of blood replacement, hypocalcemia due to citrate binding and volume dilution can be prevented by the endogenous release of calcium from bone. Only with massive transfusion and volume re-

PTH, ↓H⁺ ⟶ ↑Ca²⁺ reabsorption

↓PO₄, ↑H⁺ ⟶ ↓Ca²⁺ reabsorption

placement at rates of 100 ml/min or higher is there any need to administer supplemental calcium intravenously. to counteract the citrate the Ca²⁺ chelator.

Hypercalcemia. Hypercalcemia is defined as serum calcium values >5.5–6.0 mEq/liter (11–12 mg/dl). In the surgical patient the most common causes are primary or secondary hyperparathyroidism and metastatic bone disease, most often in women with carcinoma of the breast being treated with supplemental estrogen therapy. Mobilization of calcium from bone in bedridden patients can also be responsible for mild asymptomatic hypercalcemia.

The clinical manifestations of hypercalcemia can be vague. The first symptoms to appear are weariness, weakness, anorexia, nausea, and vomiting. As serum levels continue to rise, severe headaches, widespread musculoskeletal pain, polyuria related to impaired renal tubular concentration, and polydipsia become clinically evident. The combination of restricted oral intake, vomiting, and excessive renal fluid loss lead to hypovolemia and dehydration, both of which can become quite pronounced. Electrocardiographically, shortening of the Q-T interval and widening of the T wave are noted. When serum levels rise to 7.5 mEq/liter (15 mg/dl), weariness is replaced by somnolence, stupor, and ultimately coma. Hypercalcemia of this and greater degrees are not well tolerated and unless corrected promptly will cause death.

Treatment of Hypercalcemia The first order of therapy is to restrict calcium intake, improve hydration, and increase urinary calcium excretion. Intravenous normal or half-strength saline is administered in generous amounts, with monitoring to guard against volume overload. Loop diuretics (e.g., furosemide) also enhance urinary calcium excretion, but care must be taken to assess and replace associated electrolyte losses. Hypomagnesemia can develop with the pronounced diuresis produced by such measures. The administration of oral or parenteral phosphate supplements has been advocated as a means for complexing ionized calcium. Intravenously, phosphate can induce a precipitous fall in serum calcium, with tetany, hypotension, and renal failure reported as complications. It is thus recommended that intravenous phosphate should not be given at a rate in excess of 50 mM/12 hr and should not be given continuously for more than 48 hours. Also, phosphate should not be used in the presence of hyperphosphatemia and/or renal failure. Corticosteroid therapy, as used to suppress calcium release from bone in a variety of diseases that are associated with hypercalcemia (e.g., sarcoidosis, leukemia, lymphoma, myeloma, and vitamin D intoxication), has been advocated for use in surgical patients. However, with the doses recommended (hydrocortisone, 3 mg/kg/day) it may take 1 to 2 weeks before any appreciable reduction of serum calcium levels is apparent. This limits the use of corticosteroids in the acute situation. In urgent circumstances one can employ mithramycin, a cytotoxic drug that suppresses bone resorption and calcium release into extracellular space. Small daily intravenous doses

(25 μg/kg) given for 3 days can cause serum calcium levels to decrease within 24–48 hr and remain depressed for several days to weeks. Due to its toxic effects on bone marrow and kidneys, this agent should be used with caution in any patient who is prone to develop thrombocytopenia or has any degree of renal insufficiency.

Magnesium

The majority of total body magnesium exists in bone and soft tissues, with <1% in the extracellular space, 25% of which is protein bound. The average daily intake of magnesium is 25–30 mEq, approximately one-half of which is absorbed in the distal small intestine. Renal excretion protects against hypermagnesemia but not against hypomagnesemia, which will develop if intake is consistently <0.3 mEq/kg/day.

Hypomagnesemia. Hypomagnesemia is common in surgical patients. Inadequate enteral intake occurs with starvation, prolonged nasogastric suction, unsupplemented parenteral nutrition, inflammatory bowel disease, and any of a variety of diarrheal and malabsorption syndromes. In acute pancreatitis, hypomagnesemia can result from complexes formed in areas of fat necrosis. Loop diuretics, hypophosphatemia, diabetic ketoacidosis, and amingoglycosides cause renal wasting of magnesium. Hypomagnesemia also is seen in alcoholic patients, particularly those going through withdrawal.

Patients with low-magnesium levels are often asymptomatic but also can present with symptoms and signs similar to those seen with hypocalcemia (e.g., hyperreflexia, tremor, a positive Chvostek sign, tetany, convulsions, stupor, and coma). The more severe manifestations are seen with serum magnesium values <1 mEq/liter, at which levels hypocalcemia is often coexistent.

Treatment of Hypomagnesemia Treatment involves the replacement of magnesium. Oral doses should provide approximately 50 mEq/day. For acute symptomatic hypomagnesemia, 10–15 mEq of magnesium as either the sulfate or chloride salt can be given intravenously over 15 min, with up to 50 mEq given over a 3-hr period.

If needed, subsequent parenteral therapy can be given intramuscularly or intravenously. Special care must be taken in the treatment of hypomagnesemia in hypovolemic and oliguric patients. The common associations of hypokalemia and hypocalcemia with magnesium deficiency indicate the need for monitoring the complete electrolyte profile of patients with hypomagnesemia and treating accompanying fluid and electrolyte abnormalities.

Hypermagnesemia. Hypermagnesemia in surgical patients is most commonly a consequence of renal failure. With decreased renal function, the retention of dietery magnesium or small amounts associated with oral ingestion of magnesium-containing antacid gel can cause serum levels to increase. Under such circumstances, serum levels of magnesium and potassium ions tend to parallel each other.

Clinical findings associated with symptomatic hypermagnesemia include lethargy, weakness, and depressed deep tendon reflexes, progressing to skeletal muscle paralysis, respiratory depression, and death when serum levels rise to >10 mEq/liter. Changes in the electrocardiogram also occur (e.g., increased P-R interval, widened QRS complex, and elevated T waves).

Treatment of Hypermagnesemia   Treatment is directed at promptly reducing serum magnesium levels and controlling its clinical manifestations. Acidosis, if present, is corrected. Adequate hydration and urine output are provided by oral fluid intake or intravenous infusion of appropriate solutions. If symptoms are acute and threatening, slow infusion of 5–10 mEq of calcium (as gluconate or chloride salt) can temporarily control them. If hypomagnesemia and its clinical manifestations persist, it may be necessary to employ dialysis to clear excess magnesium from the extracellular fluid space.

Chloride → the major extracellular anion

Chloride is the major extracellular anion. It is ubiquitous in the diet, absorbed in the small and large bowel, and excreted in the urine. Chloride balance generally parallels that of sodium, except with the hypochloremic state occurring from losses of gastric acid contents. There are no symptoms or signs that are specific to abnormalities of chloride balance. However, changes in extracellular chloride content and concentration can be of significance in the genesis and/or management of fluid, electrolyte, and acid-base problems encountered in surgical patients.

Hypochloremia.   Hypochloremia is present when serum chloride concentrations fall to <95 mEq/liter. Classically it is seen with gastrointestinal fluid losses, particularly gastric. Urinary losses of chloride also can be responsible, as seen with diuretics, non-oliguric acute and chronic renal failure, and compensatory renal tubular reabsorption of bicarbonate in respiratory acidosis.

Treatment of Hypochloremia   In general, hypochloremia is treated with sodium and potassium chloride solutions, with the ratio of each determined by the underlying problem and its impact on the extracellular content and concentration of the two cations. As already discussed, the repletion of chloride deficits is necessary to the overall success of therapeutic efforts to correct hypochloremic, hypokalemic, metabolic alkalosis. Ammonium chloride infusions can be employed in such circumstances but are contraindicated in patients with advanced liver disease who are encephalopathic or at risk of becoming so. In addition, although rarely needed, intravenous solutions made up with 0.1 N hydrochloric acid have been advocated in the treatment of very severe hypochloremic alkalosis.

Another circumstance in which the importance of correcting hypochloremia is apparent is the recovery phase following an episode of severe respiratory acidosis. Renal tubular reabsorption of bicarbonate represents an important compensatory measure for minimizing the lowering of extracellular pH caused by carbon dioxide retention. When respiratory function improves and arterial blood gases return to baseline, renal excretion of the retained excess bicarbonate allows arterial pH to normalize. In the presence of hypochloremia, however, renal bicarbonate excretion is impaired. Thus extracellular bicarbonate levels remain high in the presence of lowered carbon dioxide tensions, and metabolic alkalosis results. This state will persist until chloride deficits are repleted, hypochloremia is corrected and renal excretion of bicarbonate can appropriately increase, and arterial pH can return to normal.

Hyperchloremia.   Hyperchloremia is an uncommon finding in surgical patients, occurring when serum chloride levels are elevated to >115 mEq/liter. It can be seen in association with hypernatremia or the administration of the excess of chloride in the form of potassium or ammonium salts. Hyperchloremia is a feature of renal tubular acidosis and surgical diversion of urine into segments of bowel (e.g., ileal loop or ureterosigmoidostomy). In the latter circumstances, distal small bowel and colonic mucosa can absorb excessive amounts of chloride in exchange for bicarbonate. This is especially true when mucosal contact is enhanced by delayed emptying of the intestinal segment.

Treatment of Hyperchloremia   In most instances, treatment of hyperchloremia is directed at correction of the underlying cause.

Phosphate

Only 1% of total body phosphate content is extracellular, 80% is bound in bone, and the remainder is intracellular, playing an essential role in energy metabolism. In urine, phosphate buffer systems facilitate the handling and excretion of titratable acids.

Hypophosphatemia.   Hypophosphatemia is a condition that is commonly encountered on a surgical service, particularly in critically ill patients. Total parenteral nutrition causes intracellular sequestration of phosphate in tissues undergoing rapid cell turnover and growth, a phenomenon that is most dramatic in nutritionally depleted patients. Shifts of extracellular phosphate into cells also occur with alkalosis, both metabolic and respiratory. In such instances, hypophosphatemia may become significant but does not necessarily reflect a decrease in total body phosphate content. In contrast, phosphate depletion does accompany hypophosphatemia secondary to impaired phosphate intake or absorption, as occurs with starvation, malabsorption, vitamin D deficiency, binding of phosphates in the gut lumen by ingested antacid compounds, and chronic alcoholism. Similarly, excessive renal excretion of phosphate can lead to depletion and low serum levels, as seen with renal tubular disorders, diuretic therapy, volume expansion, hypomagnesemia, and hyperaldosteronism. Other circumstances in which surgical patients can develop significant hypophosphatemia include diabetic ketoacidosis and alcohol withdrawal.

Signs Hypophosphatemia can result in muscle weakness, which in the extreme can lead to respiratory failure. Low serum phosphate levels and failure to wean from a ventilator are common clinical associations encountered in patients in surgical intensive care units. Significant consequences of hypophosphatemia also are manifest as red blood cell dysfunction secondary to decreased 2,3-DPG and ATP (i.e., limited oxygen release at tissue level and cell membrane fragility) and white blood cell dysfunction resulting from decreased ATP synthesis (i.e., decreased chemotaxis and phagocytosis). Metabolic encephalopathy associated with hypophosphatemia can become quite severe, with irritability, confusion, and weakness progressing to obtundation, seizures, and coma.

Treatment of Hypophosphatemia. Phosphate replacement should be given intravenously when serum levels fall to <1 mg/dl. A dose of 2.5–5.0 mg/kg of phosphate is repeated every 6 hr as indicated by serial serum determinations and clinical findings. Intravenous administration of phosphate must be done with great care and constant monitoring of serum levels. The main complications of phosphate therapy are hyperphosphatemia, metastatic deposition of calcium in tissues, hypocalcemia, osmotic diuresis, dehydration, and hypernatremia. The most compelling contraindications to parenteral phosphate therapy are oliguria and renal failure. In more moderate cases of hypophosphatemia, oral supplementation of phosphate is safe and effective.

Hyperphosphatemia. Hyperphosphatemia is seen in patients on a surgical service in association with severe renal insufficiency, massive trauma, severe tissue catabolism, cytotoxic drug therapy of neoplastic diseases (most often lymphomas and leukemias), and excessive phosphate administration in the management of hypophosphatemia. Although frequently asymptomatic, elevated serum phosphate levels depress serum calcium levels, raising the calcium phosphorus product to levels that can lead to metastatic calcification of soft tissue and the secondary and tertiary hyperparathyroidism of chronic renal failure.

Treatment of Hyperphosphatemia Treatment of hyperphosphatemia most often consists of dietary restriction of phosphate intake (i.e., milk, its products, and meat) and the use of phosphate-binding aluminum hydroxide antacid gels. Diuresis to enhance renal phosphate excretion also can be employed. In severe chronic renal failure, dialysis may be the only effective therapeutic option.

Disorders of Acid-Base Balance

Proper management of acid-base disorders depends on prompt recognition and evaluation of the distur-

bances involved. History and physical examination alert the physician to the nature and severity of disturbances that can occur in a particular clinical setting. Laboratory data pertinent to the fluid and electrolyte status and renal function of a patient help to identify alterations that are contributing to or are the consequences of the underlying disturbance. With the help of the above information, data provided by arterial blood gas and pH determinations are analyzed, an accurate diagnosis is made, and an appropriate course of treatment is defined. A thorough understanding and proper use of the arterial blood gas and pH information are paramount. The measured arterial pH value (pHa) makes it evident whether acidosis or alkalosis is present. The measured $PaCO_2$ value makes it clear whether a respiratory component is involved, and the derived bicarbonate concentration $[HCO_3^-]$ identifies a metabolic component. The measured PaO_2 and derived oxygen saturation values provide information concerning pulmonary alveolar gas exchange and its possible influence on the acid-base disturbance present.

The need for accurate interpretation of the blood gas data, especially when mixed disturbances are present, has prompted the introduction of a variety of methods to facilitate their analysis. Some are too complex for use at the bedside on a busy surgical service. Others, employing rules or guidelines for making simple quick calculations, seem more applicable in that setting. The information they make available is equivalent to that provided when the Henderson-Hasselbalch equation and its modifications are used. Two rules that can be found in the text used in teaching advanced cardiac life support have proven to be of particular value in practice. They provide simple means for quantitating the impact changes of $PaCO_2$ and $[HCO_3^-]$ have on pHa. In turn, that information can be used to assess the degree to which acidosis or alkalosis is caused by a respiratory or a metabolic disturbance and to quantitate the base excesses or deficits contributing to the disturbance.

| Rule 1. | An increase or decrease in $PaCO_2$ of 10 mm Hg, respectively, is associated with a reciprocal decrease or increase of 0.08 pH units. |
| Rule 2. | An increase or decrease in $[HCO_3^-]$ of 10 mEq/liter, respectively, is associated with a directly related increase or decrease of 0.15 pH units. |

Acidosis

When the pHa decreases to <7.35, acidosis is present. Whether the cause is respiratory or metabolic, the consequences of a decreased pHa can be clinically important. At pHa levels <7.2, peripheral vascular and cardiac responsiveness to catecholamines is decreased, and cardiac dysfunction due to direct myocardial depression and arrhythmia can become significant and even lethal. Ionic exchanges across cell membranes and changes in renal tubular transport of electrolytes induced by acidosis cause extracellular potassium concentrations to increase, at times to clinically symptomatic levels.

↑ PO_4 → causes ↓ serum Ca^{2+} levels, raising the Ca × PO_4 product to levels that can lead to metastatic calcification of soft tissue and the 2° & 3° hyperparathyroidism of chronic renal failure.

Respiratory Acidosis. Respiratory acidosis is the result of carbon dioxide retention due to pulmonary alveolar hypoventilation. It can be acute or chronic. When acute, its causes can be numerous, including respiratory depression due to narcotics, sedatives, anesthetic agents, and muscle relaxants; limited ventilatory effort due to painful thoracic or upper abdominal incisions, or chest wall and pulmonary parenchymal trauma interfering with mechanics of breathing (e.g., fractured ribs, flail chest, hemopneumothorax); abdominal distension and impaired diaphragmatic function; upper airway obstruction due to tumor, foreign body, edema, laryngospasm, tracheobronchial injury, and improperly positioned endotracheal tubes; and, altered pulmonary alveolar gas exchange secondary to atelectasis, pneumonia, pulmonary edema, and the adult respiratory distress syndrome. Chronic respiratory acidosis, on the other hand, most often is due to advanced long-standing disorders of the lungs, especially chronic pulmonary obstructive disease.

The clinical consequences of respiratory acidosis are due to both the effects of hypercapnea and the hypoxia commonly present with it. Acutely, mild hypertension and restlessness are evident. When $PaCO_2$ levels continue to rise to even higher levels, somnolence, confusion, and ultimately coma due to carbon dioxide narcosis will occur. In combination with hypoxemia, severe hypercapnea also can be associated with significant cardiovascular dysfunction, including cardiac arrest. In patients with chronic respiratory acidosis, carbon dioxide narcosis is the major threat, although tolerance to hypercapnea is increased. In part, this is related to the compensatory increase in $[HCO_3^-]$ due to the renal conservation of base, a phenomenon not apparent in the acute state because of the time needed for it to evolve.

Evaluation as to whether respiratory changes are responsible for an acute acidotic state can be determined by applying rules 1 and 2. If, according to rule 1, the magnitude of the $PaCO_2$ increase can account for the total pH change, a pure respiratory acidosis exists. If the pH change is greater than can be accounted for, a metabolic component of acidosis also must exist. If the pH change is less than the increase in $PaCO_2$ would predict, an element of metabolic alkalosis is present. Use of rule 2 in such a case can reveal the contribution an elevated $[HCO_3^-]$ is making to the mixed acid-base disturbance. In chronic respiratory acidosis, in contrast to the acute state, such a finding is expected as a consequence of compensatory renal retention of bicarbonate.

Treatment of Respiratory Acidosis The treatment of respiratory acidosis is directed at improving alveolar ventilation and reducing $PaCO_2$ levels, making sure that oxygenation also is adequate. In the acute state, or with acute deterioration of a chronic situation, temporary use of mechanical ventilatory support and oxygen therapy often becomes necessary. It is important that in such circumstances the rate at which acute hypercapnea is corrected should not be too rapid. Sudden decreases in $PaCO_2$ cause sudden pHa changes and

ionic shifts between cellular and extracellular fluids that can produce severe cardiac dysrhythmias, including ventricular fibrillation. The administration of bicarbonate to improve the buffering capacity of extracellular fluids in respiratory acidosis is generally not an appropriate treatment option.

Metabolic Acidosis. Metabolic acidosis can be defined as a decrease in pHa related to a decreased arterial $[HCO_3^-]$. It can be an acute or chronic alteration. Metabolic acidosis occurs for two major reasons. The first is the loss of bicarbonate from the extracellular space. This occurs acutely with certain gastrointestinal disorders (e.g., diarrhea, external pancreatic fistula) and more chronically with increased urinary bicarbonate losses occurring with renal tubular disorders, ureterointestinal anastomoses, decreased mineralocorticoid activity, and diuresis induced with the carbonic anhydrase inhibitor, acetazolamide. The second major cause for metabolic acidosis, most often as an acute process, is an increased metabolic acid load. This is seen with lactic acidemia secondary to cardiogenic, septic and hypovolemic low-flow states or ischemia of major tissue beds (i.e., mesenteric infarction), and ketoacidosis.

With both acute and chronic metabolic acidosis, respiratory compensation occurs. Ventilation is stimulated by the increased hydrogen ion concentration in arterial blood, and $PaCO_2$ is reduced. The degree of compensation can be appreciated by the extent of the hypocapnea induced, and estimates of its modifying influence on the pHa, as determined by application of rule 1. Similarly, using rule 2 to estimate whether measured decreases in $[HCO_3^-]$ can fully account for the measured changes in pHa, mixed acid-base disturbances can be identified.

Determination of the "anion gap" can help to distinguish metabolic acidosis caused by a loss of bicarbonate from that caused by an accumulation of a metabolic acid load. The *anion gap* is defined as the difference between the serum sodium concentration and the sum of the serum bicarbonate and chloride concentrations. With losses of bicarbonate, decreases in serum concentration of this anion are accompanied by reciprocal increases in chloride ion concentrations. As such the anion gap remains normal (< 12 mEq/liter). In contrast, with metabolic acid loads, chloride levels do not increase as the bicarbonate levels decrease, and the measure anion gap is greater than normal. Actually, the gap is more apparent than real, as unmeasured anions of the metabolic acids are present in amounts to account for the differences calculated solely on the basis of measured bicarbonate and chloride values.

Treatment of Metabolic Acidosis Treatment of metabolic acidosis involves the correction of the underlying disorder when possible and the intravenous replacement of bicarbonate as needed. The need to focus attention on the treatment of the underlying cause is critical in the management of metabolic acidosis due to low-flow states. Hypovolemia must be corrected, sepsis must be controlled, and cardiovascular dynamics must be enhanced to improve tissue perfusion and satisfy cellular metabolic needs. Unless this is accomplished, no amount of infused bicarbonate by itself will succeed in raising the pHa to normal. Similarly, with diabetic ketoacidosis, treatment of the pHa levels with bicarbonate will be of little value without concomitant administration of insulin and intravenous fluids.

If it is deemed desirable to use bicarbonate in the treatment of acute metabolic acidosis, the amount needed to correct the pHa to normal can be estimated in the following manner. First, using rule 1, the disparity between the pHa measured and the pHa calculated on the basis of the measured $PaCO_2$ is determined. The difference defines the pHa decrease caused by a decrease in $[HCO_3^-]$. Using Rule 2 the pHa difference can be translated into the decrease in $[HCO_3^-]$ it represents. With that information and the assumption of a bicarbonate space calculated as 25% of body weight, the amount of bicarbonate needed to correct the total body base deficit can be calculated as

$$mEq\ HCO_3^- = mEq \times liter\ [HCO_3^-]\ deficit\ (4) \times (kg\ wt \times 0.25)$$

In extreme circumstances, such as cardiac arrest, when a precipitous and life-threatening fall in pHa can impair the effectiveness of efforts to resuscitate the patient, bolus administration of the entire calculated load of the bicarbonate can be justified. Otherwise, when the disturbance is less severe and dramatic, it is better to proceed at a slower pace, avoiding the undesirable consequences of overzealous and too rapid administration of intravenous bicarbonate, which include cardiac irregularities, convulsions, metabolic alkalosis, hypokalemia, impairment of red blood cell oxygen delivery to tissues, and symptomatic hyperosmolarity due to the infusion of excessive amounts of sodium. Usually it is advisable to replace no more than one-half of the calculated bicarbonate deficit in the first 3–4 hr and then over the next 12- to 24-hr period administer the remainder until serum bicarbonate and pHa values return to more normal levels.

Alkalosis

When the pHa rises above 7.45, irrespective of cause, alkalosis is present. The nature and importance of alkalosis on fluid and electrolyte balance and oxygen carried by hemoglobin were discussed in the sections on hypokalemia, hypocalcemia, hypomagnesemia, and hypophosphatemia. Clinical features of alkalosis that are peculiar to either respiratory or metabolic alkalosis also exist.

Respiratory Alkalosis. When the increase in pHa is related to a decrease in $PaCO_2$, respiratory alkalosis is present. Often it is the consequence of pulmonary alveolar hyperventilation, which for a variety of reasons is commonly encountered in surgical patients. Apprehension, pain that does not limit respiratory effort, hypoxia, fever, central nervous system injuries, and elevated serum ammonia levels in patients with chronic liver disease are all influences that can stimulate respiration and be responsible for hypocapnea and

respiratory alkalosis. Hyperventilation, causing a decreased $PaCO_2$, is frequent in patients who are mechanically ventilated during surgery or perioperatively.

Compensatory mechanisms for acute respiratory alkalosis are relatively ineffective in surgical patients. Renal compensatory efforts do occur in the form of distal tubular excretion of bicarbonate. However, hyponatremia and increased aldosterone activity, commonly present in surgically stressed patients limit the effectiveness of this mechanism, which depends on renal excretion of sodium as the accompanying cation. Only with chronic respiratory alkalosis can any notable compensatory decrease in $[HCO_3^-]$ be appreciated.

In addition to the consequences of disturbed potassium, calcium, magnesium, and phosphate metabolism seen in all alkalotic states, the low $PaCO_2$ levels characteristic of respiratory alkalosis can, by themselves, exert significant pathophysiologic influences. Hypocapnia causes cerebrovascular arterial vasoconstriction, which can reduce blood flow to the brain by as much as 50%. Such effects can have particular significance in older patients whose cerebral arterial circulation also might be compromised by atherosclerotic disease.

Treatment of Respiratory Alkalosis. In the artificially ventilated patient, downward adjustment of the amount of ventilation being provided can correct both the reasons for and the consequences of respiratory alkalosis. In the absence of mechanical hyperventilation as a cause, however, efforts are directed at treating the underlying conditions responsible for hypocapnia.

Metabolic Alkalosis. When an elevated pHa is associated with an elevated $[HCO_3^-]$, metabolic alkalosis is present. The many ways in which gastrointestinal and renal losses of potassium and chloride ions can occur and be the cause of hypochloremic hypokalemic metabolic alkalosis were extensively discussed in the sections dealing with disorders of those ions. The accumulation of exogenously infused excesses of base also can cause metabolic alkalosis in surgical patients. This can result from overzealous infusion of bicarbonate in the treatment of metabolic acidosis or the inadvertent administration of large amounts of citrate when multiple transfusions are given.

In metabolic alkalosis, carbon dioxide retention induced by hypoventilation can help to compensate for the accumulation of base excess. In surgical patients this is not often an effective mechanism. Renal tubular excretion of bicarbonate in an alkaline urine, on the other hand, can be. However, as discussed with paradoxical aciduria appearing in the course of hypochloremic hypokalemic metabolic alkalosis, this mechanism for compensation cannot be sustained as depletions of electrolytes related to renal tubular excretion of bicarbonate grow more severe. The urine then becomes acid, as hydrogen ion is secreted and bicarbonate ion is reabsorbed, creating a situation that enhances the severity of the existing metabolic alkalosis.

In general, the clinical problems encountered with metabolic alkalosis are most often those related to the hypokalemia, hypochloremia, and volume contraction caused by gastrointestinal and/or renal losses of fluid and electrolytes. Important clinical manifestations of potassium depletion, in particular, include paralytic ileus, digitalis toxicity, and cardiac arrhythmias.

Treatment of Metabolic Acidosis   The successful treatment of metabolic alkalosis, as has been reviewed earlier, requires control of extrarenal losses of fluid and electrolytes and correction of the fluid volume, potassium, and chloride deficits that are present. Only when all of these issues are successfully addressed can appropriate renal tubular responses be restored and pHa be returned to normal.

Fluid and Electrolyte Therapy for the Surgical Patient

There are three components of fluid and electrolyte therapy for surgical patients. The first is meeting the requirements for fluid and electrolyte intake that balance daily obligatory losses. The second is recognizing and repairing imbalances and deficits that are already present. The third is providing for ongoing and additional losses occurring during the course of therapy. Each of these must be dealt with in the three phases of surgical care, i.e., pre-, intra-, and postoperative care.

Normal Daily Balance

With no unusual stresses or losses and normal renal function, fluid and electrolyte balance is maintained by the intake of adequate amounts of water, sodium, potassium, and chloride to balance daily obligatory losses. In the idealized 70-kg male, this is approximated as 2500 ml of water, 75–100 mEq of sodium (taken in as sodium chloride to satisfy chloride needs), and 40–60 mEq of potassium. Such an intake is calculated to balance outputs of 1500–1700 ml of urine, 200 ml of stool water, 0–100 ml of sweat, and 700–800 ml of combined insensible losses from lungs and skin; and, an endogenous input of approximately 250 ml of water derived from the oxidation of carbohydrate and fat. However, as these estimates are not applicable to patients of all sizes, shapes, and ages, more universal guidelines for calculating fluid and electrolyte requirements have been devised. Probably the most accurate are based on surface area, but they are cumbersome, requiring measurements of height as well as weight and a nomogram for transposing the measurements into a value for surface. Thus it is a more common practice to make determinations of water and electrolyte needs as a function of age and weight. Guidelines for employing both methods are presented in Table 6.10. If the entire intake is to be delivered intravenously, 5% dextrose in water is used to meet most of the fluid requirements, with the balance being given in sufficient volumes of 0.45% or 0.9% saline to provide the necessary sodium and chloride. The potassium supplement is added in divided amounts to the various solutions, allowing its delivery to be spread out over time.

Table 6.10
Daily Fluid and Electrolyte Maintenance

Calculated by Surface Area	
Fluid	1500 ml/m²/day
Sodium	50–75 mEq/m²/day
Potassium	50 mEq/m²/day
Chloride	50–75 mEq/m²/day
Calculated by Body Weight	
Fluid	
Children >5 kg to young adulthood	
First 10 kg	100 ml/kg
Second 10 kg	50 ml/kg
Weight >20 kg	20 ml/kg
Adults	
25–55 yrs	35 ml/Kg
55–65 yrs	30 ml/Kg
>65 yrs	25 ml/Kg
Sodium	1.0–1.5 mEq/Kg
Potassium	0.5–0.75 mEq/Kg ($\sim \frac{1}{2}$ Na$^+$)
Chloride	1.0–1.5 mEq/Kg

Overall estimates of daily needs have to be adjusted for fever and high ambient temperatures. Insensible skin and pulmonary losses increase with body temperature elevations (10–15%/°C, 8%/°F), often requiring an additional 500 ml or more of salt-free water per day in febrile patients. Similar needs for more water due to increased pulmonary insensible losses occur in tracheostomized patients inspiring unhumidified air or gas mixtures, especially with hyperventilation. In slightly different fashion, requirements for salt as well as water increase when ambient temperatures rise above 32°C (85°F). This is due to hypotonic salt losses related to sweating. Additional intravenous fluid replacement with 0.45% saline solution is appropriate in such instances.

Preoperative Therapy

Consistent with all aspects of good surgical care, management of fluid and electrolyte balance starts with assessment. A thorough history and physical examination provide the information permitting recognition of a problem that exists or that may be forthcoming and direct the surgeon to consider what laboratory data are needed to confirm what is wrong. In a patient who appears to have no special problems at the time of admission for elective surgery, the initial workup could reveal underlying cardiac, pulmonary, renal, or hepatic disease, which may significantly influence the conduct of fluid therapy during and after the operation. In such instances, if very stressful surgery is contemplated (i.e., abdominal aortic aneurysmectomy or pulmonary, pancreatic, and colonic resections) the need for central venous or pulmonary arterial pressure monitoring in the perioperative period may become apparent. A history of diuretic and digitalis therapy can direct attention to the presence of hypokalemia and/or hyponatremia. Low preoperative serum potassium levels can fall even lower during surgery, particularly in patients under general anesthesia who are hyperventilated and develop hypocapnic respiratory alkalosis. If hyponatremia is present on admission, the margin of safety between asymptomatic and symptomatic low serum sodium concentrations is reduced, making even relatively small further decreases potentially hazardous. The discovery of a patient with chronic pulmonary obstructive disease prompts arterial blood gas and pH studies as part of the preoperative workup. Similarly, BUN, serum creatinine, and electrolyte studies are indicated in a patient who has a history of chronic renal disease. With any of these disorders, any deficits and ongoing needs must be attended to in the preoperative period. This includes being aware of the need for intravenous fluid hydration in patients whose bowels are being purged in preparation for surgery and those who need volume loading prior to abdominal aortic surgery.

In patients who are acutely ill on admission, fluid, electrolyte, and acid-base imbalances must be identified and treated promptly. This becomes even more necessary in the group of patients who will need urgent operation. Again, the admitting history and physical examination should make the nature of the problems clear. Stat laboratory data should be obtained. In patients who are vomiting or who have had prolonged gastric drainage, the presence of hypokalemic hypochloremic metabolic alkalosis should be anticipated, rapidly confirmed, and treated with replacement of volume, potassium, and chloride losses. In such circumstances a profound potassium depletion present will be indicated if the urine pH is acid. Should emergency surgery be indicated, potassium replacement may have to be given in 10–20 mEq/hr boluses, with the patient being monitored electrocardiographically.

Isotonic volume depletion due to third-space fluid losses, as seen with peritonitis (bacterial or chemical), intestinal obstruction, extensive soft tissue inflammation, or trauma, is another commonly encountered problem. Like hemorrhage, such extracellular fluid losses effectively reduce intravascular volumes, which must be replaced promptly. Balanced salt solutions (Ringer's lactate) should be used to replace the isotonic losses. The indications of how much to give, however, are not always readily apparent. In such instances, clinical observations of hemodynamic changes (i.e., tachycardia, narrowed pulse pressure, hypotension), decreasing urine output (i.e., to <30 ml/hr) and laboratory data indicative of isotonic volume contraction (i.e., rising hematocrit, serum BUN, and creatinine and urine sodium concentrations <20 mEq/liter) make it clear that the losses are significant. With continuous monitoring as intravenous fluid therapy is being given, improvement of hemodynamic parameters and hourly urine outputs will indicate when volumes have been restored to more normal levels. Care must be taken to limit the intravenous administration of hypotonic fluid to patients in need of large volumes of blood or isotonic crystalloid and colloid fluid support, if clinically significant dilutional hyponatremia is to be avoided.

Intraoperative Therapy

During surgery attention is largely focused on maintaining circulating volumes and adequate tissue perfusion, as monitored by urine flow rates and central venous or pulmonary arterial pressures. Packed red blood cells, colloid, and crystalloids are used to replace whole blood losses. At least 1 liter of balanced salt solution should be used to replace third-space isotonic fluid losses in major abdominal and thoracic surgical cases. Uses of hypotonic intravenous fluids should be limited to replacement of evaporative water losses. Used freely to replace isotonic losses, such fluids will lead to the development of dilutional hyponatremia. In patients with compromise of their pulmonary function, arterial blood gas and pH studies should be performed intraoperatively to monitor their gas exchange and acid-base status.

Postoperative Therapy

In the immediate postoperative period the fluid, electrolyte, and acid-base needs of the patient, for the most part, are related to monitoring and maintaining hemodynamic stability and the adequacy of ventilation. In many patients undergoing relatively unstressful and uncomplicated elective surgical procedures (i.e., inguinal herniorraphy, cholecystectomy), in whom oral intake will be resumed within 48 hr, this is simply accomplished by physical examination and serial observations of pulse rate, arterial blood pressure, respiratory frequency, and urine output and the administration of intravenous fluids in the amount and kind as described for maintenance in Table 6.10.

In patients who have undergone more surgically stressful procedures, involving extensive tissue dissection and/or resection, and in particular those with known compromise of cardiac, renal, or pulmonary function, the needs become greater. Additional monitoring with central venous or pulmonary arterial pressures, hourly urine flows collected via an indwelling catheter in the bladder, and serial arterial blood gas and pH measurements may be necessary. Inadequate respiratory gas exchange may require use of tracheal intubation and mechanical ventilation. Colloid and crystalloid infusions will be needed to replace third-space fluid losses that can continue for 48–72 hr. In addition to daily maintenance needs, gastric intestinal, biliary, and pancreatic drainage must be replaced milliliter for milliliter with appropriate potassium-enriched solutions. Daily weights are used to help assess fluid volume depletion or retention, recognizing that gains or losses >250 gm (approximately 0.5 lb) represent changes in body fluid content. As valuable as it is to monitor extracellular fluid status, weight gains and losses relative to third-space fluid losses and their management also have to be taken into account. During the replacement of third-space losses, weight gains do not represent intravascular volume overloads. Rather they are due to replacement of needed extracellular volumes to make up for that which was lost and sequestered. Similarly, a diuresis and associated weight loss is to be expected three or more days postoperatively, when third-space fluid accumulations become mobilized. This is fluid that should be excreted and not replaced. When this fluid is mobilizing, intravascular volumes are apt to be high, making additional intravenous volume loading undesirable. In patients who are receiving parenteral nutrition with hyperosmolar glucose solutions, on the other hand, an increased urine output should not be simply interpreted as representing an appropriate excretion of excess fluids. In fact, the urine output in such instances is more apt to be caused by an osmotic diuresis occurring independently of the patient's volume status. This requires prompt recognition and intravenous fluid correction to avoid severe hyperosmolar volume contraction.

The attention to needs continues until the patient's renal and gastrointestinal function has returned to normal and all fluid, electrolyte, and nutritional requirements are being met by oral intake. At this point, with the exception of the chronically ill who may have ongoing needs, concerns for this aspect of patient care end.

SUGGESTED READINGS

Gann DS, Amaral JF: Fluid and electrolyte management. In Sabiston DC (ed): *Essentials of Surgery*, Philadelphia, WB Saunders, 1987, p 29.

Pestana C: *Fluids and Electrolytes in the Surgical Patient*, ed 3. Baltimore, Williams & Wilkins, 1985.

Shires GT, Canizaro PC: Fluid and electrolyte management in the surgical patient. In Sabiston DC (ed): *Textbook of Surgery*, ed 13. Philadelphia, WB Saunders, 1986, p 64.

Sladen A: Acid-base balance. In McIntyre KM, Lewis AJ (eds): *Textbook of Advanced Cardiac Life Support*, Dallas, American Heart Association, 1981, p X-1.

Valtin H: *Renal Dysfunction*. Boston, Little Brown & Co, 1979.

Valtin H: *Renal Function*, ed 2. Boston, Little Brown & Co, 1983.

Valtin H, Gennari JF: *Acid-Base Disorders*. Boston, Little Brown & Co, 1987.

Skills

1. Calculate sensible and insensible fluid and electrolyte losses in the febrile patients (Temp. 104 F, 40 C).

2. Write postoperative fluid orders for an unstressed, uncomplicated 70-kg patient who has had a cholecystectomy.

3. Write at least three orders that would ascertain the patient's state of hydration/dehydration.

4. Write the fluid orders for a patient with one of the following problems:
   A. Pancreatic fistula
   B. Gastric fistula
   C. Small bowel fistula
   D. Biliary fistula

5. Demonstrate the ability to draw arterial blood gases.

6. Write orders to assess and to correct the following conditions in a ventilated, postoperative patient:
   A. Acute respiratory acidosis
   B. Metabolic alkalosis
   C. Acute metabolic acidosis

Study Questions

1. Discuss the mechanisms (be sure to include renal) by which a vomiting patient develops hypochloremic, hypokalemic metabolic alkalosis. When does paradoxical urinary acidosis develop?

2. Describe the clinical signs and symptoms of progressive hypovolemia.

3. List the common etiologies of hypo- and hypernatremia. How should these be evaluated and managed?

4. Discuss the potential adverse consequences of total parenteral nutrition on fluids and electrolytes. How should these problems be treated?

5. Describe a simple bedside technique to determine whether an acidotic patient has a metabolic or respiratory cause.

6. Discuss the use of an "anion gap" to differentiate acidosis due to loss of bicarbonate from acid load.

7. Describe the method to calculate the bicarbonate needed to correct a metabolic acidosis.

8. Discuss the fluid and electrolyte losses that might occur during a major abdominal surgical procedure.

7

Nutrition

Anthony Borzotta, M.D.
Anthony L. Imbembo, M.D.

ASSUMPTIONS

The student understands the biochemistry of carbohydrate, amino acid, and fat metabolism.

The student understands the types of vitamins and their role in human metabolism.

OBJECTIVES

1. List at least four factors from a patient's medical history that might indicate the presence of malnutrition.
2. Name at least eight anthropometric and objective laboratory test measurements helpful in ascertaining a patient's nutritional state.
3. Discuss how the different types of special assessment techniques are used to determine nutritional status.
4. Describe the methods to determine a patient's protein and caloric requirements and basic considerations for meeting these requirements.
5. List at least four water-soluble vitamins, three fat-soluble vitamins, and at least four trace elements that must be replaced in a patient on long-term parenteral nutrition.
6. Briefly describe at least four metabolic changes that occur in short-term and long-term starvation.
7. Discuss the impact of injury on a patient's metabolism as it relates to nutritional status.
8. List eight indications for nutritional support and three routes for supporting nutrition in the malnourished patient.
9. Discuss the indications and contraindications of the various delivery routes for enteral feeding.
10. Contrast the risks and benefits of enteral and parenteral nutritional support.
11. List at least four gastrointestinal, four mechanical, and four metabolic complications of enteral therapy and describe appropriate prevention and/or treatment of each.
12. List four adverse sequelae of a TPN catheter and four metabolic complications of TPN. Describe appropriate treatment of each.

The surgeon frequently encounters patients who are simultaneously depleted and cannot use the normal gastrointestinal route for nutritional intake. Consequently, surgeons often find themselves caring for patients who need supplementation of their own intake or who require complete provision of nutrition to maintain body weight and normal composition. Many of the major advances in nutritional support have been made by surgeons, including the first demonstration that intravenous alimentation could support growth of beagle puppies, reported by Dudrick et al in 1969.

In this chapter the current clinical and laboratory techniques for assessment of nutritional status, the basic requirements for proteins, calories, and lipids, and the metabolic patterns found in normal, fasted, and stressed states are described and defined. The indications for beginning, and the techniques of instituting, maintaining, and monitoring, enteral and parenteral nutritional therapy are outlined. Finally, a few areas of controversy and promise for the future are mentioned.

Assessment of Nutritional Status

History

Proper history taking and keen observation usually will elicit clinical findings of malnutrition, if present. Poverty, alcoholism, and age are risk factors for malnutrition. Unplanned weight loss is identified by comparing current with earlier weights and determining whether skin or clothing have become loose.

A recent weight loss of 10% is considered significant; 15% is quite severe, and a weight loss of 20% may increase operative mortality by a factor of 10-fold.

Malnutrition can develop in a number of ways, all of which may be determined by taking a careful nutritional history. Diminished intake may occur with severely restricted diets, anorexia of depression or illness, psychologic diseases such as bulimia and anorexia nervosa, and dysphagia (e.g., due to esophageal cancer, bulbar palsy after stroke, or breathlessness while eating in people with severe obstructive pulmonary disease). Hospitalized patients maintained on 5%-dextrose solutions are on enforced fasts that may unintentionally become quite prolonged. Abnormal nutrient losses may occur in malabsorption syndromes or inflammatory bowel disease and from gastrointestinal fistulas or chronically draining wounds. Supranormal nutritional requirements unmet by usual feeding habits are seen in trauma and burns, fever, and sepsis. Catabolic medications such as glucocorticoids, immunosuppressants, or INH may alter nutrient requirements, while other therapeutic modalities such as chemotherapy or radiation therapy often have side effects that reduce the appetite or ability to eat.

Anthropometric Measurements

A variety of techniques can be used to assess body fuel depots or body composition. The simplest are anthropometric measurements. Height and weight are universally attainable and should be compared with standard tables of ideal values adjusted for age, sex, and height. (A general guide for ideal weight may be obtained by adding 5 pounds per inch over 5 feet to 100 pounds for females or 6 pounds per inch over 5 feet to 110 pounds for males.) The triceps skin fold is the thickness of a pinch of skin and fat overlying the triceps of the nondominant arm midway between the acromion and olecranon, measured using Lange skinfold calipers. When compared with standard values, this provides an estimate of subcutaneous fat stores. Skeletal muscle mass, the greatest body protein depot, can be assessed using the arm-muscle circumference. This is determined by taking the midarm circumference (mm) minus 0.314 times the triceps skin fold (mm). This measure of skeletal muscle mass, often referred to as somatic protein status, can be compared with normal values specific for sex and age. Anthropometric measurements are of only relative utility because the range of normal varies with the study population, making the data more useful in population studies and less applicable to individual nutritional assessments except over longer periods of nutritional therapy. Deviation from normal does not reliably predict a malnourished state, because the standards do not account for individual variation in bone size, hydration, or skin compressibility. These measurements respond very slowly to changes in nutritional status, and their interpretation may be complicated by simple fluid changes in hospitalized patients.

Biochemical Measurements

While skeletal muscle mass reflects somatic protein status, biochemical measurement of the plasma transport proteins is a measure of internal or visceral protein status. Long half-life albumin and transferrin and short half-life retinol-binding protein and thyroxin-binding prealbumin (Table 7.1), in the absence of nonnutritional variables, can be used to assess nutritional status and the response to feeding. Beware, however, because concentrations do not always reflect turnover rates or the production and destruction of a compound. For example, changes in the volume of distribution, such as expansion of the extracellular fluid space, can dilute albumin and lower the serum albumin level, irrespective of nutritional status. Also, the long-lived compounds don't change quickly enough to be sensitive measures of nutritional repletion; the short-lived compounds better serve that purpose.

The creatinine-height index, in the absence of increased muscle breakdown, gives an estimate of somatic protein status. Creatinine production from creatine is directly related to skeletal muscle mass. A 24-hr urine creatinine excretion value divided by that for a normal individual of the same sex, height, and ideal weight (obtained from standardized tables), multiplied by 100 equals the creatinine-height index (percentage). The normal creatine excretion is 23–28 mg/kg ideal body weight/day in men and 18–21 mg/kg ideal weight in women. These values tend to decrease with age. Creatinine-height indices of 60–80% of ideal indicate moderate depletion, while 40–50% are considered severe depletion.

Twenty-four hour urine collections for nitrogen excretion as urinary urea nitrogen (UUN) [~80–90% of total urinary nitrogen (TUN)] are necessary to measure nitrogen balance. It may be reported as grams or milligrams nitrogen per liter of urine; the total volume of

Table 7.1.
Visceral Proteins Used in Nutritional Assessment

Protein	Half-Life Days	Normal Levels[a]	Malnutrition		
			Mild	Moderate	Severe
Albumin	18	3.5–5.5 gm/dl	3.0–3.5	2.1–3.0	<2.1
Transferrin	8	200–400 mg/dl	150–190	100–150	<100
Thyroid-binding prealbumin	2–4	15.7–29.6 mg/dl	12–15	8–10	<8
Retinol-binding protein	4 hr (free) 11 hr (bound)	2.6–7.6 mg/dl			

[a]Normal ranges may vary according to laboratory.

urine must be known accurately to obtain total urine nitrogen loss. Customarily, 3 gm of nitrogen are added to the TUN value to compensate for daily skin and fecal nitrogen losses to obtain the total nitrogen output. Nitrogen intake is determined from dietary history, calorie counts, or the known composition of enteral or parenteral feedings. Nitrogen balance equals nitrogen intake minus total nitrogen losses. [Nitrogen losses or output equals either (a) TUN + 3 gm or (b) UUN × 1.15 + 3 gm.] A positive balance implies nitrogen accretion; a negative balance means more nitrogen is being lost than ingested. Zero, or balance point, varies with nutritional state, the level of intake, stress factors, and provision of adequate nonprotein calories. Nitrogen balance also depends on protein quality, that is, the proportions of essential and nonessential amino acids in a foodstuff.

Nitrogen losses are roughly proportional to the catabolic state, hence the following average losses in grams nitrogen per day: starvation adapted, 5; stable after elective surgery, 5–10; polytrauma, 10–15; and sepsis or burns, >15. Nitrogen balance measurements should be done before initiating nutritional support and weekly thereafter to assess and assure adequacy of therapy.

Immunologic Measurement

Nutrition and immunocompetence are closely linked; for example, malnutrition correlates with an increased incidence of tuberculosis, epidemics of contagious diseases, and pneumonia. Hence, immunologic functions have been used to assess nutritional state. The absolute lymphocyte count reflects visceral protein status in the absence of nonnutritional variables such as trauma, anesthesia, and chemotherapy, all of which depress the count. Low counts concurrent with hypoalbuminemia are correlated with an increased incidence of postoperative sepsis. The minimum normal level is reported to be 1500 cells/mm^3.

Delayed hypersensitivity skin tests are anamnestic immune responses to a battery of antigens placed intradermally: mumps, PPD, SK-SD (streptokinase-streptodornase), Candida, and histoplasmin. A normal response is a 5 mm or greater area of induration in response to at least one antigen. Partial responses are smaller, and nonresponders are termed anergic. Response depends on prior exposure, an adequate dose of antigen, proper technique of injection and measurement, and, perhaps, induction of a response by repeated testing. Responses are depressed by malnutrition, but also by infections, trauma, operations, anesthetics, burns, corticosteroids, malignancy, and renal failure. This testing method is increasingly being seen as an unreliable measure of nutritional status.

Comparison of Measurement Techniques

Many still rely on subjective global assessment, based on an individual surgeon's clinical experience. When history and physical examination alone were an-

alyzed in comparison with other methods of nutritional assessment, they were found to comprise the best combination of sensitivity and specificity. This indicates two things: (1) the value of close observation and personal clinical experience and (2) the lack of any independent, totally valid measure of malnutrition. The absence of a single standard is a major impediment in the analysis of the impact of nutritional therapy on acute diseases. Each of these techniques may, however, be used repeatedly in assessing the effectiveness of nutritional therapy. The goals should be positive nitrogen balance, repletion of diminished physical and chemical parameters, or their stabilization in the face of elevated metabolic demands.

Special Assessment Techniques

Nutritional researchers employ a variety of additional assessment techniques. The amine 3-methylhistidine (3MeH) is released by muscle proteolysis and excreted unchanged in the urine. Skeletal muscle contains 90% of the body 3MeH but contributes only 40–60% to excreted totals. Skin and gut contribute 9–12% and 20–30%, respectively. Increased excretion is presumed to derive from increased skeletal muscle breakdown in stress states such as sepsis and trauma.

Indirect calorimetry measures the amounts of O_2 consumed and CO_2 expired, which are quantitatively related to energy release in the body. The ratio $CO_2{:}O_2$ is the respiratory quotient (RQ) and reflects the proportions of different fuels being oxidized for energy needs. Carbohydrates produce equal volumes of CO_2 for O_2 consumed, with an RQ of 1.0. Lipids undergo β-oxidation, yielding both ketone bodies and CO_2 and are therefore associated with a lower RQ of 0.71. These techniques used in fasting, normal individuals generated the Harris-Benedict equations for basal metabolic rate (BMR), a value initially used to diagnose and monitor treatment of thyroid disease (see "Basic Nutritional Needs"). The BMR is roughly equivalent to resting metabolic expenditure (RME). Indirect calorimetry is currently being applied to stressed patients to study the composition of fuels being oxidized for energy to define optimum replacement therapy in specific clinical situations.

Amino acid analyses are done by fluorometric, autoanalytic, and high-performance liquid chromatographic techniques. The essential amino acids in animals were defined first by deleting them one at a time from the diet and observing for failure to grow. They include lysine, threonine, phenylalanine, methionine, and the branched-chain amino acids (BCAA) leucine, isoleucine, and valine. Histidine is essential in children and in the setting of renal failure. Nonessential amino acids can be produced endogenously. The identification of amino acid profiles that differ from normal postabsorptive patterns has suggested the presence of altered metabolic states in various clinical conditions, thereby providing clues for nutritional manipulation. For example, elevated aromatic amino acids (phenylalanine, tyrosine, and tryptophan) in sepsis and hepatic failure may result in synthesis of false neurotransmitters such as octopamine that have deleterious central neurologic and peripheral vascular effects. Therefore, significant restriction of their intake in these clinical settings may be appropriate. The BCAA concentrations decline in starvation and in trauma or sepsis. Their initial metabolism takes place almost exclusively in skeletal muscle, where deamination occurs. This is followed either by local oxidation by muscle branched-chain ketoacid (BCKA) dehydrogenase or by efflux of the ketoacids and subsequent oxidation in the liver. The BCAA appear to be used preferentially as energy fuels by skeletal muscle during the insulin-resistant phases of trauma and sepsis. Leucine has total body protein synthesis-enhancing properties. However, its ability to suppress protein breakdown in vitro has not been confirmed in vivo. Nutritional formulations containing enhanced amounts of BCAA are available for use in severely catabolic patients.

Isotopic tracer studies allow assessment of the relative importance of various metabolic pathways mapped out by the techniques described above. Amino acid and glucose kinetics are studied using stable isotopes (^{15}N and ^{13}C) and unstable ^{14}C in both plasma and end-product enrichment methods. Tracer studies have shown that exogenous glucose cannot suppress gluconeogenesis during acute stress responses and that increased protein breakdown can be compensated for but not reduced by nutritional supplements.

Basic Nutritional Needs

The protein requirement is the amount needed to meet physiologic needs and is the lowest protein intake at which nitrogen balance can be achieved. Proteins do not exist in a storage form: all have structural, enzymatic, immune, and transport functions. Ingestion of amino acids in excess of needs results not in storage but in deamination, nitrogen excretion as urea and ammonia, and reutilization of the carbon skeletons. When intake is insufficient, protein is mobilized, principally through skeletal muscle proteolysis, adding essential amino acids to endogenous, nonessential amino acids and providing gluconeogenic substrates. Prolonged muscle wasting is deleterious to survival. The mechanisms of compensation during starvation are discussed below.

Determination of the patient's protein requirement is the first critical step in formulating a nutritional support program. The requirements for a normal, active man are 0.9–1.5 gm protein/kg body weight daily (6.25 gm protein = 1 gm nitrogen). Requirements change with the clinical state, decreasing to 1 gm/kg/day early in refeeding after starvation and increasing to 2–3 gm/kg/day in burned or severely septic patients. Total intake may have to be limited to 40–50 gm/day in hepatic failure. The most accurate and individualized estimate of nitrogen (protein) needs comes from 24-hour urine nitrogen loss measurement.

Protein balance cannot be achieved without protein intake, but the provision of nonprotein calories significantly enhances the efficiency of protein utilization. Protein sparing is maximally achieved with 150–200 gm (700 kcal) glucose daily. This is the basis for the hypocaloric, 3% amino acid peripheral vein infusions ("protein-sparing therapy") used by some in fasting clinical situations such as repeated NPO status during prolonged diagnostic evaluation or bowel obstruction or adynamic ileus without prior weight loss. The remainder of energy requirements are met by mobilization of fat stores.

Two further concepts should be kept in mind. First, at any fixed level of protein intake, nitrogen balance improves to a maximum as calorie intake increases from levels inadequate to those exceeding energy requirements. Second, when all energy needs are met by nonprotein calories, nitrogen balance becomes increasingly negative at a fixed nitrogen intake as metabolic rate increases in disease states such as burns, peritonitis, and multiple trauma.

Caloric requirements range from 30 to 80 kcal/kg/day, depending on age (greater in childhood) and stress. The requirement can be estimated in two ways.

1. Harris-Benedict equations for RME are a good place to start because the variables are easily determined. For men, RME (kcal/day) = 664.7 + 13.75 (W) + 5 (H) - 6.76 (A). For women, RME = 655.1 + 9.56 (W) + 1.85 (H) - 4.68 (A) (W, weight in kg; H, height in cm; A, age in years). The results must be multiplied by activity factors to yield estimated total daily caloric requirements: bedrest, 1.2; ambulation, 1.3; trauma and fractures 1.8; severe sepsis and burns, 2.0; per 1°C fever, 1.13.
2. Alternatively, requirements can be based on 35 kcal/kg/day, increased by 12% after major surgery, by 20–50% during sepsis, and up to 100% with major burns.

Both of these methods are population-derived techniques and simply approximate needs. Indirect calorimetry is needed to individualize estimates.

Calories can be provided as dextrose, in concentrations based on the total caloric requirement and limitations on volume administration. Concentrations >10% require administration into a central vein to prevent phlebitis due to the hypertonicity of the solutions. A minimum of 200 g glucose daily prevents starvation ketosis.

A maximum of 60% (but usually only 40%) of calories can be given as lipid emulsions of either 10% (1.1 kcal/ml) or 20% (2.2 kcal/ml). Their combination with dextrose, known as the lipid system, is well tolerated except by patients with hyperlipidemias and possibly in septic or hypermetabolic patients. The lipid system is advantageous in glucose-intolerant patients, in cases requiring volume restriction, in very high catabolic states, for peripheral parenteral alimentation, and during weaning from mechanical ventilation in nutritionally supported patients (due to the lowered production of CO_2 from lipid as compared with glucose). Intravenous lipids do not aggravate acute pancreatitis or pancreaticocutaneous fistulas.

A minimum of 500 ml of 10% lipid emulsion must be given twice weekly to prevent essential fatty acid deficiency. Essential fatty acid deficiency in humans is due principally to a lack of linoleic acid. The clinical signs of deficiency are eczematous, desquamative dermatitis of body folds, anemia, thrombocytopenia, and hair loss. Growth retardation can occur, especially in neonates.

Micronutrients

Vitamins are compounds required in minute amounts for normal growth, maintenance, and reproduction, and which are not endogenously synthesized. Essential vitamins in humans are the four fat-soluble (A, D, E, and K) and nine water-soluble vitamins (Table 7.2). The allowances for normal persons at varying ages are well defined. The AMA Nutrition Advisory Group provides reasonable approximations of requirements during total parenteral nutrition (TPN). Needs during stress states are imprecise but have been estimated by the National Academy of Sciences.

The fat-soluble vitamins serve many functions. Vitamin A is an essential component of the visual cycle and preserves the integrity of epithelial membranes by limiting keratinization.

Vitamin D enhances gut absorption and resorption from bone of both calcium and phosphorus. Vitamin E is a family of seven tocopherols with antioxidant properties and indefinite biologic roles. Vitamin K is a cofactor for synthesis of coagulation factors II, VII, IX, and X. Vitamin K absorption in the jejunum requires the presence of bile salts, hence the abnormal coagulation times generally associated with bile duct obstruction. The destruction or alteration of colonic microflora by antibiotics also may induce vitamin K deficiency.

The water-soluble vitamins include the B complex, which contains cofactors of enzymes vital to intermediary metabolism, energy supply, and nucleic acid synthesis. Folic acid deficiency is the most common hypovitaminosis occurring in humans; it is frequently due to poor nutritional intake, such as commonly occurs with alcoholism. The B complex or multivitamin formulations must be added to TPN daily and probably should be included once daily in maintenance intravenous fluids.

Trace elements are minerals known to be essential [iron, iodine, cobalt (vitamin B_{12}), zinc, and copper] or possibly essential (manganese and chromium) (Table 7.2). In addition, animal studies indicate important roles for selenium, vanadium, molybdenum, nickel, tin, silicon, and arsenic. Zinc is lost at an accelerated rate after injury, and serum levels fall significantly during sepsis. Acute deficiency results in a wet dermatitis of the nasolabial area, progressing to involve the perineum; extensor aspects of the elbows, back, fingers, and toes; and alopecia. Chronic deficiency is more subtle; inability to heal even superficial wounds should make one suspicious.

Clinical trace element deficiency states are quite rare. In this country they appear among food faddists and severe alcoholics and elsewhere due to inadequate intake or low-quality foodstuffs. They occur with very prolonged TPN (months) when the trace elements are not routinely added but are reversible and respond rapidly to supplementation. Parenteral administration bypasses the regulatory gut mucosa, a situation exacerbated by renal insufficiency. Monitoring of serum levels may be needed.

Metabolic Patterns Affecting Nutrition

Nutrition is the study of the provision and utilization of foodstuffs in support of metabolic needs for immediate energy, protein synthesis, circulation and respiration, locomotion, energy storage, and waste product excretion. Supply and use interact in a dynamic process. Intermediary metabolism varies with absolute nutrient intake, the proportions of carbohydrate, lipid, and protein, and the homeostatic balance of the organism. Energy supply is the critical need, and metabolic adaptations serve this end; pathologic or iatrogenic maladaptations may subvert it. This section describes the broad outlines of energy flux in a variety of nutritional states (Fig. 7.1 to 7.5).

Glycogen is a carbohydrate storage form available for immediate energy needs. It is in short supply. The approximately 75 gm in the liver and 200–400 gm in adult muscle last only 1–2 days without replenishment. After glycolysis, muscle glycogen is released as lactate and pyruvate, which then are transported to the liver to be incorporated into glucose via the Cori cycle. Pyruvate can be transaminated in muscle and released as alanine, a major substrate for hepatic gluconeogenesis. Adipose tissue releases lipids, which serve immediate energy needs for nonglycolytic tissues. It is the largest storehouse of energy and is the principal energy source in long fasts. Protein, especially from skeletal muscle, is an energy source but is not a true storage form of energy. Conservation of protein does occur as a survival mechanism in long fasts.

The interprandial state exists after meals, when hepatic glycogen provides glucose for the brain. The human brain consumes 20% of RME, a proportion remarkable among mammals. The blood-brain barrier blocks the entry of large free fatty acids (FFA) or chylomicrons but allows entry of small water-soluble compounds like glucose; i.e., the brain has discriminatory energy needs. Other glycolytic tissues are erythrocytes, bone marrow, renal medulla, and peripheral nerves. The remaining tissues oxidize lipids released from adipose tissue as FFA. There is net muscle amino acid uptake.

The postabsorptive state occurs after an overnight fast. Hepatic glycogenolysis is mildly supplemented by gluconeogenesis from amino acids derived from skeletal muscle. Adipose FFA outflow continues to fuel

Table 7.2.
Micronutrients[a]

Compound	Recommended Daily Amounts Adults Usual–Stressed	During TPN	Intravenous Dosage	Function	Deficiency States
Vitamins[a-c]					
Fat-Soluble Vitamins[b-d]					
A, retinol, IU	3300–5000	1300–2900	3300	Retinal pigments; soft tissue and bone growth; functional integrity of epithelium	Xerophthalmia, night blindness, epithelial keratinization, delayed wound healing, anemia
D, cholecalciferol, IU	400	200–400	200	Mediates bone sensitivity to parathyroid hormones and gut absorption of calcium	Rickets (children); osteomalacia (adults)
E, -tocopherol, IU	10–15	2–10	10	Placental implantation; sperm mobility; antioxidant of vitamin A and unsaturated fatty acids	Male and female infertility, vitamin A deficiency, serum deficiencies of phospholipids
K, mg	2–20	2–4 mg/wk	2	Cofactor for synthesis of coagulant factors II, VII, IX, X	Bleeding disorders seen in hepatic disease, malabsorption states, certain antibiotic use
Water-Soluble Vitamins[a-c]					
B_1, thiamine, mg	1.5–10 (0.5 mg/1000 kcal)	1.2–50	3.0	Decarboxylation of pyruvate and ketoacids; coenzyme in carbohydrate metabolism	Beriberi; high-output cardiac failure; Wernicke's encephalopathy
B_2, riboflavin, mg	1.1–1.8	1.8–10	3.6	Cytochrome oxidase cofactors in cellular respiration	Cheilosis, seborrheic dermatitis, magenta tongue of pellagra, angular stomatitis
Niacin, mg	12–20	10–150	40	Cofactor in redox reactions (NAD^+ and $NADP^+$) and energy metabolism	Pellagra; photosensitive dermatitis, diarrhea, gastrointestinal hemorrhage; dementia
B_3, pantothenic acid, mg	7–40	5–25	15	Synthesis of coenzyme A involved in amino acid; carbohydrate and fat metabolism	Malaise, headache, nausea, and vomiting (only with a specific antagonist)
B_6, pyridoxine, mg	1.6–2.0	2–15	4	Coenzyme for amino acid deamination, transamination, decarboxylation, transulfuration, and glucose metabolism	CNS (irritation, depression somnolence); skin (seborrheic dermatitis, glossitis); microcytic, hypochromic anemia
Biotin	150–300	100–200	60	Coenzyme in carboxylation reactions of CHO, lipids, and amino acids	Rare; seborrheic dermatitis

[a]Requirements in specific disease states are ill-defined.
[b]*Recommended Daily Amounts,* ed 9. Food and Nutrition Board of the National Research Council, National Academy of Science, 1980.
[c]American Medical Association Nutrition Advisory Group; Multivitamin preparations for parenteral use. *J Parent Ent Nutr* 3.258–262, 1979.

liver and muscle, supplemented by products of hepatic ketogenesis also utilized by muscle.

In early starvation, glycogen stores are used up in 12–24 hours. As blood glucose concentration falls, insulin levels drop. An elevated glucagon/insulin ratio or an absolute glucagon increase plus chronic sympathetic nerve activity instigates catabolic changes. Glycogenolysis is replaced by gluconeogenesis, supplied with substrate from enhanced protein breakdown. About 300 gm wet muscle tissue per day is metabolized, and the excess nitrogen is excreted as urea. Lipolysis increases, and enhanced hepatic ketogenesis occurs. Hepatic ketogenesis is maximum after 2 to 3 days of starvation.

Prolonged starvation leads to the starvation-adapted state, a vital shift that minimizes protein breakdown.

Table 7.2.
Micronutrients[a] *(cont'd)*

Compound	Recommended Daily Amounts		Intravenous Dosage	Function	Deficiency States
	Adults Usual–Stressed	During TPN			
B₁₂, cyanocobalamin, mg	2–4	2–50	5	Coenzyme for purine and pyrimidine synthesis	Pernicious anemia; neural lesions
Folic acid, mg	100–300	200–5000	400	Purine and thymine synthesis for DNA	Leukopenia; megaloblastic anemia; steatorrhea secondary to jejunal mucosal atrophy, sprue; glossitis
C, ascorbic acid, mg	45	30–700	100	Antiscorbutic; collagen cross-linking; hydroxylation of proline	Defective sulfonated copolysaccharides and chondroitin sulfate with retarded wound healing; scurvy; wound dehiscence; chronic skin ulcers
Trace Elements[e]					
Zinc, mg	10–15		2.5–6.0	Metalloenzymes involved in lipid, carbohydrate, protein and nucleic acid metabolism	Hypogonadism; altered hepatic drug metabolism; diminished wound strength and healing rates; anorexia, diarrhea, abnormalities of taste and smell, mental depression, cerebellar dysfunction, alopecia, typical dermatitis of face
Copper, mg	1.2–3		0.5–1.5	Metalloenzymes; iron uptake in hemoglobin synthesis; normal CNS function	Anemia; skeletal defects, demyelination; reproductive failure (congenital deficiency); leukopenia
Chromium, mg	50–290		10–15	Insulin cofactor	Hyperglycemia; mental confusion; peripheral sensory neuropathy with ataxia
Iodine, mg	150		1–2 mg/kg	Thyroid hormone synthesis	Hypothyroidism; goiter
Iron, mg	10–18		Questionably useful	Constituent of hemoglobin, myoglobin, and cytochromes	Hypochromic anemia
Manganese, mg	0.7–5		0.15–0.8	Enzyme cofactor in protein and energy metabolism; fat synthesis	Sterility or diminished fertility; glucose intolerance, hypocholesterolemia, growth retardation

[d]Jeppsson B, Gimmon Z. Vitamins. In Fischer JE (ed): *Surgical Nutrition.* Boston, Little, Brown & Co, 1983, pp 241–281.
[e]AMA Department of Foods and Nutrition: Guidelines for essential trace element preparation for parenteral use. A statement by an expert panel. *JAMA* 241:2051–2054, 1979.

The peripheral (especially muscle) oxidation of ketone bodies falls, allowing β-hydroxybutyrate and acetoacetate levels to reach maximal values in 8–10 days. Their rising concentrations form a transport gradient into erythrocytes and brain, allowing ketoacids to replace glucose partially as a primary metabolic fuel. After two weeks, more than two-thirds of brain oxygen consumption is for ketoacid oxidation. The remainder is for oxidation of glucose derived from glycerol and gluconeogenesis. Muscles burn more FFA as declining insulin levels permit enhanced lipolysis. Proteolysis decreases as the need for gluconeogenic substrate falls, and thus protein is spared.

A markedly different state of affairs exists in the

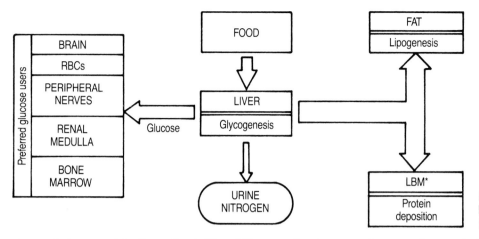

Figure 7.1. Interprandial state. **LBM,** Lean body mass; principally skeletal muscle, but includes all viscera.

stressed, hypercatabolic patient. The difference begins with the presence of an injury and the inflammation it evokes. A variety of mediators, including monokines such as interleukin 1, bacterial products such as endotoxin, and effluvia of dead and dying tissue, combined with afferent nerve stimulation, impact on the neuroendocrine system. This mediator traffic, proportionate to the severity of injury, the success of resuscitation, and organ functional reserves, induces proportional hemodynamic, hormonal, and metabolic alterations. Cuthbertson, a pioneer in metabolic studies of the injured human, described an initial ebb phase characterized by hypotension, reduced blood flow, and tissue perfusion, and a hypometabolic state lasting one or two days. The flow phase follows, marked by increased blood flow, hypermetabolism, increased energy expenditure, lean body mass wasting, and abnormal substrate utilization, lasting one to three weeks.

Resting metabolic expenditure increases minimally from normal after elective major surgery (10%) but more so after long bone fracture (10–30%), sepsis (20–45%), or burns (40–100%). Increased metabolic expenditure is needed for wound healing, synthesis of cellular and humoral immune components, and synthesis of acute-phase reactants until healing is complete. Central thermoregulation is adjusted upward (especially in burns) and increased metabolic expenditure continues unabated even if ambient temperatures are elevated.

Increased catecholamine release is the major catabolic factor. Hypercortisolemia plays a permissive role with the catecholamines. Glucagon also increases, increasing proteolysis, gluconeogenesis, and ureagenesis. Unlike starvation, the anabolic hormone insulin increases, but to a smaller degree than glucagon. Production of glucose is accelerated, is not suppressible by exogenous glucose, and is proportionate to alanine and lactate release from skeletal muscle. That is, muscle wasting provides alanine to meet increased energy needs. One theory proposes that amino acid efflux from muscle supplies the raw materials for acute-phase protein synthesis in the liver, but this is unproven. The amino acid efflux profile reflects neither muscle protein composition nor the composition of newly synthesized protein. The fate of the effluxed amino acids is reflected by urine nitrogen losses of >20 gm/day or losses of >400 gm/day of wet muscle mass. Muscle itself appears to oxidize BCAA preferentially as an energy source. Ketogenesis is blocked in the liver. Increased lipogenesis occurs. FFA continue to be released at a low rate, but triglyceride formation is accelerated and disposal impaired, resulting in septic hyperlipidemia, which is why fat emulsions are so often ineffective during fulminant infection. This "cannibalistic" situation focused on skeletal muscle breakdown continues until infection is controlled or wounds stabilized by fixation (fractures) or coverage (burns). The very late, uncontrolled state is marked by hepatic failure of gluconeo-

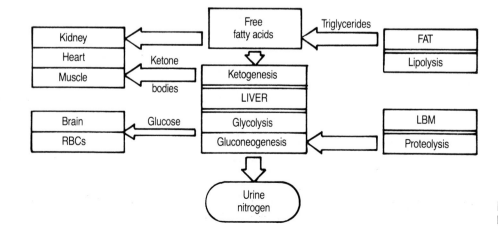

Figure 7.2 Early fasting state. **LBM,** Lean body mass.

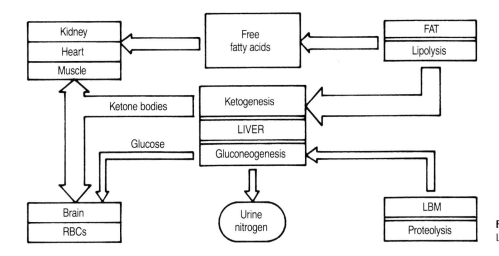

Figure 7.3. Starvation-adapted state. **LBM,** Lean body mass.

genesis, hypoglycemia, severe amino acid profile abnormalities, and death.

Techniques of Nutritional Support

The flow diagram in Figure 7.5 is a general guide to nutritional therapy, once the decision has been made that support is needed.

Choice of the Route for Administration of Nutritional Support

The route chosen for administration of nutritional support depends to a large extent on the patient. Patients with adequate appetite and a normally functioning gastrointestinal tract can usually be entirely supported with oral intake. Calorie counts can be very helpful in determining whether oral intake is adequate; supplementation with snacks and/or high-calorie liquids may be appropriate in some patients. There are other patients in whom the gastrointestinal tract is entirely normal but little or no spontaneous oral intake takes place. This group includes individuals with anorexia nervosa and depressed mental function for a variety of reasons. Tube feedings permit utilization of the functional gastrointestinal system. Short-term tube feedings are best administered through a nasoalimentary tube with the end positioned in the stomach or, in some cases, the duodenum. Such tubes may be uncomfortable for some patients or can become dislodged. For these reasons, chronic tube feedings are best administered through tubes placed operatively into either the stomach or jejunum. When gastroesophageal reflux is present, a jejunal feeding tube is generally preferred to avoid aspiration. When proximal gastrointestinal tract obstruction is present (esophageal, pyloric), the feeding tube must be placed distal to the obstruction. The parenteral route becomes necessary when the gastrointestinal tract is nonfunctional or unavailable.

Enteral Alimentation

A variety of enteral formulations is available so that an appropriate choice can be made to satisfy any given patient's specialized needs. The products fall into three broad categories based on their composition: polymeric, chemically defined, and modular formulas. The products also differ in nutrient complexity, concentration, osmolarity, caloric density, and viscosity.

Polymeric formulas are either food-based formulas or contain combinations of intact macronutrients. Blenderized food tube feedings contain intact protein and lactose. They are high in residue, viscosity, and osmolarity. These preparations are nutritionally complete and cause few gastrointestinal side effects when delivered into the stomach. The feedings are viscous and consequently may be difficult to deliver through a tube. The other polymeric formulas contain mixtures of macromolecular components, which are intact to a variable degree. They may be milk-based or lactose-free and contain protein derived from whole milk, egg, or soy; fat; and carbohydrate polymers. These polymeric formulas are also nutritionally complete, but they are low in residue, lower in osmolarity, and of only moderate viscosity. Some flavored preparations are palatable and therefore can be administered as oral dietary supplements.

The chemically defined or "elemental" formulas contain products of hydrolysis of protein and carbohydrate macronutrients. Fats are intact, and some formulas add medium-chain triglycerides. All of the chemically defined formulas are lactose-free. These products, which are characterized by relative chemical simplicity, are intended for patients with impaired digestive capacity. They contain monosaccharides and protein in the form of either amino acids or short peptides. Therefore minimal or no digestion is required. Fat content is low but sufficient to prevent essential fatty acid deficiency. The formulas are low residue and nutritionally complete but also hyperosmolar. Because they are relatively unpalatable, administration through a feeding tube is usually required.

Modular products contain only single or a few macronutrients. Protein, fat, and carbohydrate modules are available. By definition these formulas cannot provide complete nutrition. They are designed to selectively fulfill special nutritional requirements or to serve as supplements in patients who can tolerate only certain nutrients.

Access for Nutrition

Enteral Feeding. Selection of the delivery route for enteral feeding involves decisions regarding the portion of the patient's gastrointestinal tract that may be accessed, the anticipated duration of feeding, and whether the patient is an operative candidate. Either the stomach or small bowel may be used. Delivery of enteral feeding into the stomach ensures exposure to the maximal intestinal absorptive surface available, an important consideration in a patient with a limited amount of small bowel remaining. In addition, because the stomach serves as a reservoir where diets are mixed and tonicity adjusted, greater latitude in selection of diet and technique of administration results when intragastric delivery is chosen. The greater ease and flexibility with which intragastric feeding is performed must be weighed against the risks of gastroesophageal reflux, vomiting, and possible aspiration. Instillation of the diet into the small bowel virtually eliminates the problems of gastric retention, reflux, vomiting, and aspiration. In addition, jejunal motility is usually not affected by most mechanical and inflammatory processes in the upper abdomen that may inhibit gastric emptying.

Several means of nonoperative access to the gastrointestinal tract are available. Nasoenteral intubation is perhaps the simplest and most widely used method. Although individual differences exist in length and composition, most of the current feeding catheters are manufactured from silicone rubber or polyurethane. Weights are incorporated into the catheters to facilitate introduction and maintenance in the desired location. Many nasoenteral catheters use stylets to facilitate placement and, in some instances, to allow their manipulation and precise placement under fluoroscopic control. In addition, most nasoenteral catheters are of sufficient length to allow access to the proximal small bowel. Transnasal access to the small bowel is somewhat more difficult to achieve. In the ambulatory patient, the feeding catheter will spontaneously pass into the small bowel in about one-half of cases. In some instances the proximal small bowel may be successfully cannulated under fluoroscopic control, using a rigid stylet to manipulate the tip of the catheter through the pylorus. Alternatively, the tip of the catheter may be guided into the small bowel using the flexible fiberoptic gastroscope and its snare or biopsy forceps. Although nonoperative access to the small bowel is more difficult, the advantages of intrajejunal feeding can be achieved in this way. All the small, soft, nonreactive nasoenteral catheters are well tolerated over extended periods; however, nasoenteral catheters generally are used for short-term programs, because of their propensity to dislodge or cause nasal discomfort. It is essential to confirm the intra-abdominal location of the tip of the catheter by x-ray prior to institution of feedings. This prevents inadvertent feeding into the airway due to a catheter misplaced into a bronchus.

Operative access to the gastrointestinal tract for feeding can be achieved at a variety of levels. The proximal esophagus, stomach, and jejunum may all serve as sites of operative feeding enterostomies. The indications for feeding enterostomies are (1) primary: an enterostomy performed for the sole purpose of providing feeding access to the gastrointestinal tract; (2) palliative: an enterostomy performed for palliative pur-

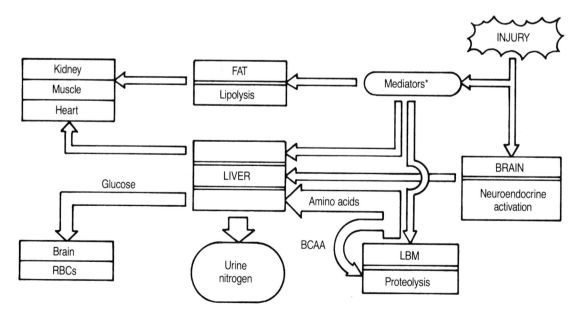

Figure 7.4 Hypercatabolic state.* Interleukin I, prostaglandins, kinins, superoxide radicals, leukotrienes, pain. **LBM,** Lean body mass. **BCAA,** branched-chain amino acids.

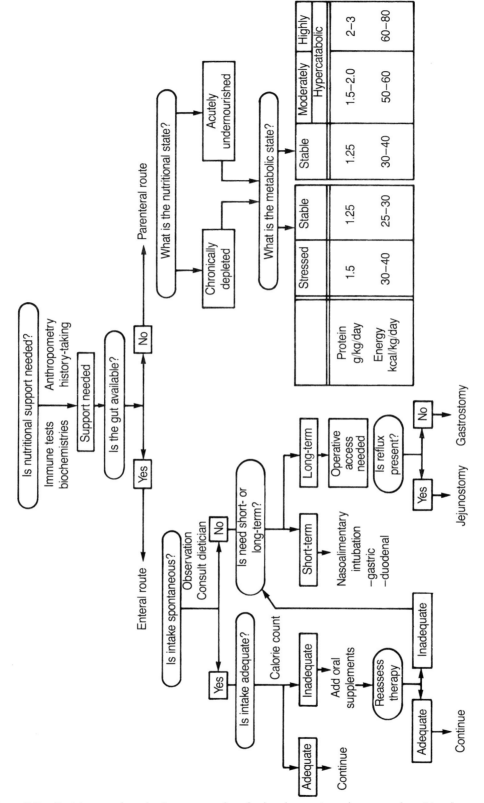

Figure 7.5. Decision-tree for selecting route and method and on estimated amount of nutritional support.

poses (for example, relief of obstruction, hydration) with the possibility of also using it for feeding; (3) preliminary: an enterostomy performed to feed the patient preoperatively before a larger major procedure; (4) adjunctive: a feeding enterostomy inserted at the time of another primary procedure for the purpose of postoperative nutritional support; and (5) supplementary: a feeding enterostomy placed in response to postoperative complications.

Implementation and Administration of Enteral Feeding Program

Orders for an enteral diet should include the name of the preparation, the strength or caloric density to be administered, the rate of administration, and any special additives to be included in the feeding formula. Order of a defined-formula diet requires selecting from a multitude of products now available. There is no single, best defined-formula diet. One must consider nutritional requirements of the patient, fluid and electrolyte needs and tolerances, tolerance of the dietary substrate, and the functional status of the gastrointestinal tract. In general, enteral feedings are started slowly with only gradual, independent daily increments in volume or caloric density until the desired intake is achieved. The formulas are best tolerated when administered continually around the clock. An overly aggressive approach to initial feeding, too rapid advancement of the diet, or simultaneous increases in caloric density and volume usually result in gastrointestinal overload, diarrhea, and poor tolerance of the enteral regimen.

For intragastric feeding, enteral formulas may be initiated at a caloric density of 1 kcal/ml with both isotonic and hyperosmolar diets. Initially, the feedings are delivered continuously at 50 ml/hr. The rate of feeding is increased daily in increments of 25–50 ml/hr until the desired or tolerated level of feeding is reached. Gastric residual should be determined periodically and feeding rate decreased if delayed gastric emptying is signaled by a residual >100 cc. Patients being fed intragastrically should be positioned with the head of the bed elevated 30° and encouraged to ambulate frequently to minimize the risk of aspiration.

Intrajejunal feeding generally utilizes continuous administration, as well. Feeding is initiated at a range of 25–50 ml/hr, using an isotonic dilution of the defined-formula diet. Feeding is advanced each day at a rate of 25–50 ml/hr until fluid and electrolyte requirements are met. The caloric density can then be independently advanced each day at a rate of 0.2–0.5 kcal/ml. Too rapid infusion of the diet or an excessive caloric density can result in abdominal distension, weakness, sweating, hyperperistalsis, cramps, and diarrhea. The diarrhea can result from several factors: osmotic overload, rapid transit through the small bowel, or incomplete absorption. Because the jejunum lacks the intact stomach's capacity to serve as a reservoir while tonicity is adjusted, there is considerably less flexibility with jejunal as opposed to intragastric feeding.

The use of mechanical pumps greatly facilitates continuous enteral feeding. Their use helps to assure even administration of the viscous formulas and prevents clogging of the tubes. There are a number of effective, efficient pumps and rate controllers commercially available.

Complications of Enteral Feeding

The possible complications of enteral therapy are listed in Table 7.3. Patient interview and examination are the most critical aspects in determining gastrointestinal tolerance of a defined–formula diet. Gastrointestinal overload may be signaled by symptoms of fullness, bloating, crampy abdominal pain, and nausea. Hyperactive bowel sounds and abdominal distension may be noted. Vomiting may follow, particularly with intragastric feeding. Significant diarrhea may also occur. Gastrointestinal side effects occur in 10–20% of tube-fed patients. Signs and symptoms of gastrointestinal intolerance should be managed by reduction of both the volume and caloric density until the patient becomes asymptomatic. Alternatively, feedings may be interrupted transiently if symptoms are severe or if gastric residual is high. Antidiarrheal medications such as paregoric or dilute tincture of opium may be added directly to the feeding in refractory cases; however, obstipation and distension may follow use of these agents.

Mechanical problems are largely related to tube size. The use of fine-bore, flexible tubes is recommended. Metabolic complications are similar to those seen with parenteral nutrition and are listed in Table 7.6.

Parenteral Nutrition

When the gastrointestinal tract is not available for use in the provision of nutritional support, the parenteral route must be used. Common indications for parenteral nutritional support are given in Table 7.4. Because of the hypertonicity of most intravenous preparations, central venous access usually is required. Delivery of the hypertonic solution into a large diameter, high-flow vein helps to avoid the phlebitis that always occurs with delivery through a peripheral vein. The most commonly used technique of central venous access is percutaneous cannulation of the subclavian vein; when the subclavian vein is unavailable because of thrombosis or if it cannot be cannulated because of local anatomical variants, the internal jugular vein may be used. With either technique, the tip of the catheter must lie in the superior vena cava before any hypertonic solution is administered. These catheters must be placed using a rigidly aseptic technique, and a chest x-ray should be obtained immediately after placement to be certain that there is no pneumothorax or hemothorax and that the catheter tip is properly positioned.

Placement of the catheter under rigidly sterile conditions and a program of regular catheter care will prevent most infectious complications. The catheter entry

Table 7.3.
Complications of Enteral Therapy

Mechanical
1. Pulmonary aspiration
2. Esophageal reflux
3. Depressed cough
4. Parotitis
5. Otitis media
6. Esophageal erosions
7. Tube obstruction
8. Inadvertent airway administration

Gastrointestinal
1. Diarrhea
2. Malabsorption
3. Abdominal cramping
4. Exacerbation of gastrointestinal disease
5. Nausea and vomiting
6. Distension

Metabolic
1. Prerenal azotemia
2. Fluid and electrolyte abnormalities
3. Hyperglycemia
4. Hyperosmolar dehydration or nonketotic coma
5. Inadvertent intravenous administration
6. Essential fatty acid deficiency

site is always covered by a sterile occlusive dressing. The dressing should be changed by trained personnel at least three times per week. The catheter should be used only for the delivery of nutrient solutions. Blood should not be withdrawn from or administered through the catheter. Medications and supplemental intravenous infusions should not be given through the catheter, because they may serve as portals for infections. Dual-lumen and triple-lumen catheters are now available (Broviac and Hickman catheters). One lumen is used exclusively for nutrition while the other can be used for drugs, specimen withdrawal, etc. However, reliable data regarding the infection rates with multiple-lumen catheters are not yet available. The tubing used for parenteral nutrition should be changed daily. The ideal system consists of a single-solution bottle connected to a drip chamber and intravenous tubing, which in turn connects directly to the catheter. Infusion pumps keep the solutions running at a steady rate and prevent accidental rapid infusion of large amounts of hypertonic fluid. Volumetric infusion pumps with an occlusion alarm, an infusion-complete alarm, and an air-in-line detector are commonly used.

Parenteral caloric requirements are most often met by the administration of dextrose as a 20–35% solution, with tonicity ranging from 1000–1500 mOsm/liter. In addition to a source of calories, parenteral nutritional programs require the administration of nitrogen in the form of pure L-amino acid solutions. Synthetic amino acid sources, as compared with natural proteins, are generally enriched in essential amino acids, as well as alanine, arginine, histidine, and proline. Concentrations range from 2.75 to 4.25% as a rule. Special formulas are available containing only essential amino acids for use in renal failure or an increased content of

BCAA with restricted amounts of aromatic amino acids and methionine, which is probably useful in hepatic failure. In addition, solutions with an enhanced content of BCAA (up to 45% of protein as BCAA) are available for use in the management of hypercatabolic states. Efficacy of these preparations is limited to the period of hypercatabolism. Following resolution of the latter, standard amino acid preparations are appropriate. A typical standard solution contains 25% dextrose and 4.25% amino acids, supplying 2700 nonnitrogen calories and 18.75 g of nitrogen when 3 liters/day are administered.

Electrolytes, vitamins, and trace elements are prescribed as well. Vitamin requirements are listed in Table 7.2. The quantities required to maintain normal serum levels vary considerably. Serum levels should be monitored frequently, particularly in the face of extraordinary losses. Hypokalemia commonly occurs after initiation of parenteral nutritional support. Utilization of glucose is associated with intracellular transport of potassium. Administration of carbohydrate and protein may result in a profound lowering of serum potassium levels if insufficient potassium is administered. However, potassium requirements may also be profoundly affected by the presence of coexistent problems such as enteral potassium losses or renal failure. Hypophosphatemia can also develop because of intracellular shifts of phosphorus. All parenteral nutrition solutions should contain phosphorus in amounts of 10–20 mM. Most preparations also contain significant amounts of acetate (40–60 mEq/liter). The initial amino acid solutions used often produced hyperchloremic metabolic acidosis because excess chloride was bound to some amino acids that, when metabolized, liberated chloride ion. The current amino acid prepa-

Table 7.4.
Indications for Parenteral Nutritional Support

Gut unavailable
1. Prolonged paralytic ileus
2. Short bowel syndrome
3. Entercutaneous and enteroenteral fistulas
4. Necrotizing enterocolitis
5. Malabsorption syndromes
6. Esophageal benign stricture or malignancy

Inadequate oral intake or "bowel rest" indicated
1. Acute pancreatitis, hemorrhagic
2. Catabolic states: burns, sepsis, polytrauma
3. Extreme prematurity
4. Tracheoesophageal fistula (infants; until gastrostomy performed)
5. Hyperemesis gravidarum
6. Intractable diarrhea
7. Wound dehiscence and evisceration

Adjunctive to other therapy
1. Cancer chemotherapy
2. Cancer radiotherapy
3. Inflammatory bowel disease
4. Acute hepatitis and hepatic failure
5. Perioperative nutritional repletion

rations substitute acetate for chloride to prevent this development. The usual desired concentrations of electrolytes for TPN are Na^+ 40–50 mEq/liter; K^+ 40 mEq/liter; Cl^- 50 mEq/liter; Mg^{2+} 4–6 mEq/liter; Ca^{2+} 2.5–5 mEq/liter; HPO_4^- 20–25 mmol/liter; acetate 40–60 mEq/liter.

In recent years it has become increasingly apparent that several trace elements are essential for humans and should be included in any complete parenteral formula. Zinc plays a key metabolic role as a component of numerous metalloenzymes, such as carbonic anhydrase, alcohol dehydrogenase, and alkaline phosphatase. Clinically, zinc is required for normal wound healing, normal immunological function, taste and smell perception, and dark adaptation. In patients maintained on TPN without zinc supplements, serial determination of zinc levels will usually show progressive decreases. About 60% of the total body zinc content is located within muscle. Therefore, conditions associated with muscle catabolism are associated with marked release of zinc and subsequent increased excretion in the urine. Zinc deficiency can also develop whenever there are prolonged enteral losses of gastrointestinal secretions. Acute zinc deficiency is manifested by diarrhea, central nervous system disturbances (including confusion and lethargy), eczematoid dermatitis, alopecia, and acute growth arrest in children. In the stable adult on TPN, the daily intravenous zinc replacement should be 2.5–4 mg/day. This should be increased by an additional 2 mg/day in the acutely catabolic patient. In adults with intestinal losses, additional zinc should be provided (12 mg/liter small bowel fluid lost; 17 mg/kg stool or ileostomy output).

Copper is a component of several important enzyme systems, such as lysoxidase (involved in maturation of collagen and elastin), ceruloplasmin (involved in iron metabolism), and tyrosinase (involved in melanin synthesis). Acquired copper deficiency can be associated with anemia, leukopenia, and bone demineralization. Copper supplementation usually amounts to 0.5–1.5 mg/day. Copper replacement should be discontinued in the presence of biliary obstruction, as the major route of copper excretion is in the bile.

Chromium is necessary in trace amounts because it acts as a cofactor for insulin. Chromium enhances the initial reaction of insulin with its receptor in insulin-sensitive tissues. Chromium deficiency in the setting of prolonged parenteral nutrition without chromium supplementation can cause weight loss, glucose intolerance, and a peripheral sensory neuropathy. Selenium is an essential trace element for many animal species and is now felt to be required for humans. It has been shown to be part of the enzyme glutathione peroxidase in human red blood cells; this enzyme protects against damage from peroxides of polyunsaturated fats. Occasional case reports of selenium deficiency have appeared; the manifestations include skeletal myopathy and/or cardiomyopathy. Selenium supplementation while on total parenteral nutrition generally is in the range of 30–100 mg/day. Selenium excess can produce central nervous system dysfunc-

tion, so serum selenium levels should be monitored when supplementation is given.

As mentioned previously, parenteral nutritional support utilizing hypertonic dextrose as a calorie source must be administered through a central venous catheter maintained according to a rigid aseptic protocol. Once such a catheter has been properly positioned, the infusion is started slowly, usually at a rate of 40–50 ml/hr. Glucose tolerance is assessed by following the patient's urinary and blood sugars. If there is no evidence of glucose intolerance, the infusion is increased at the rate of an additional liter per day until the desired level is reached. Infusion rates are kept constant through the use of an infusion pump. The patient's weight is followed daily, and urine sugars and serum electrolytes, including calcium, phosphorus, and magnesium, are closely monitored.

Parenteral Nutrition with Lipid Emulsion, Dextrose, and Amino Acids

An alternate regimen for TPN utilizes lipid as a prime, or occasionally a supplementary, calorie source. All of the lipid preparations are 10% or 20% emulsions of either soybean oil or safflower oil. These oils are mixtures of triglycerides containing predominantly long-chain fatty acids, especially linoleic acid, which is essential to humans. The solutions are relatively isotonic and contain emulsified fat particles approximating the size of a chylomicron (0.5 μm).

In general, the fat emulsion should comprise no more than 60% of the total calorie input. It is generally recommended that fat intake not exceed 2.5 gm/kg/day in adults and 4 gm/kg/day in infants and children, assuming clearance capacity is normal. The remaining calories are supplied by a 10–20% solution of dextrose, primarily to meet the requirements of the central nervous system. Fat emulsions may be infused through a peripheral vein without the rapid development of venous thrombosis, because they are relatively isotonic. To achieve positive nitrogen balance, amino acids also must be supplied, usually as a 4.25% solution. It is common practice not to mix emulsions with other nu-

Table 7.5.
Complications of Central Venous Catheterization

Upon Insertion	During Maintenance
Pneumothorax	Infection or sepsis
Tension pneumothorax	Central vein thrombosis
Subcutaneous emphysema	Thromboembolism
Subclavian or carotid artery injury	Hydrothorax
Subclavian hematoma	Hydromediastinum
Hemothorax	Cardiac tamponade
Caval or cardiac perforation	Endocarditis
Thoracic duct injury	Arteriovenous fistula
Brachial plexus injury	Air embolus
Horner's syndrome	
Phrenic nerve injury	
Improper position	

trient solutions but to administer them through a separate access site or with a Y connector near the point of entry. Containers suitable for admixture with the fat emulsion are becoming available.

The use of fat emulsions has the potential advantage of permitting nutritional support through a peripheral vein. Fat emulsions also prevent the development of essential fatty acid deficiency states and may be helpful in the patient who exhibits glucose intolerance. Because metabolism of fat is associated with a lower RQ than is the metabolism of carbohydrate, the use of fat emulsions in the provision of calories may help wean patients from ventilatory support.

Complications of Parenteral Nutritional Support

The complications of central venous catheterization are listed in Table 7.5. The most common complications are technical (secondary to insertion), central venous thrombosis, and catheter sepsis. Infusion of a hyperosmolar solution should never be started until chest x-ray confirms correct positioning of the central venous catheter in the superior vena cava and rules out complications secondary to insertion. The overall complication rate of subclavian venous cannulation varies between 3% and 10%, with experience being the major variable. The internal jugular vein can be used as an alternate site for long-term central venous cannulation. Many feel that fewer technical complications occur with internal jugular venous cannulation; however, it is more difficult to stabilize and secure this line.

Thrombosis of the central venous system has been reported occasionally secondary to long-term indwelling catheters. Endothelial damage at the time of catheter insertion may serve as a nidus for thrombus formation; alternatively, progressive aggregation of fibrin or platelets on the catheter may be responsible. This is usually a fairly acute event. The patient develops cyanosis and edema of the head, both upper extremities, and upper chest. This is frequently associated with lethargy. Treatment consists of removal of the catheter and anticoagulation, unless contraindicated by other patient problems.

Sepsis is one of the most serious complications of nutritional support using a central venous catheter. Solution contamination is rare. Catheter sepsis, defined as positive blood cultures along with microbial growth from the cultured catheter sheath, is a much more common problem. When a rigid aseptic protocol is followed for catheter maintenance, this rate is 3–5%. Therefore the infusion line is used only for parenteral nutrition, dressings are changed regularly, and skin care is provided at the entry site. The appearance of fever during TPN is an urgent problem, because of the possibility of catheter sepsis. A thorough workup for the source of fever should be performed expeditiously. If no explanation for the fever can be found, the catheter should be considered suspect, removed, and cultured. Catheter-related sepsis usually resolves within 24–48 hours after removal of the catheter, and antibiotic therapy often is not necessary.

The metabolic complications of TPN and their treatment are detailed in Table 7.6.

Frontiers and Controversies

The multiplicity of pathophysiologic states, especially when occurring against a background of chronic organ insufficiency, has stimulated the formulation of nutrient mixtures tailored to specific circumstances. Among these are BCAA-enhanced solutions recommended for use in patients with sepsis, hypercatabolism, or hepatic encephalopathy. The reasons BCAA are useful were explained earlier. Typically, enhancement is such that branched chains comprise up to 45% of all amino acids delivered. However, this amount, as well as the ratios between the three BCAA (usually favoring leucine), have not been fully worked out. The mixtures are safe, can achieve positive protein balance, and appear to stimulate protein synthesis. Use is felt to be optimal early in the acute-stress response but to have no clear advantage during the recovery phase. In acute hepatic encaphalopathy the mixtures are enriched in BCAA but also restricted in aromatic amino acid and methionine content. It has been suggested that the latter formulation reduces the degree of hepatic encaphalopathy in some patients. Whether survival is improved remains unclear.

The treatment of chronic renal failure patients with low-protein diets containing a high percentage of essential amino acids and adequate calories seems to reduce uremic symptoms, stabilize blood urea nitrogen, and increase lean body mass. In acute renal failure, histidine becomes an essential amino acid and must be added. Thus the intravenous solution for use in renal failure contains 5.4% essential L-amino acids in 70% dextrose. It is unclear whether this system has advantages over standard nutritional support during acute renal failure.

Because malnutrition increases operative morbidity and mortality, it has been reasoned that preoperative nutritional therapy should be helpful in elective surgery. The few controlled clinical trials available indicate that only prolonged (7- to 10-day) therapy in the most depleted patients combined with postoperative support reduces complications and mortality. Brief courses of therapy have no objective benefit.

Nutritional deficiencies are frequent consequences of inflammatory bowel disease. Largely retrospective studies suggest that parenteral nutrition can correct nutritional depletion in both ulcerative colitis and Crohn's disease. It is not at all certain, however, that such support is successful primary therapy or that nutritional support and bowel rest induce or prolong remissions to a greater degree than standard therapy or the natural course of disease.

Nutritional support has become, for the surgeon, an important therapeutic modality for managing many of our most complex patients. Many patients have acute or chronic nutritional problems prior to surgery, and

Table 7.6.
Metabolic Complications of Total Parenteral Nutrition and Their Treatment

Problems	Etiologies	Prevention and Treatment
Glucose Metabolism		
A. Hyperglycemia, glycosuria, osmotic diuresis, hyperosmolar nonketotic dehydration, and coma	Excessive total dose or rate of administration of glucose; inadequate insulin; glucocorticoids; sepsis with insulin resistance	Reduce or stop infusion rate; switch to lipid; add exogenous insulin; control infection (drainage, debridement, antibiotics); free-water resuscitation followed by electrolyte replacement; replace potassium
B. Ketoacidosis in diabetes mellitus	Inadequate endogenous insulin response; inadequate exogenous insulin therapy	Appropriately increase exogenous insulin; reduce glucose intake
C. Postinfusion (rebound) hypoglycemia	Persistently elevated islet cell production of insulin; decreased glycogen stores	Taper TPN slowly (over 24–48 hr); always infuse isotonic glucose for several hours after stopping hypertonic infusion
D. Respiratory failure; unable to wean from mechanical ventilatory support	Conversion of excessive glucose intake into CO_2, especially in patients with COPD	Reduce total glucose load or switch to lipid system (40% of total calories as fat emulsion)
Amino Acid Metabolism		
A. Hyperchloremic metabolic acidosis	Excessive chloride and monohydrochloride content of crystalline amino acid solutions	Administer Na^+ and K^+ as lactate or acetate salts
B. Serum amino acid imbalance	Nonphysiologic amino acid pattern of the nutrient infusion; differential amino acid uptake in various disorders	Essential amino acid only infusions (renal failure); branched-chain amino acid–enhanced/aromatic amino acid–depleted formulations (sepsis, hepatic failure)
C. Hyperammonemia (rare)	Arginine, ornithine, aspartic acid, and/or glutamic acid deficient formulations; primary hepatic disorder	BCAA-enhanced formulations in hepatic encephalopathy; reduce total amino acid intake
D. Prerenal azotemia	Excessive amino acid infusion; inadequate nonprotein calories	Reduce protein intake; evaluate other causes of prerenal azotemia; increase nonprotein calories-to-nitrogen ratio
Lipid Metabolism		
A. Hyperlipemia	Decreased triglyceride clearance; sepsis	Reduce rate of infusion or discontinue; reassess after bloodstream is cleared of fat
B. Essential fatty acid deficiency (of phospholipid, linoleic, and/or arachidonic acids); eczematous, desquamative dermatitis of body folds	Inadequate essential fatty acid administration; inadequate vitamin E administration	Administration of linoleic acid twice weekly as 500 ml of 10% lipid emulsion; cured by daily lipid emulsion infusion
Calcium and Phosphorus Metabolism		
A. Hypophosphatemia	Inadequate phosphorus administration	Monitor phosphorus levels, especially during repletion of malnourished patients, administer adequate phosphorus
1. Neuromuscular: weakness, tremor, convulsions, coma, hyporeflexia, death	Decreased CNS ATP; inhibition of muscle glycolytic pathways	
2. Hematologic: hemolytic anemia decreased oxygen release; decreased leukocyte function; decreased clot retraction and platelet survival	Decreased erythrocyte 2, 3-diphosphoglycerate; decreased cellular ATP; abnormal membrane lipids	
3. Cardiac: impaired myocardial contractility, congestive cardiomyopathy	Decreased ATP	
B. Hypocalcemia	Inadequate calcium administration; reciprocal response to phosphorus repletion without calcium; hypoalbuminemia	3–4 mEq/kg body weight in pediatric TPN; add to base solution as needed in adults
C. Hypercalcemia	Excessive calcium administration with or without high doses of albumin; excessive vitamin D administration	Withdraw calcium from future infusions; rehydration; mithramycin, corticosteroids
Miscellaneous		
A. Hypokalemia	Inadequate potassium intake relative to increased requirements for protein anabolism	Supplementary potassium added to infusion at time of preparation
B. Hypomagnesemia	Inadequate magnesium intake for increased protein and carbohydrate metabolism	Supplementary magnesium added to infusions at the time of preparation

Table 7.6.
Metabolic Complications of Total Parenteral Nutrition and Their Treatment *(cont'd)*

Problems	Etiologies	Prevention and Treatment
C. Anemia	Iron deficiency; folate deficiency; B_{12} deficiency; copper deficiency	Trace elements and multivitamin complex should be routinely included in TPN infusions; correct deficiencies when identified
D. Bleeding	Vitamin K deficiency	Weekly administration of 10 mg vitamin K; correct deficiency with parenteral vitamin K
E. Liver function test abnormalities (elevated SGOT, SGPT, alkaline phosphatase, bilirubin)	Excessive glycogen and/or fat deposition in the liver; essential fatty acid deficiency; amino acid imbalances; toxic products of tryptophan metabolism	Reduce total caloric intake; substitute lipids for up to 40% of total caloric needs; alter continuous to cyclic TPN; withdraw TPN

the procedure itself may make the gastrointestinal tract less functional or nonfunctional. Therefore the roles of enteral and parenteral feeding must be understood by all surgeons, as well as the formulation of diets in patients with specific diseases and the complications that occur secondary to nutritional support.

SUGGESTED READINGS

AMA Department of Foods and Nutrition: Guidelines for essential trace element preparation for parenteral use. A statement by an expert panel. *JAMA* 241:2051–2054, 1979.
AMA Nutrition Advisory Group: Multivitamin preparations for parenteral use. *J Parent Ent Nutr* 3:258–262, 1979.
Blackburn GL, Bistrian BR, Maini BS, et al: Nutritional and metabolic assessment in the hospitalized patient. *J Parent Ent Nutr* 1:11–22. 1977.
Cerra FB: *Pocket Manual of Surgical Nutrition.* St. Louis, CV Mosby, 1984.
Cuthbertson DP: The metabolic response to injury and its nutritional implications: retrospect and perspective. *J Parent Ent Nutr* 3:108–129, 1979.
Dudrick SJ, Wilmore DW, Vars MM, Rhoads JE: Can intravenous feeding as the sole means of nutrition support growth in the child and restore weight loss in the adult? An affirmative answer. *Ann Surg* 169:974, 1969.
Freeman JB, Egan MC, Ellis BJ: The elemental diet. *Surg Gynecol Obstet* 143:112–116, 1976.
Freund M, Yashimura N, Lunetta L, Fischer JE: The role of the branched-chain amino acids in decreasing muscle catabolism in vivo. *Surgery* 83:611–618, 1978.
Imbembo AL, Walser M: Nutritional assessment. In *Nutritional Management.* Philadelphia, WB Saunders, 1984.
Mirtallo JM, Schneider PJ, Mavko K, et al: A comparison of essential and general amino acid infusions in the nutritional support of patients with compromised renal function. *J Parent Ent Nutr* 6:109–113, 1982.
Striebel JP, Holm E, Lutz W, Storz LW: Parenteral nutrition and coma therapy with amino acids in hepatic failure. *J Parent Ent Nutr* 3:240–246, 1979.

Skills

1. List at least one reference that would identify the minimal daily requirements for trace minerals and vitamins.
2. Write orders to start an elemental diet through an enteral tube.
3. Write orders to start total parenteral nutrition.
4. Describe, in detail, a technique for central venous pressure/TPN catheter placement.
5. Pass an enteral feeding tube.
6. Change a total parenteral nutrition dressing.
7. Calculate nitrogen balance in a patient with nutritional depletion.
8. For each of the following clinical conditions, list the preferred route and type of nutritional support, the number of calories per 24 hours to be given and the type of fluid to be used: Intestinal fistula, short bowel syndrome, sepsis with ileus, inflammatory bowel disease (Crohn's), carcinoma of the esophagus, 50% 3rd degree burn, and coma following head trauma.

Study Questions

1. Discuss the nutritional support of a 26-year-old woman with ulcerative colitis who is scheduled to undergo elective colectomy. How would you determine the need for preoperative support? postoperative support?
2. Calculate the nutritional needs of a 40-year-old 70-kg man who sustains a 60% burn in a hotel fire. What route of support, composition, and caloric level would you use?
3. Write nutrition orders and appropriate laboratory tests to follow the patient in question 2.
4. Write orders for a 70-kg man who needs long-term par-

enteral alimentation. How would you change these orders in a patient with renal failure? liver failure?

5. Discuss the complications of enteral therapy and the complications of parenteral nutritional therapy.

6. Discuss the micronutrient needs of a patient on long-term total parenteral nutrition.

8

Surgical Bleeding and Blood Replacement

Hollis W. Merrick, III, M.D.
Mary R. Smith, M.D.
Bruce V. MacFadyen, Jr., M.D.
Mitchell H. Goldman, M.D.

ASSUMPTIONS

The student understands the normal physiology of blood clotting, including the extrinsic and intrinsic pathways.

The student understands the role of thrombolysis in maintaining vascular integrity.

OBJECTIVES
1. Name five etiologic factors contributing to bleeding disorders.
2. Discuss medical history and physical findings that might identify the presence and etiology of a bleeding disorder.
3. List the minimum preoperative screening tests necessary when a patient is asymptomatic.
4. Name the appropriate test(s) helpful for diagnosis for each etiologic category named in objective 1.
5. Given an exsanguinating patient who has received a massive transfusion, identify the acute etiologic factors that might be responsible for the bleeding disorder.
6. Name the common surgical conditions leading to disseminated intravascular coagulation (DIC).
7. Outline both the definitive treatment of the underlying cause and the specific component replacement therapy required for each etiologic category named in objective 1.
8. Outline the process of obtaining and transfusing blood.

Although bleeding is an accepted occurrence in most surgical procedures, the volume of blood lost is usually not large enough to create a major problem. The surgeon, however, must anticipate blood losses that might be large and could have an adverse effect on the patient's recovery. In addition, there are operations that are invariably associated with large enough blood losses that the normal hemostatic process becomes impaired.

Some patients with congenital or acquired clotting disorders will require elective or emergency surgery. Under these circumstances, a knowledge of normal and impaired coagulation is necessary to properly manage the patient. Surgeons, therefore, must be prepared to manage blood loss in their patients, knowledgeable about the components of blood replacement, and familiar with problems related to the transfusion of blood products. It has been estimated that in the United States in 1986 approximately 4 million units of blood were transfused related to surgical procedures.

The Hemostatic Process

The hemostatic process involves an interaction between the blood vessel wall, the platelets, and coagulation pathways. After injury, hemostasis begins with a brief period of vasoconstriction by those vessels with muscular layers in their walls. This vasoconstriction in the region of injury controls blood loss only for a brief time and cannot offer significant control of bleeding.

The next step is mediated by platelets, which adhere to areas of vascular injury or exposed subendothelial structures (Fig. 8.1). The term *adhesion* refers to platelets sticking to structures other than platelets. Subsequent to adhesion, a process occurs during which platelets extrude their contents (the most important of which is adenosine diphosphate), which causes platelet aggregation. This platelet-to-platelet sticking results in the initial thrombus. The process from initial injury to the white (platelet) thrombus occurs independent of the coagulation pathways; hemophiliacs, for example, can generate a normal white thrombus. However, a more permanent thrombus is required for control of bleeding and eventual healing.

There are two coagulation pathways by which one can generate fibrin to stabilize the white thrombus. (Fig. 8.2). The extrinsic coagulation pathway begins with tissue thromboplastin, which interacts with factor

PLATELETS IN THE CONTROL OF BLEEDING

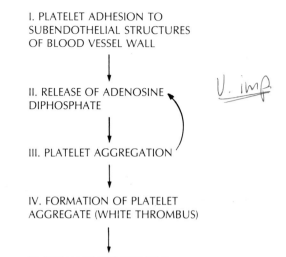

I. PLATELET ADHESION TO
SUBENDOTHELIAL STRUCTURES
OF BLOOD VESSEL WALL

↓

II. RELEASE OF ADENOSINE
DIPHOSPHATE

↓

III. PLATELET AGGREGATION

↓

IV. FORMATION OF PLATELET
AGGREGATE (WHITE THROMBUS)

↓

V. PERMANENT THROMBUS

Figure 8.1. Platelets in the control of bleeding.

VII to convert factor X to factor X^a and initiates the common pathway. The intrinsic pathway requires factors XII, XI, IX, and VIII to interact and eventually convert factor X to factor X^a. The common pathway involves factors X, V, II (prothrombin), and I (fibrinogen). The end product of coagulation is fibrin, which has a weak clot-stabilizing ability. Factor XIII (fibrin-stabilizing factor) is required to create fibrin of optimal strength (Fig. 8.2).

It is possible for bleeding to occur when a deficiency of any of the factors of the clotting pathways occurs, with the exception of factor XII. Additionally, although normal hemostasis requires calcium, hypocalcemia does not cause bleeding.

Evaluation of the Patient *(assessing bleeding risk)*

History. Obtaining a detailed bleeding history is one of the most important steps in evaluating patients with possible bleeding problems. Patients should be asked if they have had prolonged bleeding after dental extractions, minor cuts, or prior surgeries; prolonged or frequent menses; or if they have experienced bruising after minor injury. A history of "bleeders" in the family is important to obtain. For the individual patient, a history of bleeding problems is the most important preoperative information predictive of unexpected bleeding complications—even more reliable than laboratory tests.

Physical Examination. The physical examination is less helpful than the history in assessing bleeding risk. Most patients with mild-to-moderate bleeding disorders do not manifest physical signs. The examiner should seek signs of diseases such as leukemia, lymphoma, splenomegaly, hepatomegaly, hemarthroses, or liver disease that can be associated with bleeding disorders. Petechiae are said to be more typical of platelet disorders, whereas ecchymoses are more typical of abnormalities in the coagulation pathways.

Screening Tests. One should do screening tests in the presence of a history or physical examination suggestive of a bleeding disorder; also, if major bleeding

THE COAGULATION PATHWAYS

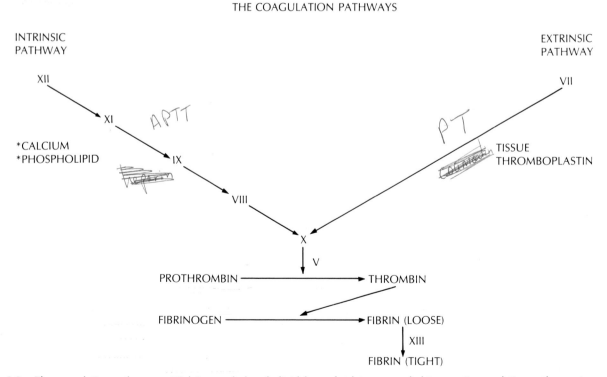

INTRINSIC PATHWAY

EXTRINSIC PATHWAY

XII

VII

XI

IX

*CALCIUM
*PHOSPHOLIPID

TISSUE THROMBOPLASTIN

VIII

X

V

PROTHROMBIN ⟶ THROMBIN

FIBRINOGEN ⟶ FIBRIN (LOOSE)

XIII

FIBRIN (TIGHT)

Figure 8.2. The coagulation pathways. *Calcium and phospholipid from platelets are needed to permit coagulation pathways to proceed at optimum rates.

is expected by the nature of the surgery planned, the patient's hemostatic capabilities should be assessed. In patients without a history of bleeding who are undergoing a major surgical procedure with an anticipated significant blood loss, a platelet count, prothrombin time (PT), and partial thromboplastin time (PTT) may be done routinely to rule out thrombocytopenia or the presence of an acquired anticoagulant.

Tests for Evaluation of Hemostasis

The bleeding time test is conducted by making two standard wounds (9 mm long, 1 mm deep) in the forearm of the patient using a spring-loaded lancet. The time from injury until bleeding stops from both wounds is then measured. A normal bleeding time requires adequate numbers and function of platelets and normal blood vessel walls. Two vascular disorders that can cause mild prolongation of the bleeding time are (1) senile ecchymoses due to aging skin and (2) long-term corticosteroid therapy.

The bleeding time may be prolonged by certain drugs (e.g., aspirin); a prolonged bleeding time often is associated with significant bleeding at surgery. An abnormal bleeding time without a patient history of drug use indicates a probable bleeding disorder.

A platelet count is done by automated methods in most institutions, but automated counters are not accurate at platelet counts below 40,000. Therefore, very low counts may need to be confirmed by manual methods. Review of the peripheral blood smear will allow one to assess whether adequate platelets are present and also to make a reasonable estimate of platelet numbers. Platelets may be present in adequate numbers and yet they may not function appropriately, as in von Willebrand's disease or with qualitative platelet defects (which require platelet transfusions).

The prothrombin time (PT) evaluates the extrinsic coagulation pathway and the common pathway; that is, it evaluates the adequacy of factors VII, X, and V, prothrombin, and fibrinogen levels (Fig. 8.3). Its most common use is monitoring oral anticoagulation by Coumadin.

The activated partial thromboplastin time (APTT) evaluates the adequacy of factors XII, XI, IX, VIII, X, V, prothrombin, and fibrinogen in the intrinsic and common pathways (Fig. 8.3). It is the most commonly used test for the monitoring of heparin therapy.

The thrombin time evaluates fibrinogen-to-fibrin conversion with an external source of thrombin. Prolongation of the thrombin time can be due to (1) low-fibrinogen levels (hypofibrinogenemia), (2) abnormal fibrinogen (dysfibrinogenemia), (3) fibrin split products, and (4) heparin (Fig. 8.3). It is used in evaluation of DIC and chronic liver disease.

Causes of Surgical Bleeding

Bleeding due to Preexisting Hemostatic Defects

Preexisting hemostatic defects can be most readily identified with an accurate history. When abnormal

TESTS OF THE COAGULATION PATHWAYS

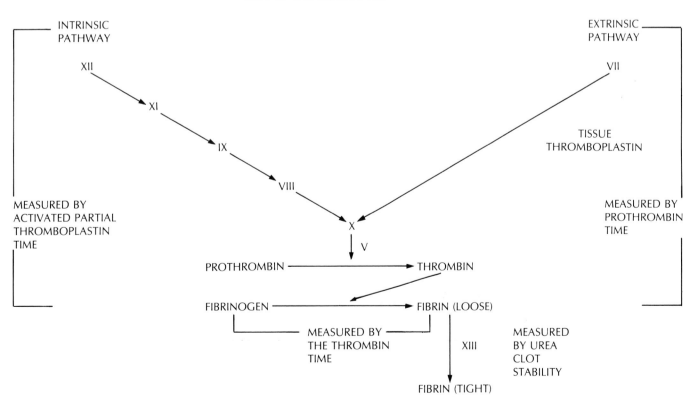

Figure 8.3. Tests of the coagulation pathways.

bleeding begins within the first 30 minutes of the operative period, a preexisting bleeding disorder should be suspected.

Congenital bleeding disorders are less common than acquired bleeding disorders. Patients may be asymptomatic even until they are quite advanced in years. Type A hemophilia and von Willebrand's disease are both characterized by deficiencies of factor VIII clotting activity (VIII_c). There are, however, differences in the two disease processes. Hemophilia is seen almost exclusively in males in whom platelet function is normal. Von Willebrand's disease affects both sexes. In addition to factor VIII_c deficiency (von Willebrand's factor), von Willebrand's disease is associated with platelet dysfunction, which is diagnosed by decreased aggregation in the ristocetin test and is corrected by pooled plasma; deficiency of factor VIII von Willebrand activity can be corrected with cryoprecipitate infusions.

Congenital platelet function disorders are uncommon and usually manifest a history of mucous membrane bleeding and easy bruising. Factor IX deficiency, Christmas disease, or hemophilia B is seen only in males and is less common than type A hemophilia. Factor XI deficiency is found almost exclusively in Jewish patients.

Acquired Bleeding Disorders

Acquired bleeding disorders are more common than congenital bleeding disorders. Liver disease is a common cause of coagulation abnormalities. Inability of the liver to synthesize proteins results in decreased prothrombin and factors V, VII, and X (but not VIII), which may cause a prolonged PT and PTT. Thrombocytopenia may occur acutely secondary to alcohol ingestion or be moderately depressed secondary to hypersplenism. However, gastrointestinal bleeding in the cirrhotic patient is usually due to varices or gastritis rather than a coagulation defect. Clotting factor deficiency secondary to obstructive jaundice can be corrected by parenteral vitamin K, whereas that secondary to hepatocellular damage (e.g., cirrhosis) does not respond as well to this form of therapy.

Anticoagulant therapy with heparin or oral anticoagulants (Coumadin) causes acquired bleeding disorders. Coumadin causes depression of clotting activity of four coagulation factors, II, VII, IX, and X. Therefore, since both the intrinsic and extrinsic pathways are affected by Coumadin, both the PT and APTT are prolonged. Heparin causes prolongation of the APTT and the thrombin time.

Acquired thrombocytopenia can be due to four mechanisms: (1) decreased platelet production in the bone marrow (aplastic anemia), (2) increased destruction of platelets in the peripheral blood [ITP (idiopathic thrombocytopenia purpura), DIC], (3) splenic pooling in an enlarged spleen (cirrhosis), and (4) any combination of these disorders (alcoholic liver failure).

Platelet function disorders are usually associated with drug therapy. Aspirin is the most common of the nonsteroidal anti-inflammatory drugs that induce platelet dysfunction. The difference between aspirin and all of the rest of the nonsteroidal anti-inflammatory drugs is that the defect aspirin induces is nonreversible. Patients should be asked not to take aspirin within one week prior to elective surgery. A second important cause of acquired dysfunctions is uremia. Patients who are uremic and are bleeding require dialysis prior to surgery to correct their platelet dysfunction.

Bleeding Associated with the Surgical Procedure

Most patients are hemostatically normal prior to entering the operating room. They have no bleeding history or evidence of bleeding by physical examination, and their coagulation screening tests are normal. However, in some patients with large blood losses, generalized oozing is noted after a period of time. In addition, there are some operations that are frequently associated with large blood losses: cardiopulmonary bypass, liver transplant surgery, prostate surgery, and portocaval shunts.

There are several common conditions that contribute to bleeding during a surgical procedure. Shock may cause or aggravate DIC. Extensive trauma may be associated with DIC. Massive transfusion of stored blood may lead to bleeding that occurs after rapid transfusion of 10 units or more of stored blood over a 4- to 6-hour period. The bleeding is due to low numbers of platelets and reduced levels of factors V and VIII in the transfused blood.

In acute hemolytic blood transfusion reaction in a patient under general anesthesia, there may be no clues that incompatible blood has been given until the onset of generalized bleeding due to DIC. The usual symptoms will not be manifested under general anesthesia. The occurrence of hemoglobinuria and oliguria are additional clinical evidence of DIC.

Bleeding in the Postoperative Period

Fifty percent of postoperative bleeding is due to inadequate hemostasis during surgery. Other causes of postoperative bleeding include the following:

1. Circulating heparin remaining after bypass surgery.
2. Shock, resulting in DIC.
3. Partial hepatectomy. If a large portion of the liver is removed, it may require 3–5 days before the remaining liver can increase its production of clotting factors enough to support hemostasis.
4. Acquired deficiency of the vitamin K–dependent clotting factors (II, VII, IX, and X). Such deficiency may develop in patients who are poorly nourished and receiving antibiotics.
5. Factor XIII deficiency. Bleeding occurs 3–5 days after surgery. The diagnosis of factor XIII deficiency is confirmed by performing a urea clot stability test.
6. DIC and fibrinolysis.

Bleeding Disorders due to Impaired Fibrinolysis

Fibrinolysis may be classified into two types. The first, primary fibrinolysis, is a disorder that occurs most commonly after fibrinolytic therapy with the drugs streptokinase or urokinase, which are used to lyse coronary artery or peripheral artery thromboses. Primary fibrinolysis may also be seen in conjunction with surgical procedures on the prostate gland, which is rich in urokinase. Primary fibrinolysis is also seen in cases of severe liver failure. Very rare disorders of inhibitors of the fibrinolytic pathway (such as congenital deficiencies of the a_2-antiplasmin) can also cause primary fibrinolysis. Treatment of these disorders is best accomplished by eliminating the precipitating drugs.

Secondary fibrinolysis is most frequently seen in response to disseminated intravascular coagulation. The coagulation pathway is activated, followed by activation of the fibrinolytic pathway. Manifestations of this in laboratory tests include hypofibrinogenemia and the presence of fibrin split products. As the disseminated intravascular coagulation is corrected, the secondary fibrinolysis resolves.

If primary fibrinolysis becomes severe, ε-amino caproic acid can be used for therapy. This drug needs to be used with caution, as it will block the fibrinolytic pathway and may predispose the patient to thrombotic events.

Disseminated Intravascular Coagulation (Consumptive Coagulopathy)

Disseminated intravascular coagulation is a disorder characterized by intravascular coagulation and thrombosis that is diffuse rather than localized at the site of injury. This results in systemic deposition of platelet-thrombin microemboli, which cause diffuse tissue injury. Some clotting factors may be consumed in sufficient amounts to lead to diffuse bleeding. DIC may appear as a very acute disorder or be clinically asymptomatic and chronic in nature.

The etiology of DIC may be any of the following: (1) release of tissue debris into the bloodstream after trauma or obstetrical catastrophes; (2) induction of intravascular aggregations of platelets due to activation of platelets by various materials, including ADP and thrombin, which may explain DIC occurring in patients with severe septicemia and immune complex disease; (3) extensive endothelial damage leading to denuding of the vascular wall and stimulating coagulation as well as platelet adhesion, which may be seen in patients with widespread burns or vasculitis; (4) hypotension leading to stasis, which prevents the normal circulating inhibitors of coagulation from reaching the sites of the microthrombi; (5) blockage of the reticuloendothelial system, which also aggravates disseminated intravascular coagulation; (6) after some types of operations involving the prostate, lung, or malignant tumors (prostate); (7) the aggravation of severe liver disease.

The diagnosis of DIC is established by detecting diminished levels of coagulation factors and platelets. The following laboratory tests may be useful in diagnosing DIC: (1) prolongation of the APTT, (2) prolongation of the PT, (3) hypofibrinogenemia, (4) thrombocytopenia, and (5) presence of fibrin/fibrogen split products. The presence of fibrin split products is secondary to the activation of the fibrolytic pathway in response to the activation of the clotting pathway.

The most important aspect of treatment of DIC is to remove the precipitating factors (e.g., treatment of septicemia). If the DIC has been severe, replacement of coagulation factors is required to correct a coagulation defect. Cryoprecipitate is the best method of replacing a profound fibrinogen deficit. Platelet transfusions may also be required. Fresh frozen plasma is useful to replace other deficits that are identified, but it must be used judiciously if volume overload is a potential problem. Rarely, it may be necessary to inhibit the coagulation pathway by using heparin or preventing platelet aggregation with drug therapy.

Blood Replacement Therapy

Whole blood is collected into plastic reservoir bags containing anticoagulant and can be stored at 4°C for up to 5 weeks. Whole blood contains many components into which it is often separated prior to use. It is preferable to administer only the specific component when it is found to be deficient. Whole blood may be separated into four major components: (1) plasma, (2) platelets, (3) white blood cells, and (4) red blood cells. Stored whole blood contains 450 ml of blood and 63 ml of anticoagulant solution. The mechanism of anticoagulation of blood is binding of plasma calcium, which prevents activation of the coagulation pathway. During storage at 4°C, platelets and leukocytes become nonfunctional within hours. There is also a gradual reduction in red cell viability related to the duration of the blood storage. Red blood cells stored for 5 weeks have a mean recovery of approximately 70%. Cellular metabolism during storage leads to progressive increases in plasma potassium and a rise in hydrogen ion concentration, thus resulting in a lowered pH. There is also a loss of coagulation factors V and VIII during storage. The level of factor VIII drops to 50% by 24 hours after collection. Factor V reaches 50% in 10–14 days.

Estimating Red Blood Cell Transfusion Needs

The following are calculations used to determine the number of units of red cell concentrate needed to raise the hematocrit of a 70-kg man from 15% to 40%.

A. Calculate the total blood volume:

Patient's weight: 70 kg
Blood volume = 7% of body weight
= 0.07% × 70 liters
= 4.9 liters

B. One unit of RBC concentrate contains approximately 200 ml of red blood cells. This will be distributed throughout the blood volume. (4.9 liters):

$$\frac{200}{4900} \times 100 = 4\%$$

C. To raise the hematocrit from 15% to 40% (i.e., 25%), we will need:

$$\frac{25}{4} = 6.25 \text{ or } 7 \text{ units of RBC concentrate}$$

Blood Component Therapy

The major indication for administration of fresh whole blood is replacement of massive blood losses. Otherwise, one should carefully consider the use of selected blood component therapy. Blood components that carry oxygen include (1) red cell concentrates, (2) leukocyte-poor blood, (3) frozen and thawed red blood cells, and (4) whole blood. Platelet-containing components include (1) platelet-rich plasma and (2) platelet concentrates. Platelet-rich plasma is obtained by gentle centrifugation of whole blood. This usually results in a suspension that is rich in platelets and has a volume of 200 ml. Platelet concentrate is obtained by recentrifugation of platelet-rich plasma. Platelet concentrates contain approximately 6×10^{10} platelets and can be stored for 3–5 days in plastic containers at 22°C. They should not be refrigerated.

Transfusion of Red Blood Cells

If transfusion of blood is expected during surgery or within 48 hours postoperatively, the patient should be typed and cross-matched preoperatively. If the probability of transfusion is low, it is usually sufficient to do a "type and screen", which means that the patient's ABO group and Rh type are determined and an antibody screen is carried out. Patients with a positive antibody screen must have blood cross-matched to minimize the risk of hemolytic transfusion reactions. With a type and screen, blood of the patient's group and type is determined to be in the blood bank but the blood has not been cross-matched for the patient. Many hospitals now allow appropriate patients to donate their own blood in advance of elective surgery for possible use during the procedure; this is the safest blood transfusion practice. It is usually possible for a healthy patient to bank 2–3 units preoperatively.

The transfusion of red blood cells is indicated when there is a decrease in the red cell mass such that oxygen transport and delivery to tissue are compromised. Generally the red cell mass should be maintained to provide a minimum hemoglobin level of 10 and hematocrit of 30 during the surgical period and immediately postoperatively. Blood group and type must be taken into consideration when red cell transfusions are given. The major blood groups are ABO and rhesus (Rh). There are numerous minor groups that generally do not complicate transfusions.

The universal donor red cells are O-negative red blood cells. The plasma from type O donors is not universal donor plasma. However, in all but the most life-threatening emergency states, at least type-specific blood, or blood that has been cross-matched, must be given.

Transfusion reactions occur with some frequency and the management depends on the type and severity of the reaction. If the patient has a febrile transfusion reaction, this can be controlled with antipyretics and antihistamines. However, if a major hemolytic transfusion reaction occurs, the blood being administered must be stopped immediately and the blood returned to the laboratory for cross-match. The subsequent management of this problem is outlined in the section on disseminated intravascular coagulation.

Plasma Component Therapy

Plasma products do not require cross-match prior to use but should be ABO compatible with the patient. Platelet-poor plasma may be fresh frozen plasma or it may be fractionated into cryoprecipitate and other plasma fractions. Fresh frozen plasma in a single plastic bag measuring 200 ml contains all the coagulation factors and can be stored up to 12 months at −30°C. Fresh frozen plasma can be used in a nonspecific manner to correct all clotting factor deficiencies. Cryoprecipitate measures 5–30 ml in a single plastic bag, is rich in factor VIII, fibrinogen, and fibronectin, and can be stored for 12 months at −30°C. Stored plasma, which is available from some blood banking centers, contains coagulation factors other than factors V and VIII and can be stored for 5 weeks at 4°C or 2 years at −30°C. Coagulation factor concentrates are also a part of plasma component therapy. The primary use of cryoprecipitate is in the treatment of hemophilia A and von Willebrand's disease. There is a small risk of hepatitis when cryoprecipitate is used. Factor VIII concentrates have the advantage of being storable at 4°C for short periods of time. There is, however, a high risk of hepatitis. Factor VIII concentrates can be used in the treatment of hemophilia A but not in the treatment of von Willebrand's disease.

Estimating Factor VIII Transfusion Requirements

One may assume that there are approximately 80 clotting units of factor VIII in each bag of cryoprecipitate and that there is a baseline factor VIII level of 3%.

In a 70-kg male the plasma volume = 4% of body weight (blood volume = 7%)

$$0.04\% \times 70 \text{ liters} = 2.8 \text{ liters}$$

A clotting unit of a coagulation factor is the amount of that factor (arbitrarily called 100%) in 1 ml of normal plasma. To raise the patient's level to 50%, we need

$$2800 \text{ ml} \times (0.50 - 0.03) = 1316 \text{ units}$$

One bag of cryoprecipitate contains 80 clotting units of factor VIII. The patient should receive

$$\frac{1316}{80} = 16.45 \text{ or } 17 \text{ bags of cryoprecipitate}$$

Recommended levels of factor VIII for management of hemophilia type A have been established for minor and major trauma. After minor trauma or during the healing period after surgery, 15–20% activity of factor VIII should be maintained. After major trauma, major surgery, or bleeding at a dangerous site (such as an intracranial bleed), 50–60% activity should be maintained. Factor VIII material (cryoprecipitate) will usually need to be transfused every 12 hours in the management of type A hemophiliacs to maintain the desired level of factor VIII.

Factor IX concentrates are used primarily for the treatment of factor IX-deficient hemophilia or factor VIII-deficient hemophiliacs with severe factor VIII inhibitors. Major side effects of factor IX concentrates include hepatitis and DIC.

Albumin is prepared from whole plasma by an ethanol fractionation method. There is no risk of transmitting hepatitis with albumin transfusion. The primary role of albumin is as an oncotic agent.

To make certain that blood transfusion products are as safe as possible, one must make every effort to avoid (1) immunologic transfusion reactions, (2) transmission of infections through bacteria or viruses (blood is routinely screened for hepatitis B virus and AIDS virus) and (3) fluid overload.

Immunologic transfusion reactions include hemolytic transfusion reactions, febrile transfusion reactions, posttransfusion thrombocytopenia, anaphylactic shock, urticaria, and graft versus host disease. Symptoms of immediate hemolytic transfusion reactions include fever, constrictive sensation in the chest, and pain in the lumbar region of the back. Signs include fever, hypotension, hemoglobinuria, bleeding (due to DIC), and renal failure. Acute hemolytic reactions occur when A and B alloantibodies in the patient's plasma bind to antigens on the transfused donor red blood cells.

If a hemolytic transfusion reaction is suspected, one should stop the transfusion immediately but leave the intravenous line in place. All the documentation and other clerical information should be checked to be sure that the patient is receiving a unit of blood that is correctly cross-matched. Blood samples should be taken from the patient to recheck the ABO blood group and Rh blood groups and also to check for free-plasma hemoglobin. One should then repeat the cross-match and Coombs test. The investigator should then retype all donor units of blood for this patient, culture the transfused blood to rule out bacterial infection, culture the patient's blood, investigate the patient for DIC secondary to microaggregates and immune complexes, and initiate close monitoring of renal function.

Treatment of acute hemolytic transfusion reaction initially involves management of hypotension with volume expanders such as Ringer's lactate and vasoactive drugs. Good renal function should be maintained with diuretic therapy such as furosemide or mannitol, bicarbonate should be given to alkalinize the urine, and any depleted coagulation factor or platelets should be replaced. Heparinization is rarely indicated, and dialysis is utilized only if acute renal failure develops.

Management of von Willebrand's Disease

Von Willebrand's disease is a complex coagulopathy characterized by prolongation of the bleeding time and by low levels of factor VIII, which lowers clotting activity (VIII_c). A slow rise in factor VIII clotting activity reaches its maximum 6–12 hours after infusion of factor VIII. However, all transfused factor VIII will be cleared from patient's circulation within 48 hours after transfusion. The bleeding time is often shortened after transfusion with factor VIII—containing material, but the interval of this shortening is difficult to predict and may be as short as 2–3 hours. One needs to individualize the transfusion support for patients with von Willebrand's disease. It may require transfusion with cryoprecipitate as frequently as every 2–3 hours or as infrequently as every 24 hours. Nonsteroidal anti-inflammatory agents should be avoided during therapy for von Willebrand's disease, as these will aggravate the coagulopathy.

Suggested Readings

Biggs R, Rizza CR: *Human Blood Coagulation, Hemostasis and Thrombosis.* Oxford, UK, Blackwell Scientific Publications, 1984.
Borzotta AP: Value of preoperative history as an indicator of hemostatic disorders. *Ann Surg* 200:648, 1984.
Bowie EJ, Owen CA Jr: The significance of abnormal preoperative hemostatic tests. *Prog Hemostasis Thromb* 5:179–209, 1980.
Colman RW, Hirsch, J, Marder UJ, Salzman EW (eds): *Hemostasis and Thrombosis.* Philadelphia, JB Lippincott, 1982.
Feinstein DI: Diagnosis and management of disseminated intravascular coagulation: the role of heparin therapy. *Blood* 60:284, 1982.
Murano G: A basic outline of blood coagulation. *Sem Thromb Hemostasis* 6(2):140–162, 1980.
Rapaport SI: Preoperative hemostatic evaluation. *Blood* 62:229, 1983.

Skills

1. Demonstrate the ability to perform a bleeding time
   A. in a normal patient:
   B. in a patient with prolonged bleeding time.

2. Demonstrate the ability to administer a unit of blood, fresh frozen plasma, and platelets.
   A. Define the specific procedural details of administering each type of blood component.
   B. Demonstrate the installation of and discuss the indications for the use of a blood filter.
   C. Demonstrate knowledge of the process of verification of the accuracy of the cross-match.
   D. Demonstrate the verification procedures of the component prior to administration.
   E. Demonstrate selection of proper intravenous tubing

and appropriate crystalloid preparations for administering packed red blood cells.

   F. Describe an infusion rate at which packed red blood cells may be safely administered.

3. Demonstrate methods of diagnosis of disseminated intravascular coagulation (DIC) and appropriate steps to establish cause.

4. Demonstrate proper interpretation of coagulation laboratory test results; e.g., abnormal PT, APTT, thrombin time, platelet count.

5. Demonstrate the ability to detect a transfusion reaction and take appropriate steps to establish cause and initiate treatment.

Study Questions

1. An 8-year-old male presents to the emergency department in an unconscious state, having been injured in a fall from a tree. He is wearing a "Medic Alert" bracelet that reads "Bleeder."
   A. What would be your initial workup for this child?
   B. What coagulation test(s) would you request?
   C. What would be the best coagulation therapy for this child? Describe how you would calculate an appropriate dose.

2. A 30-year-old female who is in labor is noted to have increased oozing from intravenous puncture sites. Her baby is also noted to be developing signs of fetal distress.
   A. What would be the most likely diagnosis?
   B. What tests would you do to attempt to confirm the diagnosis?
   C. What would be the most appropriate treatment for this patient?

3. A 78-year-old man is transferred to the SICU from the operating room after having had an abdominal aneurysm repaired. During surgery he received 16 units of stored blood and crystalloid. On arrival in the SICU he is noted to have oozing from the wound edges.
   A. What is the most likely diagnosis?
   B. What is the best test to confirm this diagnosis?
   C. What would the most appropriate therapy be?

4. A 3-year-old male infant is noted to have continued bleeding after circumcision.
   A. What is the most likely diagnosis.
   B. How would you confirm this diagnosis?
   C. How would you treat this baby?

5. You are asked to evaluate a 64-year-old man who has been in the SICU for six weeks. He has been on antibiotics and intravenous feeding the entire time. In the preceding five days his PT and PTT have risen slowly and are now two times the upper limits of normal.
   A. What is the differential diagnosis?
   B. What tests would you do to confirm your diagnosis?
   C. How would you treat this patient?

9

Shock

Kenneth W. Burchard, M.D.
Charles T. Cloutier, M.D.
Pardon R. Kenney, M.D.
Robert F. Wilson, M.D.

ASSUMPTIONS

The student knows cardiovascular physiology and understands the factors regulating blood pressure.

The student understands the principles of autoregulation and blood flow within critical organs.

The student understands the fluid compartments within the body and the composition of each.

The student understands normal sympathetic and parasympathetic nervous system anatomy and physiology.

> OBJECTIVES
> 1. Define shock.
> 2. List four categories of shock.
> 3. List at least three causes for each type on shock.
> 4. Contrast the effects of each category of shock on the heart, kidney, and brain.
> 5. List hemodynamic features (e.g., systemic vascular resistance, cardiac output), diagnostic tests, and physical findings that differentiate each type of shock.
> 6. Name and briefly describe the monitoring techniques that help in the diagnosis and management of shock.
> 7. Outline the general principles of fluid, pharmacologic, and surgical intervention for each category of shock.

Introduction

Broadly defined, shock is a condition where total body cellular metabolism is malfunctional, usually because of inadequate delivery of oxygen to meet cellular needs and occasionally because of inability of cells to utilize oxygen. When treated aggressively, this cellular metabolic dysfunction is reversible. When allowed to continue, shock results in cellular death, organ damage, or death of the patient.

Although commonly associated with hypotension, shock may be present without hypotension and may not be present with hypotension. Because most forms of shock represent inadequate oxygen delivery to tissues, it is useful for diagnostic and therapeutic reasons to consider the various etiologies of shock in terms of each condition's effect on oxygen delivery (Table 9.1). Therefore, for each of the four common etiologies of shock described here, particular attention is paid to the physiologic mechanisms that impair oxygen delivery or utilization and the therapeutic modalities used to enhance oxygen delivery.

Before each etiology of shock is discussed in detail, the reader should review the commonly measured and derived hemodynamic and oxygen delivery parameters that are presented in Table 9.1. Table 9.2 describes the common differences noted in these hemodynamic and oxygen delivery variables in the various forms of shock.

Hypovolemic Shock

Definition

Hypovolemic shock is present when marked reduction in oxygen delivery results from diminished cardiac output secondary to inadequate vascular volume. Hemorrhage is the most common cause of hypovolemic shock. Because surgeons are frequently involved in controlling massive bleeding, this is a problem seen frequently on a surgical service. However, a loss of plasma or other body fluids such as occurs in burns, peritonitis, protracted diarrhea, vomiting, and acute pancreatitis can also cause hypovolemic shock.

Because hemorrhagic shock has been studied more frequently than any other etiologies of hypovolemic shock, the following discussion addresses primarily hemorrhagic shock. The principles pertaining to hemorrhagic shock can generally be applied to other etiologies of hypovolemic shock.

Table 9.1.
Hemodynamic and Oxygen Delivery Variables

Item	Definition	Normal
CVP	Central venous pressure; CVP = RAP; in the absence of tricuspid valve disease, CVP = RVEDP	5–15 mm Hg
LAP	Left atrial pressure; in the absence of mitral valve disease, LAP = LVEDP	5–15 mm Hg
PCWP	Pulmonary capillary wedge pressure; PCWP = LAP, except sometimes with high PEEP levels	5–15 mm Hg
MAP	Mean arterial pressure, mm Hg; MAP = DP + $\frac{1}{3}$ (SP − DP)	80–90 mm Hg
CI	Cardiac index; CI = CO/m² BSA	2.5–3.5 l/min/m² BSA
SI	Stroke index; SI = SV/m² BSA	35–40 ml/beat/m² BSA
SVR	Systemic vascular resistance; $SVR = \frac{(MAP - CVP) \times 80}{CO}$	1000–1500 dyne-sec/cm⁵
PVR	Pulmonary vascular resistance; $PVP = \frac{(MPA - PCW) \times 80}{CO}$	100–400 dyne-sec/cm⁵
CaO₂	Arterial oxygen content (vol %); CaO₂ = 1.39 × Hgb SaO₂ + (PaO₂ × 0.0031)	20 vol %
Cv̄O₂	Mixed venous oxygen content (vol %); Cv̄O = 1.30 × Hgb × Sv̄O₂ + (Pv̄O₂ × 0.0031)	15 vol %
C(a−v̄)O₂	Arterial venous O₂ content difference; C(a−v̄)O₂ = CaO₂ − Cv̄O₂(vol %)	3.5–4.5 vol %
O₂D	O₂ delivery; O₂D = CO × CaO₂ × 10; 10 = factor to convent ml O₂/100 ml blood to ml O₂/liter blood	900–1200 ml/min
O₂C	O₂ consumption; O₂C = (CaO₂ − Cv̄O₂) × CO × 10	250 ml/min 130–160 ml/min/m²

BSA, body surface area (m²); CO, cardiac output; DP, diastolic pressure; LVEDP, left ventricular end-diastolic pressure; PaO₂, arterial PO₂ (mm Hg); Pv̄O₂, mixed venous PO₂; RAP, right atrial pressure; RVEDP, right ventricular end-diastolic pressure; SaO₂, arterial oxygen saturation (%); Sv̄O₂, mixed venous oxygen saturation; SP, systolic pressure.

Pathophysiology

In hemorrhagic shock, oxygen delivery to the tissues is diminished by two mechanisms: (1) diminished cardiac output or fluid flow secondary to decreased venous return and (2) diminished hemoglobin or oxygen carrying capability. The pathophysiological response to hemorrhage is related to not only the amount of intravascular fluid loss but also the rate at which the fluid

is lost (Table 9.3). In an attempt to preserve and maintain cellular perfusion, the body initiates homeostatic defense mechanisms at the hemodynamic and metabolic levels.

In response to hemorrhage, venous return to the heart is diminished. This results in decreased cardiac output and a drop in systemic arterial pressure. A low systemic arterial blood pressure stimulates sympathetic receptors in the arterial wall of the carotid sinus. These receptors send diminished afferent impulses to the central nervous system, resulting in increased activity of the sympathetic nervous system. Subsequent elaboration of norepinephrine produces constriction of arterioles and venules. Sympathetic stimulation of the adrenal medulla leads to epinephrine release. Tachycardia develops and myocardial contractility increases. Elevated catecholamines result in peripheral hyperglycemia and suppression of insulin release.

Acting simultaneously with the hemodynamic and sympathetic response is an outpouring of antidiuretic hormone, adrenal cortical hormone, and growth hormone. The renin-angiotensin axis is activated, producing increased amounts of aldosterone.

Blood flow to vital organs such as the heart and the brain must be maintained at all costs if the patient is to survive. To accomplish this, the cardiac output is redistributed, with decreased flow to the skin, abdominal contents, and skeletal muscles. The fall in renal blood flow is marked by redistribution of flow within the kidney, favoring the medulla, with resulting cortical ischemia.

At the metabolic level there is a shift from aerobic to anaerobic energy pathways, resulting in a rapid accumulation of lactic acid. Although this represents an attempt by the body to continue energy production, the rate at which energy is produced is much less efficient with anaerobic metabolism than with aerobic metabolism. Although this may help over the short term, it eventually leads to cell death. A further attempt at compensation by the organism is an increase in respiratory rate in an attempt to improve blood oxygenation as well as to promote filling in the right heart.

Almost immediately following hemorrhage, plasma shifts from the interstitial space into the intravascular space. This attempt to increase plasma volume is a hemeostatic defense mechanism that, if the red cell volume is not replaced, can contribute to the perfusion deficit at the cellular level.

Diagnosis

Despite technological advances in monitoring capabilities and the ability to perform sophisticated laboratory tests, shock remains a clinical diagnosis based on an assessment of tissue perfusion. No single laboratory or physiologic measurement is adequate to establish the diagnosis of shock. Laboratory tests for the most part are confirmatory and aid in the differential diagnosis. Although they may be useful in determining the adequacy of resuscitation, they should not be relied on to establish the diagnosis of shock. In the diagnosis of

Table 9.2.
Hemodynamic Parameters as Aids in Diagnosis

Condition	BP, mm Hg	P	PCWP, mm Hg	CI, liters/min/m²	SVR, dyn/sec/cm⁻⁵	O₂D, ml/mm	O₂C, ml/mm
Normal (N)	120/70	80	5–15	2.5–3.5	1000–1500	900–1200	200–300
Hypovolemia	↓	↑	↓	↓	↑	↓	↓
CHF	↑	↑	↑	↓	↑	↓	↓
Cardiogenic Shock	↓	↑	↑	↓↓	↑↑	↓↓	↓↓
Sepsis	↓	↑	↓ or N	↑	↓	↑	↑ or N
Neurogenic	↓	↑ or N	↓ or N	↑ or N	↓	↑ or N	N

BP, arterial blood pressure; P, pulse; PCWP, pulmonary capillary wedge pressure; CI, cardiac index; SVR, systemic vascular resistance; O₂D, oxygen delivery; O₂C, oxygen consumption.

shock, the various etiologies must be differentiated. Table 9.2 lists parameters useful in confirming the etiology of shock.

Classically, the blood pressure level has been used to diagnose shock. This parameter is not an accurate diagnostic index of shock and is often misleading. In the normal steady state, blood pressure merely reflects the balance between cardiac output and peripheral resistance. With a loss of intravascular volume, there ensues a reduction in cardiac output; if this loss is slow enough, compensatory hemeostatic mechanisms can increase peripheral vascular resistance without a resultant drop in blood pressure. For instance (Table 9.3), hypotension in a supine patient often requires a 30% blood volume loss. Therefore a significant reduction in cardiac output may occur without a significant drop in blood pressure. Patients with long-standing hypertension may reach the shock state with low-normal blood pressure.

In arriving at a diagnosis of hemorrhagic shock, the following factors should be considered singly or in combination: the general status of the patient; the magnitude and site of trauma, if present; pallor; skin temperature; level of consciousness; air hunger; cuff blood pressure; peripheral pulse rate; and the quality of the pulse as a reflection of intravascular volume. Classically, the patient in hemorrhagic shock is hypotensive, exhibits tachycardia and tachypnea, is oliguric, and has a look of anxiety. He appears tired and, de-

pending on the degree of shock, can be extremely restless or frankly comatose. The skin is pale and cool with decreased core temperature. There is a delay in capillary refill. Patients frequently have nausea and vomiting.

Laboratory Determinations

Ideally, a laboratory test for a patient in shock would be diagnostic, an accurate measure of the adequacy of cellular perfusion, and an indicator of the adequacy of resuscitation. Unfortunately, no such test is available. However, the following tests may provide valuable information for both diagnosis and therapy.

The first test is arterial blood gases. Arterial pH is considered normal in the range of 7.35–7.45. The PaCO₂ is considered normal in the range of 35–45 mm/ml. An arterial pH <7.35 associated with a normal or less than normal PaCO₂ establishes the diagnosis of metabolic acidosis. However, a pH in the normal range when associated with marked hyperventilation (PaCO₂ <30 mm/ml) should arouse suspicion of an associated metabolic acidosis. Hyperventilation of such a magnitude should result in an elevation of pH above the normal range. Therefore the presence of significant metabolic acidosis may not be immediately apparent unless a careful evaluation of the relationship to pH and PaCO₂ is undertaken.

The second test is serum electrolytes. Early in hem-

Table 9.3.
Hemodynamic Effects of Intravascular Volume Loss in Supine Subjects

Amount	Rate	BP	P	Mentation	Skin Vaso-constriction	Urine Output
10% or less	5 min	NL	NL	NL	NL	NL
10% or less	1 hr					
20%	5 min	↓	↑	NL	↑	↓
20%	1 hr	NL	↑	NL	NL	↓
30%	5 min	↓↓	↑↑	↓	↑↑	↓↓
30%	1 hr	↓	↑	↓	↑	↓
50%	5 min	↓↓↓	↑↑↑	↓↓	↑↑↑	↓↓↓
50%	1 hr	↓↓	↑↑	↓↓	↑↑	↓↓

NL, normal.

orrhagic shock, serum electrolytes are nearly always normal, but it is important to establish baseline values so that subsequent electrolyte abnormalities can be quickly identified and appropriately corrected. With acidosis, electrolytes reveal a drop in total CO_2 as a reflection of decreased bicarbonate buffer. This results in an increase in the anion gap [anion gap = serum sodium - (serum bicarbonate + serum chloride)] and when elevated (>12 mEq/liter) indicates the presence of an anion such as a lactate and ketoacids. Again, in hypovolemic states, elevated lactic acid would be the most likely etiology of an increased anion gap.

The third test is the serum lactic acid level. Although arterial lactic acid levels are perhaps more sensitive indicators of perfusion, this test may not be readily available in many clinical laboratories and therefore may not be practical in a rapidly changing resuscitation scenario.

Creatinine is useful as an evaluation of renal function, and clearance determinations are possible when coupled with urine volume and creatinine excretion. The hematocrit is a useful estimate of red cell mass. However, hematocrit may be close to normal early in hemorrhagic shock and may fall only after resuscitation and/or capillary refill. A subsequent drop in hematocrit is a more useful indication of how much hypoperfusion is secondary to hemorrhage.

Treatment

Because patients in hemorrhagic shock have impaired perfusion secondary to reduced volume, the principles of treatment are straightforward—restore volume and control hemorrhage. The patient in hemorrhagic shock has lost blood; there is no question that blood is needed as part of the resuscitative regimen. By replacing vascular volume and hemoglobin, oxygen delivery is improved both by the resultant increase in cardiac output and an increased oxygen carrying capacity. The question is, "What type of fluid does one use until blood is available?" The preferred solution should be readily available and similar to plasma in electrolyte composition. Ringer's lactate or normal saline is most frequently used. Restoration of circulating volume can be achieved by the infusion of 3 ml of balanced electrolyte solution for each milliliter of blood lost. There is no conclusive evidence that colloid solutions (albumin, plasma, protein fraction) improve the rate of resuscitation or eventual outcome. Fluids are infused through two large-bore intravenous lines. Additional measures include the administration of supplemental oxygen, pressure dressings to control obvious external blood loss, and a Foley catheter to monitor renal function. The establishment of urine output at approximately 50 cc/hr for the adult has proven to be a very sensitive indicator of the adequacy of resuscitation.

Obviously, after resuscitation, the most important therapeutic intervention is to arrest hemorrhage. This may be accomplished by the administration of drugs (e.g., vasopressin in esophageal varices hemorrhage),

surgery (e.g., repair of ruptured abdominal aneurysm), or through techniques of interventional radiology (e.g., embolization of pelvic arteries after pelvic fracture). The goal of resuscitation is to maintain adequate circulation and oxygen delivery to the tissues until definitive therapy arrests hemorrhage or interrupts the loss of fluid from the vascular tree in other etiologies of hypovolemic shock.

Early operative intervention to correct intra-abdominal or intrathoracic blood loss is desirable. Although some people have recommended the use of sodium bicarbonate and osmotic diuretics in the treatment of patients in hemorrhagic shock, there is no benefit to be gained from the use of these agents. Vasoconstrictors should be avoided. The use of Swan-Ganz catheters and arterial lines to monitor pulmonary artery pressure and systemic arterial pressure, respectively, although helpful in following the operative and postoperative course of these patients, in most instances is not required during the early resuscitative period. Central venous catheterization should be performed only for monitoring purposes and should not be considered a resuscitation line.

Septic Shock

Definition

Septic shock is shock that develops as a result of the systemic effects of infection, primarily with bacterial or fungal organisms. Septic shock is the second most common etiology of shock in surgical patients. As described below, the organ dysfunction that accompanies sepsis and septic shock can be particularly perplexing, especially because this organ dysfunction may occur in the face of what appears to be normal or supernormal oxygen delivery to the tissues. This has variously been attributed to inadequate oxygen delivery in the face of supernormal oxygen demand by the increased metabolism of septic cells or by metabolic derangement of cellular metabolism such that cells cannot utilize oxygen, even though normal or supernormal delivery is provided. Still, as with other etiologies of shock, management includes measures to provide increased oxygen delivery to the tissues.

Pathophysiology

Table 9.4 describes common hemodynamic and oxygen delivery parameters associated with increasing degrees of sepsis. While classically described for Gram-negative sepsis, septic shock may also be seen with Gram-positive and fungal organisms.

Early Septic Shock (Warm Shock). The typical patient in early septic shock, despite having a low systolic blood pressure, tends to have a relative normal pulse pressure and stroke volume with a normal or high cardiac output. Because these patients tend to be vasodilated and have a low systemic vascular resistance, the skin is usually warm (or even flushed) and dry. Vaso-

Table 9.4.
Typical Hemodynamic Changes with Increasing Sepsis

Stage Sepsis	Description	Arterial BP, mm Hg	HR	CI, liters/min/m²	CVP, mm Hg	PAP, mm Hg	PAWP mm Hg	SVR, dyn/sec/cm⁻⁵	PVR, dyn/sec/cm⁻⁵	O₂C, ml/min/m²
0	Normal	120/80	72	3.3	3.0	20/7	5.0	1200	70	145
I	Mild-mod sepsis	125/75	100	3.5	3.0	21/7	5.0	1000	80	165
II	Mod-severe sepsis	100/50	120	3.7	3.0	22/7	5.0	800	120	200
III	Early (warm) shock	78/40	130	4.0	3.0	25/8	5.0	600	160	95
IV	Late (cold) shock	70/50	130	1.8	5.0	30/10	5.0	1300	280	50

BP, blood pressure; HR, heart rate; CI, cardiac index; CVP, central venous pressure; PAP, pulmonary arterial pressure; PAWP, pulmonary arterial wedge pressure; SVR, systemic vascular resistance; PVR, pulmonary vascular resistance. O₂C, oxygen consumption.

dilation results in a ''relative'' hypovolemia. Tachycardia and tachypnea are generally quite marked, with a minute ventilation often twice normal. Left and right atrial filling pressures, pulmonary artery pressures, and pulmonary vascular resistance may be normal. Despite a normal or increased cardiac output and oxygen delivery, oxygen consumption may be less than normal. When such is the case, impaired oxygen extraction may be secondary to impairment of cellular metabolism by a wide variety of toxins or substances released by the septic process. Arterial blood gases usually reveal a moderate respiratory alkalosis, with relatively little change in bicarbonate. Lactate levels are usually normal or only mildly increased initially.

Late Septic Shock (Cold Shock). As septic shock progresses, there is an increasing tendency for the patient to have impaired organ function. The hypovolemia is compounded by an increasing capillary permeability (largely due to bradykinin) and increasing cell membrane dysfunction. Increased capillary permeability diminishes or abolishes the normal intravascular-extravascular oncotic pressure difference, which favors intravascular fluid retention. Impaired cell metabolism allows sodium, calcium, and water to enter the cytoplasm, depleting the functional extracellular fluid volume. Intracellular potassium leaves the cell, resulting in intracellular depletion and, as plasma ionized calcium levels may fall below 1.6 mEq/liter, myocardial function may become further impaired.

Cardiac index usually falls below normal, and this, together with the reduced cellular oxygen extraction, results in an oxygen consumption that is often less than normal. Lactate levels begin to rise rapidly and bicarbonate levels fall so that even with an increasing minute ventilation and very low PaCO₂ levels, the pH becomes increasingly acidotic. This results in increasing vasoconstriction and an increase in systemic vascular resistance, which may rise to normal levels or higher. The skin becomes cold, clammy, mottled, and cyanotic. In extreme cases the tips of fingers or ears may become necrotic. Pulmonary arterial pressures and pulmonary vascular resistance rise. Consequently the central venous pressure may be high despite relatively low pulmonary artery wedge pressures.

Organ function becomes increasingly impaired, and the patient may become increasingly lethargic and confused. However, some patients with Gram-negative sepsis stay surprisingly alert until just prior to death. With increasing activation of the proteolytic stress cascades, blood levels of coagulation factors, complement, antithrombin, prekallikrein, and fibronectin may fall.

If septic shock continues, the organs that acutely demonstrate dysfunction are the cardiovascular system, the lungs, the kidneys, and the brain. The cardiovascular changes have been described. The lungs demonstrate diminished ability to oxygenate the blood. Oliguria and depressed mental status are common accompaniments of severe sepsis.

Diagnosis

Temperature elevation is a common phenomenon in surgical patients. There are many etiologies of temperature elevation in surgical patients, and the diagnosis of severe sepsis, therefore, is not simply dependent on elevation in body temperature (in fact, severe sepsis may be associated with hypothermia) but is dependent more on the interpretation of several clinical parameters. Most septic shock is caused by Gram-negative enteric bacteria. It is uncommon below the age of 40 y, except in septic abortions and neonates. In older individuals, septic shock is most frequently associated with urinary tract infections, particularly after instrumentation of the urinary tract. Other frequent causes of sepsis include pneumonia, peritonitis, intra-abdominal abscess, intravenous catheter infection, wound infection, infected burn wounds, and opportunistic infections in patients undergoing immunosuppressive or antineoplastic therapy.

The onset of the sepsis is often heralded by a shaking chill and rapid rise in rectal temperature to 39°C (102.2°F), often within 24 hours of a surgical procedure. An early clue may be an abrupt increase in tachypnea and confusion. The blood pressure may rise as the sepsis begins but usually falls to < 80 mm Hg systolic as shock ensues. In early warm sepsis, the skin may appear flushed and will be warm and dry. There may be physical examination evidence suggesting localization of the septic process (e.g., findings consistent with pneumonia, peritonitis, pyelonephritis). In more severe sepsis, vasoconstriction will result in cold, cyanotic extremities. Hypotension may be more marked, and the patient may be frankly comatose.

Although the presence of severe sepsis is usually fairly obvious, we are seeing an increasing number of critically ill patients with severely impaired host defenses. These anergic patients often cannot develop the fever, leukocytosis, or localized inflammatory changes characteristic of sepsis. In such individuals the sepsis may be manifested primarily as a dysfunction of one or more of the following organs: lungs, heart, kidney, liver, central nervous system, and gastrointestinal tract. As stated previously, severe sepsis is associated with a malfunction of several organs, which has been termed *multisystem organ failure* (MSOF). The sequence of MSOF is variable but usually involves the lungs first, then gastric mucosa, kidneys, and liver. Therefore a significant change in the function of any of these organs in a patient considered at high risk for sepsis should alert the clinician to the possibility of underlying sepsis that, again, may be manifested without temperature elevation.

Laboratory Determinations

Typical laboratory findings include a leukocytosis with a marked shift to the left, respiratory alkalosis, and metabolic acidosis. Blood sugar is elevated secondary to increased levels of catecholamines, glucagon, and glucocorticoids. Arterial blood gases may reveal metabolic acidosis, low PaO_2, and usually a low $PaCO_2$. Creatinine and BUN may be elevated as a reflection of poor kidney function, and bilirubin and alkaline phosphatase may be elevated as a consequence of impaired liver function.

In at least half the patients with septic shock, repeated blood cultures will be negative. The etiology of septic shock and localization of the septic focus usually requires a careful review of epidemiologic, physical examination, and laboratory data, along with tests that may help rule in or rule out specific diagnoses (e.g., chest x-ray for pneumonia).

The platelet count commonly falls with sepsis, and blood levels of other coagulation factors may also be depressed, resulting in prolonged prothrombin and partial thromboplastin times.

Table 9.5.
Septic Shock Treatment

I. **Correct Primary Process**
   A. Antibiotics
   B. Drainage
II. **Resuscitation**
   A. Ventilatory support and O_2 as needed
   B. Fluids
   C. Inotropes
   D. Vasodilators or vasopressors

Treatment

The treatment of septic shock should be directed at eradicating or controlling the primary infectious process and resuscitation or restoration of adequate vital organ function (Table 9.5).

Controlling the Primary Process. Controlling the primary process depends on the etiology. Some diseases, such as pneumonia or pyelonephritis, are usually adequately treated with antibiotics. Other diseases, such as intra-abdominal abscess and empyema, require surgical drainage.

Antibiotics. Appropriate antibiotic therapy may increase the chances of survival 2- to 10-fold. If a preexisting infection has been diagnosed, it can generally be assumed that the organism(s) identified previously is involved. Utilizing the available sensitivity studies, the appropriate antibiotic(s) can be selected.

If information is not available from a prior Gram stain or culture, cultures of blood and all other possible sites of infection must be obtained immediately. The empiric antibiotics started will depend on the clinical situation and organisms most likely present.

Whenever possible, bactericidal antibiotics should be used. Once information is obtained about specific organisms, antibiotic therapy should be tailored. The overall goal should be to use the least number and narrowest spectrum of antibiotics appropriate for the organism(s) involved. The potential risk of each antibiotic should be recognized (e.g., renal failure with aminoglycosides) and appropriate steps taken to monitor and adjust the dosage (e.g., peak and trough levels for aminoglycosides).

Resuscitation

In contrast to hemorrhagic shock, in septic shock oxygen delivery may be impaired by both impaired lung function and impaired circulation. Therefore, resuscitation in sepsis will frequently require institution of mechanical ventilation and increased inspired oxygen concentration [sometimes with positive end-expiratory pressure (PEEP)] to provide 90% arterial saturation. The first step in restoring circulation in sepsis is to increase vascular volume. As a consequence of increased capillary permeability and the inability of oncotic forces to maintain fluid in the vascular tree, septic patients may require extremely large volumes of fluid to maintain vascular volume. With increased capillary permeability, the effectiveness of colloid solutions (albumin, dextran, hetastarch) has been questioned and, in general, crystalloid solutions are preferred for raising intravascular volume. One colloid—red cells—is large enough to stay in the intravascular compartment and, in addition, increases oxygen delivery by raising hemoglobin levels. In severe sepsis, hemoglobin levels should be kept at 12–14 g/dl. Because severe acidosis may impair cardiac function if the arterial pH is <7.1, bicarbonate may be required.

If the cardiac index is <3.0–3.5 liters/min/m² despite volume loading (an increase in central venous pressure or pulmonary capillary wedge pressure to 15–18 mm Hg), inotropic support may be necessary. Dopamine in doses of 5–15 μg/kg/min seems ideal for improving myocardial contractility and cardiac output in hypotensive vasodilated patients. If the blood pressure is relatively normal, the patient is vasoconstricted, and filling pressures are elevated, dobutamine may be preferable.

Severe vasoconstriction may impede cardiac function by increasing afterload. In such situations, a vasodilator, such as nitroprusside, added to volume replacement, may result in improved cardiac output. On the other hand, severe vasodilatation from sepsis may result in low mean arterial pressure despite large cardiac output. When such a low mean arterial pressure is considered dangerous (<50 mm Hg), the administration of low doses of norepinephrine (1–5 μg/min) may be useful to raise systemic vascular resistance and blood pressure.

Cardiogenic Shock

Definition

Cardiogenic shock is present when severe reduction in oxygen delivery is secondary to marked impairment of cardiac output (cardiac index <1.8 liters/min/m²), which is accompanied by elevated left ventricular end-diastolic volume. Simply stated, cardiogenic shock is lack of perfusion from pump failure. The final common pathway for patients in shock is similar. Cardiogenic shock is related to the inability of the myocardium to produce sufficient flow and/or pressure to maintain adequate tissue perfusion.

Etiology

The etiologies of cardiogenic shock are broadly categorized into four groups (Table 9.6): 1) ischemic heart disease, 2) valvular heart disease, 3) arrhythmias, and 4) trauma. In each case, only severe impairment of cardiac function will result in hypotension from reduced

Table 9.6.
Etiologies of Cardiogenic Shock

I. Ischemic Heart Disease
   A. Acute myocardial infarction, usually anteroseptal
   B. Ventricular septal defect rupture
   C. Papillary muscle rapture
   D. Ventricular aneurysm
II. Valvular Heart Disease
   A. Acute mitral or aortic insufficiency
   B. Severe aortic stenosis
III. Arrhythmias
   A. Supraventricular
   B. Ventricular
IV. Trauma
   A. Tension pneumothorax
   B. Pericardial tamponade, may include nontraumatic causes
   C. Cardiac contusion

cardiac index. Cardiogenic shock is a distinct clinical entity from congestive heart failure.

With diminished cardiac output of any etiology, the normal neuroendocrine response results in systemic vasoconstriction. This is true for both congestive heart failure and cardiogenic shock. In congestive heart failure, with mild-to-moderate reductions in cardiac output, this vasoconstriction produces a proportionally greater increase in systemic vascular resistance, usually resulting in increased arterial pressure. This usual elevation of arterial pressure in congestive heart failure (Table 9.2) distinguishes congestive heart failure as a diagnostic entity from cardiogenic shock, wherein the depression in cardiac output is of such a magnitude that even severe vasoconstriction cannot maintain a normal arterial pressure.

The severe impairment in cardiac output results in hypotension, tachycardia, tachypnea, severe vasoconstriction, oliguria, acidosis, and mental obtundation. If not reversed, such severe hypoperfusion and diminished oxygen delivery result rapidly in progressive organ failure and death.

Diagnosis

The first step in making the correct diagnosis of cardiogenic shock is to distinguish it from congestive heart failure. The maintenance of a normal or, more commonly, an increase in arterial pressure in congestive heart failure separates congestive heart failure as a diagnostic entity from cardiogenic shock. Cardiogenic shock is usually easily distinguished from septic shock and neurogenic shock. This is particularly true because hypotension in these circumstances is commonly associated with warm extremities, exemplifying diminished systemic vascular resistance rather than an increase (Table 9.2). More problematic is distinguishing cardiogenic shock from hypovolemic shock because, in both cases, there is hypotension associated with increased systemic vascular resistance. First of all, hypovolemic shock is a much more common entity than cardiogenic shock. Secondly, the marked depression in cardiac function seen in cardiogenic shock most often results from an acute, major insult to cardiac function (Table 9.6). These sudden, catastrophic events produce equally sudden changes in the clinical condition of the patient. Cardiogenic shock does not "brew" and develop as a subtle finding from such etiologies as excessive fluid administration by a physician or fluid ingestion by a patient. Cardiogenic shock is not present simply because a patient has a history of heart disease. The history, physical examination, and laboratory data obtained from a patient in cardiogenic shock should easily allow a clinician to distinguish cardiogenic shock from hypovolemic shock and to distinguish between the four broad categories of etiologies listed in Table 9.6.

The patient with antecedent ischemic heart disease or a history consistent with acute myocardial infarction would most likely fit into the ischemic heart disease category. A patient with a history of rheumatic heart disease or known mitral or aortic valve disease would be likely to fit into the valvular heart disease category. A patient with the history of trauma would most likely fit into the trauma etiologies, and a patient with any history of previous heart disease or severe metabolic diseases (e.g., metabolic acidosis, hyperkalemia, metabolic alkalosis) will be a candidate for arrhythmias.

In most cases physical examination will reveal tachycardia, tachypnea, severe vasoconstriction, and distended neck veins. Other signs of cardiac dysfunction include rales, wheezes, and an S3 gallop. A ruptured ventricular septal defect (VSD) or papillary muscle dysfunction will produce a loud holosystolic murmur. Valvular heart disease may produce physical findings consistent with severe mitral or aortic regurgitation or aortic stenosis. Tension pneumothorax will demonstrate absence of breath sounds in one chest associated with tracheal deviation to the opposite side. Pericardial tamponade will demonstrate muffled heart tones and pulsus paradoxus. Arrhythmias will be evident by alterations in the peripheral pulse, either by brady- or tachyarrhythmias.

Laboratory Determinations

Laboratory tests that confirm the presence of cardiogenic shock include elevated central venous pressure or pulmonary capillary wedge pressure (>18 mm Hg), severe reduction in cardiac index (<1.8 liters/min/m²), chest x-ray consistent with pulmonary edema, hypoxia, metabolic acidosis, and rising BUN and creatinine levels. Calculated pulmonary and systemic vascular resistance will be elevated. An ECG demonstrating an acute myocardial infarction and an elevation in myocardial enzymes will support the diagnosis of ischemic heart disease. An echocardiogram demonstrating valvular damage would support that etiology. A chest x-ray demonstrating a tension pneumothorax would confirm this etiology. An echocardiogram demonstrating pericardial fluid and an ECG demonstrating low voltage would support the diagnosis of pericardial tamponade. Cardiac contusion is very difficult to diagnose but may be supported by elevated myocardial enzyme serial ECG demonstrating arrhythmias, and a MUGA scan demonstrating a reduction in right ventricular ejection fraction. Arrhythmias are diagnosed by ECG.

Treatment

The first step in management is to make the correct diagnosis. Because the most common cause of hypotension is hypovolemia rather than cardiogenic shock, the decision not to administer fluid to a hypotensive patient should be supported by ample evidence that cardiogenic shock is present. This requires more than simply a history of heart disease. The diagnosis and management of cardiogenic shock requires invasive monitoring. Cardiogenic shock does not respond simply to reducing intravenous fluid administration. Aggressive support of the severely impaired heart is required.

Table 9.7.
Determinants of Myocardial Oxygen Consumption

I.   Heart Rate
II. Contractility
III. Wall Tension, Preload
IV. Afterload

The primary goal in the management of cardiogenic shock is the same as in all other forms of shock, i.e., improving oxygen delivery to tissues. Although oxygen delivery may be depressed by arterial hypoxia secondary to cardiogenic pulmonary edema, the main determinant of decreased oxygen delivery in cardiogenic shock is diminished cardiac output. Cardiac function should be improved without significantly increasing the metabolic demands of the heart itself. The determinants of myocardial oxygen consumption are 1) heart rate, 2) contractility, 3) preload, and 4) afterload (listed in Table 9.7). As described next, the pros and cons of each of the methods of managing cardiogenic shock relate primarily to the effects of management on myocardial oxygen consumption.

Cardiogenic shock cannot be managed appropriately without the measurement of right and left ventricular filling pressures, cardiac index, and arterial blood pressure and the ability to calculate oxygen delivery, oxygen consumption, and pulmonary and systemic vascular resistance. The pulmonary artery catheter, therefore, is mandatory.

The "Physio-Logic" of Cardiogenic Shock Management

The therapy of cardiogenic shock is broadly based on four methods: 1) increasing contractility, 2) altering preload and afterload, 3) mechanical support, and 4) arrhythmia control.

Increasing Contractility. Drugs that increase contractility (inotropic) improve the performance of cardiac muscle. The three drugs most commonly used to increase cardiac contractility are dobutamine, dopamine, and isoproterenol. All drugs that increase contractility increase myocardial oxygen consumption. This is based both on the increased heart rate (chronotropic effect) and the increase in oxygen consumption associated with increased contractility. In certain types of

Table 9.8.
Hemodynamic Effects of Inotropic Drugs and Vasodilators

	Hemodynamic Parameters			
	HR	Contractility	Preload	Afterload
Dopamine	↑↑	↑	↑	↑ or NC
Dobutamine	↑	↑↑	↓	NC or ↓
Isoproterenol	↑↑	↑↑	↓	↓
Nitroprusside	±	NC	↓	↓↓
Nitroglycerin	±	NC	↓↓	↓

cardiogenic shock, particularly ischemic heart disease, increasing oxygen consumption may aggravate the ischemic insult. The relative hemodynamic effects of the three inotropes are listed in Table 9.8. Of particular importance is the propensity of dopamine to increase preload as cardiac output improves, making it a less than optimal choice compared with dobutamine for cardiogenic states.

Reducing Preload and Afterload. In congestive heart failure, diuretic administration is a common therapy employed to reduce preload and increase cardiac output. However, in cardiogenic shock, the marked reduction in cardiac output results in such severe reduction in renal perfusion that diuretic therapy may be ineffective in promoting diuresis and reducing preload. Diuretics may be used as an adjuvant in the treatment of cardiogenic shock but not as a primary agent. Vasodilator therapy may improve cardiac output by reducing both preload and afterload. As cardiac output improves, heart rate usually falls. Because vasodilator therapy does not enhance contractility, the resultant reductions in heart rate, preload, and afterload all diminish myocardial oxygen consumption, a distinct advantage when dealing with the ischemic heart.

Coronary artery perfusion depends primarily on diastolic blood pressure; thus the provision of vasodilator therapy to a patient already hypotensive is somewhat problematic. To avoid aggravating hypotension, inotropic therapy may be begun initially to provide an increase in cardiac output and blood pressure at some cost to myocardial oxygen consumption. Subsequently vasodilator therapy may be added to reduce preload and afterload, thereby enhancing cardiac output and reducing myocardial oxygen needs (Fig. 9.1).

Mechanical Interventions. With tension pneumothorax, relief of tension in the chest cavity should immediately improve cardiac hemodynamics. Similarly

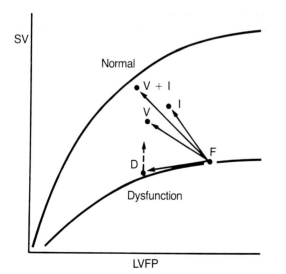

Figure 9.1. Expected hemodynamic response in severe left ventricular dysfunction to administration of diuretics (**D**), inotropic drugs (**I**), vasodilators (**V**), and a combination of vasodilators and inotropics (**V + I**). **SV**, stroke volume. **LVFP**, left ventricular filling pressure.

Table 9.9.
Complications of the Intra-Aortic Balloon Pump

1. Injury to femoral vessels
2. Ischemic extremity
3. Hemolysis and/or thrombocytopenia
4. Infection

pericardiocentesis will markedly improve cardiac function in the case of pericardial tamponade. Because the right-sided cardiac chambers have the least amount of muscle mass and are the most compromised, at least initially, by the restriction in distensibility, some improvement in cardiac function may be achieved by volume infusion to increase the right-sided filling pressure.

Another mechanical method of improving cardiac output in cardiogenic shock is the intra-aortic balloon pump. This device is usually passed through a femoral artery, either percutaneously or via a Dacron graft anastomosed to the femoral artery, into the descending thoracic aorta. This pump, which inflates in the descending thoracic aorta during diastole and deflates during systole, provides for increased cardiac output, increased coronary perfusion, and decreased afterload for the severely compromised left ventricle. The major limitations to intra-aortic balloon pumping are complications associated with its use and include vascular injury, extremity ischemia, hemolysis, thrombocytopenia, and infection (Table 9.9).

Arrhythmias. Common drugs used for arrhythmia control are listed in Table 9.10 with their most common indications. In addition, direct current countershock may be required for arrhythmia control when an acute cardiogenic shock state is associated with arrhythmias. For bradyarrhythmias, pacemaker therapy may be required to improve cardiac output.

Neurogenic Shock

Definition

The term *neurogenic shock* is widely used to describe hypotension secondary to central nervous system dysfunction. However, unlike the other forms of shock de-

Table 9.10.
Common Drugs for Arrhythmias

Supraventricular tachycardia	Digitalis
	Verapamil
	Propranolol
	Procainamide
	Quinidine
Ventricular ectopy	Lidocaine
	Procainamide
	Bretylium
	Quinidine

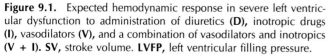

scribed in this chapter, the hypotension associated with neurogenic shock is rarely associated with diminished oxygen delivery and/or utilization. In fact, as described next, cardiac output and oxygen delivery may be normal or even elevated. Therefore the use of the term *shock* to describe this condition is a misnomer.

Because neurogenic shock is most commonly seen in trauma, patients may also be suffering from hypovolemia and/or tension pneumothorax or cardiac tamponade. Such combinations of disease states may make initial recognition of a neurogenic shock state difficult. The discussion that follows is pertinent only for the pure neurogenic shock state.

Pathophysiology

Neurogenic shock results primarily from the disruption of the sympathetic nervous system. The sympathetic nervous system originates in the hypothalamus and subsequently passes down through the brain stem, through the cervical spinal cord, and exits the spinal cord throughout the thoracolumbar region. Sympathetic ganglia (the sympathetic trunk) reside outside the spinal cord in the thoracolumbar region and are connected to both the afferent and efferent fibers. Postganglionic nerves innervate most tissues. Norepinephrine release results primarily in vaso constriction in the periphery. The release of norepinephrine innervating the heart produces increased force of contraction. Sympathetic innervation of the adrenal medulla stimulates the release of epinephrine. The release of epinephrine from the adrenal medulla results in increased heart rate and increased myocardial contractility.

Hypotension in neurogenic shock is primarily secondary to loss of sympathetic nervous system function, either through interruption of the sympathetic nervous system close to its origin (hypothalamus and brain stem) or, more commonly, secondary to interruption of the cervical or thoracic spinal cord. The resultant loss of sympathetic tone results in vasodilatation and decreased peripheral vascular resistance. Such vasodilation may result in an increased capacitance of the venous vasculature and diminished venous return. If hypovolemia accompanies the neurogenic shock state, such diminished venous return will be aggravated. However, if vascular volume is well maintained, venous return may be normal or higher than normal because of decreased vascular resistance. Therefore, only when venous return is diminished, usually in association with accompanying hypovolemia, would neurogenic shock result in decreased oxygen delivery and potential injury.

Diagnosis

Most trauma patients with hypotension exhibit a response consistent with stimulation of the sympathetic nervous system, e.g., tachycardia, vasoconstriction, and agitation. Any hypotensive trauma victim with a normal or slow pulse rate, warm extremities, and little or no agitation should be suspected of having neurol-

ogic injury. Commonly, the hypotensive trauma victim with warm feet cannot move the feet. The mechanism of injury (e.g., the driver of an automobile who broke the windshield), a depressed level of consciousness, and loss of gross motor function (inability to move the legs and/or arms) should alert the clinician to the possibility of a neurogenic etiology of hypotension. A severe head injury with loss of the brain stem function (midposition, fixed pupils, no corneal reflexes, no oculocephalic or oculocaloric reflexes) may be associated with severe cardiovascular instability and profound hypotension. Despite evidence of neurologic injury, however, no patient should be presumed to be in neurogenic shock, and other etiologies of shock (hypovolemia, cardiac tamponade, tension pneumothorax) should be ruled out.

Laboratory Determinations

In pure neurogenic shock, no significant abnormalities in acid-base status, indices of renal function, or hemoglobin concentration should be noted. If such abnormalities are noted, another etiology of hypoperfusion is more likely and should be pursued.

Treatment

Once other potential etiologies of hypoperfusion are either ruled out or treated, the treatment for neurogenic shock may require neurosurgical intervention (relief of epidural or subdural hematomas causing hypothalamic brain stem malfunction, surgery on the spinal column to relieve epidural pressure on the spinal cord). More commonly, simple attention to maintaining adequate vascular volume is the only therapy possible or required. Sympathomimetic agents are rarely indicated. When considered necessary, the drug of choice is phenylephrine hydrochloride (Neo-Synephrine®). This drug is a pure vasoconstrictor with little, if any, effect on the myocardium. More potent vasoconstrictors such as norepinephrine may result in more intense vasoconstriction and diminished renal vascular blood flow.

SUGGESTED READINGS

Hypovolemic Shock

Shires GT, Canizaro PC, Carrico CJ: Shock. In Schwartz SI, Shires GT, Spencer FC, Storer EH (eds): *Principles of Surgery*. New York, McGraw-Hill, 1984, pp 115–164.
Carey LC, Lowery BD, Cloutier CT: Hemorrhagic shock. *Curr Prob Surg* 3–48, January, 1971.
Powers SR: Renal response to systemic trauma. *Am J Surg* 119:603–605, 1970.
Cloutier CT, Lowery BD, Carey LC: The effect of hemodilutional resuscitation on serum protein levels in hormones in hemorrhagic shock. *J Trauma* 9:514–521, 1969.
Lowery BD, Cloutier CT, Carey LC: Lactated Ringer's solution versus unbuffered saline in restoration of severely wounded humans in shock. *Surg Gynecol Obstet* 133:273–284, 1971.
Carrico CJ, Canizaro PC, Shires GT: Fluid resuscitation following injury: rationale for the use of balanced salt solutions. *Crit Care Med* 4(2):46–54, 1976.

Poole CV, Meredith JW, Pennell T, Mills SA: Comparison of colloids and crystalloids in resuscitation from hemorrhagic shock. *Surg Gynecol Obstet* 154:577–586, 1982.

Claybaugh JR, Share L: Vasopressin, renin and cardiovascular responses to continuous slow hemorrhage. *Am J Physiol* 224(3):519–523, 1973.

Trunkey DD, Sheldon GF, Collins JA: The treatment of shock. In Zuidema GD, Rutherford RB, Ballinger WF (eds): *The Management of Trauma*. Philadelphia, WB Saunders, 1979, pp 80–101.

Septic Shock

Kaufman B, Rackow EC, Falk FL: The effect of fluid resuscitation on oxygen consumption in patients with hypovolemic and septic shock (Abstract). *Crit Care Med* 10(3):207, 1982.

Weil MH: Current understanding of mechanisms and treatment of circulatory shock caused by bacterial infections. *Ann Clin Res* 9:181–191, 1977.

Visner MS, Cerra FB, Anderson RW: Hemodynamic and metabolic responses. In Simmons RL, Howard RJ (eds): *Surgical Infectious Diseases*. New York, Appleton-Century-Crofts, 1982, pp 313–338.

Powers SR, Saba TM: Organ failure in sepsis. In Simmons RL, Howard RJ (eds): *Surgical Infectious Diseases*. New York, Appleton-Century-Crofts, 1982, pp 339–358.

Gelin LE, Dawidson I, Haglund U, Heideman M, Myrvold H: Septic shock. *Surg Clin N Am* 60(1):161–174, 1980.

Groeneveld ABJ, Bronsveld W, Thijs LG: Hemodynamic determinants of mortality in human septic shock. *Surgery* 99(2):140–152, 1986.

Cardiogenic Shock

Cohn JN, Franciosa JA: Vasodilator therapy of cardiac failure (Part I). *N Engl J Med* 297(1):27–31, 1977.

Forrester JS, Diamond G, Chatterjee K, Swan HJC: Medical therapy of acute myocardial infarction by application of hemodynamic subsets (Part I). *N Engl J Med* 295(24):1355–1362, 1976.

Forrester JS, Diamond G, Chatterjee K, Swan HJC: Medical therapy of acute myocardial infarction by application of hemodynamic subsets (Part II). *N Engl J Med* 295(25):1404–1412, 1976.

Goldberg LI: Dopamine—clinical uses of an endogenous catecholamine. *N Engl J Med* 291(14):707–710, 1974.

Hill NS, Antman EM, Green LH, Alpert JS: Intravenous nitroglycerine: a review of pharmacology, indications, therapeutic effects and complications. *Chest* 79(1):69–76, 1981.

McCabe JC, Abel RM, Subramanian VA, Gay WA: Complications of intra-aortic balloon insertion and counterpulsation. *Circulation* 57(4):769–773, 1978.

Sibbald WJ, Calvin JE, Holliday RL, Driedger AA: Concepts in the pharmacologic and nonpharmacologic support of cardiovascular function in critically ill surgical patients. *Surg Clin N Am* 63(2):455–482, 1983.

Snow N, Lucas AE, Richardson JD: Intra-aortic balloon counterpulsation for cardiogenic shock from cardiac contusion. *J Trauma* 22(5):426–429, 1982.

Sonnenblick EH, Frishman WH, LeJemtel TH: Dobutamine: a new synthetic cardioactive sympathetic amine. *N Engl J Med* 300(1):17–22, 1979.

Leier CV, Heban PT, Huss P, Bush CA, Lewis RP: Comparative systemic and regional hemodynamic effects of dopamine and dobutamine in patients with cardiomyopathic heart failure. *Circulation* 58(3):466–475, 1978.

Colucci WS, Wright RF, Braunwald E: New positive inotropic agents in the treatment of congestive heart failure: mechanisms of action and recent clinical developments (Part I). *N Engl J Med* 314:290–299, 1986.

Colucci WS, Wright RF, Braunwald E: New positive inotropic agents in the treatment of congestive heart failure: mechanisms of action and recent clinical developments (Part II). *N Engl J Med* 314:349–358, 1986.

Neurogenic Shock

Shires GT, Canizaro PC, Carrico CJ: Shock. In Schwartz SI, Shires GT, Spencer FC, Storer EH (eds): *Principles of Surgery*. New York, McGraw-Hill, 1984, pp 115–164.

Shires GT, Carrico CJ, Canizaro PC: Major problems in clinical surgery. In: *Shock*. Philadelphia, WB Saunders, 1973, vol XIII, pp 149–150.

Youmans JR: *Neurological Surgery: A Comprehensive Reference Guide to the Diagnosis and Management of Neurosurgical Problems*. Philadelphia, WB Saunders, 1982, pp 2504, 2509–2510.

Skills

1. Given a patient with shock, interpret the cardiac output, left atrial (wedge) pressure, blood pressure, pulse, and urine output. Using these values, determine the category of shock.

Study Questions

HYPOVOLEMIC SHOCK

1. A 27-year-old male driver of an automobile is involved in a head-on collision at high speed. On arrival in the emergency department, he is awake and oriented but complains of abdominal pain. He is noted to have bruises across his upper abdomen consistent with having been thrown forward against a steering wheel. Discuss how you would initially evaluate this patient.

   Based on your initial evaluation you determine that this patient is in shock. Discuss how you arrived at this diagnosis. Discuss your initial therapeutic intervention.

2. A 46-year-old male sustains a close-range small-caliber gunshot wound to the midabdomen. Entrance wound is to the right of the umbilicus; there is no exit wound. On arrival at the emergency department he is in profound shock with the following parameters: blood pressure 60 palpable, heart rate 140, his skin is cold and clammy, he is profusely diaphoretic and is belligerent and somewhat combative. There is a strong odor of alcohol on his breath. Discuss what resuscitative measures you would immediately institute on this patient. Discuss what laboratory tests and diagnostic procedures you would order, why, and what results you would anticipate. Discuss in sequence, giving rationale for each, additional diagnostic and therapeutic measures that you would institute.

SEPTIC SHOCK

1. A 65-year-old female, in previous good health, comes to the emergency room with a complaint of increasing (gradually over 24 hours) left lower quadrant abdominal pain, anorexia, and two loose bowel movements. In the emergency room the patient is noted to have a blood pressure of 90/60, a pulse of 120, and a temperature of 102.4°F. Abdominal examination reveals slight abdominal distension, percussion, referred tenderness to the left lower quadrant, and involuntary guarding in the left lower quadrant. Rectal examination reveals no tenderness and stool negative for occult blood. Examination of the extremities reveals that they are warm and fingers and toes are pink.

   What are the priorities in the initial management of this patient? What diagnostic studies would you consider necessary?

2. A 55-year-old male is brought to the surgical intensive care unit following an abdominal operation for a leaking sigmoid colon anastomosis. During the operation there was noted to be contamination of the entire abdominal cavity with feculent material. The patient was severely hypotensive and tachycardiac during the operation, with systolic blood pressure recorded at 60 mm Hg. Upon arrival in the surgical intensive care unit, the patient has a systolic blood pressure of 80, pulse of 130, and temperature of 97°F. He is vasoconstricted, with cyanotic hands and feet. The last recorded urine output was 15 cc for the previous hour. Review of his record reveals that he suffered an anterior septal myocardial infarction 6 months prior to this surgery.

   What hemodynamic monitoring parameters should be measured in this patient? From what types of shock may this patient be suffering? Which is most likely? What monitoring parameters would help distinguish these potential etiologies of shock?

CARDIOGENIC SHOCK

1. Earlier this day a 65-year-old man with a 3-year history of angina that was stable on propranolol and nitroglyc-erin therapy underwent an abdominal aneurysm resection. During the resection hypotension to a blood pressure of 60 developed for 10 minutes after removal of all vascular clamps. Subsequent to the surgery he arrives in the intensive care unit with a blood pressure of 80/60, a pulse of 120, and a temperature of 97°F, with severe vasoconstriction evident peripherally.

   How would you initially evaluate this hypotension? If 24 hours later the patient again develops hypotension and an electrocardiogram reveals an acute anterior septal or a myocardial infarction, how would you initially treat this patient?

2. A 25-year-old male driver of an automobile accident arrives in the emergency room with a blood pressure of 70/40, pulse of 130, respirations 30. The steering wheel was crushed in the accident.

   How would you distinguish hypovolemic shock from a traumatic cardiogenic etiology of hypotension? What are the etiologies of traumatic cardiogenic shock and how is each managed?

NEUROGENIC SHOCK

1. A 24-year-old man is admitted to the emergency room following a 30-foot fall from scaffolding at work. The initial blood pressure is 80/50, but the pulse is 64 and the patient appears warm and well perfused. He is awake and oriented and cannot move his legs. What are the initial steps in management of this patient?

2. A 59-year-old white female is brought to the emergency department following a motor vehicle accident. She is unconscious but can be aroused with painful stimuli. Chest x-ray does not show any evidence of intrathoracic hemorrhage, and peritoneal lavage to assess for intra-abdominal bleeding is also negative. Hypotension persists despite 4 liters of crystalloid solution. What would be the next step in management of this patient?

10 Wounds and Wound Healing

Martin C. Robson, M.D.
Talmage Raine, M.D.
David J. Smith, Jr., M.D.

ASSUMPTION

The student has successfully completed a basic science curriculum of biochemistry, physiology, and pathology dealing with the mechanisms of tissue repair and wound healing.

OBJECTIVES

1. Define a wound and describe the sequence and approximate time frame of the phases of wound healing.
2. Describe the essential elements and significance of granulation tissue.
3. Describe the three types of wound healing and the elements of each. Describe the phases of wound healing distinct to each type of wound.
4. Describe clinical factors that decrease collagen synthesis and retard wound healing.
5. Define a clean, a contaminated, and an infected wound and describe the management of each.
6. Describe the rationale for the uses of absorbable and nonabsorbable sutures.
7. Discuss the functions of a dressing.

A wound, in the broadest sense, is a disruption of normal anatomic relationships as the result of an injurious process. The injury may be intentional, such as in an elective surgical incision, or accidental after trauma. Regardless of the cause, the biochemical and physiologic processes of healing are identical in character, although the time course and intensity of the process may vary. The closure of wounds may be classified into three distinct types: primary, secondary, and tertiary, based on the timing of replacing epithelium over the wound. Wound healing may also be divided by physiologic process into stages or phases: the substrate phase, the proliferative phase, and the remodeling phase. Biochemical and physiological events can be correlated with gross morphologic changes in the wound. A knowledge of these events and changes al-lows the physician to maximize the chances of successful healing while minimizing the resultant scar deformity.

Stages or Phases of Wound Healing

Inflammation is the basic physiologic process that is common to all wounds. Clinically, inflammation is identified by the cardinal signs of redness (rubor), heat (calor), swelling (tumor), pain (dolor), and loss of function. These same signs of inflammation are also seen in wound infections, which ultimately may result in wound disruption. They differ only in degree and time course from the primary sequence of events that leads to normal wound healing. The physiology underlying these clinical signs is a complex amalgam of biochemical and cellular events.

Biochemical Aspects

Trauma activates a cascade of chemoattractants and mitogens that recruit phagocytes, fibroblasts, and endothelial cells. These chemoattractants are produced during the clotting of blood by degradation of the surrounding tissue and by the cells entering the wound. These substances regulate the numbers and types of cells in the wound and control the rate of wound healing.

One such factor, the platelet-derived growth factor (PDGF), is released only at the site of injury and has both chemotactic and mitogenic activity toward fibroblasts and smooth muscle cells. PDGF appears to be primarily a wound hormone. Addition of PDGF to an experimental wound model increases the entry and proliferation of cells and the rate at which collagen is deposited. Arachidonic acid (AA) is contained in the walls of the cells, and when cells are injured, this substance is released. Degradation of AA into prostanoid derivatives of prostaglandins and thromboxanes elicits a number of responses associated with the inflammatory response, including vasodilatation (rubor), swelling (tumor), and pain (dolor).

Physiologic Aspects

At the same time that these biochemical events are developing, leukocytes are marginating, sticking to vessel walls, and emigrating through the walls toward the site of injury. Venules are dilating and lymphatics are being blocked. This inflammatory response in the wound occurs for a variable period of time, depending on local tissue and host factors. Some of these factors are responsive to manipulation by the knowledgeable physician.

Substrate Phase

The substrate phase is the first phase of wound healing. It is also known by the terms *inflammatory* phase, *lag* phase, or *exudative* phase. This phase is characterized by a continuation of the inflammation described above. The main cells involved in this process are polymorphonuclear leukocytes (PMN) and macrophages. Shortly after wounding, PMNs appear and remain the predominant cell for approximately 48 hours. Induced selective neutropenia has not been shown to alter normal wound healing. The activated leukocyte may be the origin of many inflammatory mediators, including complement and kallikrein. Small numbers of bacteria are handled by the macrophages present in the wound. However, large numbers of bacteria cannot be controlled and in the neutropenic state will lead to a clinical wound infection.

The neutrophil is not crucial for normal wound healing; the macrophage is. Monocytes enter the wound after the PMNs and reach maximum numbers approximately 24 hours later. They evolve into macrophages, which are the main cell involved in wound debridement. Experimental wounds depleted of macrophages and monocytes exhibit marked inhibition of fibroblast migration, proliferation, and loss of collagen production. Macrophages secrete substances that cause *(1)* fibroblasts to replicate [macrophage-derived growth factor (MDGF)] and *(2)* blood vessels to approach the wound [wound angiogenesis factor (WAF)].

At the time that clot, debris, and bacteria are being removed, substrates for collagen synthesis are being arranged. In primary wound healing, this process occurs over approximately 4-day period. The wound appears edematous and erythematous at this time, and it may be difficult to distinguish this normal process from early signs of a wound infection. In healing by secondary or tertiary intention, this phase continues indefinitely until the wound surface is closed by ectodermal elements (epithelium for skin or mucosa in the gut).

Proliferative Phase

The second and third phases of wound healing are relatively constant, regardless of the type of wound healing that is occurring. These phases begin only when the wound is covered by epithelium. The proliferative phase is the second stage in the healing wound. It is characterized by the production of collagen in the wound. The wound appears less edematous and inflamed than before, but the wound scar itself may appear raised, red, and hard. The main cell in this phase is the cell that makes the collagen, the fibroblast.

Collagen is the principal structural protein of the body and is ubiquitous through all of its varied tissues. It is a complex, three-dimensional structure. The process of collagen synthesis begins with the production of amino acid chains in the cytoplasm of the fibroblast. These α-chains are unique in that each third amino acid is glycine (Gly-x-y). Two amino acids, hydroxyproline and hydroxylysine, are found only in collagen and require hydroxylation in their synthesis by specific enzymes, which in turn require cofactors of ferrous ion, α-ketoglutarate, and ascorbic acid. The absence of ascorbic acid leads to the production of defective, unhydroxylated collagen, of which very little is excreted from the fibroblast. This is scurvy. It develops as normal collagen turnover is not replaced by adequate new collagen.

Three α-peptide chains are woven into a right-handed triple helix, and the entire structure is then twisted into a left-handed "super helix." A galactose unit attaches to the triple helix and the molecule is excreted from the fibroblast. This molecule is called procollagen. Removal of several terminal amino acids from the α-chains produces tropocollagen. Tropocollagen aggregates to form collagen fibrils, and these aggregates are held together by cross-links created by conversion of lysine to an aldehyde and then reaction with another aldehyde from an adjacent tropocollagen molecule. In the primary wound (which has been closed immediately after the wound occurred), production of collagen begins about day 7 after wounding and continues until approximately day 60. The production of collagen is not a constant event; it begins slowly at first, then there is a rapid spurt of production from day 18 to approximately day 50 after wounding (Fig. 10.1). The increased proliferation of collagen is reflected in the rapid gain in tensile strength during this period.

Remodeling of collagen is the process whereby randomly arranged collagen fibers and aggregates are gradually replaced by a more organized formation of fibers in response to local stress factors in the wound. The laying down of collagen is a dynamic process that involves production and remodeling.

Maturation Phase

The third and final phase of wound healing is the remodeling or maturation phase. It is characterized by the maturation of collagen by intermolecular cross-linking. The wound scar appears to gradually flatten out and become less prominent and more pale and supple. This phase remains a time of great metabolic activity, although there is no net collagen production. The maturation process clinically corresponds to the flattening of the scar and requires approximately nine months to

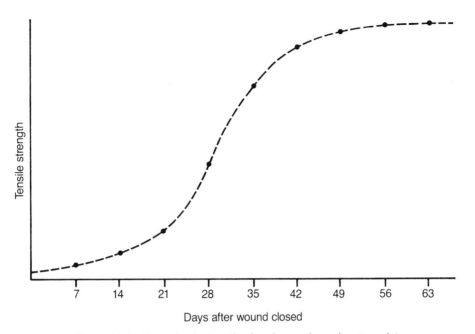

Figure 10.1. Strength of primarily closed wound as a function of time.

take place in the adult. The proliferative and maturation phases of wound healing are divided into categories to describe the predominant physiologic process occurring at a particular time.

Classification of Healing Wounds

Primary Healing

In primary healing (healing by first intention) the wound is closed by direct approximation of the wound edges. In larger defects, pedicled flaps or skin grafts are used to close the wound. This is still primary wound healing—wound healing that occurs by immediate coverage with epithelial elements in some form.

Secondary Healing

Secondary healing (spontaneous wound closure) is characterized by leaving the wound open and allowing it to heal spontaneously. Spontaneous wound closure is a bimodal process of wound contraction and epithelialization. Contraction occurs by a centripetal force in the margin of the wound that is generated by myofibroblasts.

The myofibroblast appears to have special contractile properties. The term *myofibroblast* is derived from observations concerning this specialized cell and its internal structure. Under light microscopy, the cell appears as any other fibroblast. However, under transmission electron microscopy, myofibrils identical to those found in smooth muscle cells are seen at the periphery. These myofibrils respond appropriately to smooth muscle stimulants. Contraction is believed by some investigators to be controlled by these myofibroblasts, as they are seen in great numbers near the edges of contracting wounds. Other investigators believe the

myofibroblast is not a functioning cell but only a skeleton and that the actin and myosin in the wound margin are responsible for contraction. This contraction is a normal process. Contracture, a pathologic deformity caused by contraction of scar, is not desirable and must be considered in the healing of all wounds (Fig. 10.2).

Epithelialization is the other component of healing by secondary intention. The epithelium proliferates from the wound margins to the center at the approximate rate of 1 mm/day. This occurs only in a wound that is not infected (see "Management of the Contaminated and Infected Wound").

In the middle of the open wound that is healing by secondary intention, the inflammatory phase continues unabated. The product of this prolonged inflammatory process is granulation tissue. Granulation tissue consists of inflammatory cells and a proliferation of capillaries. This is the "proud flesh" that our surgical forefathers welcomed as a sign of healthy wound healing. The modern surgeon should view this merely as a prolonged inflammatory phase of a wound that is in need of closure. There are a number of options in most of these wounds that are granulating. The informed physician will choose among these options and may elect to excise all this wound granulation and perform a delayed primary (tertiary) closure. Another option is to allow healing by secondary intention to proceed. A third option is to skin graft the wound and thereby close it.

Tertiary Healing

Tertiary wound healing (healing by third intention) is closure of a wound by active means after a delay of days to weeks. This process occurs when a granulating, open wound is closed with sutures or sterile tape before it has healed. The process of closing the wound

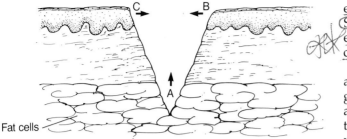

Fat cells

Figure 10.2. Wounds that heal by secondary intention. **A,** Granulation tissue forms at base. **B,** Wound margins contract. **C,** Epithelium migrates.

interrupts the secondary healing process. Delayed closure should be performed only in wounds that are in bacterial balance (see "Management of the Contaminated and Infected Wound").

Factors Affecting Wound Healing

Proper wound closure is the sine qua non of successful wound management. The goal of all wound closure is expedient, precise, and definitive tissue approximation while, at the same time, preventing infection, fibrosis, and secondary deformities (wound contracture). The ability of the surgeon to achieve this goal depends on his or her knowledge of local and systemic factors that affect this process and the willingness and ability to control them.

Several local factors are extremely important and should be considered each time the physician is presented with a wound problem. The amount of tissue trauma that the wound has sustained is extremely important. A laceration with a knife is minimally damaging to any tissue except directly in the wound margin. Crush or avulsion injuries are much more difficult to evaluate and thus manage successfully. In a crush, large areas of tissue adjacent to the wound itself are tenuous and difficult to assess for ultimate viability.

Hematoma is the bane of unimpeded wound healing. A collection of clot in the wound does not allow for orderly removal of debris and laying down of collagen. The hematoma is a perfect medium for promoting bacterial proliferation and fostering clinical wound infection.

Bacterial contamination and wound infection are factors of extreme importance in local control of the wound and proper closure. All wounds contain bacteria to a greater or lesser amount. A relationship exists between the bacteria in the wound and the patient who is wounded; this relationship can best be described as a biologic balance (or equilibrium). There are a number of factors that affect this equilibrium: blood supply to the wound, necrotic debris present, local wound care requirements, and the use of systemic or topical antimicrobial agents. A wound can usually tolerate contamination of up to 100,000 (10^5) organisms per gram of tissue and still be closed successfully without infection developing. If more than 10^5 bacteria/gm are pres-

ent, closure will lead to clinical wound infection. Streptococci are the only exception to this. The presence of streptococci in the wound in any quantity is a contraindication to wound closure.

The proper management of a wound will depend on a number of factors, including the type of injury, degree of contamination, time from injury to treatment, and the patient's host defense mechanisms. A carefully taken history will reveal much about the nature of a wound and the amount of contamination present. Proper assessment of the contamination will dictate the subsequent care and ultimate success of wound management.

In addition to an assessment of the contamination with common pathogens, the student should be aware of the possibility of tetanus in many wounds. Tetanus prophylaxis is an important consideration in all wounds. The best means of preventing tetanus is with toxoid immunization combined with a thorough cleansing and debridement. The Committee on Trauma of the American College of Surgeons has established guidelines that should be carefully reviewed (see Chapter 11).

General Management of the Clean Wound

The clean wound is one that is relatively new (less than 12 hours) and has minimal contamination. Clean wounds may be classified according to the method of injury and how the wound presents. An abrasion is superficial loss of epithelial elements with much of the dermis and deeper structures intact. Usually, only cleansing of the wound is required, as the remaining epithelial cells will regenerate and migrate to close the wound. Careful cleansing is critical to prevent traumatic tattoos. Traumatic tattooing can occur with trapping of dirt particles beneath newly regenerated epithelial cells. A surgical scrub brush is often helpful in removing the debris. For large abrasions with traumatic tattooing, general anesthesia is often required to adequately scrub and properly care for the wound. Epithelial migration has been shown to occur most rapidly in a moist environment. Therefore, desiccation of an abrasion should be avoided.

A contusion is a soft tissue swelling and hemorrhage without a violation of the skin elements. Evacuation of a hematoma with aspiration may be required. Otherwise, management consists of cold compresses early (less than 2 hours from injury) to minimize swelling, then warm, moist compresses for comfort and to speed the absorption of blood.

Lacerations are the classic wound and are managed with debridement of ragged edges and devitalized tissue followed by atraumatic suture closure. An avulsion injury is more difficult to manage than a simple laceration because of the extensive undermining that creates a flap. Partial avulsions should be debrided and sutured into place if viable. Total avulsions are generally not replaceable except as a skin graft after the fat has been removed. If the avulsed part has an adequate

Table 10.1
Steps in Wound Care

1. Sterile prep and drape
2. Administration of local anesthetic
3. Hemostasis
4. Irrigation and debridement
5. Closure in layers
6. Dressing and bandage

single artery and vein in it (greater than 0.5 mm), it may be sometimes replanted with microsurgical technique. Puncture wounds generally do not require closure per se. Management consists of assessment of damage to underlying vital structures and examination for a foreign body. X-rays and xeroradiographs are often helpful in assessing the presence or absence of a foreign body.

Crush injuries often are accompanied by loss of significant amounts of tissue that may initially appear viable. The extent of injury in this particular wound may be evaluated with intravenous flourescein, which diffuses into the interstitial tissue from capillaries in the immediate area that are patent. Flourescence under an ultraviolet lamp will indicate blood flow in the area and predicts survival of the tissue.

Technique of Wound Debridement and Closure

Care of the wound requires debriding the wound and then approximating the tissue in physiologic and anatomic order. Almost all nonmilitary wounds can be managed by primary closure if prepared properly (Table 10.1). Sedation of the patient may help to allay anxiety. This should be done only after assessment of any possible central nervous system injury.

Anesthesia and Wound Cleaning

The wounded area is prepared by washing with an antibacterial solution. If the wound is extensive, local anesthetic may be required prior to this step to reduce patient discomfort. An adequate working area must be prepared around the wound to prevent contamination of suture material and instruments. Sterile gloves are worn, and frequently the physician wears a surgical mask and gown. Sterile towels are then draped around the wound to provide the sterile field. Some wounds may require ingenuity in draping, particularly in areas that are difficult to reach. It is helpful to take a few extra minutes in considering draping plans to ensure that drapes do not cover the patient's face, interfere with breathing, or confine the patient in such a way that the draping promotes a feeling of claustrophobia. This is particularly true if closure may take some time. Patients may become restless, frightened, or uncooperative, making it difficult for the patient and frustrating for the physician. Particular thought should be given when preparing a child for wound closure.

Local anesthesia is generally adequate for smaller wounds. Patients should be questioned about known sensitivity or adverse reactions to anesthetic agents.

Xylocaine® 1% or 0.5% is usually sufficient. An anesthetic agent with longer action, Marcaine®, may be occasionally useful. A new vial of anesthetic agent should be opened. Agents containing epinephrine should be used with caution. Chemical vasoconstriction is often helpful in tissue with a rich blood supply but may produce detrimental ischemia in other areas, e.g., digital blocks of fingers or toes. When administering the agent, use as small a needle as practical, 23–26 gauge, and inject slowly. Tell the patient what you are doing and what he or she can anticipate, such as the stick and the burning sensation with the injection. The difference between a good and a poor local anesthetic is five minutes. Be patient and give the drug the opportunity to work for you and most importantly for the patient. The toxic dose of lidocaine is approximately 7 mg/kg. A 1% solution contains 10 mg/ml, a 0.5% solution 5 mg/ml, etc. A 10 ml dose of 1% Xylocaine® in a 20-kg child approaches the toxic dose.

Irrigate the wound copiously with normal saline and remove all debris. Sharply debride necrotic tissue and freshen the skin edges with a scalpel if needed. Hemostasis is achieved by cautery or ligation of bleeding points. The wound should be dry prior to beginning closure.

Wound Debridement and Closure

The best way to cleanse the wound is sharp debridement to remove clot, debris, and necrotic tissue and then irrigation with a physiologic saline solution. A 20-cc syringe with an 18-gauge needle is ideal for this (Fig. 10.3). Hematoma should be evacuated and all active bleeding controlled. Hemostasis is achieved with cauterization or absorbable ligature. Closure of the wound is undertaken in layers, with absorbable sutures placed in those layers that provide the greatest strength, i.e., dermis and fascia. The epithelium is approximated with superficial placement of nonabsorbable, monofilament suture to seal the wound (Fig. 10.4).

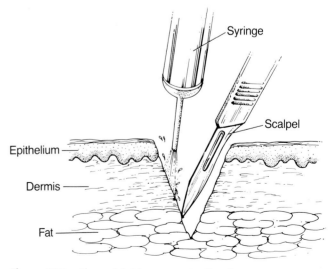

Figure 10.3. Sharp debridement and saline lavage to prepare the wound for closure.

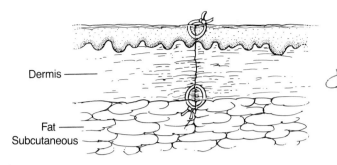

Figure 10.4. Dermis approximated for strength. Epidermis closed to seal wound and align surface cells.

Closure of "dead space" is usually not necessary, given proper closure of the strong layers of the wound, skin, or fascia. Needless sutures placed in the subcutaneous layer only serve to necrose fat cells and introduce an unneeded foreign body that promotes infection. Handling of the tissue with atraumatic technique will favorably affect wound healing. Proper, atraumatic technique involves using instruments that will grasp but not crush the tissues.

Suture Material

Great emphasis is often placed on the suture material used for closure, but it is less important than attention to adequate debridement and hemostasis. Suture material may be classified as synthetic or biologic, absorbable or nonabsorbable, mono- or multifilament. Gut sutures, usually derived from sheep intestine, are examples of biologic sutures, lasting 7–10 days, and are absorbed by proteolysis and phagocytic action. They induce an inflammatory reaction in the tissue and therefore are not usually utilized for closure of the skin.

Newer absorbable sutures include synthetic material of polyglycolic acid. Dexon® and Vicryl® are examples. These are polyfilament sutures that are absorbed by hydrolysis and are useful for reapproximation of tissue below the skin surface. The braided nature of the suture make them less desirable for skin closure.

Nylon is an excellent example of synthetic suture material. It is usually monofilament but may be woven or braided. This material is biologically inert; therefore it cannot be broken down or absorbed. Monofilament nylon induces little inflammatory reaction and is useful for skin closure.

Silk is a complex suture material. It is biological and eventually broken down and absorbed, but this takes so much time (years) that it is considered permanent. Silk suture is woven or braided and therefore has small spaces in the strand (interstices) that can trap bacteria and serous exudate, promoting an inflammatory reaction around the suture. Otherwise, it is considered biologically inert. Silk remains the suture to which all others are compared, especially in terms of strength.

Suture size is graded by the number of "0s"; the more "0s" the smaller the suture, i.e., "0" is very large, "0000" (4-0) is smaller. Number 1 suture is even larger. A 3-0 or 4-0 suture is used for skin on the extremities or torso, while 5-0 or 6-0 is appropriate for

the more delicate tissues of the face. A 2-0 to 4-0 suture is appropriate for closure of deeper tissues.

Suture material, size, and type, should be chosen based on the type of reapproximation that is needed. Usually absorbable synthetic suture is preferred for closure of the deep layers. Muscle is very friable and will not hold sutures; therefore the fascial covering of the muscle must be used for approximation. Subdermal tissue is closed, then the skin. For simple closure, wound drains are not required. The need for drainage usually suggests the need for better hemostasis. Small monofilament sutures are ideal for the skin. Knots should be tight enough to approximate, not strangulate, the tissue. Swelling of the tissue will occur over 24–48 hours and tighten the suture naturally. Excessive tension produces ischemia of the wound edge and additional inflammation. This exaggerates the suture marks across the wound and accounts for the "railroad track" appearance of the scar. Although cosmesis is the last element to consider in wound closure, avoidance of excessive tension produces a more desirable result. If the wound will not close without tension, consideration should be given to some other management plan, e.g., rotational flaps, skin graft.

Dressings

A dressing is usually placed over the closed wound. The functions of a wound dressing are many. To be maximally functional the dressing should *(1)* protect the wound, *(2)* immobilize the area, *(3)* compress the area evenly, *(4)* absorb any secretions, and *(5)* be aesthetically acceptable. Proper wound dressing should fulfill all of these criteria. The dressing should consist of sufficient bulk to afford protection from inadvertent trauma. The bulk provided by fluffed gauze and ABD pads will allow for adequate absorption of wound secretions and help to immobilize the area. Further immobilization may be provided by a plaster splint or cast. An outer layer of firmly wrapped, rolled gauze and a loosely, but evenly, applied elastic roll will provide even compression and aesthetic appearance.

Suture Removal

Sutures used for skin closure are removed when they have done the job for which they were placed. If dermal sutures were placed properly, the epidermal sutures may be removed within several days of placement. If skin is closed in a single layer, the sutures may not be removed for 7–10 days. Sterile forceps and fine scissors are the basic instruments used to remove sutures. The use of sterilized supplies is important in infection control procedures. The suture is grasped with forceps and cut, then gently removed.

Management of the Contaminated and Infected Wound

All wounds are contaminated to a greater or lesser extent. Even the wounds considered "clean" have a

Common Ambulatory Skin And Soft Tissue Problems

11

Patricia J. Numann, M.D.

ASSUMPTIONS

The student knows basic anatomy of the skin and digits.
The student knows basic pathophysiology of wounds and infection.

OBJECTIVES

1. Evaluate a wound to determine the need for suturing and wound care.
2. Outline the procedure for wound suturing and wound care of simple surgical wounds.
3. Describe the indications and dose of local anesthesia.
4. Describe the use of local anesthesia for simple surgical wounds, abrasions and digital blocks.
5. Describe the care of animal and human bites on the face and other areas of the body.
6. List the indications for tetanus prophylaxis and the administration of tetanus prophylaxis.
7. List the indications and methods for removal of foreign bodies, rings and fish hooks.
8. Describe the treatment for puncture wounds of the foot.
9. Describe the removal of small skin lesions.
10. Describe the treatment of subungual hematomas, paronychia, and felons.
11. Describe the management of ingrown toenails and fungal infections of the toes.

Evaluation and Care of Soft Tissue Injuries

The first step in wound management is the careful evaluation for damage to important underlying structures. When wounds occur in the vicinity of major nerves, arteries, and tendons, the integrity of these nerves, arteries, and tendons should be evaluated prior to the use of local anesthesia or any manipulation of the wound. The inexperienced surgeon should not attempt to repair damaged functional structures, as additional injury may occur. Most of these injuries require repair in the operating room. Hemostasis should be obtained with care not to clamp and further injure nerves or vessels; the skin should be closed over complex injuries involving these tissues. These patients should be referred to an appropriate surgical specialist.

Once the extent of the injury has been assessed, the wound should be injected with local anesthetic. The wound should be carefully cleaned and the interior of the wound carefully examined for injury to deeper structure prior to repair. Wounds should rarely be closed if they are more than six hours old, if they were caused by blast or missile injuries or electrical burns, or if they contain debris and dirt that cannot be easily debrided. Human and animal bites should rarely be closed. When bites occur on the face they may sometimes be closed with care not to use deep sutures, with antibiotic coverage, and with careful follow-up. For most wounds, injection into the subcutaneous tissue will provide adequate local anesthesia, if care is taken not to exceed the toxic dose of Xylocaine® (7 mg/kg). For the majority of wounds, the use of epinephrine in the local anesthetic is unnecessary and may cause symptoms of anxiety and tachycardia in the already apprehensive patient. For small areas on the head and face, epinephrine may facilitate wound closure by decreasing bleeding. Epinephrine should never be used adjacent to a terminal artery, particularly distal to the distal palmar or the distal plantar crease, as the epinephrine may produce ischemic necrosis of the digit. Although intradermal injection of Xylocaine® produces the most rapid anesthetic effect, this may be difficult in an open wound. If there are large abraded areas, topical anesthesia can be applied by soaking 4 x 4 gauze sponges in Xylocaine® or applying a small amount of viscous Xylocaine® to the abraded wound. This works particularly well for large open areas of abrasion that are dirty and require vigorous cleansing, such as occur in children who have fallen on gravel. Care must be taken to use a total volume of local anesthetic less than the toxic limit. In patients who are very apprehensive, who have large wounds, or in small children, a sedative and/or systemic pain control may be helpful. With large wounds or wounds requiring complicated repair, general anesthesia may be necessary. This is particularly true for children. If general anesthesia is used or there is a delay before the patient is taken to the operating room, the wound should be dressed with topical antibiotic and covered.

Once adequate local anesthesia has been achieved, the wound should be vigorously cleaned by irrigating the wound, picking out with a forceps all foreign bodies, and debriding obviously devitalized tissue. The careful use of cautery for hemostasis and minimal use of absorbable suture in the depths of the wound where it may act as a foreign body is advisable. The decision to suture the wound or to appose the wound with wound closure strips (such as Steristrips®) depends on several circumstances. A wound that is on a pressure-bearing area and is long enough to separate when pressure is put on that area should be sutured. If the wound is on a nonpressure-bearing area, is small, and can be adequately apposed with a wound closure strip, this type of closure may be acceptable. Prior to putting wound closure strips on the wound, the wound must be dry to allow the closure strips to stick and approximate the wound edges precisely. Pressure on the edges of the wound will achieve hemostasis in most cases and allow the strip to be placed. If exact apposition cannot be achieved, the wound should be sutured. A nonabsorbable fine suture should be used to attain the best cosmetic results. In many wounds, where the suture must remain for a week or more, the best cosmetic result can be achieved with a running subcuticular pullout suture. The best wound closure depends on the exact apposition of the epidermal layer. In certain areas of the body the wound should be sutured, even if it is very tiny. This is most true on areas of the face, where exact anatomic lines must be preserved. Examples include the ala of the nose, the edge of the eyelid, the pinna of the ear, and when the injury is perpendicular to the vermilion border of the lip or the eyebrow. Where the wound has extended deep into structures such as the muscles, the fascia of the muscles should be closed.

A dry sterile dressing should be placed on the wound and maintained for 48 hours. At that point the wound is sealed and further contamination should not occur. A small amount of antibacterial ointment may be applied to the wound and may reduce bacterial contamination at the suture site. After 48 hours the patient may remove this dressing, cleanse with soap and water gently, and reapply a bandage if desired. Generally sutures in the area of the face should be removed in 3–5 days; sutures in areas of tension and weight-bearing areas should be removed at 2 weeks; all other sutures can usually be removed at 7–10 days. The longer the suture is left, the more likely there will be a scar where the suture penetrates the skin. In areas of tension, if the suture does not help to appose the wound until the period of healing has occurred, the wound edges may separate. Wounds that separate should be vigorously cleaned, and frequent dressing changes should be carried out to see that the wound is not contaminated. Quantitative wound cultures may be used to determine when the wound can be secondarily closed.

Bite Wounds

Wounds resulting from either human or animal bites require special care. All bites, human and animal, are contaminated with bacteria that can quickly cause wound infection. A human or animal bite should be treated with antibiotics in addition to the local wound care measures discussed. Penicillin is generally adequate coverage and should be instituted immediately, either as oral penicillin or an intramuscular injection at the time of wound evaluation. Oral erythromycin is a good substitute when penicillin allergy exists. Bites on areas of the body where the cosmetic result is of less concern should not be closed, but treated with dressing changes until they heal by secondary intention. Many bite wounds are on the face and the hands. Bite wounds on the hand should always be treated open with dressings. Deep hand space or tendon sheath infection is a serious complication of a hand wound. The wound should be examined regularly to see that a tendon sheath infection or deep-space infection is detected early if it occurs. If the tendon sheath becomes infected, the earlier it is drained, the less the functional loss. Such complications require urgent care by a surgical specialist.

Bite wounds on the face create a serious cosmetic defect if they are not closed. It is reasonable to assume the risk of infection in order to reduce the cosmetic defect in many cases. Vigorous wound irrigation is essential if this approach is chosen. Antibiotics specific to the common oral bacteria are important adjuncts to management. Absorbable suture material buried in the wound may increase the risk of infection because of the presence of the foreign body. The skin should be ap-

Table 11.1.
Immunization Recommendations

History of Immunization	Tetanus Prone		Nontetanus Prone	
	Tetanus Toxid	Tetanus Immune Globulin	Tetanus Toxid	Tetanus Immune Globulin
Unknown or incomplete	0.5 ml[a]	250 units	0.5 ml[a]	No
Complete, last booster >5 yr ago	0.5 ml	No	No[b]	No
Complete, last booster <5 yr ago	No	No	No	No

[a]In unimmunized children, DT (diptheria, tetanus) DPT (diptheria, pertussis, tetanus) is used. Completion of immunizations is necessary.
[b]Yes, if booster >10 years ago.

Table 11.2.
Wound Classification

	Tetanus Prone	Nontetanus Prone
Age	>6 hr	<6 hr
Type	Crush	Sharp/clean
	Avulsion	
	Extensive abrasion	
	Burn/frostbite	
Contaminants (soil, saliva)	Present	Absent

posed with a nonabsorbable suture. This wound should be reevaluated at 48 hours and again at five days if all is well. Early, streptococcal species cause the majority of the problems while staphylococcal organisms are the offending agents after 48 hours. Patients should be informed of the risk of infection and the signs of infection so that the wound may be opened immediately.

Tetanus Prophylaxis

Patients should receive tetanus prophylaxis in accordance with the recommendations of the Committee on Trauma of the American College of Surgeons (Tables 11.1 and 11.2). The wounds that are tetanus prone should be given tetanus toxoid. The only contraindication to the use of tetanus is a history of neurologic or severe hypersensitivity reaction from a previous dose of tetanus toxoid.

Embedded Foreign Bodies

Many wounds are caused by foreign bodies. All foreign bodies that are porous or contain organic material should be removed, as they are sources of bacterial contamination that may cause wound infections, tetanus, or gas gangrene. Metallic or nonporous, nonorganic materials may occasionally be left as foreign bodies within the wound. Foreign bodies on weight-bearing surfaces become chronically irritated, encapsulated, and painful; therefore, foreign bodies on the palms of the hands, the soles of the feet, and in areas such as the knees, the buttocks, and other pressure-bearing areas should be removed. If the wound had contained organic porous material, it should be vigorously cleaned (once the foreign body is removed), packed open, and allowed to close by secondary intention or closed secondarily when quantitative wound cultures indicate it is safe. If the wound was caused by a nonporous material, contamination was minimal, and the wound was in an area of cosmetic importance, the wound may be closed primarily. Bullet wounds should never be closed primarily, as the surrounding blast effect from the bullet causes dead and devitalized tissue, which is hard to identify at the time of initial evaluation. Grossly devitalized tissue should be removed at the time of initial wound treatment. The wound should be packed open to allow drainage.

Difficulty locating a foreign body such as a needle, BB, or radiopaque substance is common, and x-ray localization may be helpful. A radiopaque marker placed either on the skin or in the open wound can help locate the object as it relates to this marker. If location of the object continues to be difficult, fluoroscopy may be helpful. After removal of the object, x-rays are generally not indicated, particularly if it can be determined that the entire foreign body has been removed. Certain wounds require special mentioning. Patients who step on needles that break off within their foot should have the needle removed. If there is thread hanging from the foot, this should not be pulled, as the needle may be lost (under the thick callous of the foot). If a small incision is made next to the thread, the needle can be grasped and easily removed. The eye of the needle should be inspected once it is removed, as a residual piece of needle can serve as an irritant. Frequently the needle may go through the foot in a heavily calloused area, causing minimal bleeding without an obvious wound. If the patient is certain he or she has stepped on a needle and a wound is not obvious, an x-ray should be obtained. A radiopaque marker over the area of tenderness on the foot may be helpful. Larger foreign bodies that may penetrate a major body cavity should only be removed in the operating room under direct visualization. A small foreign body in the soft tissues of the extremities may be removed under direct visualization in the outpatient setting. One must pay careful attention to the proximity of important neurovascular structures, so that these are not further damaged during the removal of the foreign body. If hemorrhage does occur, direct local pressure should be applied to the vessel. Clamps should not be applied until one can ascertain the nature of the bleeding and the size of the vessel from which the hemorrhage is occurring. Applying clamps to minimally injured major arteries can cause further injury and difficulty in suturing the vessel.

Fishhooks with barbs require special consideration. To properly remove the fishhook, the barb should be advanced through the skin, cut off with a wire cutter, and the remainder of the fishhook should be withdrawn through the original entrance site.

Puncture wounds by nails in the feet should be carefully debrided to prevent a subdermal abscess. As the dirty nail punctures the shoe and the callous of the foot, it deposits dirt on the outside of the callous, but as it is withdrawn from the foot, it deposits a layer of debris just beneath the callous. These wounds can be adequately debrided by picking up the corners of the wound with a small forceps and cutting off the corners of the wound with a #11 scalpel.

Common Benign Skin Lesions

Patients frequently have small skin lesions they wish removed. The most common are small papillomas, or skin tags, attached to the skin by a narrow base. These are viral in etiology and usually occur around the neck or underneath the breast or arms, where the skin is warm and moist. The small papillomas may be treated effectively by cauterizing the very tip of the lesion without local anesthesia. If the lesion is large, it is advantageous to inject local anesthesia into the base of the lesion. These lesions may also be removed by snipping them off at the base, followed by cauterization at the base after excision.

Warts, particularly plantar warts, aggravate patients. The amount of keratin and dense callous covering the wart should be removed with a scalpel to expose the base of the wart. The softer base can then be cauterized, and the wart will generally fall off. The patient should be advised to return if any wart tissue remains. Repeat treatment early will improve the success rate. Other remedies, such as salicylic acid pads and liquid nitrogen, are also appropriate means of treatment. The salicylic acid pads are cut to the size of the wart and taped in place directly over the wart. Liquid nitrogen is touched directly to the lesion. Podophyllin, although very effective on venereal warts, is not generally effective on plantar warts. It may be effective on softer warts on the hand. It is important to surround the wart with Vaseline® so that the podophyllin does not burn the surrounding normal skin. The podophyllin is then placed on the wart and allowed to dry. The patient can be given a small amount of podophyllin to use in this same fashion if the wart does not disappear with one treatment. Generally, treating the wart every three to four days is adequate.

Sebaceous cysts are commonly identified by the patient as a small lump appearing beneath the skin. Frequently the patient's real concern is whether this lump could be cancer. A sebaceous cyst can be identified by the pore where the cyst started. Sebaceous cysts should generally be removed electively, as they frequently become secondarily infected. The skin incision should be made along the naturally occurring anatomic lines to leave a minimal cosmetic scar. An elipse should be made around the cyst pore. The cyst should be gently dissected from the surrounding tissue. The cyst will generally pop out quite easily if dissection is carried out beside the plane on the white, outer capsule of the cyst. The skin incision should be made to the level of the cyst capsule, otherwise excision will be difficult. This is particularly true on the back, where the skin is very thick (the entire cyst capsule should be excised). The wound should be irrigated with saline and then closed. On the back, the suture should be left in for two weeks.

If the cyst has become tender and is somewhat reddened, then secondary infection is suspected. The appropriate treatment for an infected cyst is drainage. Antibiotics without drainage are not beneficial, as the cyst will not be penetrated. If untreated, chronic inflammation will eventually result. The cyst will continue to smoulder along ultimately draining spontaneously. This usually results in additional discomfort for the patient and a poor cosmetic result. The cyst can generally be incised and drained by quickly puncturing it with the point of a #11 scalpel. The cyst material can be expressed by pressing along the edges of the in-

flamed area. This will evacuate the debris within the cyst, allowing the cyst to close and heal. This generally is done without local anesthesia. Local anesthesia may not be effective in inflamed, infected areas. Local anesthetics are pH specific and are not active in the acid medium of an infected wound. Also, blood flow is increased in this area. The local anesthetic may be carried away too quickly to be effective. Patient education in this area may allay any misunderstandings or reservations. The wounds should be loosely packed. The patient should be instructed so that the edges of the wound remain open until drainage has ceased. The cyst may be excised one month to six weeks later, when the inflammation has subsided. Systemic antibiotics are usually unnecessary.

Subcutaneous Lesions

The majority of subcutaneous lesions are lipomas. They are freely movable, are deep to the skin, and therefore will not move when the skin is moved over them. If they move with skin motion, then they are either a sebaceous cyst or a dermatofibroma. Usually lipomas are diagnosed clinically. Many patients wish them removed because of local pain. A small incision should be made along skin lines down to the capsule of the lipoma. The lipoma then can be freed by blunt dissection and is easily removed through the wound. The incision only has to be the width of the smallest diameter of the lipoma. If the lipoma is very large, a small incision can still generally be made. The lipoma can be broken up and removed through the small incision. Larger lipomas or lipomas in anatomic areas adjacent to important anatomic structures may require surgical expertise.

Minor Injuries and Infections of the Digits

Hands frequently are the recipients of minor trauma. These injuries frequently can be cared for by the general physician. One common injury is a subungual hematoma, which occurs when the patient slams a finger in a door or window. Care must be taken to evaluate these patients for underlying boney injury. A black spot will develop underneath the fingernail. These injuries are extremely painful and should be drained. A simple method is to straighten a paper clip. The end should be heated in a flame until it is red hot. The red hot end of the paper clip is touched to the middle of the nail directly over the hematoma. It will burn quickly through the nail and the blood will drain. The clip may need to be reheated to puncture the nail. Once the blood is drained, the patient will experience immediate relief. If an open flame is not allowed, a small drill used specifically for this purpose may be available. If neither the hot paper clip nor the small drill is available, local anesthesia is administered and the nail is drilled with a needle. A digital nerve block is usually satisfactory.

The digital vessels run in a line along the top of the

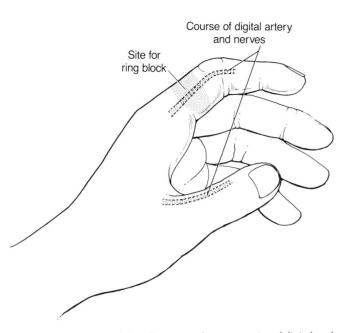

Site for
ring block

Course of digital artery
and nerves

Figure 11.1. Course of digital artery and nerves as site of digital and ring nerve block.

interphalangeal creases (Fig. 11.1). By injecting approximately 0.5 cc of 2% Xylocaine® anesthesia just beneath the skin, the digital bundle will be anesthetized. This must be done on both sides of the finger. A digital block will give good anesthesia distal to the midfinger. If anesthesia is required in an area near the proximal interphalangeal joint, a ring block may be performed. A ring block is done by injecting local anesthetic around the circumference of the finger. Care must be taken not to overdistend the tissue or the block can produce a tourniquet effect on the finger. The needle is placed in the same area as the digital bundle and then is advanced anteriorly beneath the skin as a wheel of local anesthesia is injected. The posterior half of the finger is injected similarly (Fig. 11.1).

Avulsion of the very distal end of the fingertip not to the level of the bone is another common traumatic problem. The majority of these need only be dressed with antiseptic dressings and a light pressure bandage. The wound should be cleaned and debrided as previously discussed. The dressings should be changed daily. If the top of the bony phalanx is not exposed, this is adequate treatment. If the tip of the phalanx is exposed, then it may need to be shortened with a small bone rongeur so that the skin can close over the tip of the finger easily. Reimplantation distally is generally not indicated. The patient who has a specific need for sensitivity at the end of the finger should be referred to a hand surgeon.

Avulsion of fingernails is also a common minor traumatic injury. If the fingernail is completely avulsed, a protective dressing should be placed over the nailbed. The nailbed should be repaired if injured. There are small protective devices that can be taped on by the patient until the nail regenerates. (The nail, if present, may serve to protect the distal phalanx after it is cleaned and replaced in its normal position.) As long

as the nail matrix at the base of the nail has not been disturbed, the nail will regenerate. If the nail is only partially avulsed, the nailbed should be carefully examined to see that it is intact. If the nailbed is not intact, it should be sutured so that it can heal and be flat. The nail may be replaced as a dressing. With a cutting needle, the parts of the nail can be sutured together again to serve as a protective dressing. The new nail will push out the old nail. The nail can be lifted off once it has loosened. (Anatomic repair of the nailbed is necessary to provide a functional distal phalanx as well as one that is not exquisitively sensitive.)

Frequently patients have rings on their fingers when injured, which produce constriction. Occasionally the ring cannot be removed manually and must be removed by cutting the shank of the ring. There are ring cutters in essentially every emergency room for this purpose. Permission from the patient is necessary to do this, as the repair of these rings may be difficult or impossible. Compressing the edematous area over the proximal interphalangeal joint may be of benefit in ring removal. This can be done by passing an ''O'' silk beneath the ring, then wrapping the silk tightly around the finger toward the tip of the finger. This compresses the tissue around the interphalangeal joint and the ring can be pushed over the compressed area. If this does not work, then the ring must be cut off. Unless the patient is inordinately cooperative, is willing to keep the hand elevated, use ice on the hand, and return if there is progressive swelling or numbness in the finger, it is very dangerous to leave a constricting band around any digit.

Two common infections of the fingernails are paronychia and felons. A paronychia is an infection just at the base of the nail, which is usually caused by infection occurring beneath the cuticle. If only slight erythema and tenderness is present, the infection can be treated by elevating the cuticle from the nail. If there is already a small abscess, the abscess should be incised and drained. If the abscess has extended beneath the base of the nail, then the nail may require drainage beneath the nail. The infection at the base of the nail has generally loosened it so that a drain can be inserted or a window made in the nail to facilitate drainage. These wounds should be treated with gauze dressings so that they do not reaccumulate pus. Systemic antibiotics are reserved for those at increased risk for infection.

The felon is an infection of the pulp of the nailbed. The etiology is usually from a puncture wound with a contaminated instrument, such as occurs in young mothers who are changing diapers and stick their fingers with diaper pins. Once the fingerpad is red, tender, and swollen, it is infected and requires drainage. Antibiotics alone are insufficient. A digital block is usually required. The incision should be made laterally and extend beneath the tuft of the finger on either side to adequately drain all of the little pulp spaces. The larger abscesses require placing a small drain through and beneath the tuft of the finger, leaving it in place for 48 hours. Warm soaks and dressing changes then follow until the process resolves. These are inordinately painful infections and delay in diagnosis increases the risk of osteomyelitis of the finger tuft.

The most common problem seen in toes requiring care by the general physician is ingrown toenails. If the ingrown toenails exhibit erythema and are tender at the corner, they may be treated by making a V in the nail back to the level of the nailbed and placing cotton under the corners of the nail. The nail should then be allowed to grow out beyond the end of the toe and should be cut straight across so that it does not continue to pierce the skin. If the nail is already deeply embedded, with an abscess at the corner of the nail, then the lateral edge of the nail must be removed. A digital block can be carried out in the toe, just as in the finger. The edge of the toenail is removed from the abscess by grasping it with a heavy clamp, such as a small Kocher clamp, and cutting the nail down to the corner of the nailbed with sharp scissors. The corner of the nailbed should then be curetted so that the lateral aspect of the nail does not grow again. Wet-to-dry dressings can be used until this heals. If the nail is very thick and deeply embedded, the entire nail should be removed. The base of the nail should be curetted, and the patient should be informed that the nail will not regrow. Usually this very deep difficult toenail is caused by chronic fungal infection. Fungal infections, if treated early, can be eradicated. Occasionally a very local area of fungal infection can be treated by just applying nailpolish regularly to that area until the nail grows out. Keeping the nails from being chronically moist is also helpful in preventing recurrence. Chronic fungal infection requires the application of dilute potassium permanganate solution. A teaspoon of potassium permanganate crystals in a quart of water is sufficient. The toes are soaked in this solution daily for about 15–20 minutes, washed, and dried. The solution is poisonous and should be kept out of the reach of children. Generally treatment requires a month to 6 weeks. The toes will have a purple discoloration from the potassium permanganate. Topical 5-fluorouracil is also useful and is applied regularly until the toenail has grown out. It is rarely necessary to treat the patient with systemic antifungal agents, as the risk of the toxicity and the cost of the treatment are generally not warranted by the nature of the disease. In doing anything to the feet or the toenails, one must be very careful to ensure that the patient does not have vascular disease or diabetes mellitus. The patient who has vascular disease should be referred to a vascular surgeon or someone who has experience in the treatment of diabetic or ischemic feet.

SUGGESTED READING

Committee on Trauma. American College of Surgeons: *A Guide to the Initial Therapy of Soft Tissue Wounds.* Chicago, June, 1983.

Study Questions

1. Describe the management of
   A. A 4-cm laceration from a knife to the left cheek, 30 minutes old
   B. An avulsion injury with a stellate laceration to the dorsal aspect of the left forearm, 1 hour old
   C. A puncture wound to the left calf from a pitch fork, 1½ hours old
   D. A dog bite causing a 1-cm laceration of a child's cheek

2. Describe in detail the management of a classmate who slices the tip of his left index finger, removing 4 mm of the distal tip in the anatomy laboratory.

3. Discuss the management of multiple abrasions in a 3-year-old unimmunized child after a tricycle accident.

4. Differentiate between a paronychia and a felon and the management of each.

12

Surgical Infections

Richard N. Garrison, M.D.
Donald E. Fry, M.D.
Louis F. Martin, M.D.
John Mihran Davis, M.D.

ASSUMPTIONS

The student understands the basic categories of bacteria and their pathologic potential in humans.

The student understands the general classes of antibiotics, indications for use, and common complications of each.

OBJECTIVES

1. List the factors that contribute to infection after a surgical procedure.
2. List the types of surgical infections.
3. Describe the diagnostic features and indicated treatment for common skin infections.
4. Discuss four common hand infections and describe the treatment for each.
5. Describe the clinical features and treatment of anaerobic and synergistic gangrene.
6. List the causes of postoperative fever and discuss the diagnostic steps for evaluation.
7. Describe the indication and method for providing routine and reverse isolation.
8. Describe the diagnostic evaluation for an intraabdominal abscess.
9. Identify the antibiotic of choice for acute cholecystitis, perforated sigmoid diverticulitis, empyema of the lung, and a vascular graft infection.
10. Describe principles of prophylactic antibiotic use.

Pathogenesis of Infection

Planned surgical procedures, traumatic injury, and nontraumatic local invasion can each result in a severe bacterial insult. Regardless of the anatomic site, bacterial soilage of host tissues initiates well-defined processes of host defense to combat the microorganisms. Potent mediators of the inflammatory response (e.g., kinins, histamine) are released that alter capillary permeability in the area of injury and contamination. Plasma proteins then permeate the area of contamina-

tion as the inflammatory process evolves. Complement, fibrinogen, and specific or nonspecific opsonins are delivered into the area of the bacterial invaders. Circulating neutrophils then "marginate" at the site of vascular permeability alteration and move by the process of diapedesis out of the intravascular compartment and into the interstitium. Neutrophil movements are directed toward the site of contaminations by chemoattractants, with the cleavage products of activated complement being the most potent. Neutrophils subsequently make contact with the foreign particles or bacteria. Opsonins previously bound to the foreign particle facilitate the adherence to the neutrophil plasma membrane, and phagocytosis is initiated. The engulfed organism or foreign particle is then surrounded within the phagosome and intracellular killing and digestion are started by the release of lysosomal enzymes, hydrolases, superoxide compounds, and other enzymes. Ingestion of microorganisms in excess of the ability of the phagocyte to achieve intracellular killing will result in death and dissolution of the phagocytic cell. Dead phagocytic cells, fibrin, and densities of microorganisms become the essential components of pus. Thus the primary determinant of infection for a given level of contamination, whether the consequence of trauma or surgical incision, is the density of bacteria present versus the efficiency and effectiveness of the host in disposing of the organisms.

Numerous adjuvants affect either bacterial virulence or cellular host response and thus may alter the host-pathogen interaction in favor of the bacteria. Hemoglobin has been repeatedly shown to potentiate bacterial virulence. Ferric iron may enhance bacterial growth, and hemoglobin may alter the efficiency of the neutrophil in eradication of the microorganism. Regardless of the cause, hemoglobin facilitates the infection over the host, so it is advisable to rid the wound of blood before closure.

Dead tissue and foreign bodies are likewise potent adjuvants. Dead tissue is not readily penetrated by host defense mechanisms and serves as a haven for bacterial proliferation. Foreign bodies in surgery are numerous,

121

and whether they are suture material in the surgical wound, Foley catheters in the urinary bladder, or intravenous cannulae, they provide protection for bacteria against the host response.

Systemic factors such as shock, hypovolemia, and hypoxia work to the detriment of host defense. Hemorrhagic shock results in tissue hypoperfusion and thus increases septic complications in patients with traumatic injury or emergent surgical procedures. Oxygen is an essential metabolic component of phagocytosis and intracellular killing. Inadequate oxygenation at the site of contamination significantly enhances the likelihood of subsequent infection.

Other coexisting systemic problems with the host may also prove deleterious. Diabetics have impaired neutrophil mobility. Obesity facilitates local wound infection, presumably because of the poor blood supply of adipose tissue. Starvation with protein-calorie malnutrition renders the host more vulnerable to infection. Acute and chronic alcoholism impairs the host response and has implications for both emergent and elective surgical procedures. Systemic drug therapy with corticosteroids or cancer chemotherapeutic agents is well established for rendering the host vulnerable to invasive infection.

In summary, the interaction between the pathogen and the host determines whether contamination has no sequelae or whether clinical infection is the result. Numerous local and systemic variables swing the biologic ''balance of power'' in favor of the bacterial invaders. The objective of surgical therapy is to reduce the bacterial concentration and alter the tissue environment so that supremacy of the host defense is established.

Prevention of Surgical Infection

The prevention of infections in patients with traumatic injury or in those patients undergoing elective procedures is essential for quality surgical care. Traumatic injuries of the soft tissue have numerous local adjuvant factors that must be managed mechanically to avoid infection. Debridement of nonviable tissue, copious irrigation to remove bacteria-laden clot and fibrin, and meticulous removal of dirt and other foreign bodies are mandatory. Closure of the wound can then

be undertaken with a reasonable prospect for uncomplicated healing. In multiple trauma, restoration of systemic oxygenation and tissue perfusion are important for numerous reasons, of which prevention of infection is one.

Surgical wounds are at different degrees of risk for infection. Infection in these wounds is primarily a consequence of contamination and adjuvant factors that are present in the wound at the time of closure. Recognition of these different degrees of risk has resulted in several classification schemes to allow stratification of similar operations. Only when operative wounds at similar risk are examined can the impact of different preventive measures be assessed. The classification system most commonly used for surgical wounds is listed in Table 12.1.

In clean procedures, surgical asepsis is of paramount significance in the prevention of operative site infection. The frequency of clean wound infections is the most sensitive indicator and surveillance tool to judge overall sterile technique in the operating room. Preoperative hospitalization should be limited to avoid colonization of the patient with resistant, hospital bacteria. Preoperative showers with specific cleansing of the proposed operative site is useful. Hair removal with either a razor or mechanical clippers should not be performed the night prior to operations, because small nicks and cuts are colonized overnight and increase clean infection rates. Depilatory creams, however, may be used the evening prior to operation. Otherwise, hair removal is performed immediately prior to the procedure in the operating room. Adhesive plastic skin drapes have been advocated to reduce infection rates but actually increase clean wound rates of infection. Reducing the operative time is associated with a lower wound infection rate. Operations lasting more than 2 hours have a 40% greater infection rate than those lasting less than 1 hour.

Intraoperative efforts should be designed to minimize the introduction of bacteria but should also be focused on the reduction of adjuvant factors. Hemostasis is important, but it is also important to minimize the excessive use of suture material and the indiscriminate use of electrocautery that may leave large areas of devitalized tissue. Wound drains are seldom indi-

Table 12.1
Classification of Surgical Wounds

Wound	Bacterial Contaminants	Source of Contamination	Infection Frequency	Examples
Clean	Gram positive	OR environment, surgical team, patient's skin	3%	Inguinal hernia, thyroidectomy, mastectomy
Clean-contaminated	Polymicrobial	Endogenous colonization of the patient	5–15%	Common duct exploration, elective colon resection, gastrectomy for carcinoma
Contaminated	Polymicrobial	Gross contamination	15–40%	''Spill'' during elective GI surgery, perforated gastric ulcer
Dirty	Polymicrobial	Established infection	40%	Drainage of intraabdominal abscess, resection of infarcted intestine

cated and should be closed-suctioned drains when used. Drains should not exit through the surgical wound but rather should have a separate stab wound to exit the subcutaneous space. The purpose of drains is to remove the adjuvant material, such as blood; they should only be used when they are actively removing debris or fluid. They are a two-way street; a drain that is not functioning may allow bacteria into the area that is being drained. At the time of closure of the wound, the patient's fate is sealed with respect to wound infection. The postoperative dressing is generally used but probably serves no purpose with respect to the prevention of wound infection after the first few hours.

Although most surgical infections stem directly from the patient's own endogenous microflora and the degree of contamination present at the time of the procedure, the operating room environment does contribute to wound infections. Personnel (surgeons, anesthetists, nurses, and students) are the most common source of bacterial contamination in this setting. Bacteria-laden droplets from respiration and mouth secretions, along with the bacteria shed from exposed skin and hair, are a measurable threat to clean incisions. Operating room attire, with clean operating room clothes, head covers, masks, and shoe covers, is designed to minimize this source of contamination. To prevent contamination of the wound or operative field by direct body contact from operating room personnel, two other methods are employed. Scrubbing of the hands and arms with an antiseptic solution and the donning of sterile gowns and gloves are the last barriers used to prevent contamination. When infections occur following clean operative procedures, a break in this routine should be suspected. The techniques of scrubbing and sterility (described in Chapter 4) should be utilized for all procedures done within the operating room.

Several very expensive devices have been advocated for the prevention of wound infection. Ultraviolet irradiation of the operating room and laminar flow air-handling devices have both had their advocates. They can only be expected to reduce infection rates in those operations where the contaminant is secondary to airborne organisms. Controlled prospective data to support the use of these devices are presently not available.

Perioperative Antibiotics

Since the introduction of antibiotics in the 1940s, these drugs have been used to prevent infection in patients undergoing elective operations. Early efforts to document the effectiveness of antibiotics failed because cases were not classified by risk and the timing of antibiotic administration was not controlled.

Experimental studies have shown that antibiotics must be present in the tissue at the time of bacterial contamination if the natural history of soft tissue infection is to be altered. Antibiotics given after the contamination has occurred are not effective. Clinical studies during the last 15 years have documented the effectiveness of preoperative systemic antibiotics. The important issues in surgical prophylaxis with antibiotics, regardless of the clinical setting, are to give the drug preoperatively and to select a drug with activity against anticipated pathogens. Long half-life antibiotics (e.g., cefazolin: half-life = 2 hours) are preferable to short half-life drugs (e.g., cephalothin: half-life = 30–40 minutes). The most commonly used regimen is cefazolin 1 hour preoperatively and 6 hours later.

Because elective colon surgery has been associated with wound infection rates of 30–50%, it has been a special area for antibiotic utilization for prophylaxis. Orally administered, poorly absorbed antibiotics will reduce the numbers of aerobic and anaerobic species

Table 12.2.
Antibiotic Selections for Common Infections

Infection Site	Anticipated Organism	Antibiotic Choice
Soft tissue cellulitis	Group A *Streptococcus, Staphylococcus*	Nafcillin/oxacillin
Breast abscess	*Staphylococcus*	*Nafcillin/oxacillin*
Synthetic vascular graft	Usually *Staphylococcus*	Nafcillin/oxacillin
Hip prosthesis		
Heart/valve prosthesis	*Staphylococcus, Streptococcus Viridans, Enterococcus,* etc.	Specific sensitivity needed
Biliary tract infection	*E. coli, Klebsiella, Enterococcus* [a]	Cefazolin
Peritonitis; Intraabdominal abscess	*E. coli,* other Enterobacteriaceae, *B. fragilis,* other obligate aerobes	Clindamycin/aminoglycoside, metronidazole/aminoglycoside, third-generation cephalosporin [b]
Hospital-acquired pneumonia	*Pseudomonas, Serratia,* resistant Enterobacteriacea	Amikacin (and/or expanded spectrum penicillin)
Catheter-associated bacteremia	*Staphylococcus,* Enterobacteriaceae	Specific sensitivities (beware methicillin-resistant *S. epidermidis*)
Urinary tract (postcatheterization)	*Pseudomonas, Serratia,* Enterobacteriaceae	Specific sensitivity
Candidiasis	*Candida*	Amphotericin
Pneumocystosis	*Pneumocystis carinii*	Trimethoprim/sulfamethoxazole

[a] *Enterococcus* is not specifically covered primarily in either the biliary tract or in intraabdominal infection. Consideration for treatment should be given when the *Enterococcus* emerges as a secondary pathogen or when isolated in blood culture.
[b] Includes cefotaxime, cefoperazone, moxalactam, ceftizoxime, ceftriaxone.

that reside in the bowel and ultimately contaminate the surgical wound during colon resection. If the common colonic organisms are known, the types of antibiotics that are most likely to be beneficial can be determined. Oral antibiotics have been shown to be effective in reducing wound infection rates to less than 10% for elective colon resections. Oral neomycin and erythromycin base have been the antibiotics most commonly used, along with a mechanical bowel preparation. Whether systemic antibiotics for prophylaxis are equal to preoperative oral neomycin-erythromycin base or whether the two methods together are superior to either used individually, remains controversial.

When dealing with contaminated wounds or dirty procedures, the risk of a wound infection exceeds 15–20%. Therefore, many surgeons will close only the fascial layers, with the skin and subcutaneous tissues left open. The open wound can then be managed with wet-to-dry saline dressings and may be closed by delayed primary closure on postoperative day 4 or 5. Small open wounds rarely become infected when the underlying tissue is viable, although the wound surface may become colonized. Prolonged postoperative systemic antibiotics will not facilitate the process of delayed primary closure.

Management of Established Infection

For the purpose of organization, established surgical infections are divided into community-acquired infections and postoperative (nosocomial) infections. Community-acquired infection refers to all active processes that were initiated prior to presentation of the patient for treatment. Postoperative infections include all that occur after surgical procedures. Thus peritonitis is usually a community-acquired infection, but intraperitoneal abscess is most commonly a postoperative

problem. Potential choices for antibiotic selection for each type of infection are indicated in Table 12.2.

Community-Acquired Infections

Skin–skin Structure Infections. Soft tissue infection, usually following a minor cut or puncture, ordinarily presents with spreading cellulitis. The blanching erythema of cellulitis is usually group A streptococci and responds to penicillin therapy. Staphylococci may also be the culprit of cellulitis, particularly if gross suppuration (pus) is present at the injury site.

Necrotizing streptococcal gangrene may rarely be seen in these patients. These infections are characterized by nonblanching erythema with blisters and frank necrosis of the skin. The nonblanching erythema indicates the subdermal thrombosis of the nutrient blood supply of the skin. Extensive surgical debridement of the affected area in combination with high-dose penicillin is the treatment of choice. A gram stain of blister fluid will be useful in differentiating this infection from other necrotizing infections of the skin and subcutaneous tissue.

Severe staphylococcal soft tissue infections are usually readily identified by the gram stain of the pus. Nafcillin and oxacillin are first-line antibiotics to be used in addition to surgical drainage and debridement of the primary focus of infection. Because staphylococci are readily passed to other patients by health care personnel or by objects passed between patients, it may be desirable to place these patients in isolation.

Isolation is commonly applied to bacterial (e.g., staphylococcal) infections or selected viral infections (e.g., hepatitis) to prevent the organism being carried out of the quarantined room where the patient is kept. Gowns and gloves are worn and then removed upon leaving the patient's room, and traffic into the patient's room is restricted. The objective is to prevent nurses

Table 12.3.
Common Soft Tissue Infections

	Etiology	Usual Organism	Physical Findings	Treatment
Cellulitis	Break skin barrier	*Streptococcus*	Diffuse nonblanching erythema, tenderness	Systemic antibiotics usually, local wound cleansing
Furuncle, carbuncle	Bacterial growth within skin glands and crypts	*Staphylococcus*	Localized induration, erythema, tenderness, swelling, creamy pus formation	I + D; systemic antibiotics for carbuncle
Hidradenitis suppurativa	Bacterial growth within apocrine sweat glands	*Staphylococcus*	Multiple abscesses; drainage; thick pus from axilla, groin regions	I + D small lesions; wide debridement; excision and grafting, large areas
Lymphangitis	Infection within lymphatics 2° to distal infection	*Streptococcus*	Swelling and erythema distal extremity, inflamed streaks along involved lymphatic channels	Local wound cleansing, removal of any foreign body, systemic antibiotics
Gangrene	Destruction of healthy tissue by virulent microbial enzymes	Synergistic *Streptococcus/Staphylococcus*, mixed aerobic-anaerobic organisms, *Clostridium perfringens*	Necrotic skin/fascia, extremity swelling, grayish liquid discharge, crepitation/gas formation within tissue planes	Radical debridement of all involved tissues, parenteral antibiotics

galactocele = retention cyst caused by occlusion of a lactiferous duct.

and physicians from serving as vectors in transmission of the organism to others. Isolation is contrasted with reverse isolation, where the objective is to prevent pathogens being introduced into contact with severely immunosuppressed patients. In the latter circumstance, masks may be desirable for persons attending these patients to prevent airborne organisms being introduced into the controlled environment. Common soft tissue infections are outlined in Table 12.3.

Breast Abscess → staphylococcus

A particularly important staphylococcal soft tissue infection is the breast abscess. Postpartum women with galactoceles are particularly at risk for this infection. These abscesses are characterized by localized pain, swelling, and redness associated with a mass that may or may not be fluctuant. If suspicious but not sure, aspirate with a 19-gauge needle. These abscesses must be recognized (severe tenderness and fluctuance) and must be drained. Antibiotics alone will not suffice. A delay in drainage awaiting unrealistic results from antibiotics may risk subcutaneous necrosis of large amounts of the patient's breast tissue.

Perirectal Abscess

Another commonly encountered cutaneous infection is the perirectal abscess. These abscesses result from infection within the crypts of the anorectal canal that subsequently suppurate and are identified as tender masses in the perianal area. Because both perirectal and breast abscesses are exquisitely tender, they usually need to be drained under general anesthesia. Antibiotics for the perirectal abscess patient are usually broad spectrum for both anaerobes and aerobes but are probably only necessary to protect the patient from the bacteremia associated with the drainage process.

Gas Gangrene

Clostridial soft tissue infections usually include both cellulitis and myonecrosis. This combination is usually referred to as gas gangrene. These infections commonly follow soft tissue wounds with contaminated objects. These infections commonly have a brown, watery drainage from the wound site and are associated with marked tenderness about the wound. Palpable crepitance is commonly present but may be quite subtle when the myonecrosis extends along the subfascial plane. Roentgenograms may be necessary to demonstrate the soft tissue gas in selected cases.

Prevention is achievable for most patients at risk for clostridial myonecrosis or cellulitis with tetanus toxoid immunization along with adequate surgical debridement without primary wound closure. Tetanus antitoxin may be administered to selected patients with high-risk wounds who have an uncertain history of prior immunization. When clostridial gas gangrene is diagnosed, immediate and radical surgical debridement is necessary to achieve survival. Massive doses of penicillin are necessary for killing the organism,

Clostridium perfringens, but will not be useful in the absence of aggressive debridement of the affected tissue.

Tetanus

Tetanus (lockjaw) is caused by the exotoxin produced by the organism *Clostridium tetani.* After an incubation period of from two days to several weeks, a prodromal symptom complex of restlessness, headache, stiffness of the jaw muscles, and muscular contractions in the area of the wound evolves. Violent generalized tonic muscle spasms usually follow within 24 hours, resulting in respiratory arrest in untreated cases. The keystone in management of these patients is prevention by debridement and cleansing of all wounds where devitalized, contaminated tissue is present, along with a program of immunization. All patients with traumatic wounds should receive intramuscular injection of tetanus toxoid, and those who have not been immunized within the past 10 years should receive additional therapy with tetanus immune globulin (human). The use of systemic antibiotics specific for *Clostridia* species should be considered for all tetanus-prone wounds.

Hand Infections

Hand infections are relatively common and are outlined in Table 12.4. Although not life-threatening, severe morbidity in the loss of function of the hand can occur. The paronychia is usually a staphylococcal infection of the proximal fingernail that ordinarily ''points'' in the sulcus at the nail border. Simple drainage and hot soaks are usually sufficient for these infections. Felons occur as deep infections of the pulp space of the terminal phalanx. These usually occur after penetrating injuries of the distal phalanx and are treated by drainage. Subungual abscess represents the extension of a deep paronychia that can be identified by fluctuance beneath the nail. Removal of the nail is usually necessary to effect adequate drainage of these infections. Neglected infections of the fingers may result in tenosynovitis. This represents infection that extends along the tendon sheath of the finger. Drainage requires opening of the sheath along its entire length to prevent the necrosis of the tendon with its functional implications. Finally, human bites of the hand are quite common but should not be underestimated in terms of their potential infectious nature. Such infections are commonly due to contamination by polymicrobial mouth flora. Deep-space infections, including tenosynovitis, may be consequences of these bites. Copious irrigation and debridement are required initially to prevent the infection. Human bites may be the only penetrating injury of the hand where primary closure is not employed.

Biliary Tract Infections

Biliary tract infections are usually a consequence of obstruction within the biliary tree, involving either the cystic or the common bile duct. The bacteria likely to

Table 12.4.
Common Hand Infections

	Location	Signs	Treatment
Felon	Pulp space of digits	Swollen, indurated, tense, throbbing distal finger; point tenderness	I + D the length of phalanx along side of finger
Paronychia	Skin over mantle of nail and lateral nail folds	Swelling/induration of nail folds, point tenderness, purulent drainage	I + D at base of nail, removal of nail if infection beneath
Tenosynovitis	Tendon sheath	Throbbing, pain with movement, entire finger swollen, tenderness over sheath, finger held semiflexed	I + D entire length of sheath and bursa; systemic antibiotics usually indicated
Fascial space	Spaces of the hand/thenar regions	Tenderness of involved space, swelling over region involved, limited motion	I + D along surface lines of projection; systemic antiotics indicated
Human bites	Point of skin penetration and underlying regions	Injury site wound, induration and swelling, purulent drainage, limited motion	Wide debridement and irrigation; systemic antibiotics and tetanus immunization indicated

be involved include *Escherichia coli,* *Klebsiella* species, and the enterococci. Anaerobes are not commonly encountered. Antibiotics to cover these anticipated organisms are usually employed, but surgical intervention in the biliary tract is often necessary for effective drainage and resolution.

Acute cholecystitis is the most common inflammatory process in the biliary tract. Acute cholecystitis is initially a nonspecific inflammatory process that begins secondary to obstruction of the cystic duct. Entrapped bacteria may give an invasive infectious character to the process, although early cholecystitis may not have culturable bacteria within the gallbladder lumen.

With acute cholecystitis, several potential outcomes may occur. The stone obstruction may be dispelled into the common duct (with the sequelae discussed in detail in Chapter 19) or the stone may be dislodged back into the gallbladder with temporary resolution of the process. Empyema of the gallbladder occurs when infection in the gallbladder is undrained, eventually leading to a purulent distension and often severe systemic sepsis. Increased intraluminal pressure may eventually lead to perforation. The increased intraluminal pressure combined with invasive bacterial infection may embarrass the blood supply of the gallbladder, resulting in gangrene and perforation. Prevention of these complications of acute cholecystitis can best be achieved by early operation for these patients.

Infection proximal to a common duct obstruction results in ascending cholangitis. Patients present with fulminant fever, leukocytosis, and jaundice. These patients are usually quite toxic and frequently have hemodynamic instability. It is imperative that these individuals have prompt surgical intervention if mortality is to be avoided. At operation, or by percutaneous radiologic methods, the common duct must be drained, usually via a T tube.

Acute peritonitis. Acute peritonitis results when bacteria are present within the peritoneal cavity, usually following a mechanical perforation of a hollow viscus. Primary peritonitis may occur without a perforation but is a very uncommon event, usually seen in

alcoholics or the immunocompromised patient. The diagnosis of gram-negative peritonitis cannot be established without a laparotomy, since occult perforations far exceed the likelihood of primary peritonitis.

Peritonitis is diagnosed by the presentation of patients with acute abdominal pain, usually accompanied by fever and leukocytosis. Palpation of the abdomen usually demonstrates marked tenderness with rebound and may show a board-like rigidity. An upright chest roentgenogram will commonly demonstrate free air beneath the diaphragm from the perforated viscus.

Peritonitis is variable in severity among patients. Different segments of the intestine that may perforate have very different bacterial and chemical compositions and densities of microorganisms; therefore it is probably inappropriate to consider all these illnesses classified as peritonitis as a single disease entity.

Perforated gastroduodenal ulcers usually occur as precipitous events with acute abdominal pain. Approximately 80% will have free air on the upright chest film (Fig. 12.1). The patients may or may not have antecedent symptoms of peptic ulcer disease. In younger patients, the peritonitis may be of only a chemical nature with no bacteria culturable from the peritoneal cavity in the first 12 hours after the perforation. Bacterial peritonitis becomes increasingly severe when the perforation persists for longer than 12 hours. Operative repair of the perforation, usually with a definitive ulcer operation (e.g., vagotomy and pyloroplasty), is the treatment of choice (Chapter 16). Antibiotics for common gram-negative bacteria are usually employed but are of minimal benefit except in the elderly and achlorhydric patients or patients with delayed operation.

A perforated appendix is another common cause of peritonitis that usually starts as acute appendicitis. In the absence of an appropriate operation, perforation may occur after 24 hours of symptoms. (Patients usually have diffuse tenderness and generalized rebound tenderness.) Antibiotic therapy is directed against both aerobic (*E. coli*) and anaerobic (*Bacteroides fragilis*) enteric organisms. Treatment requires appendectomy and debridement of the right lower quadrant of the peritoneal cavity. When a localized abscess is identified, external

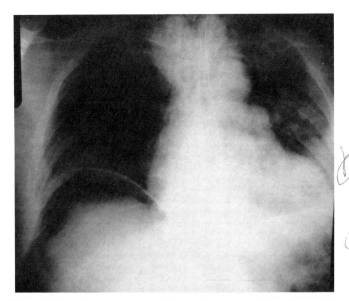

Figure 12.1. A large amount of free air is seen in this patient with a perforated duodenal ulcer of 12-hours duration.

drainage is indicated. External drainage is unnecessary and ineffective for diffuse peritoneal spillage.

Colonic perforations from either carcinoma or diverticular disease are the most virulent causes of peritonitis. Colonic microflora consist of high densities of both aerobic and anaerobic bacteria. Patients usually have marked peritoneal signs and will ordinarily be systemically toxic. After volume resuscitation and the initiation of broad-spectrum systemic antibiotics, operation is required for management of the perforation, drainage of pus, and debridement of nonviable tissue within the peritoneal cavity (Chapter 18). Left colon perforations usually require division of the fecal stream as part of their management because of the high frequency of anastomotic failure when primary repair is attempted.

Peritonitis can occur from other sources as well. It is important to appreciate that it is only necessary to be convinced that sufficient findings are present to justify celiotomy (a surgical abdomen). Exploration will define the specific diagnosis.

Hospital-Acquired Infections

The discussion of hospital-acquired infections in surgical patients is by definition a discussion of postoperative fever. The onset of fever usually heralds an evolving infectious problem and requires that the student of medicine understand the pathogenesis of fever and its many causes.

Fever is a consequence of the synthesis and release of the endogenous pyrogen, interleuken 1. Macrophages come into contact with foreign particles, usually bacteria, and this stimulates the synthesis of interleuken 1. Interleuken 1 is released into the inflammatory environment, is transported via the circulation, and by virtue of actions at the hypothalamus results in increased body temperature. This body temperature increase is attended by neutrophilia, hypoferremia, hypozincemia, hypercupremia, and the synthesis of acute-phase proteins by the liver (e.g., C-reactive protein). All acute responses mediated by interleuken 1 are adaptive responses mediated by the host to presumably bolster defenses against evolving infections.

To manage fever in surgical patients, the source of pathogen-macrophage interaction must be identified. Empirical use of antibiotics should not be a customary practice; the primary focus must be identified and then disrupted by mechanical means (e.g., drainage of infected sites).

Pulmonary Infection. Pulmonary infection in the postoperative patient may be from three pathologically distinct causes. First, nonrespirator-associated pneumonia results from atelectasis. Poor postoperative tidal volumes resulting from anesthesia, analgesia, and painful abdominal or thoracic incisions provoke collapse of small airways. Entrapped organisms plus alveolar macrophages result in fever usually within the first 48 hours after operation. Prevention and management of atelectasis require early ambulation, coughing, deep breathing, and even nasotracheal suctioning (in refractory cases) of postoperative patients. Intermittent positive-pressure breathing and various incentive spirometers represent expensive, and probably less effective, alternatives to the prevention and management of atelectasis. When a new fever and suspected atelectasis are present in the first 48 hours after surgery, laboratory and radiographic studies are usually unnecessary. If fever persists despite aggressive pulmonary chest physical therapy, the chest roentgenogram is often beneficial. When infiltrates are identified on chest roentgenograms, and leukocytosis evolves, then invasive infection has occurred and systemic antibiotics are warranted. Drug selection requires culture and sensitivity data. Organisms in this setting may be either gram positive or gram negative.

Second, postoperative pneumonitis may be respirator associated. Critically ill patients are very vulnerable to infection while on the ventilator. The lung has usually been assaulted by large volumes of intravenously administered fluids. The endotracheal tube represents a foreign body that injures tracheal mucosa and permits bacterial proliferation. The ventilator then serves as a reservoir to "shower" the vulnerable pulmonary tissues with multiresistant hospital microflora. Weaning the patient from the ventilator promptly is the most important preventive measure. When infection occurs, opportunistic gram-negative species (e.g., *Pseudomonas, Serratia*) predominate and usually require aminoglycosides for treatment. Pharmacokinetic dosing of the aminoglycoside will usually be necessary, and addition of a later generation of penicillin (e.g., ticarcillin, piperacillin) may achieve improved results because of presumed synergism of this combination.

Third, aspiration is an ever present risk in the postoperative patient. The patient at risk for aspiration will usually have gastric distension and altered mental status. Head-injured and elderly patients are particularly at risk. Gastric decompression will not totally obviate the risks of aspiration but will certainly reduce the probabilities. Once aspiration has occurred, bronchoscopy will be diagnostic and may also permit evacuation of particulate matter from the tracheobronchial tree. If hypoxemia is present after aspiration, bronchoscopy must be approached with caution lest cardiopulmonary arrest be provoked. Management of aspiration requires support of systemic oxygenation. Antibiotics should be withheld until clinical and culture evidence identifies an organism for specific therapy. Although many testimonials advocate the use of massive doses of corticosteroids for these patients, the management of severe aspiration is not a religious activity. Steroids are unproven, perturb stress metabolism, and are adversaries to normal host responses.

Urinary Tract Infection. Postoperative urinary tract infections are usually consequences of an antecedent indwelling Foley catheter. These catheters traumatize the bladder and urethral tissues and provide ready access for pathogens. To-and-fro movements of the catheter provide a "sump" effect to translocate catheter and urethral microorganisms into the bladder. Prevention requires aseptic placement of the catheter, firm fixation of the catheter after placement, maintenance of the closed drainage system, daily catheter care, and removal of the catheter when its specific purpose has been served. Systemic antibiotics will not prevent postoperative urinary tract infection but only modify the microflora that are potential pathogens.

The diagnosis of postoperative urinary tract infection has traditionally been the quantitative bacterial culture. When more than 100,000 organisms/ml of urine are identified, surgeons usually have the mistaken confidence that the source of postoperative fever has been located. The astute scholar of the surgical sciences must beware. Bacteriuria does not in itself indicate invasive urinary tract sepsis, and bacteriuria does not cause fever. Most positive cultures after Foley catheterization will clear with removal of the catheter and an adequate "flush" by a volume-induced diuresis. Systemic bacteremia from the urinary tract in surgical patients without functional or anatomic obstruction to urine flow is uncommon. Significant postoperative fever from the urinary tract is always a presumption, even with positive cultures. Constant surveillance for other sources of fever must be pursued.

Urinary infections that develop after catheterization will not be the usual urinary tract pathogens (e.g., *E. coli*). One can expect *Pseudomonas, Serratia,* and other resistant gram-negative organisms. Treatment almost always requires culture and sensitivity data. *Candida* and enterococci are being cultured from the urinary tract in more and more patients. Systemic treatment for these presumed urinary tract pathogens should be deferred in the absence of positive blood cultures.

Wound Infections. Wound infection and its prevention have been discussed. Postoperative fever should sensitize the clinician to look where "the hands of man" have been. The wound is always a prime suspect, especially when tenderness, redness, heat, or a mass effect are noted when inspecting the wound. The discharge of pus from the wound is definitive. The absence of a "healing ridge" in one portion of the incision is also a useful clinical sign of wound infection.

A wound infection requires the wound to be opened. Pus is evacuated, fibrin is debrided, and subcutaneous suture material is removed. Systemic antibiotics are not an alternative to drainage. Antibiotics are only necessary for those patients with severe or progressive cellulitis and for those patients with necrotizing infection. In the latter cases, frequent wound debridement is an essential component of management.

Intraabdominal Infection. Postoperative intraabdominal infection generally occurs in two settings. First, complications of elective gastrointestinal or biliary surgery may result in postoperative peritonitis or abscess. Major dehiscence of anastomoses is usually associated with florid sepsis, and reoperation for management of this complication is usually based on clinical criteria. Abdominal tenderness and pain, fever, leukocytosis, and the toxic septic state rather than roentgenograms, contrast studies, or other sophisticated diagnostic methods are the most important indicators of a need for reoperation. Patients who have had an initial laparotomy for infection or penetrating trauma will commonly have a degree of bacterial contamination that makes a subsequent abdominal abscess a frequent event. The majority of postoperative intraabdominal infectious complications are abscesses.

The diagnosis of intraabdominal abscess is quite difficult. Physical examination is markedly compromised by the painful abdominal incision of a prior procedure. Localized tenderness is only useful in about one-third

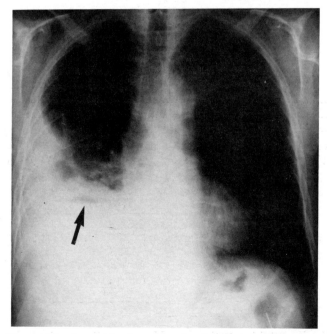

Figure 12.2 An upright chest x-ray showing an air-fluid level below the right hemidiaphragm and a reactive pleural effusion in a patient with a subphrenic abscess (**arrow**).

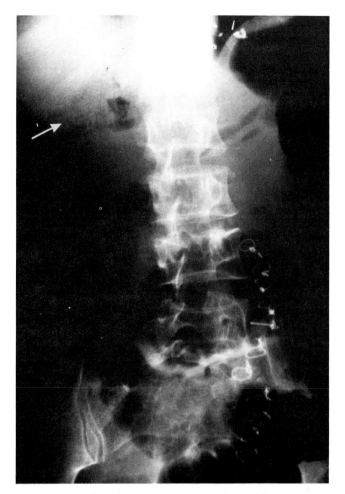

Figure 12.3. A plain abdominal film shows stippled free air (**arrow**) beneath the liver in a patient with a subhepatic abscess.

of patients, and palpable masses are of benefit in less than 10% of patients with abscess. The rectal examination continues to be a particularly valuable method when pelvic abscess is a concern.

Roentgenograms of the abdomen are helpful when positive findings are identified but are unfortunately not commonly present. The so-called "three-way" abdominal series (an upright chest film, upright abdominal film, and lateral decubitus film) is frequently ordered but is useful in less than 20% of patients (Figs. 12.2 and 12.3). Upper or lower gastrointestinal gastrographin studies may show filling defects or intestinal leaks (Fig. 12.4) but may be undesirable in patients who have had recent anastomoses constructed. Under fluoroscopic guidance, installation of water-soluble contrast agents through drain sites may also help identify undrained collections within the abdomen.

Ultrasound has been a popular diagnostic method used in identification of intraabdominal abscess. It is inexpensive, allows for immediate interpretation, and equipment can be taken to the bedside rather than having to transport critically ill patients to another area of the hospital for evaluation. However, the receiver surface must make direct contact with the skin of the abdomen. In patients with dressings, open wounds, and

stomas, the ultrasound may not give a complete examination. Anatomic detail is rather poor with ultrasound; and intestinal gas, as is commonly encountered in septic postoperative patients, will result in limited anatomic detail and outline of abscesses.

Gallium-67 scans have generated considerable interest as a diagnostic tool for the patient with a suspected abscess. Gallium-67 citrate is preferentially localized in areas of inflammation and theoretically should provide diagnostic information. However, the scan may require 48 hours for completion and requires a mechanical intestinal preparation before scanning, since gallium is excreted into the gastrointestinal tract. In the postoperative patient, cathartics may be contraindicated because of postoperative ileus and recent suture lines. Gallium localizes in all areas of inflammation, which includes the surgical wound. This latter characteristic severely compromises the use of the gallium scan in the postoperative patient.

With accuracy better than 90%, computed tomography (CT) is the fastest and most useful diagnostic study for suspected intraabdominal abscess (Fig. 12.5). Water-soluble contrast agent is given orally and intravenously to help distinguish abscesses and fluid collections from gastrointestinal, vascular, and urinary structures. When adynamic ileus prevents filling of the gastrointestinal tract or contrast agent is contraindicated or when the patient has ascites (making identification of specific fluid collections difficult) or when CT results are equivocal, diagnosis can be made by radionuclide scanning after injection of indium-111–labeled autologous leukocytes. Total body scanning can be done within one day after injection and *all* sites of infection can be shown. If indium-111 leukocyte scanning is added to CT in equivocal cases, abdominal abscess can be accurately diagnosed in nearly all instances.

Drainage is the primary treatment of an intraabdominal abscess. Drainage allows removal of the bacteria, fibrin, and debris that are fueling the septic process. When the abscess has been precisely located in those patients that are tolerating the septic process, then localized drainage via CT or other radiologically guided percutaneous methods or limited operative procedure is justified. However, those patients with severe metabolic and physiologic decompensation as a result of the septic process, particularly those with associated organ failure, need to have a comprehensive reexploration to ensure total and complete surgical drainage and debridement.

Infection in the peritoneal cavity is usually polymicrobial. These infections usually have lipopolysaccharide-laden organisms (e.g., *E. coli*) and obligate anaerobes (e.g., *B. fragilis*). The organisms appear to have a synergistic relationship that is quite complex. Conventional antibiotic coverage for the patient with peritonitis or intraabdominal abscess is to cover both halves of the synergistic pair. Usually aminoglycosides have been used to cover the facultative *E. coli*, while clindamycin or metronidazole is used for the treatment of *B. fragilis*. Increasing information suggests that

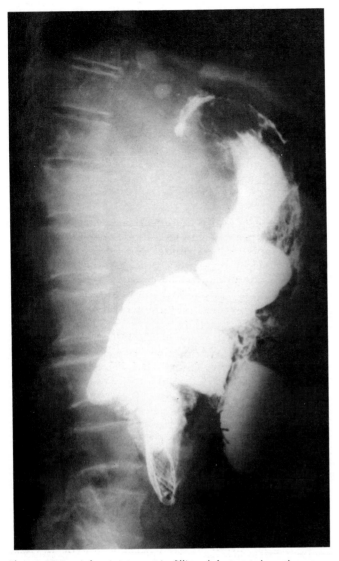

Figure 12.4. A large retrogastric filling defect noted on the upper gastrointestinal barium study represents a lesser sac abscess after a penetrating injury to the abdomen.

newer broad-spectrum cephalosporins (e.g., cefoxitin) may be of comparable benefit to the clindamycin-aminoglycoside combination. Regardless of antibiotic selection, treatment is destined to failure without adequate drainage and debridement.

Pleural empyema. Empyema may be a complication in the postoperative period after thoracotomy or chest tube placement. It may occasionally occur spontaneously or in association with a pneumonic process. Endogenous flora from pulmonary or esophageal resection or from technical failures of these resections may cause empyema. Chest tubes represent ''two-way'' streets that may allow blood and fluid to exit the pleural space but may also permit exogenous bacteria into the pleural space. The chest roentgenogram will show an effusion, usually in the dependent portion of the pleural space. Because patients may be lying down

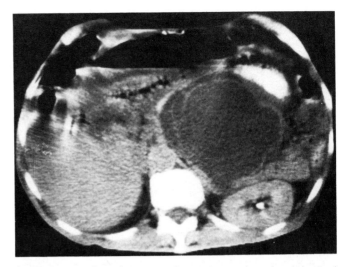

Figure 12.5. A large lesser sac abscess is noted on the abdominal CT scan of a patient with severe pancreatitis.

most of the time, a loculated empyema cavity may be very posterior. Thus a lateral chest film, CT, or ultrasound may be very valuable in diagnosis. CT is particularly useful for distinguishing between loculated empyema, lung abscess, and combinations thereof. The diagnosis of empyema is confirmed by aspiration of pus by needle thoracentesis. Ultrasound guidance during needle placement is very helpful. CT guidance is invaluable to depict the anatomy when there are multiple loculations requiring tube drainage.

Pathogens in an empyema are highly variable, and gram stain of the pus is quite useful in antibiotic selection. In patients with empyema after a prior chest tube, gram-positive staphylococcal organisms predominate. Antibiotic failure in patients with appropriate coverage usually reflects inadequate drainage. In this latter case, rib resection to marsupialize the empyema may be necessary.

Intravascular Device-Associated Bacteremia. Surgical patients are inundated with invasive intravascular catheters and devices. Peripheral intravenous cannulae, Swan-Ganz catheters, percutaneous pacemakers, and arterial lines are but a few of the devices that currently are used in patients within the intensive care unit. These portals of entry into the intravascular compartment are being recognized with increasing frequency as sources of postoperative nosocomial bacteremia.

Indwelling lines permit organisms to migrate from the skin level into the intravascular compartment of the device. Bacteremia then occurs from the catheter. Intimal injury with localized clot formation may serve as an additional growth media for bacteria. Likewise, contamination of this clot may allow suppurative thrombophlebitis to evolve with persistent bacteremia after the catheter has been removed.

Prevention of this complication requires that peripheral intravenous cannulae, Swan-Ganz catheters, arterial lines, etc., not be left in place more than 72 hours. Only hyperalimentation catheters should be maintained for a longer period of time, and they must be handled with meticulous sterile technique. Casualness in the day-to-day care of intravascular devices is primarily responsible for the increasing frequency of these complications. Asepsis must be exercised in the care of all intravascular lines.

The diagnosis of intravascular device bacteremia is suspected in any postoperative surgical patient with positive blood cultures, particularly when either *Staphylococcus aureus* or *Staphylococcus epidermidis* is recovered. A semiquantitative culture of the suspected catheter tip may help to confirm the diagnosis.

Treatment of intravascular device-associated bacteremia is the removal of the foreign body. The patient's clinical response to removal will usually confirm the diagnosis. Persistent fever, leukocytosis, and bacteremia suggest suppurative thrombophlebitis; therefore, the sites of previous intravascular devices must be examined carefully. Local incision and drainage may be necessary to identify pus within the vein. The entire length of involved vein then needs to be excised. Antibiotics specific to the bacteremic organisms are used until clinical resolution occurs. When patients have had staphylococcal bacteremia, metastatic foci of staphylococcal infections do occur. Therefore many clinicians continue parenteral antibiotics for 10–14 days in patients with staphylococcal bacteremia. Any recurrence of the bacteremia, regardless of organism, should alert the surgeon to reevaluate the adequacy of local excision of suppurative vein.

Postoperative Fever. It is estimated that one-third of patients undergoing a major operative procedure will experience a postoperative fever. The evaluation of fever in this setting is based on a careful repeat history and physical examination along with selected laboratory studies. The workup entails the evaluation of the "four Ws" (wind, wound, water, walk). The lungs (wind) are the most common culprit, especially in the early postoperative period, as atelectasis and/or pneumonia frequently follow general anesthesia and operative procedures. Lung auscultation and a chest roentgenogram will usually lead to the diagnosis; specific therapy may be instituted after cultures have been obtained.

The operative incision (wound) should be examined by removal of all dressings and the careful palpation and inspection of the wound edges. Any evidence of inflammation or drainage should be cultured and the skin sutures removed to facilitate drainage and debridement. The urinary tract (water) is evaluated routinely by a urinalysis and subsequent culture if pyuria is present. Extremity tenderness and swelling (walk) and all intravenous catheter sites should be carefully inspected, as both thrombophlebitis and suppurative phlebitis can have very subtle causes of fever yet serious consequences. All central intravenous lines and invasive monitor devices such as Swan-Ganz catheters

should be removed and/or changed and cultured. Should the above patient evaluation fail to yield a plausible explanation for the elevated temperatures, blood cultures should be drawn and repeated physical examinations done. Empiric antibiotic coverage should be avoided if possible until the source of infection is identified. Occasionally drugs will cause a fever, but this should only be considered in the surgical patient after all other possibilities have been excluded.

The Future of Surgical Infection

The character of the pathogen in surgical infection has undergone a constant evolution since the introduction of antibiotics. All evidence suggests that this evolution is continuing. Instead of bacterial pathogens, fungi, viruses, and protozoans are now being identified. As critically ill patients are sustained for longer periods of time in the contemporary intensive care unit, the host will be vulnerable to all manner of microorganisms. The pattern of bacteria and other organisms to adapt to various kinds of antimicrobial chemotherapy suggests that treatment modalities beyond those that are available currently are going to be necessary in the next decade. Until that time, the common thread of treatment of all infections in surgical patients is to ensure that local mechanical treatment has been optimized and that systemic antibiotic therapy has been timely and appropriate.

SUGGESTED READINGS

Cruse PJE, Foord R: A five-year prospective study of 23,649 surgical wounds. *Arch Surg* 107:206, 1973.
Fry DE, Garrison RN, Heitch RC, Calhoun K, Polk HC Jr: Determinants of death in patients with intra-abdominal abscess. *Surgery* 89:517–523, 1980.
Garrison RN, Fry DE, Berberich S, Polk HC Jr: Enterococcal bacteremia: clinical implications and determinants of death. *Ann Surg* 196:43, 1982.
Johanson WG Jr, Pierce AK, Sanford JP, Thomas GD: Nosocomial respiratory infections with gram-negative bacilli: the significance of colonization of the respiratory tract. *Ann Intern Med* 77:701, 1972.
Maki DG, Weise CE, Sarafin HW: A semiquantitative culture method for identifying intravenous-catheter-related infection. *N Engl J Med* 296:1305, 1977.
Martin LF, Asher EF, Casey JM, Fry DE: Postoperative pneumonia: determinants of mortality. *Arch Surg* 119:379, 1984.
National Research Council Division of Medical Sciences, Ad Hoc Committee of the Committee of Trauma: Postoperative wound infections: the influence of ultraviolet irradiation of the operating room and various other factors. *Ann Surg* 160 (Suppl 2):1, 1964.
Polk HC Jr, Fry DE, Flint LM: Dissemination of causes of infection. *Surg Clin N Am* 56:817–829, 1976.
Polk HC Jr, Lopez-Mayor JF: Postoperative wound infection: a prospective study of determinant factors and prevention. *Surgery* 66:97, 1969.
Stamm WE: Guidelines for prevention of catheter-associated urinary tract infections. *Ann Intern Med* 82:386, 1975.
Stone HH, Kolb LD, Currie CA, et al: *Candida* sepsis: pathogenesis and principles of treatment. *Ann Surg* 179:697, 1974.

Skills

1. Scrubbing technique: In preparing for a surgical procedure done in the operating room environs, the student should demonstrate proper scrubbing and drying of the hands and arms. Particular attention should be placed on the proper sequence of washing so as not to contaminate the part that has been previously cleansed.

2. Contaminated wound dressing: The student should replace a dirty dressing with a sterile dressing in a patient with an open contaminated wound. Emphasis should be placed on the actual inspection of the wound, with the removal of any loose or necrotic tissue, and the proper disposal of the contaminated material.

3. Drainage of superficial abscess: The student should be able to diagnose, incise, and drain a superficial abscess. The student should apply a local anesthetic and obtain a specimen of the material for bacteriologic identification. Complete evacuation of the cavity should be assured prior to the application of a clean dressing.

Study Questions

1. Outline the classification of surgical wounds and give two examples of each type. In which of these wounds would you recommend prophylactic systemic antibiotics be used? Why?

2. Discuss which antibiotics are indicated and the rationale for their use in a patient with diffuse peritonitis secondary to perforated sigmoid diverticulitis.

3. Discuss abdominal wound management after exploration and established peritonitis.

4. List the factors that affect the host-pathogen interaction in the development of clinical wound infections.

5. Discuss the elevation of a 101°F temperature that occurs 8 hours after an abdominal surgical procedure for closure of a perforated duodenal ulcer. What would be the most frequent etiology for fever in this situation?

13

Trauma and Burns

A. Craig Eddy, M.D.
David M. Heimbach, M.D.

ASSUMPTION

The student knows the basic anatomy and physiology of the skin and subcutaneous tissue.

OBJECTIVES

1. Describe the conditions, signs, and symptoms commonly associated with upper airway obstruction.
2. Describe the risks associated with the management of an airway in the traumatized patient.
3. Outline the options available and the sequence of steps required to control an airway in the traumatized patient, including protection of the cervical spine.
4. List the identifying characteristics of patients who are likely to have upper airway obstruction.
5. Define shock, including the pathophysiology.
6. List four types of shock and outline the management of a patient in hemorrhagic shock.
7. List the indications and contraindications for use of a pneumatic antishock garment in patients with hemorrhagic shock.
8. List six thoracic injuries that are immediately life threatening and should be identified in the primary survey and six that are potentially life threatening and should be identified in the secondary survey. Outline a treatment plan for each injury.
9. List the indications for chest tube insertion, pericardiocentesis, and needle thoracentesis. Outline the technique for each.
10. List three common thoracic injuries that, although not life threatening, need skilled care.
11. Define the limits of the abdominal cavity, demonstrate the abdominal examination for trauma, and outline the tests that are of use in abdominal trauma.
12. Differentiate between blunt and penetrating trauma.
13. List the indications, contraindications, and limitations of peritoneal lavage. Describe a positive peritoneal lavage.
14. Outline the pathophysiologic events leading to decreased levels of consciousness, including the unique anatomic and physiologic features of head and spinal injuries.
15. List the three functions assessed by the Glasgow coma scale and outline the point scale.
16. Outline the initial management of the unconscious patient and the patient with suspected spinal cord injury.
17. List the test results and assessment results that should be passed to neurologic consultants.
18. Outline the differences between non-life-threatening and life-threatening extremity injuries and the management of each.
19. Describe a thorough examination of the extremities in a traumatized patient.
20. Outline the factors of significance when applying the ABCs to burn patients.
21. Describe burn depth and size in a patient with a major burn.
22. Outline the initial stabilization and resuscitation of burn patients, including a list of injuries that are frequently associated with burn patients.

Urban violence, industrial equipment, and more automobiles have resulted in a progressive increase in the amount of trauma each year. Trauma now is the most common cause of death in children and adults who are under 35 years old. In 1986 there were approximately 2.8 million trauma-related deaths in the United States, and the morbidity associated with trauma costs society approximately $84 billion. Management of a patient with major trauma requires adequate facilities (e.g., radiologic, operating room, blood banking) and individuals with expertise in care of the trauma patient. Often there is not time for an inexperienced clinician to read about the management of a trauma problem; consequently, the physician must be prepared for and ready to treat most trauma problems prior to the severely injured patient's admission to the hospital.

The most crucial aspect in the care of the trauma victim is the initial examination and treatment performed in the emergency room. To facilitate a rapid and thorough assessment and ensure prompt institution of appropriate treatment of the multiply injured patient, the American College of Surgeons has developed a treatment algorithm that is promulgated in the Advanced Trauma Life Support course. In this chapter, we outline and expand this algorithm to prepare the student to handle the complex problems that these patients present.

Care of the trauma victim can be divided into four parts: primary survey, resuscitation, secondary survey, and formation of a definitive care plan.

The primary survey consists of sequential evaluation of the airway, breathing, circulation, and neurologic function. It is designed to identify all immediately life-threatening injuries. Each of these injuries is treated in sequence before advancing to the next stage.

Resuscitation occurs simultaneously with the primary survey. The airway is secured and the patient is ventilated. Intravenous lines are established with balanced crystalloid solution to ensure adequate volume resuscitation. External hemorrhage is controlled with direct pressure. Gross neurologic injury is identified and the patient fully exposed.

The secondary survey consists of a detailed physical examination, beginning at the patient's head and working to the toes. The goal of the secondary survey is to identify all potentially life-threatening injuries and to uncover any occult injuries. Baseline laboratory studies are drawn at this time and include the tests listed in Table 13.1.

After completing the secondary survey, the physician should recheck the vital signs and confirm that the patient remains stable. If at any point the patient is judged unstable, the physician should begin the examination again from the beginning of the algorithm. The physician should then prioritize the injuries that have been identified and make a plan for definitive care.

This algorithm forms the basis of treatment for the multiply injured patient. It offers a well-thought-out plan of management to systematically identify all life-threatening and potentially life-threatening injuries and

smoothly guide the multiply injured patient into definitive care. This chapter discusses the initial assessment and secondary survey, going through the body by systems and outlining for the student the injuries commonly seen after severe trauma.

Airway Management

Providing, protecting, and maintaining an adequate airway is the physician's first priority in managing the trauma victim. Failure to obtain an airway is a common cause of early and preventable death. Conditions as simple as a fractured mandible or drug intoxication may compromise the airway. Although airway obstruction is usually apparent on the initial examination, it may also develop at any time during the evaluation. Trauma victims are often unstable due to multiple injuries, and a sudden deterioration must always prompt reevaluation of the airway.

In general, patients at risk for airway problems have either sustained an injury to the head or neck that causes mechanical obstruction or they have an altered level of consciousness. The latter may be secondary to a central nervous system injury or to intoxication with drugs or alcohol. Victims of motor vehicle accidents frequently strike their heads on the windshield or dashboard, causing trauma to the midface or mandible, which may lead to fracture of the supporting facial structures and cause upper airway collapse. In addition, the fractures may be associated with hemorrhage into the pharynx and increased secretions, which may also cause or exacerbate mechanical obstruction. Neck injuries may directly damage the trachea or cause hematomas that extrinsically compress the airway.

The airway obstruction should be identified and localized systematically. An awake patient who answers appropriately a simple question such as, ''Are you all right?'' is clearly oxygenating well with an unob-

Table 13.1.
Baseline Laboratory Tests

Complete blood count	Hct, WBC, platelets
Basic chemistries	Sodium
	Potassium
	Chloride
	Carbon dioxide
	BUN
	Creatinine
	Glucose
Arterial blood gases	
X-rays	Lateral C-spine films
	Chest films
	Pelvis films
Blood sent for type and cross match	

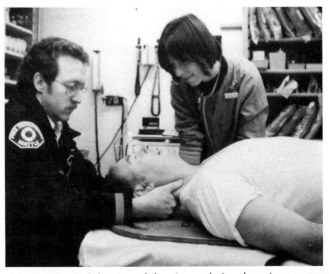

Figure 13.1. Stabilization of the airway during the primary survey of the injured patient.

structed airway. Lack of appropriate response should prompt a search for the injuries discussed above or for evidence of an altered level of consciousness. The physician should listen for abnormal airway sounds such as stridor, snoring, or gurgling, which suggest a supraglottic injury. Dysphonia or pain on speaking implies obstruction at the laryngeal level. The physician should carefully listen and feel for movement of air at the patient's mouth with expiratory effort.

Management of Airway Obstruction

If the airway is not patent, it must be cleared immediately. The major risk in providing an airway is inadvertent extension or flexion of the neck in the presence of a cervical spine injury. Therefore the neck must be completely immobilized in the neutral position. A soft or rigid cervical collar does not adequately protect against cervical spine injury. Immobilization of the neck is best accomplished by designating an individual to kneel at the head of the stretcher and grasp the patient's cervical spine and occipital ridges with his or her hands, while immobilizing the neck with both forearms (Fig. 13.1).

Once the neck is immobilized, the physician should correct the obstruction and establish an adequate airway with the simplest method possible. This sequence is graphically illustrated in Figure 13.2. The first maneuver is the chin lift or jaw thrust. While placing the thumbs behind the lower incisor and the second and third fingers in the submental area, the chin is lifted anteriorly and inferiorly. Alternatively, with the jaw thrust, both hands may be used to grasp the angles of the mandible and displace it forward. The disadvantage of the jaw thrust is that it requires the use of both hands. These maneuvers must be done carefully to prevent any hyperextension of the neck. The physician should then illuminate the oropharynx, look for an obstruction, and listen for movement of air. Blood and secretions should be removed with a rigid suction device under direct visualization (Fig. 13.3). Soft suction devices should not be used, as they cannot be adequately controlled and may result in iatrogenic injury.

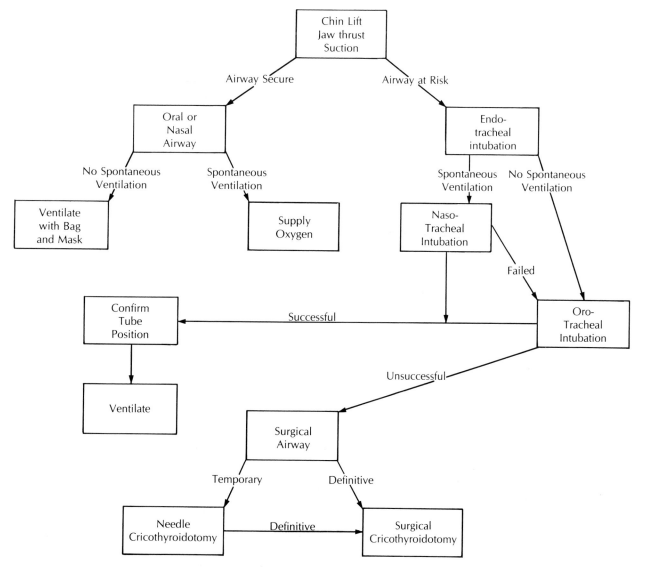

Figure 13.2. Airway management.

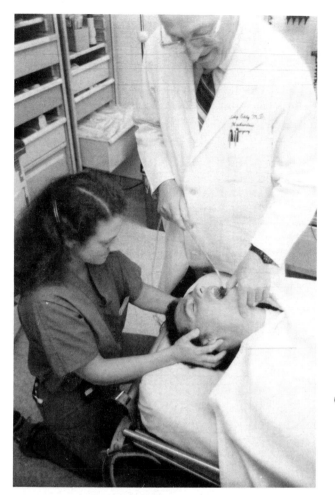

Figure 13.3. Rigid suction device.

If the airway is patent after suctioning, it can usually be maintained by inserting an oropharyngeal airway (Fig. 13.4). While the nondominant hand lifts the chin, the dominant hand inserts the inverted airway to the soft palate. The airway is then rotated 180° until it slips into place over the tongue. This should be done gently, to avoid damaging dentition. Although the oropharyngeal airway provides a very good airway, it is often poorly tolerated by fully conscious patients because of the gag reflex. If the patient is fully conscious, a nasopharyngeal airway is a reasonable alternative. This device should be first well lubricated and passed through a nostril into the hypopharynx. If an obstruction is encountered, the airway can be placed in the opposite nostril. If obstruction is bilateral, attempts to use the nasopharyngeal airway should be abandoned. Once the airway has been established, if the patient can ventilate spontaneously, a face mask supplying 100% oxygen should be applied.

Tracheal Intubation

If the methods outlined above do not successfully secure the airway and allow ventilation, endotracheal intubation is indicated. This can be difficult in a severely injured patient who is combative, and it may

require multiple attempts. The patient must be adequately ventilated with 100% oxygen, using an anesthesia bag and face mask prior to and between attempts at intubation. The endotracheal tube may be placed in a nasal or oral passage.

Nasotracheal intubation is possible only if the patient is spontaneously ventilating. It should not be performed on patients with midface injuries. A further drawback of the nasotracheal intubation is that awake patients often find it uncomfortable and may move abruptly, placing their cervical spine at risk. For this reason, orotracheal intubation is the method of choice. However, this must be done with meticulous care to immobilize the cervical spine. Immediately after placement of the tube, the chest should be carefully auscultated for symmetric breath sounds to ensure the tube is not in the esophagus or has not been advanced into the right main stem bronchus. The tube position must be confirmed as soon as possible by a chest x-ray.

Cricothyroidotomy

If an adequate airway is not secured using these methods, a surgical airway must be considered. There are two types of surgical airways: the needle cricothyroidotomy and the surgical cricothyroidotomy. The needle cricothyroidotomy is the procedure of choice in children less than 12 years of age and is a temporizing maneuver for adults. Performance of a needle cricothyroidotomy entails placing a 12- or 14-gauge plastic cannula through the cricothyroid membrane into the trachea. The cannula is connected to wall oxygen at 40–50 lb in², using a Y connector or mechanical valve (Fig. 13.5). Intermittent ventilation is performed using a 1-second interval for inhalation and 4-second pause for exhalation. A patient can be ventilated for approximately 30 minutes using this method, allowing time for a more secure airway to be established. This method may also generate sufficient intratracheal pressure to expel an obstructing foreign body in the glottic area. Surgical cricothyroidotomy consists of a single incision through the skin and cricothyroid membrane with a #11 blade. The blunt end of the scalpel is then inserted through the incision and turned 90 degrees to open the airway, allowing the insertion of a small endotracheal or tracheostomy tube (Fig 13.6 and 13.7). The patient can then be allowed to ventilate spontaneously or, if unable to ventilate spontaneously, may be mechanically or manually ventilated.

Circulation

Shock is defined as inadequate cellular perfusion. The diagnosis of shock is not based on laboratory results but on the clinical recognition of a constellation of symptoms and signs that result from inadequate organ perfusion.

Hypoperfusion for any reason produces characteristic cellular and metabolic responses. These responses can be divided into early and late changes. The first

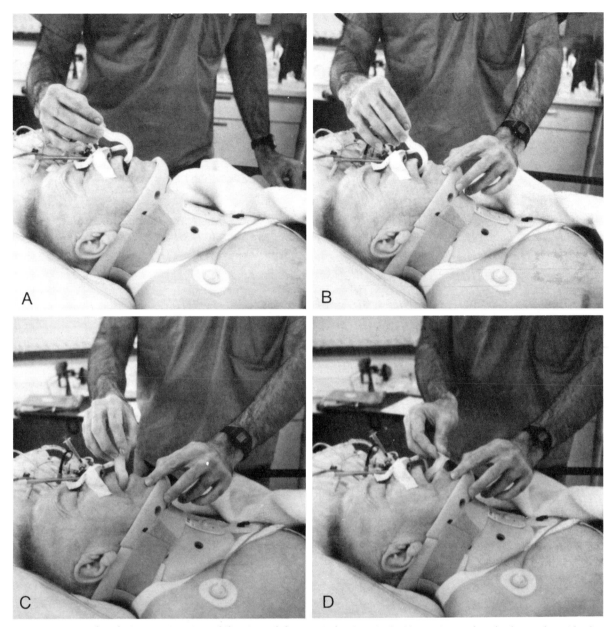

Figure 13.4. Insertion of oral airway. Note immobilization of the cervical spine. **A–B,** Airway inserted and advanced upside down. **C–D** Once inserted, the airway is rotated 180°.

response is a compensatory vasoconstriction and a shift from aerobic to anaerobic metabolism in the nonessential organ systems. This affects primarily the cutaneous, visceral, and musculoskeletal circulation. Adequate perfusion of the heart and brain are maintained by this mechanism. Later, as hypoperfusion persists, oxygen delivery to nonessential and essential organs may be inadequate to maintain cellular function. The inadequately oxygenated cells shift to anaerobic metabolism and produce lactic acid. The transcellular membrane potential difference falls and the energy-dependent sodium-potassium pump fails. Fluid shifts into the cells and leads to intracellular swelling. This causes a further decrease in efficiency of the cellular metabolic processes and, if oxygenation and perfusion are not restored, this leads to a vicious cycle, resulting in progressive organ failure and death.

There are essentially four clinical syndromes that produce shock: hemorrhage, neurologic injury, myocardial failure, and sepsis. Hemorrhagic shock is the most common cause of hypoperfusion in the immediate period after trauma. Hemorrhage should be assumed to be the etiology of shock until proven otherwise. It is vital to estimate the magnitude of blood loss to initiate appropriate therapy and monitor progress. The clinical criteria listed in Table 13.2 can be used to accomplish this estimation. With these criteria it is possible to divide hemorrhagic shock, according to its severity, into four classes. Class I hemorrhage is defined as loss of approximately 15% of the circulating blood volume. The clinical manifestations are minimal and consist of a slight tachycardia, with no measurable change in blood pressure, pulse pressure, capillary refill, or respiratory rate. Urine output remains normal.

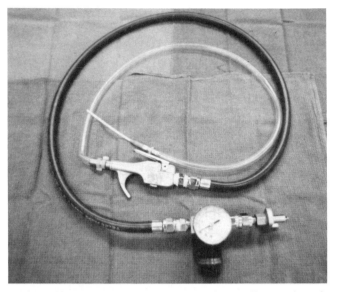

Figure 13.5. Cannula for jet ventilation for needle cricothyroidotomy.

Class II hemorrhage is defined as loss of 15–30% of the circulating blood volume. This results in tachycardia and tachypnea and, while the systolic blood pressure remains normal, the diastolic pressure is high and results in decreased pulse pressure. There may be central nervous system excitation manifested as anxiety, fear, or combativeness. Capillary refill time, measured by depressing the fingernail and timing the interval until return of normal color, is usually prolonged. Normal capillary refill time should be approximately 2 seconds or the time required to say capillary refill. Capillary refill time cannot be accurately estimated in patients who are hypothermic.

In class I and class II hemorrhage, intravascular losses may usually be replaced with crystalloid solution alone. However, if ongoing blood loss is suspected, administration of blood products becomes necessary.

Class III hemorrhages are defined as loss of 30–40% of the circulating blood volume. These patients have the classical signs and symptoms of hypoperfusion, including tachycardia, tachypnea, decreased systolic blood pressure, a narrowed pulse pressure, and altered mental status.

Losses exceeding 40% of the circulating blood volume constitute a class IV hemorrhage and may be rapidly lethal. These patients are tachycardic, hypotensive, cold, and clammy. The urine output is markedly reduced and the patients are generally obtunded.

The initial step in the management of hemorrhagic shock is intravascular volume replacement. This requires adequate intravenous access. At the least, these patients need two intravenous catheters (16 gauge or larger) placed in the upper extremity. Catheters should not be placed in an extremity if it has been injured, or venous flow may be altered. Ideally, lines are placed percutaneously, but if this is not possible, cutdowns may be placed. If a peripheral line cannot be established quickly in an upper extremity, femoral or saphenous veins may be used for rapid fluid infusion. Subclavian or internal jugular lines may be used for central venous pressure monitoring but are unsuitable for delivering large volumes rapidly.

Once access is secured, the volume of fluid replacement needed should be estimated. In adults, normal circulating blood volume constitutes approximately 7% of the total body weight. This amounts to almost 5 liters in a 70-kg man. In children this percentage is

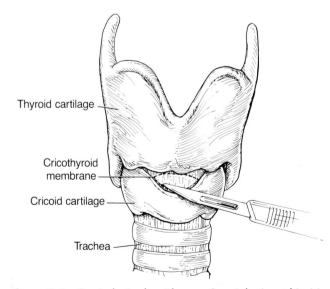

Figure 13.6. Surgical cricothyroidotomy. Step 1, horizontal incision through skin and criocothyroid membrane.

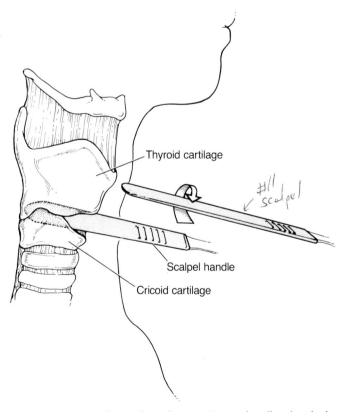

Figure 13.7. Surgical cricothyroidotomy. Step 2, handle of scalpel is inserted through cricothyroid membrane into the airway and rotated 90° to keep the airway open.

Table 13.2.
Classification of Hemorrhagic Shock

	Class 1 (15%↓)	Class 2 (15-30%↓)	Class 3 (30-40%↓)	Class 4 (>40%↓)
Level of consciousness	Normal or mildly anxious	Anxious	Anxious or combative	Anxious, combative
Heart rate	Normal	Mildly increased	Increased	Markedly increased
Respiratory rate	Normal	Slightly elevated	Elevated	Markedly elevated
Blood pressure	Normal	Normal	Slightly decreased	Markedly decreased
Pulse pressure	Normal	Decreased	Decreased	Markedly decreased
Urine output	>30 cc/hr	>20 cc/hr	>10 cc/hr	0-10 cc/hr
Capillary refill	Normal	Slow	Prolonged	Markedly prolonged

slightly higher at 8–9%, with younger children tending to have higher percentages. By estimating the patient's normal blood volume and percentage lost, a rough calculation of the blood loss is possible.

Fluid therapy with an initial bolus of balanced crystalloid solution is given immediately. Fluid should always be given in boluses to rapidly assess the initial response and potential need for additional fluids. In the normal-size adult, the initial bolus is usually 1 liter. In children the initial bolus should be 20 cc/kg of body weight. In patients with class I, II, or early class III hemorrhages, the response is carefully monitored and, if clinical criteria do not improve, a second bolus is infused. If the response to the second bolus is inadequate, type specific or O-negative blood is transfused. Patients in late class III or class IV shock should start receiving blood in addition to crystalloid fluid as soon as intravenous access is obtained. The majority of patients in class III shock and nearly all patients in class IV shock will require surgical intervention. In those patients, the general surgeon should be involved early.

An adjunct to fluid resuscitation of patients in hemorrhagic shock is the pneumatic antishock garment (PASG). This is an inflatable garment that is placed under the patient and buckled into place around both the patient's lower extremities and pelvis. The legs of the garment are first inflated and then the waist panel, to a pressure sufficient to increase the patient's central blood pressure to 90 mm Hg. This garment should not be used as a replacement for adequate fluid therapy. However, it can be used to maintain the patient's blood pressure until adequate intravenous access is established. Table 13.3 lists the indications and contraindications for their usage.

After the patient's circulatory status has stabilized, the PASG should be deflated, beginning with the abdominal panel. Panels are gradually deflated until the patient's blood pressure falls by 5–10 mm Hg. At this time, deflation is stopped and fluid resuscitation is continued until blood pressure returns to normal. Deflation is then resumed and this sequence continued until the garment is fully deflated.

The goal of fluid resuscitation is to restore adequate perfusion of all tissues. The parameters outlined previously must be carefully monitored, identifying trends and adjusting the resuscitation as necessary. Aiming for a particular blood pressure or central venous pressure is less important than stabilizing each parameter and following its trends. If the anticipated response does not ensue, it is vital to search for the cause of this discrepancy. If hemorrhagic shock is absolutely excluded, other causes must be considered. Neurogenic shock occurs when brain stem dysfunction or spinal cord injury causes denervation of the sympathetic nervous system. A head injury without brain stem injury is not sufficient to produce neurogenic shock. Unlike other shock states, tachycardia and cutaneous vasoconstriction are unusual in neurogenic shock. After traumatic injury, this diagnosis must not be made until the presence of hemorrhagic shock has been excluded.

Cardiogenic shock occurs when myocardial dysfunction precludes adequate tissue perfusion. In the setting of acute trauma, this can occur from direct myocardial injury such as myocardial contusion or more rarely from myocardial infarction. Distended jugular veins in the presence of hypotension suggest cardiogenic shock. In this instance an abnormal electrocardiogram may be of little benefit in differentiating cardiogenic shock from other causes. Hypovolemia alone may produce ischemic changes on the electrocardiogram. Measurement of central venous pressure in combination with systemic pressure allows the most accurate diagnosis of cardiogenic shock.

Septic shock requires a minimum of several hours to develop and is not commonly seen in the immediate

Table 13.3.
Use of the Pneumatic Antishock Garment

Indications
  Maintenance of tissue perfusion until intravenous lines can be started
  Tamponading of soft tissue hemorrhage
  Stabilization of leg fractures
  Stabilization and tamponade of hemorrhage in pelvic fractures until definitive treatment can be initiated
Absolute Contraindications
  Myocardial dysfunction
  Pulmonary edema
Relative Contraindications
  Pregnancy
  Head injuries
  Intrathoracic bleeding
  Ruptured diaphragm

Table 13.4.
Thoracic Injuries Often Rapidly Fatal

Airway obstruction
Open pneumothorax
Tension pneumothorax
Massive hemothorax
Flail chest
Cardiac tamponade

postinjury period. This syndrome is characterized by loss of vasomotor tone, thought to be the result of circulating endotoxin.

Neurologic injury will be dealt with in a separate section. However, it is important to remember that hypotension should never be attributed to an isolated head injury.

Thoracic Injury

Injury to the chest wall and the structures within the thoracic cavity can cause complex cardiopulmonary alterations and rapidly precipitate death. Although the mechanism of injury may vary, the common denominator causing death in thoracic injury is hypoxia. The most exciting aspect of treating thoracic injuries is that rapid intervention of thoracic injuries with simple techniques can provide definitive care for the vast majority of patients: 85% of thoracic injuries can be treated with techniques that every graduating medical student should be able to perform. This leaves only 15% of patients who will need further definitive care.

There are 15 common thoracic injuries that can be divided into three groups. The first group includes those injuries that are likely to be rapidly fatal if not identified immediately. These injuries (listed in Table 13.4) must be committed to memory so that they are carefully considered and excluded during the primary survey.

The first in this group, airway obstruction, has already been discussed. An open pneumothorax or sucking chest wound occurs if there is an open defect in the chest wall larger than two-thirds of the tracheal diameter. In this situation, inspiratory and expiratory efforts simply move the air in and out of the pleural space through the chest wall defect rather than the trachea. The treatment for an open pneumothorax is intubation with positive-pressure mechanical ventilation and closure of the defect in the chest wall. If the defect is small, it may be covered with a flap valve, using a sterile occlusive dressing with a nonpermeable material such as Vaseline gauze or plastic drape, which is then taped on three sides (Fig. 13.8). This occludes the wound during inspiration, while allowing the air to escape as intrathoracic pressure increases during expiration. It is crucial not to tape the dressing on all four sides, as this may convert the open pneumothorax to a tension pneumothorax if there is underlying pulmonary injury.

Tension pneumothorax and cardiac tamponade are considered together because it is frequently difficult,

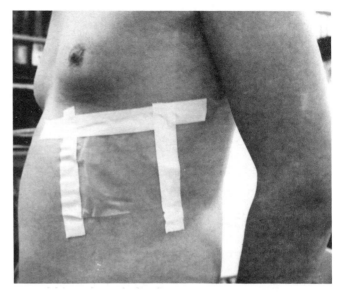

Figure 13.8.   Three-sided dressing for open pneumothorax.

yet vital, to differentiate between these diagnoses. Tension pneumothorax occurs when air is forced into the pleural space without a means of escape, causing complete collapse of the affected lung. In addition, increased intrathoracic pressure shifts the mediastinum and trachea to the opposite side and inhibits venous return to the heart, while compromising ventilation of the opposite lung. This results in respiratory distress and hypotension. Cardiac tamponade occurs when the pericardial sac fills with blood and interferes with diastolic filling of the heart.

Both conditions are associated with hypotension and distended neck veins. In the busy emergency room it may be difficult to auscultate the hypertympanic percussion note over the chest in a tension pneumothorax or appreciate the muffled heart sounds and pulsus paradoxus characteristic of cardiac tamponade. These injuries are immediately life threatening and must be identified from clinical information, as there is rarely enough time to obtain definitive studies, such as a chest x-ray or echocardiogram. Tension pneumothorax occurs more commonly than cardiac tamponade and is more likely to occur after blunt trauma than after penetrating injury. Tamponade is most likely to occur after a penetrating injury near the heart. Even if a definitive diagnosis cannot be determined, the physician must decide which is the most likely diagnosis in the individual patient at hand and initiate therapy.

The treatment of tension pneumothorax is needle thoracentesis. A 10 to 12-gauge needle is inserted into the second intercostal space in the midclavicular line just superior to the third rib. This allows escape of the pressurized air from the pleural space and restores normal hemodynamics. This must be followed by insertion of a chest tube.

Cardiac tamponade is treated with pericardiocentesis. A 12-gauge plastic catheter is introduced in a subxyphoid position and aimed at a 45° angle to the right and posterior while aspirating with a syringe. Aspiration of as little as 10 cc of blood is enough to re-

Table 13.5.
Potentially Fatal Thoracic Injuries

Pulmonary contusion
Traumatic aortic rupture
Injuries to the tracheobronchial tree
Esophageal injury
Traumatic diaphragmatic hernia
Myocardial contusion

verse the tamponade. Once the catheter is in place in the pericardial sac, it should be secured with tape and a stopcock placed on the end of the plastic cannula so that repeat aspiration may be performed as needed.

Occasionally the physician may be faced with a situation in which it is not possible to clinically differentiate between these two diagnoses. In this case, a needle should be inserted into the pleural space, as outlined above, on the side most likely to be affected. If this does not produce a rush of air and rapid hemodynamic improvement, the procedure should be repeated on the opposite side. If the patient remains hypotensive, a pericardiocentesis must be done.

Massive hemothorax is defined as loss of 1000–1500 cc of blood into the thoracic cavity. This problem nearly always requires emergent thoracotomy. Initial management is aimed at ensuring that there is adequate volume replacement prior to decompression of the chest cavity. After large-bore intravenous lines are placed and fluid resuscitation is begun, a chest tube is inserted. If 1000–1500 cc are evacuated and it is obvious that the blood loss is ongoing, the patient will need to be taken immediately to the operating room. However, if this quantity of blood is evacuated and there is no further blood loss, chest decompression may be the only treatment that is necessary. After placement of the chest tube (tube thoracostomy), chest x-ray is necessary to ensure that all the blood has been removed and the lung is fully reexpanded.

Flail chest occurs when the ribs are broken in multiple places and a segment of the chest wall loses its bony continuity. This produces a detached or ''flail'' segment that moves paradoxically to the rest of the chest wall during respiration. A tremendous amount of force is necessary to produce this type of injury, and generally a severe pulmonary contusion is concomitant. The combined result is inadequate ventilation and oxygenation. If hypoxia cannot be corrected with sup-

Table 13.6.
Roentgenographic Signs Suggesting Injury to the Thoracic Aorta

Mediastinum wider than 10 cm on upright PA film
Loss of the aortic knob
Pleural cap
Deviation of the trachea to the right
Fracture of the first or second ribs or scapula
Elevation of the right main stem bronchus
Depression of the left main stem bronchus
Obliteration of the aortopulmonary window
Deviation of the esophagus to the left

plemental oxygen therapy, endotracheal intubation and positive-pressure ventilation with positive end-expiratory pressure may be necessary. In addition, it is important to place a central monitoring line and try to avoid inadequate or overzealous fluid replacement.

The second category of injuries consists of six thoracic injuries that usually become manifest during the secondary survey. These injuries are listed in Table 13.5.

Pulmonary contusion is simply a hemorrhage into the pulmonary parenchyma. It generally requires 1–4 hours to develop. Particularly in children, a pulmonary contusion may develop in the absence of flail chest or even rib fractures. Thus a patient thought to have relatively minor chest injury may develop progressive hypoxemia several hours after the injury. Judicious use of fluids guided by central pressure monitoring during the initial resuscitation phase may minimize respiratory compromise.

Traumatic aortic rupture is the most common cause of immediate death after an automobile accident or a fall from a great height. Up to 90% of these people are found dead at the scene of the accident. The remaining 10% can frequently be salvaged if the injury is rapidly identified. Angiography is the only test that can reliably identify traumatic rupture to the aorta. All other radiologic findings are indirect. To successfully identify these patients and intervene, the physician must maintain a high index of suspicion. A combination of suggestive history and one or more of the findings listed in Table 13.6 should prompt the physician to order an aortogram.

An aortogram should be obtained in all patients who are at risk for aortic rupture as soon as possible after the patient has been stabilized. Aortic rupture usually occurs at the ligamentum arteriosum (Fig. 13.9). These injuries can rupture at any time and should be surgically repaired as soon as possible.

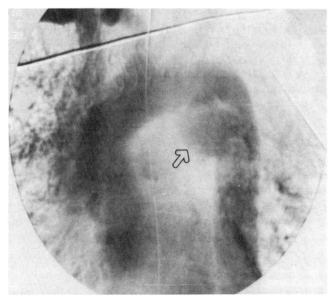

Figure 13.9. Traumatic rupture of thoracic aorta, demonstrated by thoracic angiography.

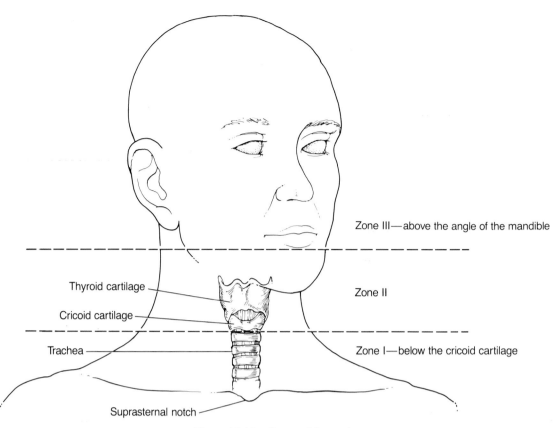

Zone III—above the angle of the mandible

Thyroid cartilage

Cricoid cartilage

Zone II

Trachea

Zone I—below the cricoid cartilage

Suprasternal notch

Figure 13.10. Zones of the neck.

Traumatic disruption of the tracheobronchial tree is relatively uncommon. Penetrating injuries are usually obvious and may be associated with injuries to the great vessels, esophagus, or trachea. To evaluate penetrating injuries to the neck, it is helpful to divide the neck into three zones (Fig. 13.10). Injuries to zone 2 can be taken directly to surgery because, if a vascular injury is present, proximal and distal vascular control can be obtained without difficulty. Penetrating injuries occurring in zones 1 and 3 require further preoperative evaluation. In zone 3, an arteriogram must be obtained because distal control of the carotid artery can be very difficult in this area. If the arteriogram is normal, local exploration can be performed and any injuries encountered can be repaired. Injuries in zone 1 can affect the great vessels, esophagus, or trachea. In this instance, an aortogram should be performed, and, if the aortogram is normal and the patient exhibits no signs of hemodynamic instability, a contrast study of the esophagus should be performed. If this demonstrates no injury, bronchoscopy and esophagoscopy should be performed prior to exploration of the neck wound. Penetrating injuries to the tracheobronchial tree require surgical repair.

Blunt injuries to the tracheobronchial tree are more subtle. Blunt injuries to the trachea and neck may fracture the larynx, an injury that presents with abnormal phonation, subcutaneous emphysema, or palpable crepitus on motion of the thyroid cartilage. Blunt injury to a major bronchus usually occurs within 1 inch of the carina. These patients present with hemoptysis, sub-

cutaneous emphysema, and pneumothorax. After performance of a tube thoracostomy, there is often a persistent air leak. The injury is confirmed by bronchoscopy, and these injuries should be acutely repaired surgically.

Another potentially life-threatening injury is myocardial contusion. This injury is caused by a direct blow to the myocardium that results in myocardial cell dysfunction. This diagnosis requires a high index of suspicion based on the history of the injury and signs of central chest injury such as contusion or fracture of the sternum. When the heart is contused due to a direct injury, it is usually the right ventricle that is primarily involved. Unlike myocardial infarction, this involvement is usually diffuse and patchy and frequently not transmural. Arrhythmias after a blow to the anterior chest suggest a myocardial contusion but are not diagnostic. The weaker right ventricle electrical activity is frequently overshadowed by the activity of the left ventricle, making diagnosis by electrocardiogram difficult. An elevation of CPK (myocardial band isoenzyme) is sometimes seen. Careful examination of the heart by echocardiography is the most reliable test, and ventricular wall motion abnormalities are diagnostic of myocardial contusion. Any patient who suffers a myocardial contusion should be monitored in the intensive care unit for 48–72 hours to identify and treat arrhythmias. Repeat echocardiography should be performed at one and three months to detect a slowly developing ventricular aneurysm.

Most esophageal injuries are penetrating and can

most accurately be identified by a combination of esophagography and esophagoscopy. Once the injury is identified, it should be surgically repaired and well drained. Blunt injury to the esophagus is much more rare and usually occurs after a forceful blow to the upper abdomen. This produces a linear tear in the left posterior aspect of the esophagus. These patients frequently present with severe epigastric or left chest pain and shock. Fluid may be seen in the left chest, and, if a tube thoracostomy is performed, particulate matter may be found in the fluid. Diagnosis is again made by esophagoscopy or esophagography, and once the diagnosis is established, surgical repair with wide drainage is performed. If an esophageal injury is missed and mediastinitis develops, the result is frequently fatal.

Traumatic diaphragmatic hernia can also occur after blunt or penetrating trauma. Penetrating trauma usually results in small holes in the diaphragm, which may be easily overlooked. Often these will increase in size over several years and present in a delayed fashion with herniation of abdominal contents into the chest. A severe blow to the upper abdomen may cause large linear tears in the diaphragm. These occur more often on the left side; the diagnosis is suggested on chest x-ray and confirmed with upper gastrointestinal contrast studies. Diaphragmatic injuries should be closed surgically.

The remaining category of injuries is made up of non-life-threatening injuries that include simple pneumothorax, nonmassive hemothorax, and rib fractures. Traumatic pneumothorax can develop into a tension pneumothorax and therefore is always treated with a tube thoracostomy. Because traumatic hemothorax can result in restrictive pulmonary disease if not evacuated, this is also treated with a tube thoracostomy. Rib fractures are the most commonly seen injury of the thoracic cage. Fractured ribs are a clinical and not a radiologic diagnosis. Any person who has had thoracic injury should have their ribs carefully palpated to identify areas of fracture. Areas of fracture are identified by crepitation or localized tenderness on palpation. Patients who have rib fractures frequently have trouble ventilating due to pain and, because of their small tidal volumes, are prone to develop atelectasis and pneumonia. Patients with a small number of rib fractures who are able to generate adequate tidal volumes can be instructed in coughing and deep breathing and sent home from the emergency room with a mild systemic analgesic and seen daily to ensure that pneumonia does not develop. Elderly patients and patients with multiple rib fractures should be admitted for pulmonary toilet. Fractures of the first three ribs are associated with severe trauma and should alert the physician to other possible intrathoracic injuries. These patients should always be admitted to the hospital for a period of observation. Rib belt binders and taping of the rib should be avoided because they only increase pulmonary complications.

Indications for tube thoracostomy include pneumothorax, hemothorax, and prophylaxis in patients with thoracic trauma who will undergo operative procedures where they cannot be assessed for long periods of time. In trauma, tube thoracostomy is performed in the fifth intercostal space in the anterior axillary line with the tube directed posteriorly and superiorly. This should always be done under sterile conditions and, if time permits, an intercostal nerve block should be performed prior to insertion of the chest tube.

Abdominal Trauma

Evaluation of the abdomen in trauma occurs during the secondary survey after the trauma victim has been stabilized. Patients who have sustained abdominal trauma or who are suspected to have sustained abdominal trauma should be evaluated early by a general surgeon. Abdominal injury, although its presentation may be subtle, often is life threatening, and the treatment of intraabdominal injury usually takes precedence over other less life-threatening injuries. Prompt recognition of intraabdominal injury is the most important factor affecting the outcome of this injury. The diagnosis may be difficult, because associated injuries may overshadow the presence of abdominal injury. The patient may have an altered state of consciousness due to drug or alcohol ingestion or associated head injury. Because of these factors, anyone who is suspected of having abdominal injury must be aggressively assessed with physical examination and diagnostic tests until the absence of such injury is clearly established.

The physician attending a trauma victim does not necessarily need to identify precisely the intraabdominal injury that is present. Rather, the physician needs to address in a logical fashion the questions noted below:

1. Is the patient hemorrhaging into the abdominal cavity?
2. Does the patient have an intraabdominal injury that will require an operation?
3. Does the patient have an injury to the abdominal cavity that warrants further investigation and observation?

With these three questions in mind, the physician should begin a careful assessment of the abdomen. The abdominal cavity begins superiorly at the nipple line and extends inferiorly to the pubic symphysis. Laterally, it extends from midaxillary line to midaxillary line (Fig. 13.11). Although the liver and spleen are well protected by the ribs and are largely above the costal margin, these two organs are the most commonly injured in blunt trauma. The abdomen can be further divided into the intraperitoneal and retroperitoneal organs. Damage to intraperitoneal organs is often easily assessed, while the clinical presentation of injury to the retroperitoneal organs is often more subtle and can be easily overlooked.

Abdominal examination should include a thorough history. Physical examination of the abdomen is divided into four parts: inspection, auscultation, percussion, and palpation. The abdominal wall should be

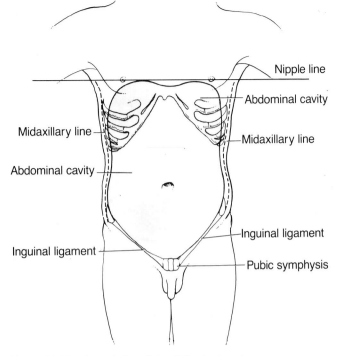

Figure 13.11. Boundaries of the abdominal cavity.

carefully inspected for any abrasions or contusions that may suggest blunt injury. Any break in the skin or laceration suggests a penetrating injury. These wounds may be small and should not be overlooked. The presence or absence of bowel sounds should be noted but does not accurately correlate with the presence or absence of acute injury. Tenderness to percussion or other signs of peritonitis anywhere in the abdomen are suggestive of peritoneal inflammation and mandate celiotomy. Palpation should proceed in a systematic fashion and should include palpation of the ribs in the lower half of the thorax, followed by palpation of the ribs in the lower half of the thorax, followed by palpation of each of the four quadrants of the abdomen. Tenderness to palpation is the most consistent symptom in intraabdominal injury, and a patient who has findings of significant tenderness to palpation on two or more examinations over a 10- to 30-minute period will need a celiotomy and therefore does not need further diagnostic testing. No abdominal examination is complete without a rectal examination. The perineum should be visually inspected, then a finger inserted into the rectum. Sphincter tone, position and mobility of the prostate, and the presence of rectal lacerations should be carefully assessed. The examining finger should then be carefully inspected for the presence of bright red blood and tested for occult blood.

Bimanual examination of the vagina and pelvic organs should also be performed. Vaginal lacerations secondary to pelvic fractures or penetrating injury are easy to overlook. When the patient is fully stable, if there is any question on bimanual examination speculum examination of the vagina should be performed. Patients who have been sexually assaulted require specialized examination and tests, which vary according to local laws. The local sexual assault center may provide information in this area.

After the abdominal examination is performed, patients can be triaged based on their hemodynamic stability and the results of the abdominal examination. Abdominal trauma can be divided into blunt or penetrating. Patients with blunt trauma who are hemodynamically unstable and who have no extraabdominal source of hemorrhage to explain their hemodynamic instability should be taken directly to the operating room for celiotomy. Patients who are stable but demonstrate signs of ongoing hemorrhage, unstable patients who have other injuries that could explain their hemodynamic instability, and patients who have an altered mental status for any reason need further diagnostic workup to exclude intraabdominal injury.

Penetrating abdominal trauma can be subdivided into abdominal trauma caused by gunshot or penetration with a sharp instrument. Gunshots require celiotomy. Even if the missile did not actually penetrate the peritoneal cavity, damage to peritoneal contents can occur from blast injury, and the abdomen must be carefully explored to rule this out. Wounds to the abdominal wall caused by sharp instruments may initially be carefully explored in the emergency department. The wound should be explored under sterile conditions and using local anesthesia to determine if anterior abdominal wall fascia has been penetrated. If there is no penetration of the fascia, the wound can be irrigated and sterilely closed. If there is penetration of the anterior abdominal fascia, two options are available. The first option is to take the patient to the operating room to undergo exploratory celiotomy. This is a common approach to penetrating injury but results in a significant number of negative abdominal explorations. Another option is to perform peritoneal lavage.

Diagnostic options to consider in abdominal trauma include plain roentgenographs, peritoneal lavage, computed tomography and (CT) scan. Plain roentgenographic examination of the abdomen has no place in the evaluation of trauma victims. A plain film of the pelvis is important to rule out bony pelvic injury, but plain abdominal films take up a large amount of time and the diagnostic accuracy from these films is too low to be of value.

Peritoneal lavage is an invasive test that can be performed in the emergency room and should be considered a surgical procedure. The advantages to this test are that it is highly sensitive and specific for identifying blood in the peritoneal cavity, which correlates well with the presence of intraabdominal injury. Further advantages are that it can be performed quickly without removing the patient from the emergency department, and, if gross blood is aspirated from the abdominal cavity, celiotomy is indicated. In skilled hands, it can be performed in less than 5 minutes. The main disadvantage is that it is an invasive procedure and may be associated with complications, including perforation of intraabdominal viscus or laceration of intraabdominal blood vessels.

The CT scan is slightly less sensitive and specific

than peritoneal lavage for identification of intraabdominal injury but has the added advantage that it may identify the actual organ that is injured or bleeding. In addition, the CT scan provides information about the retroperitoneal structures that cannot be found using peritoneal lavage. The disadvantage of CT scan is that it requires removal of the patient from the immediate area of resuscitation and it takes 20–30 minutes to perform. For this reason, it can be performed only on absolutely stable patients who are able to tolerate removal from the resuscitation area.

If it is decided that peritoneal lavage will be performed, it is imperative to decompress the stomach. A nasogastric tube or an oral gastric tube must be inserted prior to the lavage. A nasogastric tube should never be inserted if there is any question of facial fractures, because the nasogastric tube could pass through a fractured ethmoid plate into the cranial vault. An oral gastric tube is the safest option in this case. The urinary bladder must also be emptied prior to peritoneal lavage by placing a Foley catheter. Before passing a Foley catheter, a rectal and genitourinary examination must be done to rule out the presence of urethral injury. In females, the urethra is so short that urethral injury is very rare. However, in males with pelvic fractures, urethral injuries are common, and it is important that they be recognized so that injuries are not aggravated by inserting a Foley catheter. Indications of possible urethral injury include blood at the tip of the penile meatus, scrotal or perineal hematoma, or a mobile prostate gland on rectal examination. If there is any question about urethral injury, a retrograde urethrogram should be performed before placing a Foley catheter. In the presence of urethral injury, a percutaneous suprapubic cystostomy is an alternate route to urethral catheterization to drain the bladder prior to peritoneal lavage. This must be performed by an experienced physician.

Peritoneal Lavage

After decompressing the stomach and draining the urinary bladder, peritoneal lavage may be performed. This is usually performed below the umbilicus but can be performed anywhere in the abdominal wall. A small incision is made just below the umbilicus and rectus abdominis fascia is identified. A small nick is made in the midline fascia and the peritoneum is identified and grasped. A small nick is made in the peritoneum, and the peritoneal lavage catheter is introduced into the abdomen. The catheter is then connected to a syringe and aspirated. If 10–20 cc of blood is obtained, this is considered a ''grossly'' positive lavage and the patient should be surgically explored. If gross blood is not obtained, 10 cc/kg of warm Ringer's lactate (generally 1 liter in adults) is instilled into the peritoneum through the dialysis catheter. The abdomen is then gently shaken to distribute the fluid throughout the peritoneal cavity, then the fluid is siphoned off. Two-thirds of the fluid must be removed for the test to be accurate. The lavage fluid is then sent to the laboratory for cell count, microscopic, and chemistry examination. Positive findings in blunt trauma include greater than 100,000 erythrocytes/mm^3 or 500 white blood cells/mm^3 on cell count, amylase greater than serum amylase, bilirubin greater than serum bilirubin, or the presence of bacteria or fecal material on microscopic examination. A negative peritoneal lavage does not rule out injuries to the retroperitoneal organs such as the pancreas, duodenum, aorta, vena cava, or kidneys. In penetrating trauma, if more than 1,000 erythrocytes/mm^3 are found, the lavage is considered positive and celiotomy should be performed.

Complications of peritoneal lavage include bleeding from the abdominal wall resulting in a false-positive examination without intraabdominal injury or perforation of intraabdominal or retroperitoneal organs or vessels. Wound complications such as infection or hematoma may also occur. After the lavage has been performed, midline rectus fascia must be closed and the skin incision must be closed.

The indications for CT examination are essentially the same as for peritoneal lavage, except that the patient must be absolutely stable before being taken to the CT scanner. Combative patients and young children may require sedation before CT examination can be performed.

Figure 13.12 graphically demonstrates the decision process leading to laparotomy, diagnostic tests, or observation in patients with intraabdominal injury.

Patients with suspected genitourinary trauma require special consideration. Urethral injury has been discussed. If no urethral injury is present but the patient has gross hematuria or microscopic hematuria that is present on two determinations 10-20 min apart, further evaluation is indicated. A urologist should be consulted and an intravenous pyelogram and cystogram or CT scan and cystogram should be performed based on the preference of the urologic consultant.

Patients requiring immediate celiotomy who have gross or microscopic hematuria or blunt or penetrating injury to the flank should undergo a single exposure intravenous pyelogram (IVP) in the emergency department or operating room prior to surgery to establish whether the patient has two functioning kidneys.

Head and Spinal Cord Injuries

The object of this section is to acquaint the student with the principles of evaluation and initial management of patients who have sustained injury to the central nervous system or supporting structures. A detailed description of the anatomy and physiology of the central nervous system is beyond the scope of this chapter. However, it is important that students become familiar with a few simple precautions and interventions that can greatly improve the prognosis of these patients.

The most sensitive sign of central nervous system trauma is an alteration of mental status. Though drug or alcohol ingestion may also produce these changes, the etiology of altered consciousness in the multiply injured patient should be considered traumatic until

Management of Abdominal Trauma

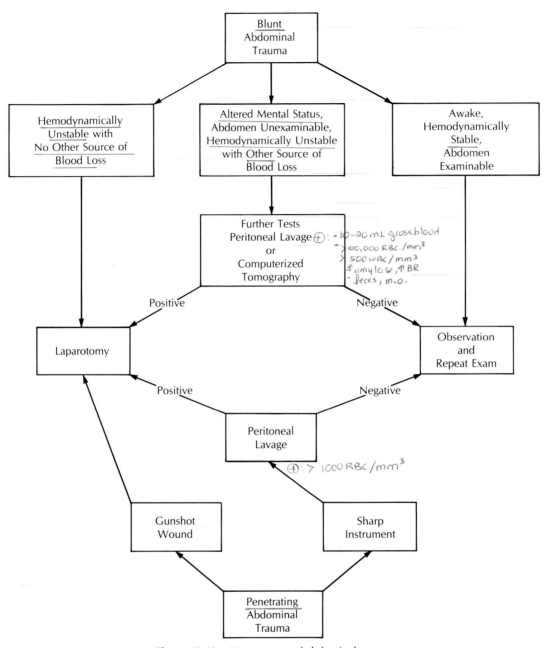

Figure 13.12. Management of abdominal trauma.

the examining physician proves otherwise. The four fundamental mechanisms through which central nervous system trauma causes altered consciousness are bilateral cerebral cortical injury, reticular activating system injury, increased intracranial pressure, and decreased cerebral blood flow.

The brain and spinal cord are unique in that they are surrounded by the rigid skull and vertebral column. Therefore, injury to these organs causing edema and swelling will increase the pressure within these bony chambers and cause decreased perfusion pressure. As perfusion deteriorates, the delivery of oxygen and nutrients to this metabolically active tissue is re-

duced, causing tissue ischemia and additional swelling. This cycle must be identified and interrupted as early as possible. Therefore, if the patient is to survive, all physicians must be alert for possible neurologic injury and familiar with the interventions used to arrest this cycle.

Patients who have sustained multiple injuries frequently have injuries to the cervical spine and spinal cord. In patients with an altered level of consciousness, there is a 10% chance of bony cervical spine injury, and it is imperative to avoid additional iatrogenic injury. The patient should be placed on a long rigid backboard with a semirigid cervical collar. These collars only offer

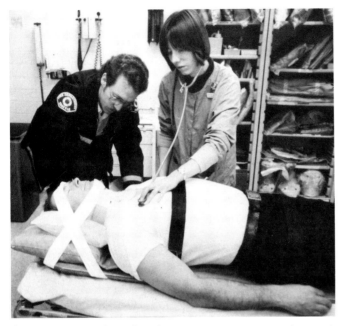

Figure 13.13. Head taped in place to prevent movement of cervical spine.

Table 13.7.
Glasgow Coma Scale

Eye opening	
Spontaneous	4
Verbal stimulus	3
Painful stimulus	2
None	1
Verbal response	
Oriented	5
Confused	4
Inappropriate	3
Incomprehensible sounds	2
No response	1
Intubated	IT
Best motor responses	
Obeys commands	6
Localizes painful stimulus	5
Withdraws from painful stimulus	4
Flexion response	3
Extensor response	2
No response	1
Score range	
Extubated	3–15
Intubated	3T–11T

partial protection, particularly if the patient is combative. The rigid collar can be reinforced with sandbags placed on both sides of the patient's head and the head taped securely into place for added protection (Fig. 13.13).

Once the cervical spine has been adequately protected and airway, breathing, and circulation have been stabilized, an abbreviated neurologic examination is done using the Glasgow Coma Scale. This is a rapid graded examination assessing these functions: eye opening, verbal response, and motor response. The maximum number of points is assigned for a normal examination and one point is assigned for no response (Table 13.7). If a patient is intubated, "1-T" is assigned for verbal response. The student should memorize the Glasgow Coma Scale so that it can be accomplished in a matter of seconds. Central nervous system injury may also be associated with several nonneurologic signs. Increased intracranial pressure and brain stem injuries frequently alter respiratory drive, blood pressure, and pulse. The first evidence of an acute increase in intracranial pressure is slowing of respiration. As intracranial pressure continues to rise, tachypnea and abnormal breath sounds may occur. Hypertension and bradycardia, the Cushing reflex, occur with further increases in intracranial pressure. A rapid change from bradycardia to tachycardia and hypertension to hypotension is usually a sign of brain stem herniation and is a terminal event.

Treating a suspected head injury is second in priority to maintaining an adequate circulating blood volume. However, if the history and physical examination suggest a head injury and the patient is hemodynamically stable, measures to minimize cerebral edema and intracranial pressure should be initiated immediately. The patient should be placed in the head-up position

and hyperventilated to reduce $PaCO_2$ to 26–28 torr. If the patient does not require intubation simply to protect the airway, it is reasonable to perform intubation solely for hyperventilation. Intubation should be performed with C-spine stabilization, as previously outlined.

The physician should then perform the secondary assessment, starting at the head and working inferiorly. Using sterile gloves, any cranial lacerations should be carefully palpated to look for depressed skull fractures. Periorbital ecchymoses (raccoon's eyes), perimastoid ecchymoses (Battle's sign), and hemotympanum all indicate basilar skull fracture. The physician should carefully check for otorrhea or rhinorrhea secondary to CSF leakage. This may be difficult to detect if there is bleeding from these sites. In these cases, it is helpful to allow a drop of the fluid to fall on a piece of filter paper and observe its movement. The presence of cerebrospinal fluid in the fluid is suggested by a "double ring sign"; the blood in the fluid moves slowly and forms a dark ring in the center, while cerebrospinal fluid diffuses more rapidly, forming a larger clear ring.

While exerting traction on the cervical spine manually, the cervical collar is removed and the neck is carefully examined. The spine should be carefully palpated for tenderness, deformity, or stepoff. A careful motor and sensory examination of the extremities and torso should include testing for light touch, pain, and two-point discrimination and reflexes. Any abnormalities or asymmetry should be carefully noted and rechecked later. At the completion of the secondary assessment, the patient is carefully logrolled onto one side and the entire thoracic and lumbar spine palpated.

Lateral cervical spine film should be obtained as previously discussed. In addition, AP and odontoid films should be taken. The absence of abnormality on x-ray does not absolutely rule out injury to the ligamentous supporting structures. Any patient who is not fully conscious must be treated as if neurologic injury exists until a full roentgenographic series can be completed and examined by a radiologist. If there is a question of injury, a neurosurgeon or other surgeon should be consulted.

After completion of the secondary assessment, a definitive care plan must be made. If any neurologic injury has been identified, neurosurgical consultation must be obtained early. The examining physician should have the results of three neurologic examinations; the first one performed by the paramedical personnel in the field, the second abbreviated neurologic examination performed during the initial assessment, and a complete neurologic examination performed during the secondary survey. These results, along with an assessment of the respiratory and cardiovascular status, vital signs, and a summary of all injuries, should be communicated as rapidly as possible to the neurosurgeon. Patients with an altered state of consciousness should undergo CT examination of the head as soon as possible after injury. Neurologic intervention is generally based on findings at CT scan.

It is imperative to ensure that the trauma patient has been adequately fluid resuscitated after injury, but hypervolemia must be avoided, as it may augment cerebral edema. If the level of consciousness deteriorates, addition of mannitol, loop diuretics, or steroids may be considered at the discretion of the neurosurgeon. If CT scanning is not available, the neurosurgeon may consider surgical decompression with burn holes.

Seizures are a frequent and dangerous complication of head injury, because a convulsive patient may become hypoxic and hypercapnic. Moreover, the violent movements may cause spinal cord damage if there is preexisting bony injury. Convulsions should be treated promptly, initially with intravenous diazepam, followed by longer-acting anticonvulsive agents such as diphenylhydantoin or phenobarbital.

If spinal cord injury has been identified on the secondary assessment, the spine must be carefully immobilized until definitive neurosurgical treatment can be performed. It is important to distinguish between incomplete and complete spinal cord lesions, because the former have a more favorable prognosis. The anal, perineal, and scrotal areas should be examined carefully for sensory perception and voluntary motor function. Sacral sparing, the preservation of these functions, indicates an incomplete cord transection. These patients have a higher likelihood of regaining cord function.

Extremity Trauma

The evaluation and stabilization of the traumatized extremity is discussed in this section. Although injury of the extremities is rarely life threatening, it is a source of permanent disability if not properly managed. In the primary survey, these injuries are addressed only to the extent of controlling hemorrhage by applying direct pressure to bleeding vessels. In the secondary survey, each extremity is carefully examined thoroughly and systematically to assess neurologic function, perfusion, deformity, and range of motion.

The patient must be completely undressed for adequate physical examination. Each extremity is carefully observed for deformity or swelling, noting the color of the limb and any soft tissue wounds. Next the extremity is carefully palpated to look for tenderness or crepitance and grossly determine the temperature. The patient should be asked to move each extremity, and the range of motion of each individual joint should be checked. If the patient is unconscious, the physician should gently move every joint and palpate every long bone. Obvious fractures or dislocations should not be moved. It is important to assess the joint above and below the sites of any fracture for signs of dislocation.

Table 13.8.
Recommendation for Tetanus Prophylaxis

Immunization Status	Wound Classification	Recommendation
Previously fully immunized Last booster within 10 yr	Nontetanus prone	No therapy
Previously fully immunized Last booster more than 5 yr ago	Tetanus prone	0.5 cc of absorbed toxoid
Previously received 2 injections of absorbed toxoid Last booster more than 10 years ago	Tetanus prone and nontetanus prone	0.5 cc of absorbed toxoid
Previously received 0–1 injections of absorbed toxoid, or	Nontetanus prone	0.5 cc of absorbed toxoid
Immunization history unknown	Tetanus prone	0.5 cc of absorbed toxoid and 250 units of tetanus human immune globulin given at 2 separate sites with separate syringes and needles

Lastly, a careful neurovascular examination is performed. Each pulse is checked manually or with a Doppler instrument; pain, light touch, and two-point discrimination are evaluated. Pain or motion on palpation and compression of the pelvis are suggestive of pelvic fractures. Areas of suspicion on physical examination should be evaluated radiographically.

Serious extremity injuries are divided into fractures, dislocations, amputations, and compartment syndromes. Potentially life-threatening injuries include crush injuries to the abdomen and pelvis, major pelvic fractures, traumatic amputations proximal to the hand or foot, and massive open femoral fractures. Pelvic fractures can be associated with severe hemorrhage if they involve sacral fractures or disruption of the sacroiliac joint. Pelvic fractures associated with signs of major blood loss can be stabilized by application and inflation of the pneumatic antishock garment. All fractures should be assessed for deformity and open wounds. Open fracture wounds should be carefully irrigated and covered with moist saline dressings. A broad-spectrum antibiotic effective against staphylococcus and streptococcus should be administered intravenously as promptly as possible. Tetanus prophylaxis should be given as outlined in Table 13.8. If there is any uncertainty about immunization status, the patient should be considered unimmunized.

Displaced fractures should be aligned and immobilized. It is critical to immobilize the extremity one joint above and one joint below the fracture. After alignment and immobilization, neurovascular examination should be repeated to ensure that these manipulations have not caused additional injury. Often in extremities with absent or diminished pulses, alignment and immobilization are accompanied by marked improvement of the pulses. Although an abnormality of distal pulses strongly suggests a vascular injury, a normal examination does not rule this injury out. Whenever a vascular injury is suspected clinically, an angiogram should be performed. Dislocations and fracture dislocations, particularly if the elbow and knee are involved, can result in arterial and neurologic injury and have a high priority for treatment. Prompt orthopedic consultation should be obtained for all dislocations and relocation performed as soon as possible. Occasionally, reduction of a dislocation will require general anesthesia.

Trauma to the lower leg and forearm may result in the compartment syndrome, particularly if associated with a crush injury. Neurovascular compromise is secondary to hemorrhage and edema within a compartment bounded by fascial planes. Classically, the syndrome presents as a painful pale extremity with decreased pulses and sensation; in the late stage, paralysis develops. These manifestations may be subtle, yet limb viability is threatened. The diagnosis of the compartment syndrome is confirmed by measuring intracompartmental pressures. Pressures exceeding 30 mm Hg indicate the need for emergent fasciotomy to preserve the limb.

Traumatic amputation requires immediate consultation with and transfer to a facility at which microsurgical reimplantation is possible. Amputated parts should be carefully cleaned with sterile saline, wrapped in a moistened sterile towel, placed in a sterile plastic bag, and transported in an insulated cooling chest filled with crushed ice. The ice should not come into direct contact with the amputated part, as this will cause further tissue damage. (Some centers differ in the preservation of the amputated part; it is prudent to consult with the center regarding the management prior to transportation.) Any amputated part should always be transported with the patient. The decision regarding the feasibility of replantation should be made by the physicians who will perform the surgery.

Burns

Burn injuries should be approached like any major traumatic injury, and the resuscitation of a burn patient should follow the same orderly progression of primary survey and resuscitation followed by secondary survey and definitive care. However, there are several unique features of thermal injury that slightly modify the basic resuscitation algorithm, and the student should become familiar with these changes.

Initially the physician must determine that the burning process has been arrested. Synthetic fabric still adherent to the patient can smolder and burn without obvious signs. Once the burning process has been stopped, attention is turned to the airway and breathing. Although the subglottic airway is protected from direct thermal injury and can only be burned through exposure to super-heated gas or steam, the supraglottic area is highly susceptible to thermal injury. Pharyngeal injury may produce significant upper airway edema, which may not be apparent clinically until several hours after the injury. Thus a patient with an intact airway on initial evaluation may later develop airway obstruction. Therefore the physician must be alert for signs of inhalation injury and secure the airway early, before the edema develops. Factors that are commonly associated with inhalation injury are listed in Table 13.9. If any of these clinical signs are present, the patient should be considered for early endotracheal intubation and mechanical ventilation.

After controlling the airway and breathing, the physician should focus on supporting the circulating blood volume. Two large-caliber intravenous lines should be placed immediately in the upper extremities. An un-

Table 13.9.
Signs Suggesting Inhalation Injury

History of confinement in a burning building
History of explosion
History of decreased level of consciousness
Carbon deposits around the mouth or in the oropharynx
Inflammatory changes in the oropharynx
Carbonaceous sputum

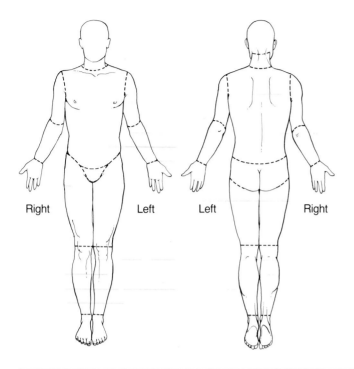

Right   Left   Left   Right

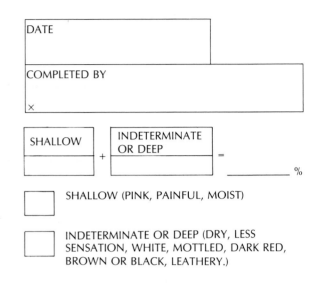

DATE

COMPLETED BY

×

| SHALLOW | + | INDETERMINATE OR DEEP | = | _____ % |

☐ SHALLOW (PINK, PAINFUL, MOIST)

☐ INDETERMINATE OR DEEP (DRY, LESS SENSATION, WHITE, MOTTLED, DARK RED, BROWN OR BLACK, LEATHERY.)

Percent Surface Area Burned
(Berkow Formula)

AREA	1 YEAR	1–4 YEARS	5–9 YEARS	10–14 YEARS	Y 15 YEARS	ADULT	SHALLOW	INDETERMINATE OR DEEP
Head	19	17	13	11	9	7		
Neck	2	2	2	2	2	2		
Ant. Trunk	13	13	13	13	13	13		
Post Trunk	2½	2½	2½	2½	2½	2½		
L. Buttock	2½	2½	2½	2½	2½	2½		
Ganitalia	1	1	1	1	1	1		
R. U. Arm	4	4	4	4	4	4		
L. U. Arm	4	4	4	4	4	4		
R. L. Arm	3	3	3	3	3	3		
L. L. Arm	3	3	3	3	3	3		
R. Hand	2½	2½	2½	2½	2½	2½		
L. Hand	2½	2½	2½	2½	2½	2½		
R. Thigh	5½	6½	8	8½	9	9½		
L. Thigh	5½	6½	8	8½	9	9½		
R. Leg	5	5	5½	6	6½	7		
L. Leg	5	5	5½	6	6½	7		
R. Foot	3½	3½	3½	3½	3½	3½		
L. Foot	3½	3½	3½	3½	3½	3½		
TOTAL								

HOSP. NO. _____   PATIENT NAME _____   WARD _____

IMPRINT HERE

HARBORVIEW MEDICAL CENTER
INITIAL BURN CHART

HMC 0653   REV DEC 85

Figure 13.14. Initial burn chart.

burned site is preferable but, if unavailable, peripheral lines may be placed through burned skin. Any patient with burns covering more than 20% of the total body surface area will require intravenous fluid support with a balanced crystalloid solution. The remainder of the primary survey and resuscitation are carried out as previously outlined.

The secondary survey is next, beginning with a thorough history, which should include the mechanism of injury and concurrent medical problems. This is followed by a careful physical examination to assess any concomitant injuries. It is imperative to remove any rings, bracelets, or other jewelry, when encountered on physical examination, to prevent circulatory compromise.

After completing the standard secondary survey, the burns are then evaluated for extent and depth. Burn wounds are divided into three categories, according to their depth. First-degree burns produce skin erythema that is very sensitive to the touch but does not blister. These burns do not permanently damage the dermis. An example of a first-degree burn is the common sunburn. Second-degree or "partial-thickness" burns are characterized by as red or mottled appearance, with edema and blister formation. The surface is usually weeping and is painfully hypersensitive. Third-degree, or "full-thickness burns," can appear waxy-white or dark and leather-like. The surface is generally dry and, because all dermal elements have been destroyed, is painless.

In estimating the extent of burns, first-degree burns are ignored, and second- and third-degree burns are grouped together. The most accurate method of estimating burn size is by drawing on a burn chart (Fig. 13.14). By drawing and comparing two charts, one indicating the burned area and the other indicating the unburned area, a very accurate estimate of the percent of surface area burned can be reached. The body surface area of infants and children differs considerably from that of adults, with the head accounting for a much larger proportion of surface area and the extremities a much smaller proportion (Fig. 13.14). If a burn chart is unavailable, two useful guides for estimating the extent of a burn are the Rule of nines (Fig. 13.15) and the observation that the area of an individual's palm represents approximately 1% of body surface area.

Once the extent and depth of the burn have been accurately estimated, a definitive care plan can be constructed. The most important part of the initial therapy of the burn patient is adequate early fluid resuscitation. In general, during the initial 24 hours, the burn patient requires approximately 4 ml of balanced crystalloid solution per kilogram of total body weight multiplied by the percent of body surface area burned. Half of this requirement should be given in the first 8 hours and the second half over the next 16 hours. For example, a 70-kg male with a 50% total body surface second-degree burn will require 14 liters of fluid in the first 24 hours. Therefore the fluid should infuse at 875 cc/hr for the first 8 hours and 435 cc/hr for the next 16 hours.

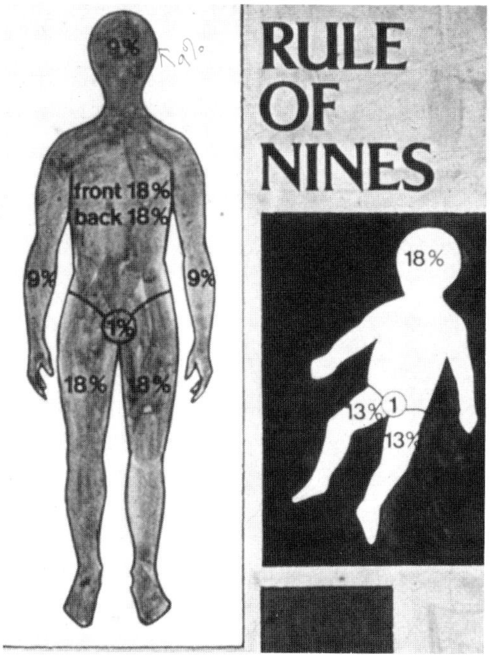

Figure 13.15. Rule of nines. Estimation of burn size by the rule of nines.

This formula provides only an estimate of fluid requirements. It is critical to place a urinary catheter and monitor the urine output to confirm adequate resuscitation. A normal adult should put out 30–50 cc of urine per hour and a child should put out 1–2 cc/kg/hr. If the urine output is inadequate despite what appears to be an adequate fluid resuscitation, a central venous catheter should be placed for further monitoring.

Any patient burned over more than 20% of their body surface area requires a nasogastric tube to prevent abdominal distension, nausea, and emesis, which occur secondary to a reflex ileus.

At the end of the secondary survey, an assessment of the circulation distal to burned areas should be performed. A Doppler instrument is used to confirm pulsatile flow in the digital, palmar, and pedal vessels. Circulatory compromise secondary to a circumferentially burned limb is an indication for escharotomy. Escharotomy is also occasionally required in patients who have circumferentially burned torsos to allow for adequate ventilation. In general, a surgeon's help is useful if an escharotomy is needed.

Topical antibiotics and creams should not be applied in the emergency room, as they will have to be removed during subsequent debridement. For burn wounds less than 10% of the body surface area, cold soaks may be applied for 10–15 minutes to help reduce pain. If a greater percentage of the body has been burned, cold soaks will only produce hypothermia and should not be used.

Chemical and electrical burns require special consideration. Chemical burns are caused by topical, acidic, or alkaline exposure. Burns secondary to alkali tend to cause more serious tissue damage and penetrate more deeply. The extent of chemical burns is determined by

Table 13.10.
Burn Transfer Criteria

Burns > 25% of the body surface area in 10- to 40-yr-old
Burns > 20% of the body surface area in children < 10 yr and adults > 40 yr
Full thickness burns involving > 10% of the body surface area
All burns involving the face, eyes, ears, hands, feet, or perineum
Burns associated with other major injuries
Electrical burns
Chemical burns
Inhalational injury
Any burn in a patient with significant preexisting disease

the duration of contact and the concentration and type of chemical. No attempt should be made to neutralize chemical burns. Instead, they should be irrigated with warm water for at least 20–30 minutes.

Electrical burns are usually more serious than the surface of the body indicates. The severity of electrical burns depends on the voltage and current of electricity. As the current passes through the body, muscles, nerves, blood vessels, and bone may be destroyed. Extensive muscle destruction can liberate sufficient myoglobin to cause acute renal failure. Patients with significant electrical burns must be placed on an ECG monitor and urinary output should be maintained at greater than 100 cc/hr. If there is visible discoloration of the urine despite an output of greater than 100 cc/hr, 25 gm of mannitol should be administered immediately and 12½ mg of mannitol given with each subsequent liter of fluid. In addition, 50 mEq of sodium bicarbonate can be given with each liter of fluid to prevent precipitation of the myoglobin pigment.

Patients with partial thickness burns less than 5% of their total body surface area, excluding burns of the face, hand, feet, and perineum, may be treated as outpatients unless social circumstances indicate otherwise. Any burn treated as an outpatient should be seen by a general surgeon familiar with burn care. Patients with uncomplicated partial-thickness burns of between 5 and 20% of total body surface area may be treated at community hospitals. Larger burns and complex burns, particularly electrical and chemical burns, should be treated at specialized facilities. Table 13.10 lists the criteria established by the American Burn Association for transfer to specialized facilities.

The transfer of any patient to a burn unit must be coordinated with the physician in charge of that unit, and all pertinent information gathered at the initial care facility must be communicated in an accurate and orderly fashion.

SUGGESTED READINGS

Baker SP, O'Neill B, Karpf RS: *The Injury Fact Book*. Lexington, MA, DC Heath, 1985.

Carter DC, Polk HC: *Trauma*. Stoneham, MA, Butterworths, 1981.

Collicott PE, Aprahamian C, et al: *Advanced Trauma Life Support Course for Physicians*. Subcommittee on Advanced Trauma Life Support (ATLS) of the American College of Surgeons Committee on Trauma, 1983–1984.

Department of Defense. *Emergency War Surgery*. United States Revision 1, NATO Handbook, 1975.

Federle MP, Brant-Zawadzki M: *Computed Tomography in the Evaluation of Trauma*, ed 2. Baltimore, Williams & Wilkins, 1986.

Jennett B, Teasdale G: *Management of Head Injuries*. Philadelphia, FA Davis, 1984.

Moore E, Eiseman B, Van Way CW: *Critical Decisions in Trauma*. St. Louis, Mosby, 1984.

Sabiston DC: *Textbook of Surgery. The Biological Basis of Modern Surgical Practice*, ed 13. Philadelphia, WB Saunders, 1986.

Schwartz SI, Shires GT, et al: *Principles of Surgery*, ed 4. New York, McGraw-Hill, 1983.

Shires GT: *Care of the Trauma Patient*, ed 2. New York, McGraw-Hill, 1979.

Trunkey DD, Lewis FR: *Current Therapy of Trauma*, ed 2. BC Decker, 1986, vol 2.

Wiener SL, Barrett J: *Trauma Management For Civilian and Military Physicians*. Philadelphia, WB Saunders, 1986.

Worth MH: *Principles and Practice of Trauma Care*. Baltimore, Williams & Wilkins, 1982.

Zuidema GD, Rutherford RB, Ballinger WF: *The Management of Trauma*, ed 3. Philadelphia, WB Saunders, 1979.

Skills

1. Conduct an initial assessment and management survey on a simulated or actual multiply injured patient, using the correct sequence of priorities and explanation of the management techniques for primary treatment and stabilization.

2. Conduct a mini-neurological examination and determine the Glasgow Coma Scale on a simulated or real patient with head trauma.

3. Demonstrate your ability to immobilize the spine on a real or simulated patient with a back injury.

4. Demonstrate your ability to immobilize a fractured extremity of a real or simulated patient.

5. Interpret a chest x-ray in a patient with severe closed chest trauma.

6. Observe the performance of peritoneal lavage in a traumatized patient; order and interpret the resulting tests.

7. Demonstrate your ability to place large (< 20-gauge) intravenous lines in a simulated or real traumatized patient.

8. Given a patient with a 45% deep second degree burn of the legs and trunk, calculate the fluid resuscitation requirements for the first 24 hours.

9. Describe the necessary steps in the outpatient treatment of a patient with a small burn on the forearm.

Study Questions

1. Describe the sequence of events necessary for evaluation of the multiply injured patient after a motor vehicle accident who is brought to the emergency department by the life squad with a blood pressure of 80/–, pulse 130, and respiratory rate of 36 and very shallow.

2. Calculate the fluid requirements (milliliter/hour) for a 42-year-old male who sustained full-thickness burns to the left side of his face and head, both hands, and anterior chest as the result of a house fire. Describe what special problems could develop and how they should be evaluated and managed.

3. Discuss the advantages and disadvantages of nasotracheal intubation over oral intubation.

4. A multiply injured patient is brought to the emergency department after a high-speed single-car accident. He is responsive to painful stimuli by withdrawing, and he moves all four extremities. He has an obvious left femur fracture with a good distal pulse. Breath sounds are symmetrical. After 30 min in the emergency department, no other injuries are apparent by physical examination. He has received 3000 of balanced saline solution, but his pressure has gradually fallen to 70/– mm Hg. Discuss how you would evaluate this problem.

5. A 17-year-old motorcyclist riding without a helmet is thrown from his bike. He is brought to the hospital 10 minutes later by his friends. His vital signs are normal, but he is combative and restless. Shortly after being placed in the trauma room he has a seizure. Describe how you would manage this patient.

6. Describe the advantages of computed tomography over diagnostic peritoneal lavage in the evaluation of the abdomen, or vice versa. If you had to choose only one of these procedures to be available in your hospital, which would you choose? Defend your position.

14

The Abdominal Wall, Including Hernia

D. Byron McGregor, M.D.
Richard A. Bomberger, M.D.
L. Beaty Pemberton, M.D.
Dan C. English, M.D.

ASSUMPTION

The student understands the normal anatomy of the inguinal and femoral regions.

OBJECTIVES

1. Define indirect inguinal hernia, direct inguinal hernia, and femoral hernia.
2. List the factors that predispose the development of inguinal hernias.
3. Discuss the relative frequency of indirect, direct, and femoral hernias by age and sex.
4. Define incarcerated inguinal hernia, strangulated hernia, and "sliding hernia."
5. Define incarcerated femoral hernia, strangulated femoral hernia, and Richter's hernia.
6. Outline the principles of management of patients with groin hernias, including the surgical treatments for repair and indications for their use.
7. Define an umbilical hernia and relate to the embryological origin of the umbilicus.
8. List the factors that predispose the development of umbilical hernia, including congenital factors.
9. Outline the principles of management of patients with umbilical hernias.
10. Define Spigelian hernia, Morgagni's hernia, Bochdalek's hernia, and Petit's hernia.
11. List three etiologies for the development of incisional hernia.

This chapter deals with the structure, function, and common abnormalities of the soft tissue layers comprising the abdominal wall. We intend that completion of this chapter will enable the reader to ascribe specific abdominal wall symptoms to common intraabdominal diseases, describe common abdominal incisions, and display a broad understanding of the etiology, significance, and management of hernias.

Anatomy

Surface Relationships

There are few useful anatomical landmarks. Only the coastal margins, anterior superior iliac spines, and umbilicus break the otherwise flat plane of an all-too-well upholstered abdominal wall. Where anatomy has failed, verbiage has been substituted. *Hypochondriacal* (below the ribs), *periumbilical* (around the belly button), and *epigastric* (high abdominal) are all examples of such colorful but imprecise terms. Other attempts have been made to define abdominal regions by drawing imaginary lines across the abdominal wall. The abdomen has thus been halved, trisected, even divided into as many as nine separate imaginary compartments in attempts to provide reliable topographic characteristics. The most useful of these is the creation of simple vertical and horizontal lines through the umbilicus, dividing the abdomen into four imaginary quadrants (Fig. 14.1). In this format, the right upper quadrant covers such symptom-prone intraabdominal organs as the gallbladder, the duodenum, the right pleura, and the liver; the left upper quadrant protects the spleen, stomach, left pleura, and tail of pancreas; the left lower quadrant obscures the sigmoid colon and left ureter; and the right lower quadrant overlies the right ureter, cecum, Meckel's diverticulum, and that typifier of right lower quadrant pain, the appendix.

Cutaneous Nerves

Sensory innervation of the anterior abdominal wall is supplied by the sensory branches of the lower intercostal nerves down through L-1. They appear first on the anterior abdominal wall as the lateral cutaneous nerves that appear at the anterior axillary line. They proceed anteriorly, dividing into anterior and posterior branches, and supply the anterior and posterior abdominal walls in a dermatome-like fashion, with rela-

154

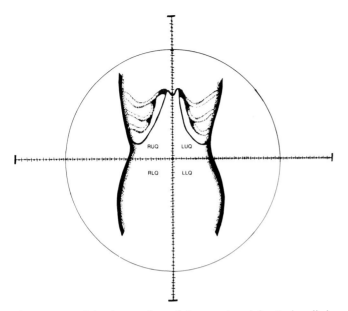

Figure 14.1. Sniper's eye view of the anterior abdominal wall defining descriptive sectors of anatomy.

tively transverse distribution in the upper abdomen and a more oblique pattern in the groins (Fig. 14.2). The intercostal nerves also provide the anterior cutaneous branches that run in the anterior abdominal wall between the transversus abdominus muscle and the internal oblique muscle toward the midline, where they pierce the rectus sheath, supply the rectus muscle, and proceed anteriorly to innervate the midline and contribute to the segmental pattern started by the lateral cutaneous branches (Fig. 14.2B).

The result of this rich cutaneous innervation is a series of dermatome-related clues to intraabdominal diagnoses. For example, visceral afferent fibers from the appendix follow the same nerve distribution as that of the small intestine back to their T-10 origins. It is therefore not surprising that the early picture of appendicitis is that of a central abdominal pain in the T-10 dermatome distribution. Later in the course of the disease, if the inflammatory process from the appendix develops anteriorly and irritates the peritoneum beneath the right lower quadrant of the abdomen, this irritation is sensed by somatic afferent fibers of the T-12 nerve route and reflected back in the appropriate lower cutaneous distribution as hyperesthesia. The disease can be well

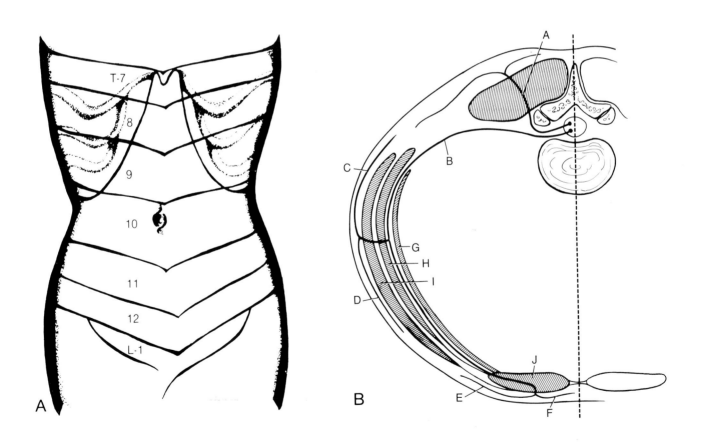

Figure 14.2. **A,** Cutaneous nerve distribution to anterior abdominal wall. **B,** Schema of cutaneous nerves: **A,** posterior primary division; **B,** anterior primary division; **C,** posterior division of lateral cutaneous nerve; **D,** anterior division of lateral cutaneous nerve; **E,** lateral division of anterior cutaneous nerve; **F,** medial division of anterior cutaneous nerve; **G,** transversus abdominus muscle; **H,** internal oblique muscle; **I,** external oblique muscle; **J,** rectus abdominus muscle.

described by abdominal wall findings alone, without knowing anything about the appendix.

Despite this apparent degree of segmental precision, considerable overlap of cutaneous nerves exists. This is fortunate for the surgeon who must occasionally sacrifice cutaneous nerves in the course of abdominal incisions. Because of this overlap, the cutting of any single cutaneous nerve usually results in no permanent sensory loss. This safety factory is less pronounced in the lower sensory nerves (ilioinguinal and iliohypogastric), which, if injured, can leave permanent numbness in the groin, scrotum, and anterior thigh.

Layers of the Abdominal Wall

A brief review of the seven individual layers making up the abdominal wall is pertinent prior to any discussion of the use of these layers to explain surgical disease or design surgical repairs. The following discussion presents the anatomy of the seven individual layers, with particular attention to the origins and reflections of fascial continuity for each. The most notable of the reflections occurs in the groin, where all of the layers of the abdominal wall are reflected into the scrotum, much as the layers of a shirt, jacket, and overcoat are reflected off the chest wall and onto a sleeve, while maintaining constant relationship to each other.

Skin

As elsewhere, the skin over the abdominal wall is transgressed by Langer's lines of cleavage. These lines of skin tension are produced by the course of fibrous bundles and the disposition of elastic fibers in the cornium. Across the anterior abdominal walls these lines are dispersed transversely. In the lower abdomen, like the cutaneous nerves, Langer's lines assume a slightly more oblique pattern as they course into the groins.

The skin, its cleavage lines, and its superficial cutaneous innervation all are continuous into the scrotum. In describing the continuity of layers, it must first be said that skin becomes skin.

Superficial Fascia

The superficial fascia of the abdominal wall is present as two layers. The more superficial of these and the more fatty of the two is Camper's fascia. The deeper, more fibrous, denser layer is Scarpa's fascia. There is considerable disagreement regarding precise definition and fascial connection of these two adipose layers, and in general they can be freely transgressed in any plane with no adverse effect. They are generally conceded to be contiguous into the perineum as the superficial perineal fascia of Colles of the penis and the tunica dartos of the scrotum. It is along this fascial continuity that infections and urinary extravasations proceed out of the perineum and onto the abdominal wall.

External Oblique Muscle

The major functioning muscles of the abdominal wall are broad, flat constricting layers that in general overlap throughout their course and join symmetrically in the midline. The most superficial of these is the external abdominal oblique muscle. This muscle arises broadly from the lower six ribs and interdigitations of the serratus anterior muscle. In the flank, it forms a thick broad muscle whose fibers run obliquely downward, but, as it courses over the anterior aspect of the abdominal wall, the fibers of its aponeurosis (its flat tendon) run essentially transversely. Above the umbilicus, this aponeurosis fuses with half of the aponeurosis of the internal oblique muscle at the lateral margin of the rectus abdominus muscle to form the anterior rectus sheath (Fig. 14.3). Below the umbilicus, this fusion occurs very close to the midline. In the groin, the

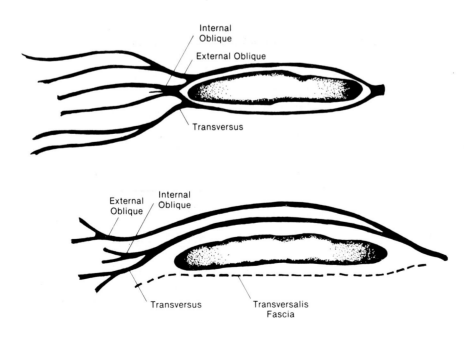

Figure 14.3. Midline fascial relationships above (**top**) and below (**bottom**) the semicircular line of Douglas.

aponeurotic fibers of the external oblique muscle angle downward, taking the direction of your fingers if placed comfortably in your jeans. Further laterally this aponeurosis rolls on itself to form the inguinal ligament. This ligament is a free margin suspended between the anterior superior iliac spine and the pubic tubercle, with no muscular origins or insertions. Medially the fibers of the inguinal ligament rotate and attach onto the most medial portion of Cooper's ligament as the lacunar ligament, which forms the final medial buttress of a femoral hernia. The external oblique aponeurosis is contiguous into the scrotum as the external spermatic fascia and onto the anterior thigh as the fascia lata. Finally, near the medial attachment of the external oblique aponeurosis onto the pubic tubercle, the aponeurosis divides, forming a triangular orifice through which the spermatic cord and testicle descend. This aperture persists as the "external" or "superficial" inguinal ring.

Internal Oblique Muscle

The internal oblique muscle also arises broadly from the iliac crest, the lumbodorsal fascia, and the psoas fascia, as well as from continuity with its homologue, the internal intercostal muscles of the lower chest wall. Its fibers are directed obliquely upward in the high flank, transversely in the midflank, and obliquely downward in the low flank. Like the external oblique muscle, the internal oblique forms a broad aponeurosis that fuses into the midline and contributes to the anterior rectus sheath throughout the abdomen as well as the posterior rectus sheath in the upper abdomen (Fig. 14.3). The internal oblique remains muscular in the groin, where it has no attachments, and its fibers reflect the spermatic cord as the cremasteric muscle.

Transversus Muscle

The transversus abdominus muscle, the deepest of the three muscular layers, has similar origins and attachments to the internal oblique, arising from the lower six ribs, the thoracolumbar fascia, and the iliac crest and fusing medially to form the rectus sheaths and the linea alba. The fibers of its aponeurosis again run transversely, except in the groin, where the clinical importance of this aponeurosis is realized as it curves medially and downward to attach onto the pubic tubercle, the pectineal (Cooper's) ligament, and continues down the thigh as the anterior femoral sheath. It is in the groin that the aponeurosis of the transversus abdominus and its fused underlying transversalis fascia are the posterior inguinal wall, through which (via its triangular orifice, the "abdominal" or "deep" or "internal" inguinal ring) the spermatic cord descends. It is through this layer that all groin hernia pathology develops.

Transversalis Fascia

The transversalis fascia forms a complete uninterrupted envelope of fascia around the interior of the abdominal cavity. Being a true fascial layer, the transversalis fascia has little intrinsic strength but through its fusion to aponeurotic layers establishes continuity between such seemingly unrelated areas as the diaphragm, the obturator internus, and the aforementioned layers of the anterior abdominal wall. It is separated from the underlying peritoneum by a variable layer of preperitoneal connective tissue and fat. With the descent of the testicle, the transversalis fascia establishes continuity with the internal spermatic fascia of the spermatic cord.

Peritoneum

The peritoneum is a serous membrane lining the entire peritoneal cavity and investing the intraabdominal structures. Details of the intraabdominal reflections of the peritoneum and the formation of the greater and lesser peritoneal sacs are discussed in Chapters 16–18; the peritoneum is best thought of here as only the exquisitely sensitive final lining layer of the anterior abdominal wall. With the descent of the testicle, a portion of the peritoneum is also advanced into the scrotum (Fig. 14.4). With complete development, this peritoneal

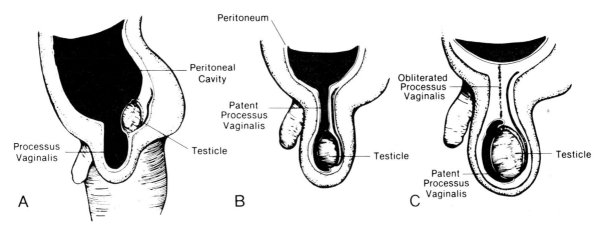

Figure 14.4. Peritoneal accompaniment of testicular descent. **A,** Prior to descent of testicle. **B,** Full patency of processus vaginalis after descent. **C,** Patent remnant or noncommunicating hydrocele.

remnant remains as the tunica vaginalis of the testicle. In normal development, the remainder of the peritoneal connection is obliterated and the peritoneal cavity is once again a sealed space within the abdominal cavity (with the exception of the fallopian tube orifices). Failure to complete this obliteration process results in varying degrees of persistence of an open communication between the peritoneal cavity and the tunica vaginalis. These varying degrees of patency result in either a communicating or noncommunicating hydrocele or a mere persistent patency of the processes vaginalis, inviting herniation.

Central Relationships Across Midline

All the layers of the abdominal wall are continuous across the anterior midline. The skin, subcutaneous tissues, transversalis fascia, and peritoneum are simple continuations, but the fusions and attachments of the abdominal muscles, the umbilicus, and the umbilical cord remnants deserve special attention.

To understand these midline structures, the sheaths and locations of the rectus abdominus muscles must be described. In comparison to the other abdominal muscles, these are narrow, thick bands of muscle that parallel the midline from coastal cartilages to the pubic symphysis. Each muscle is divided along its course by a variable number of tendinous inscriptions, which essentially divide the muscle into a series of interconnected muscles. They are separated in the midline above the umbilicus by a condensation of the aponeuroses of the other abdominal muscles, called the linea alba. The formation of that linea alba and of the rectus sheaths is of some anatomical interest and surgical importance (Fig. 14.3). Approximately midway between the umbilicus and the symphysis pubis exists an anatomical landmark, the semicircular line of Douglas. Above this line the anterior sheath is formed by a fusion of the external oblique aponeurosis and the anterior leaf of the internal oblique aponeurosis. The posterior sheath in this position is formed by a fusion of the posterior leaf of the internal oblique aponeurosis and the aponeurosis of the transversus. Below the semicircular line, all three aponeuroses cross anterior to the rectus muscle, leaving only the peritoneum and the transversalis fascia between the rectus muscles and the abdominal contents. Below the semicircular line, the exact point of fusion of the aponeurotic layers to form the rectus sheath is variable. The external oblique usually joins far medially. The internal oblique and transversus fuse close to the lateral edge of the rectus muscle. Wherever the latter fusion occurs, the anterior rectus sheath is born. No fusion of these layers occurs along the inguinal canal, so the often mentioned, but seldom present, ''conjoint tendon'' normally does not exist.

Umbilicus

By the start of the second trimester, the omphalomesenteric duct has disappeared, the gut has rotated and reentered the peritoneal cavity, and the body walls have formed, with the exception of a ring of variable size in the middle of the abdomen. Through this ring pass the umbilical arteries, the left umbilical vein, and the allantois. These three atrophy into fibrous cords at the time of birth. With healing of the transected cord, the force of retraction of those vessels modifies the formation of scar of the umbilical ring. These forces result in weak portions of the scar, usually at the superior portion of the umbilical defect, where later herniations can develop.

Remnants of this physiological closure yield structures that are of occasional surgical interest. The left umbilical vein persists as the ligamentum teres of the liver, coursing in the falciform ligament from the umbilicus to the hepatic margin. Though it physiologically closes and fibroses after birth, this vessel is frequently available for cannulation in the newborn (and even occasionally in the adult) for venous access. Remnants of the omphalomesenteric duct persist as vitelline duct cysts, duct patency with stooling at the umbilicus, or Meckel's diverticulum. Finally, failure of allantois closure may result in urachal cysts or total urachal fistula with urinary soiling at the umbilicus.

Abdominal Incisions

As important as a house's front door is for energy conservation, security, and appearance, most of the use of the doorway is to get through it. So surgeons see the abdominal wall. Access through this hingeless, knobless, abdominal wall is via surgical incisions. The ideal incision provides adequate access to the intraabdominal organ under investigation, reestablishes the

Incisions

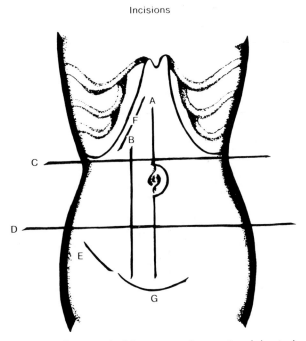

Figure 14.5 Common incisions across the anterior abdominal wall. **A,** Midline; **B,** paramedian; **C** and **D,** two of multiple planes of transverse incisions; **E,** McBurney incision; **F,** subcostal incision; **G,** Pfannenstiel incision.

strength and form of the abdominal wall postoperatively and leaves a cosmetically acceptable surgical scar. The commonly used surgical incisions are few (Fig. 14.5) but deserve individual mention.

Vertical incisions are the most widely used of all abdominal incisions. They are directed through the fused aponeurotic midline anywhere from the xiphoid to the pubic tubercle. This incision has multiple advantages, including the speed at which it can be made (since no vascular structures cross the midline), its ability to provide access to all portions of the abdomen, and its extendability. This is the incision of choice in trauma or when lack of a preoperative diagnosis may require exposure of all portions of the abdomen.

Transverse incisions are preferred by some surgeons as more "physiologic" incisions. These skin incisions are made in line with Langer's lines, so a more cosmetic scar results. More importantly, they are made in line with the direction of muscle tension, so postoperative coughing or exercise tends to close the incision rather than open it, as in vertical incisions. Incidence of wound dehiscence and late herniation are, therefore, minimized. The transection of the rectus abdominus muscle is not a significant problem, since a fibrous union the equivalent of an additional tendinous inscription results. Intraabdominal exposure, however, is compromised by transverse incisions. Misdiagnosis can result in awkward, cumbersome exposure or may necessitate the creation of a second appropriate incision once the diagnosis is made.

Paramedian incisions have fallen into some disrepute in recent years. They add very little to the exposure provided through a midline vertical incision and have several disadvantages: 1) they are time consuming to create and close, 2) they may denervate portions of the rectus muscle and overlying skin, and 3) because of inherent weakness, they are the most prone to herniation or disruption. The farther lateral a paramedian incision is fashioned, the more detrimental it is.

Subcostal incisions are advocated for reasons of improved visibility for certain diseases in the upper abdomen. Although they combine some of the better aspects of the previous incisions, subcostal incisions offer the disadvantages of both. Lines of muscular pull, cutaneous innervation, and skin tension are all traversed, as in the vertical incision, while the possibility of extension in the case of misdiagnosis is compromised, as for the horizontal incisions.

The Pfannenstiel incision, commonly used in gynecologic procedures, provides the strength of a transverse incision with the added cosmetic benefit of placing the skin incision in the pubic hairline.

Specific incisions for specific diseases are occasionally useful. The best example of this is the right lower quadrant Rocky-Davis incision for approach to the appendix. When such a localized preoperative diagnosis is made, all the benefits of this well-planned surgical incision can be realized. The transverse skin incision is in line with Langer's lines, and none of the cutaneous nerves (including the ilioinguinal and iliohypogastric) are disturbed. The precise location of McBurney's point

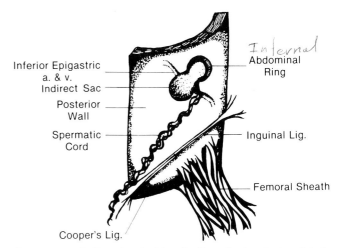

Figure 14.6. Indirect inguinal hernia. Posterior inguinal wall is intact. Hernia develops in the patent processus vaginalis (sac) on the anteromedial aspect of the cord. (In this figure and Figs. 14.7 and 14.8 the external oblique and internal oblique layers have been deleted since they have no role in the development or repair of inguinal hernias.)

(two-thirds of the distance from umbilicus to anterior iliac spine) allows formation of a small incision immediately over the disease. The muscle layers are divided bluntly in line with their direction of pull, so herniation and disruption are rare. Once the peritoneum is closed, some claim no further approximation of soft tissues is necessary for strong and cosmetic healing.

Hernias

A hernia is the protrusion of any organ, structure, or portion thereof through its normal anatomical confines. With respect to the abdominal wall, hernias represent the protrusion of all or part of any intraabdominal structure through any congenital, acquired, or iatrogenic defect. Commonly used, "hernia" refers to any of the three groin hernias, and any other hernias (such as umbilical or diaphragmatic hernias) require special designation.

Groin Hernias

Indirect Inguinal Hernia

The indirect inguinal hernia occurs when bowel, omentum, or some other intraabdominal organ protrudes through the abdominal ring within the continuous peritoneal coverage of a patent processus vaginalis (Fig. 14.6). The indirect inguinal hernia is a congenital lesion; if the processus vaginalis does not remain patent, an indirect hernia cannot develop. Since 20% of male cadaver specimens retain some degree of processus vaginalis patency, patency of the processus vaginalis is necessary, but not sufficient, for hernia development. The medical history will often yield the immediate reason for herniation. A 20-year-old workman hoisting a refrigerator is adequate cause for increased

Table 14.1.
Approximate Incidence of Hernia Type

	Direct	Indirect	Femoral
Males	40%	50%	10%
Females	Rare	70%	30%
Children	Rare	All	Rare

intraabdominal pressure, but it is equally valid to ask a 60-year-old man, who has had a congenital patency since birth, why this congenital lesion should appear at this late date. All too often, a chronic cough from a bronchial carcinoma, straining at micturition from prostatism, or straining at defecation from a sigmoid obstruction present as an inguinal hernia. Despite this, most authors feel that extensive invasive investigation of these organ systems at the time of hernia diagnosis is inappropriate in the absence of related symptoms. Indirect hernias are the most common hernia in both sexes and all age groups (Table 14.1). They occur more commonly on the right because of delayed descent of that testicle.

Because indirect inguinal hernias originate through a relatively small aperture in the posterior inguinal wall (the abdominal ring), there is a significant risk that bowel that slipped rather easily into the processus vaginalis can become swollen, edematous, engorged, and finally entrapped outside of the abdominal cavity. This process is referred to as incarceration and is the most common cause of bowel obstruction in persons without previous abdominal surgery and the second most common cause of all small bowel obstruction (see Chapters 17 and 18 for details of small and large bowel obstruction, respectively). This entrapment can become so severe that blood supply to or return from the bowel is compromised (a process called strangulation), and necrosis can follow. While it is possible to have omentum or even loops of bowel chronically incarcerated outside the abdominal wall for months or years and never proceed to strangulation, it is to prevent this complication that surgeons recommend hernia repair whenever the diagnosis is made. When an incarceration is encountered, a few gentle manual attempts at reduction (returning the entrapped organ to the confines of the abdominal cavity) are warranted. Though such attempts are only successful in 60–70% of cases and are associated with some risk to the entrapped structure, the benefits of patient comfort, relief of obstruction, prevention of strangulation, and the diagnostic information obtained justify a few gentle attempts.

With the passage of time, repeated protrusion of abdominal organs sufficiently dilates the abdominal ring so that incarceration and strangulation become less likely. This process, however, also implies greater destruction of the posterior inguinal wall, more difficult repair, and greater likelihood of recurrence.

The indirect hernia has two close cousins in the groin, the hydroceles. The communicating hydrocele differs from the indirect hernia only in that no bowel

has yet protruded into the groin. Instead, serous peritoneal fluid fills this peritoneal peninsula to whatever level the patency exists. Since there is free communication between the hydrocele and the peritoneal cavity, the fluid collection is greater after standing and less after recumbency and is significantly augmented by pathologic formation of ascites within the abdominal cavity. The noncommunicating hydrocele occurs when a small portion of the processus vaginalis adjacent the testicle fails to obliterate while the remainder of the processus vaginalis between it and the peritoneal cavity has been obliterated (Fig. 14.4).

Direct Inguinal Hernia

The *direct* inguinal hernia, contrary to the serpentine course of the indirect hernias, proceeds *directly* through the posterior inguinal wall (Fig. 14.7). As opposed to the indirect hernias, these protrude medial to the inferior epigastric vessels. Because there is no sac, they tend not to protrude with the cord into the scrotum and are generally felt to be an acquired lesion, though considerable congenital variation in the strength of posterior walls has been established. A spectrum of abnormality exists from very small-necked pedunculated herniations of preperitoneal fat, referred to as diverticular direct hernias, to large bulging protrusions destroying the entire posterior inguinal wall.

Femoral Hernia

The third category of herniation in the groin is the femoral hernia. Like the direct hernia, it is an acquired lesion and has no hernia sac. Its etiology lies in a short medial attachment of the transversus abdominus muscle onto Cooper's ligament, resulting in an enlarged femoral ring, inviting herniation (Fig. 14.8). On physical examination these hernias present as bulges much lower in the groin than other hernias, below the inguinal ring and onto the anterior thigh. Despite maximal

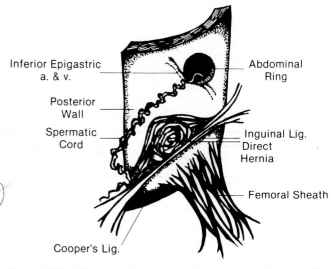

Figure 14.7. Direct inguinal hernia. Abdominal ring is intact. Hernia defect is a diffuse bulge in the posterior inguinal wall medial to the inferior epigastric vessels.

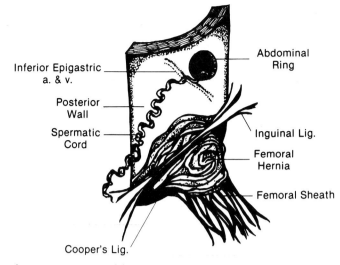

Inferior Epigastric a. & v.

Posterior Wall

Spermatic Cord

Cooper's Lig.

Abdominal Ring

Inguinal Lig.

Femoral Hernia

Femoral Sheath

Figure 14.8. Femoral hernia. Defect is through the femoral canal but otherwise involves similar structures and insertions as direct inguinal hernia.

dilatation from repeated protrusion, the femoral hernia ring is finally limited by rigid structures (the inguinal ligament with its lacunar attachments and Cooper's ligament); this hernia is, therefore, very susceptible to incarceration and strangulation. While femoral hernias comprise only 1–2% of hernias in men, they represent nearly 30% of the hernias in women.

Surgical Repair of Hernias

The repair of all groin hernias is conceptually simple: (1) reduce any abdominal viscus to the abdominal cavity; (2) complete Mother Nature's process of obliterating the processus vaginalis at a point high against the abdominal wall; and (3) reform a snug abdominal ring around the spermatic cord by anchoring the nondiseased remnants of the posterior wall back to their normal anatomic insertions into Cooper's ligament and the anterior femoral sheath. That simple concept, which took you 20 seconds to read, took anatomists and surgeons 100 combative years to develop.

During that development, many different concepts of hernia repair have arisen, then fallen from favor, leaving only an eponymic trail of past surgical masters. Evolution of that process has left us with a handful of surgical treatments for groin hernia repair.

Marcy Repair. The Marcy repair is popular in very small or early indirect hernias. Since these hernias represent only a dilatation of the abdominal ring, the Marcy repair simply snugs that aperature by sewing the transversus aponeurosis on the lateral side of the ring to the transversus aponeurosis on the medial side of the ring until that layer is snug around the cord.

McVay Hernia (Cooper's Ligament Repair). The McVay hernia requires an anatomical repair (like the Marcy operation) used for larger indirect hernias and direct hernias. The principle of this repair is that when the posterior inguinal wall has been destroyed by the hernia, the surgical repair of that wall ought to be as close as possible to the original anatomy. This involves

sewing any remaining strong transversus aponeurosis to that tendon's natural lateral insertions, the Cooper's ligament and the anterior femoral sheath.

Bassini Repair. The Bassini repair is a more superficial repair in which margins of transversus and internal oblique muscles are anchored laterally to the inguinal ligament.

Shouldice Repair. The Shouldice repair incorporates a series of four running suture lines approximating and imbricating the transversus aponeurosis to several lateral structures, in a sense combining a deep repair similar to McVay's with a superficial repair similar to Bassini's.

Pediatric Repair. Since in children the patent processus vaginalis has not had time to grow and dilate the abdominal ring, only this peritoneal protrusion, now called the hernia sac, needs to be addressed. Its obliteration, such that all peritoneum is returned to within the abdominal wall, is all that is required for a successful hernia repair.

Truss. A truss is a fist-sized ball formed of leather, rubber, or fabric that is positioned by the patient over his protruding hernia bulge and strapped in place with variously designed belts and straps. Hernia defects never close spontaneously. Truss application only increases scarring and the risk of incarceration. These two facts speak for early diagnosis and treatment of all hernias. Despite this caution, there is occasionally a patient at such high risk to any invasive procedure that the application of a truss may represent the better portion of valor.

Umbilical Hernias

Like the groin hernias, umbilical hernias come in three types. By far the most common of these is fortunately of least significance and threat to the patient. It is the small (usually less than 1 cm) defect in the abdominal wall resulting from incomplete umbilical closure. Through this fascial defect can protrude small portions of omentum, bowel, or other intraabdominal organs. Because the developmental process of the abdominal wall continues into extrauterine life, small protrusions of this type are very common in infants. Unless incarceration occurs, these are best ignored until preschool years and most will resolve spontaneously. Commonly used folk remedies, such as stuffing cotton balls into the umbilicus or taping coins over it to prevent protrusion only delay developmental closure or complicate the hernia with necrosis of the overlying skin. Despite their innocuous nature in infancy, however, umbilical hernias are some threat in adulthood, in that the rigid surrounding walls of the linea alba predispose to strangulation and incarceration of protruded organs.

The other two types of abdominal wall herniation are much more severe, affect only the newborn, and are fortunately very uncommon. An omphalocele results when, after incomplete closure of the abdominal wall by the time of birth, a portion of abdominal contents herniates into the base of the umbilical cord. Unlike the simple umbilical hernia, which is covered by all layers of skin, in omphalocele the abdominal contents are separated from the outside world by only a thin membrane of peritoneum and the amnion. Gastroschisis represents an even more severe failure of abdominal wall closure and results in a full-thickness abdominal wall defect lateral to the umbilicus. The hernia of gastroschisis is into the amniotic cavity, so there is no sac; there is no covering of any kind over the intestinal contents, which protrude from the lateral edge of the umbilicus.

The treatment for the umbilical hernias is as straightforward in concept as it was for the groin hernias: *(1)* reduce the abdominal contents and *(2)* establish abdominal wall continuity. The surgical procedures with a simple umbilical hernia are as simple in execution as they are in concept. Surgical therapy for omphalocele and gastroschisis has by necessity been more intricate and complex, including bowel resections and the formation of extraanatomic compartments fashioned of prosthetic materials. Despite such efforts, the mortality for these lesions remains high.

Other Hernias

A surgery clerkship is usually not complete without someone asking the student for a definition of or details about some of the more obscure hernias. Although not exhaustive, the following definitions should place you in good stead for such taunts and maybe even allow you to turn the tables.

Spigelian Hernia

Spigelian hernias are herniations through the semilunar line (lateral margin of rectus muscle) at or just below the junction with the semicircular line of Douglas. These hernias lie cephalad to the inferior epigastric vessels, thus distinguishing them from groin hernias. The tight aponeurotic defect predisposes to incarceration.

Grynfelt's Hernia

Grynfelt's hernia is a wide-mouthed hernia protruding through the superior lumbar triangle, which is bounded by the sacrospinalis muscle, the internal oblique muscle, and the inferior margin of the 12th rib. Diagnosis is hampered by the protrusion of these hernias under the latissimus dorsi muscle.

Petit's Hernia

Petit's hernia protrudes through the inferior lumbar triangle, which is bounded by the lateral margin of latissimus dorsi, the medial margin of the external oblique, and the iliac crest. Like the superior lumbar hernia, these hernias tend to be broad, bulging hernias without tendency to incarcerate.

Richter's Hernia

Richter's hernia is a hernia at any site through which only a portion of the circumference of a bowel wall (usually jejunum) incarcerates or strangulates. Since the entire lumen is not compromised, symptoms of bowel obstruction can be absent, despite gangrene of the strangulated portion.

Littre's Hernia

Any of the groin hernias containing a Meckel's diverticulum are Littre's hernias and are usually incarcerated or strangulated.

Obturator Hernia

Obturator hernias are deceptive hernias, often of Richter's type, through the obturator canal. They are much more common in women and usually present in the seventh and eighth decades. An obturator hernia is classically diagnosed by symptoms of intermittent bowel obstruction and paresthesias on the anteromedial aspect of the thigh from obturator nerve compression (the Howship-Romberg sign).

Hesselbach's Hernia

Hesselbach's hernia is described as protruding onto the thigh like a femoral hernia beneath the inguinal ligament, but coursing lateral to the femoral vessels.

Hesselbach's Triangle

That portion of the posterior inguinal wall through which direct herniation occurs is Hesselbach's triangle. Its classical boundaries are the rectus sheath, the inferior epigastric vessels, and the inguinal ligament. Since the inguinal ligament has no attachments to the posterior wall, it is increasingly popular to define the lateral margin as Cooper's ligament.

Pantaloon Hernia

The pantaloon hernia is the simultaneous presentation of a direct and an indirect hernia, presenting as two bulges straddling the inferior epigastric vessels.

Sliding Hernia

A sliding hernia is any hernia in which a portion of the wall of the protruding peritoneal sac is made up of some intraabdominal organ (usually sigmoid, cecum, ovary, or bladder), which, as the sac expands, gets drawn out into the hernia. Its repair involves only the careful return of that organ to the abdominal cavity, followed by the traditional sequence of obliteration of the sac and closure of the fascial defect.

Incisional Hernia

The protrusion of abdominal contents through defects acquired from incomplete closure of previous abdominal incisions is an incisional hernia. While orientation of incision, suture materials chosen, and various technical details can be implicated, the most common reason for formation of an iatrogenic hernia is the development of an infection in the previous wound.

SUGGESTED READINGS

Anson BJ, McVay CB: The anatomy of the inguinal region. *Surg Gynecol Obstet* 111:707, 1960.

Bassini E: Sulla cura radicale dell'ernia inguinale. *Arch Soc Ital Chir* 4:380, 1887a. [Summarized by G Lusena in *La Societa Italiana di Chirurgia Nei Suio 30 Congressi (1883–1923)*. Rome, Manuzio, 1934, p 284.]

Condon RE: Surgical anatomy of the transversus abdominis and transversalis fascia. *Ann Surg* 173:1, 1971.

Shouldice EE: Surgical treatment of hernia. *Ont Med Rev* 4:43, 1945.

McVay CB, Chapp JD: Inguinal and femoral hernioplasty: the evaluation of a basic concept. *Ann Surg* 148:499, 1958.

Skills

1. Demonstrate the ability to perform a thorough exam for inguinal hernia.

2. Describe the examination of a patient with incarcerated hernia.

Study Questions

1. What diagnostic tests or other workup is appropriate for
   A. A newborn with an umbilical hernia;
   B. A longshoreman with recent onset of a groin bulge;
   C. An elderly obstipated woman with a firm groin mass and hemoptysis.

2. What postoperative parasthesias might be expected from
   A. A vertical midline incision from xyphoid to pubis;
   B. A 10-cm subcostal incision for cholecystectomy;
   C. A 4-cm groin incision for hernia repair.

3. Discuss the named anatomic structures involved in
   A. Incisional hernia repair of a previous appendectomy incision;
   B. McVay repair of a direct inguinal hernia;
   C. Umbilical hernia repair.

15

Diseases of the Esophagus

Hiram C. Polk, Jr., M.D.
Richard M. Bell, M.D.
James W. Pate, M.D.
James F. Lind, M.D.

ASSUMPTION

The student knows the anatomy and physiology of the normal esophagus and esophagogastric junction.

OBJECTIVES

1. Describe esophageal hiatal hernia with regard to anatomical type (sliding and paraesophageal) and need for treatment.
2. Describe the anatomical and physiological factors predisposing to reflux esophagitis.
3. Describe the symptoms of reflux esophagitis and discuss the diagnostic procedures used for confirmation.
4. List the indications for operative management of esophageal reflux and discuss the physiologic basis for the antireflux procedure used.
5. Describe the pathophysiology and clinical symptoms associated with achalasia of the esophagus. Briefly outline the management options.
6. List the common esophageal diverticula, their location, symptomatology, and pathogenesis.
7. With particular reference to etiologic factors, differentiate pulsion and traction diverticula of the esophagus.
8. Describe and recognize the radiologic findings that characterize motility disorders of the esophagus, including achalasia and manometric evaluation of the lower esophageal sphincter.
9. List the symptoms suggestive of an esophageal malignancy.
10. Outline a plan for diagnostic evaluation of a patient with a suspected esophageal tumor.
11. Describe the natural history of a malignant lesion of the esophagus and list treatment options, indicating the order of preference.
12. List the common types of benign esophageal neoplasms and briefly describe how they are differentiated from malignant lesions.

13. Describe the etiology and presentation of traumatic perforation of the esophagus and the physical findings that occur early and late after such an injury.

The function of the esophagus is to provide a muscular conduit for the appropriate passage of orally ingested material from the mouth, through the negatively pressurized thorax, and into the upper stomach. An important secondary function is to provide for the emesis of material, based on its own toxic nature or due to the inability of the distal alimentary tract to provide for timely prograde passage. The esophagus is a muscular tube that originates at the cricoid cartilage and pharynx in the neck. It transverses the posterior mediastinum behind the aortic arch and left main stem bronchus to enter the abdominal cavity through the esophageal hiatus of the diaphragm. In most adults there is only a very short, less than 3-cm segment of true esophagus within the celomic cavity before it joins with the fundus of the stomach (Fig. 15.1).

The esophagus is composed of two layers, the mucosa, which consists of stratified squamous epithelium, and occasional mucous glands and a muscular layer. The inner muscular layer is oriented in a circular fashion, while the outer layer is oriented longitudinally. In contrast to the remainder of the gastrointestinal tract, there is no serosal layer. The significance of this anatomical relationship becomes apparent when considering the extension of neoplasms that originate in the esophagus, the relative ease with which the esophagus can be perforated during instrumentation, or the difficulty with surgical reconstruction after resection. The musculature of the upper one-third of the esophagus is skeletal, while the lower two-thirds is smooth muscle. While the division between striated and smooth muscle cannot be determined precisely by histologic examination, the entire esophagus functions in a coordinated fashion. There is one physiologic sphincter

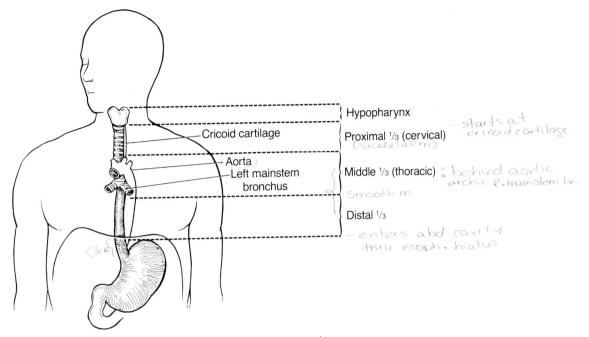

Figure 15.1. Clinical divisions of the esophagus.

at the level of the diaphragm, and although distinct muscle fibers with specialized sphincter function cannot be identified at this position, the peritoneal reflection that surrounds the esophageal hiatus and the phrenoesophageal ligament function to produce an area of relative high pressure with respect to the remainder of the esophagus and stomach just distally. Like all sphincter mechanisms in the gastrointestinal tract, the purpose of this lower esophageal sphincter is to prevent the reflux of gastric content, but unlike other sphincter mechanisms with well-defined circular muscle fibers (like the pyloris), this sphincter relies on a unique anatomical relationship to accomplish this. Disturbances of this rather precarious relationship allow for the reflux of acid gastric content on to a very sensitive, unprotected epithelial surface rich in sensory innervation. Failure of this lower sphincter to "relax" appropriately can result in proximal dilatation of this muscular tube, which is not confined by a serosal layer, and eventually result in disordered contractility.

The motility of the distal esophageal sphincter is increasingly being studied, and our understanding of this physiology is rapidly growing. The esophagus is an active organ, rather than a passive tube. When food en-

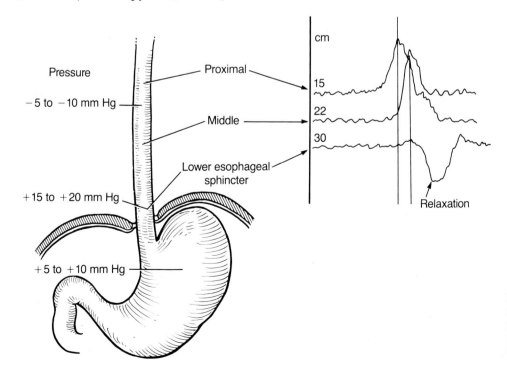

Figure 15.2. Manometry of a normal swallow. Note the progression of the primary peristaltic wave and the appropriate "relaxation" of the lower esophageal sphincter.

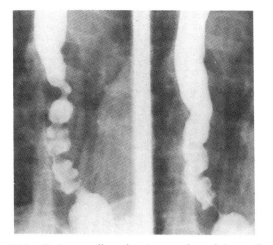

Figure 15.3. Barium swallow showing esophageal dysmotility with tertiary contractions in association with sliding hiatal hernia.

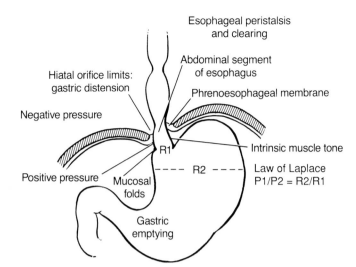

Figure 15.4. A summary of the anatomical and physiologic factors that are thought to prevent reflux of gastric content into the lower esophagus. (From Skinner DB: *Ann Surg* 202:533, 1985.)

ters the upper esophagus, it is propelled down the esophagus by a peristaltic wave. Fluids may fall faster than the peristaltic wave by gravity when an individual stands upright. Coordination of contraction and relaxation is shown in the manometric tracing in Figure 15.2. The lower esophageal sphincter relaxes in anticipation of the food bolus, allowing the food to enter the stomach. The lower esophageal sphincter then returns to its normal high resting pressure of 15–25 cm H_2O above the pressure in the stomach to prevent reflux.

Manometry and fluoroscopy can frequently be used to diagnose abnormalities in esophageal motility. Normally, swallowing a bolus of food results in a primary peristaltic wave. Secondary waves occur if the food has not been cleared from the esophagus. Tertiary waves are abnormal and represent nonpropulsive "fibrillation" of the esophagus (Fig. 15.3). In addition to assessing peristalsis, manometry can identify the normal cricopharyngeal and gastroesophageal sphincters, as well as determining whether they function normally.

The concept of acid reflux into the lower esophagus deserves special comment, as it has only been within recent years that an understanding of the concept has begun to emerge. Since a definite anatomical sphincter cannot be demonstrated in humans in the distal esophagus to account for the high-pressure zone measured by clinical and research studies, other mechanisms of this sphincteric action must be proposed. Theories to explain this observation, or the lack of it in individuals symptomatic from reflux, include the fact that the smooth muscle in the distal esophagus may respond differently than the rest with regard to the hormonal environment. Furthermore, while atropine administered to normal individuals ablates the high-pressure zone by manometric measurement, reflux does not occur. The length of the intraabdominal segment of the esophagus may play a significant role in limiting reflux. A shortened intraabdominal segment, defined as the distance between the insertion of the phrenoesophageal membrane into the wall of the esophagus to the flare of the gastric pouch, correlates well with symptomatic reflux. Additional evidence for this theory is

derived from the fact that following surgical antireflux procedures or esophageal replacement with reversed gastric tubes or colonic segments, a high-pressure zone can be measured that functions quantitatively as well as qualitatively as the normal distal esophagus. Basic physical laws, specifically the law of Laplace, may have some bearing on reflux. Simply stated, the pressure required to distend a pliable tube is inversely related to the diameter of the tube. Applied to the problem of reflux, it is easy to see how the larger diameter stomach would distend more than the small esophagus in response to pressure, unless the anatomical relationship had been altered. Consider this in view of the anatomical relationships demonstrated in Figures 15.2 and 15.4. Other considerations in preventing reflux include other anatomic relationships involving the angle of His and gastric mucosal folds, as well as a role for gastric emptying. A summary of these mechanisms is shown in Figure 15.4.

While it is tempting to ascribe reflux to the presence of hiatal hernia, they are truly separate conditions. Although 80% of patients with reflux have hiatal hernia, the remainder do not. Qualitative investigation of reflux and the quantitation of its severity have become relatively sophisticated, combining several independent invasive tests, including prolonged pH monitoring of the distal esophagus, with correlations of patient symptomatology and delays in acid clearance (Fig. 15.5). Such investigations have implied that all reflux symptoms are not exclusively related to an acidic environment and that alkaline reflux may occur as well. Pressures are recorded manometrically from three positions. Perfusion of the distal esophagus alternatively with hydrochloric acid and with normal saline is correlated with the patient's symptoms. Acid reflux is assessed by injecting a 15-cc bolus of hydrochloric acid to the midesophagus and monitoring pH levels 5 cm above the high-pressure zone. Additionally, an indication of how rapidly an individual clears acid from the

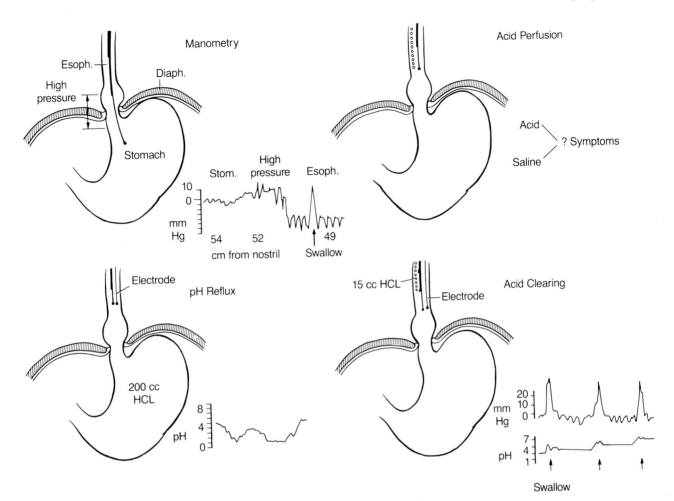

Figure 15.5. Various esophageal function tests. Catheters are passed into the esophagus through the nose or mouth. Pressure measurements are then made, or the catheters are used to infuse hydrochloric acid or saline to reproduce symptoms of acid reflux. pH electrodes can also be inserted to determine the presence of endogenous acid reflux. (From Skinner DB: *Ann Surg* 202:548, 1985.)

esophagus can be measured. A normal individual can restore the pH to normal with less than 10 swallows. Common problems that affect the esophagus and frequently require a physician's attention are hiatal hernia reflux esophagitis, esophageal motility disorders, cancer of the esophagus, and occasional esophageal disruption.

Hiatal Hernia and Relux Esophagitis

Pathogenesis

There are two major types of hiatal hernia, the type I or "sliding" hiatal hernia and the paraesophageal hiatal hernia type II (Fig. 15.6). A sliding hernia allows the gastroesophageal junction and a portion of the stomach to "slide" into the mediastinum. It is physiologically significant only when this hernia is associated with the reflux of gastric acid into the lower esophagus. The paraesophageal hiatal (rolling) hernia has an esophagogastric junction that is located in a normal position, and reflux is uncommon. The portion of the gastric fundus that herniates alongside the esophagus is prone to incarceration and/or strangulation,

much like inguinal hernias. Like a true hernia, the fundus of the stomach is inside a sac of peritoneum. The medical treatment and/or surgical repair of type I hiatal hernia is a function of the degree of acid reflux and resulting symptoms. In contrast, the paraesophageal, or type II hiatal hernia, should, like any other hernia, be treated promptly on discovery to preclude incarceration and/or strangulation. Some texts describe a type III hiatal hernia. This represents a combination of the elements of types I and II and usually represents a very large defect in the esophageal hiatus. Other abdominal organs may be found in the mediastinum with the stomach in this defect. These require surgical repair to preclude necrosis.

Clinical Presentation

Sliding hiatal hernia are the most common by over 100:1. The loss of the anatomical relationship between the diaphragmatic hiatus and the esophagus disrupts the lower esophageal sphincter mechanism, rendering it incompetent. Reflux of acid gastric juice produces a chemical burn of the susceptible esophageal mucosa. The degree of mucosal injury is a function of the duration of acid contact and not a disease of hyperacidity.

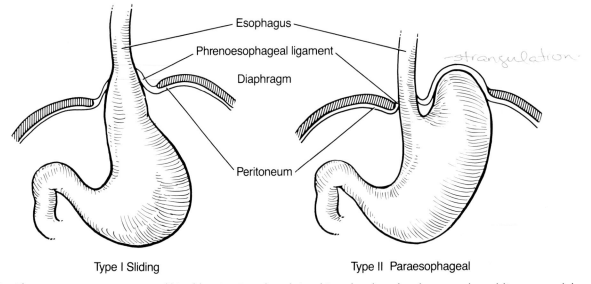

strangulation.

Type I Sliding   Type II Paraesophageal

Figure 15.6. The two most common types of hiatal hernia. Note the relationships of each to the phrenoesophageal ligament and the peritoneum.

It is a disease of normal acid in the wrong place. Continued inflammation of the distal esophagus may lead to mucosal erosion, ulceration, and eventually scarring and stricture. In the Western population, hiatal hernia occurs predominantly in women who have been pregnant or in men and women with increased intraabdominal pressure. It is more than coincidental that type I hiatal hernia with reflux is frequently found in patients who are overweight. Most investigators believe that increased intraabdominal pressure predisposes to reflux of gastric acid into the distal esophagus. Many patients with type I hiatal hernia have no symptoms. Individuals with significant reflux classically complain of a burning, epigastric or substernal pain or tightness. Usually the pain does not radiate. It may be described as a tightness in the chest and can be confused with the pain of myocardial ischemia. A characteristic feature is that the intensity of the pain is positional, worse when the patient is supine or leaning over. Antiacid therapy frequently improves the symptoms. Patients may also complain of a lump or feeling that food is stuck beneath the xyphoid. This is generally due to muscular spasm of the esophagus. All common gastric irritants and stimulants, such as alcohol, aspirin, tobacco, and caffeine have been reported to exacerbate the symptoms. Occasionally the only indication of re-

flux is a chronic aspiration pneumonitis. Late symptoms of dysphagia and vomiting usually suggest stricture formation. Even in this circumstance, nearly all patients will describe reflux symptoms prior to the onset of dysphagia. Type II hernias generally produce no symptoms until they incarcerate and become ischemic. Dysphagia, bleeding, and occasionally respiratory distress are the presenting symptoms.

Diagnosis

The diagnosis of reflux esophagitis is usually suspected based on the patient's history. Physical examination is generally unrewarding, unless weight loss is a feature due to distal esophageal stricture and the resultant nutritional depletion. The diagnosis of hiatal hernia and reflux esophagitis can be confirmed by fluoroscopy during a barium swallow (Fig. 15.7). Sometimes barium reflux from the stomach into the distal esophagus is not observed radiographically but inferred by the presence of other anatomic abnormalities, such as dysmotility, stricture, or ulceration. In addition, local signs of esophageal irritation and/or ulceration are frequently present. The diagnosis of reflux esophagitis can also be made by esophagogastric endoscopy and biopsy of the inflamed esophagus. Most experienced endoscopists recognize esophagitis visu-

history
- fluoroscopy (Ba swallow)
- endoscopy
- bx (inflam'n)
- manometry: ↓ LES tone.

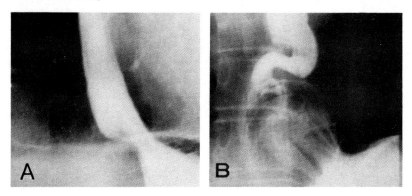

A   B

Figure 15.7. A, Normal distal esophagus shown by barium swallow. **B,** Small sliding hiatal hernia shown by barium swallow.

ally, and biopsy is seldom necessary to confirm the clinical findings. Manometry may show a loss of the lower esophageal high-pressure area or nonspecific disordered contractions if the disease is long-standing.

Treatment

Medical Therapy. Primary treatment for esophagitis is medical and includes all of the following:

1. Avoidance of gastric stimulants (coffee, tobacco, and alcohol).
2. Elimination of tight garments that raise intraabdominal pressure, such as girdles or abdominal binders.
3. The regular use of antiacids (particularly those that coat the esophagus), as well as the use of antiacid mints (such as Tums and Rolaids) to provide a steady stream of protection. By increasing the pH of the refluxed gastric juice, H₂ blockers may also be beneficial and, in selected cases, metoclopramide may be helpful when poor gastric

emptying is a component of the symptom complex.

4. Abstinence from drinking or eating within several hours of sleeping.
5. Sleeping with the head of the bed elevated at least 6 inches to reduce nocturnal reflux.
6. Weight loss in obese patients.

Approximately two-thirds of patients will respond to medical treatment, and half of them will respond so completely that surgery is unnecessary. About one-third of patients fail to respond to initial medical treatment, and half of those who initially respond will ultimately relapse and require surgery.

Surgery Therapy. The principles of surgical treatment are relatively straightforward: 1) correct the anatomic defect and 2) prevent the reflux of gastric acid into the lower esophagus by reconstruction of a valve mechanism (Fig. 15.8). There are several eponyms for the common surgical procedure for reflux esophagitis (Nissen, Hill, Belsey); each one has its advocates, and

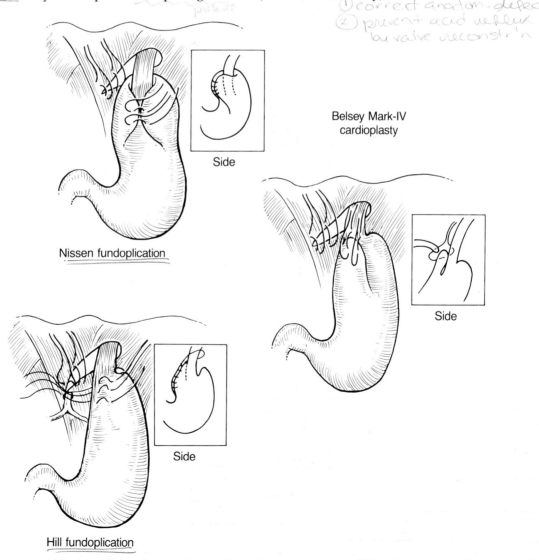

Figure 15.8. Three common hiatal hernia repairs. In each case the defect at the esophageal hiatus is repaired and a valve mechanism is constructed using all or part of the gastric fundus.

each varies in its approach to repairing the defect and creating the valve. However, all procedures combine these two principles.

The results of these surgical procedures provide greater than 90% relief of symptoms, a surgical mortality under 1%, and a morbidity rate that is typical for clean, major abdominal procedures. The route of repair is important; it may be accomplished through a transthoracic or transabdominal approach. The abdominal procedure is slightly less morbid and allows access to other intraabdominal pathology that might require repair at the same time. On the other hand, esophageal shortening is best approached with a transthoracic exposure.

Postoperative complications include inability to belch or vomit, frequently referred to as the "gas-bloat" syndrome. This is generally due to making the valve too tight and can be minimized by the use of intraoperative calibration of the size of gastroesophageal junction with mercury bougies. Dysphagia may result from making the gastroesophageal junction too narrow. Disruption of the repair with recurrent symptoms, intraabdominal infection processes, and esophageal perforation are complications. Splenic injury is always a possibility when performing procedures in this area.

Esophageal Motility Disorders

Esophageal motility disorders occur due to abnormalities of peristalsis at various levels in the esophagus. They may also lead to other disorders, such as diverticula, which occur as a result of distal obstruction.

Achalasia

Pathogenesis. The most common motility disorder affecting the esophagus is achalasia, which literally means "failure to relax" and occurs at the distal esophageal circular muscle segment. Contrary to common belief, it is not due to spasm but rather to failure of the high-pressure zone sphincter to relax, resulting in painless dysphagia and a slow but progressive dilatation of the proximal esophagus. The precise mechanism for the distal circular muscle abnormality is not known.

Clinical Presentation. Dysphagia, regurgitation of undigested food, and weight loss are the classic symptoms of achalasia. Unlike reflux esophagitis, pain in this condition is uncommon. Patients will often report consuming large quantities of liquids to force their food down. Aspiration pneumonia is common. Patients will frequently complain of spitting up foul-smelling secretions when simply leaning forward.

The diagnosis of achalasia is generally first confirmed roentgenographically by contrast studies of the esophagus, frequently using cineradiography. Dilatation of the proximal esophagus is classic, and esophageal diverticula may be present at any level. While endoscopy is frequently performed, one needs to be particularly careful to avoid diverticular perforation,

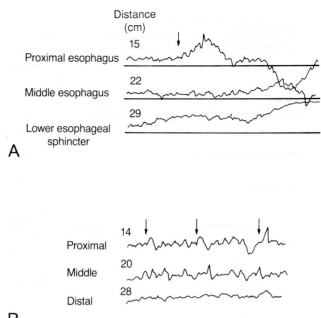

Figure 15.9. Manometric findings in achalasia. **A,** Manometry shows the lack of effective peristaltic activity and failure of the lower esophageal sphincter to relax (cf. Fig. 15.2). **Arrow,** patient swallowed. **B,** Manometry shows total lack of coordinated muscular activity, described as fibrillation. Lower esophageal sphincter does not demonstrate any evidence of relaxation with repeated swallowing (**arrows**). Numbers represent distance in centimeters from the nostril.

since it is sometimes easier to pass the endoscope into the diverticulum than the main channel of the esophagus. In complicated cases, esophageal manometry may be extremely helpful, particularly in those patients who have undergone previous operations. The manometric pressures are characteristic, showing tertiary waves with diffuse spasm and evidence of hypertonic activity of the esophagus at the high-pressure zone of the distal esophagus (Fig. 15.9).

Treatment. Medical treatment has generally not been helpful, although calcium channel blockers have not been adequately studied in proper trials. The treatment of choice lies between an invasive endoscopic procedure and surgical transection of the muscle. The endoscopic procedure involves the placement of a balloon at the region of high pressure in the esophagogastric junction and rapid inflation ("forceful dilatation") to rupture the distal esophageal circular muscle, without full-thickness mucosal rupture. The response to forceful dilatation is variable. About 80% of patients are cured by this procedure, but the complications, when they occur, are quite severe. The procedure is not widely practiced or readily learned.

The surgical procedure, esophageal myotomy, is carried out over the distal 2 inches of the esophagus and extended 1 cm onto the stomach, producing the same end as forceful dilatation. Presently, surgical treatment is the most reliable, since more than 95% of patients have complete relief of symptoms. The procedure involves a surgical incision in the muscular layer

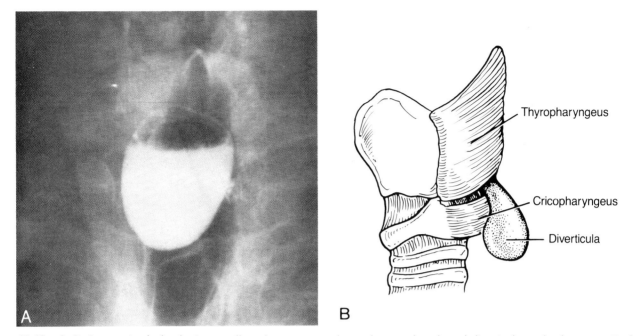

Figure 15.10. **A,** Barium retained after barium swallow demonstrates a large pharyngealesophageal diverticulum, also known as Zenker's diverticulum. **B,** Artist's conception. Diverticulum is a mucosal hernia between the two muscles of the pharyngeal constrictor mechanism. It is a false diverticulum, as it does not contain all layers of the esophagus, only mucosa.

of the lower esophagus (myotomy). Its only disadvantage is the occasional development of reflux, due to an overly lengthy myotomy. Consequently, most surgeons accompany the myotomy with a modified fundoplication. A complete 360-degree wrap of the lower esophagus may exacerbate dysphagia in the occasional patient and therefore should be avoided.

Esophageal motility disorders are commonly found in association with a number of collagen vascular diseases, most notably scleroderma, a disease in which systemic smooth muscle is replaced by fibrosis. While scleroderma is a disease whose etiology is not understood, esophageal involvement is so common in these patients (up to 70%) that the determination of esophageal abnormalities constitutes a major role in the diagnosis. Patients show marked abnormalities of esophageal motility, with a progressive decline in muscular contractility toward the lower esophageal sphincter. At this level ineffective, poorly coordinated simultaneous contractions are recorded. These findings occur before the classic changes are noted by standard barium swallow radiographs. Patients complain of the constitutional symptoms of general malaise and fatigue and, if the esophagus is involved, may complain of dysphagia or the necessity to force down their food with large volumes of liquids. With progressive reflux, extensive ulceration of the distal esophagus may occur. Medical therapy with antiacids and H_2 blockade may offer only partial relief. Stricture formation is common. While there is no known cure for the disease itself, surgical therapy to provide relief from severe esophageal symptoms may offer significant palliation in these individuals.

Esophageal Diverticula

The second most common manifestation of esophageal motility disorders is the development of diverticula or an outpouching of all or part of the wall of the organ. Diverticula have been termed either *pulsion* or *traction*, depending on the mechanism that leads to their development. Cervical diverticula, or Zenker's, (Fig. 15.10) are pulsion and are closely related to dysfunction of the cricopharyngeal muscle, though the precise abnormality of motility has not been resolved. Anatomically, they occur between the oblique fibers of the thyropharyngeal muscle and the more horizontal fibers of the cricopharyngeus, an area of potential weakness. Patients with symptomatic Zenker's diverticula complain of regurgitation of recently swallowed food or pills, choking, or a putrid breath odor. These diverticula are best treated by excision of the diverticula and myotomy of the cricopharyngeal muscle.

Diverticula of the distal third of the esophagus are generally associated with dysfunction of the esophagogastric junction as a result of chronic stricture from acid reflux, antireflux surgical procedures, achalasia, or other uncommon disorders. Excision of these diverticula should always be accompanied by correction of the underlying pathological process. The results of such therapy yield better than 90% symptomatic relief, with a surgical morbidity and mortality of less than 1%.

Middle-third esophageal diverticula are almost always traction and therefore not related to an intrinsic abnormality in esophageal motility. They are usually the result of mediastinal inflammation (usually inflammatory nodal disease from tuberculosis) or histoplasmosis, which results in scar formation and subsequent contracture that places "traction" on the esophagus. They are usually asymptomatic and do not warrant treatment.

Esophageal Neoplasms

Benign Tumors. Benign tumors of the esophagus are exceedingly rare and are mentioned only for the sake of completeness. They arise from the various anatomical layers of this organ and are most commonly found in the middle and distal thirds. Leiomyomas are the most common intramural tumors, and the potential for malignant degeneration appears to be quite low. They have a characteristic smooth surface seen to indent the lumen of the esophagus on contrast radiography. Although they are usually asymptomatic, many surgeons recommend excision, as they tend to grow progressively and cause dysphagia and to exclude the possibility of malignancy.

Malignant Tumors. Carcinoma of the esophagus usually arises from squamous epithelium, and in the United States it most commonly occurs in black men in association with alcohol and/or tobacco abuse. In other parts of the world the etiology has been related to diet, vitamin deficiency, poor oral hygiene, surgical procedures, and a number of premalignant conditions, including caustic burns, Barrett's esophagus, radiation, Plummer-Vinson syndrome, and esophageal diverticula. Occasionally, adenocarcinoma occurs in the esophagus, but more commonly these tumors originate in the fundus of the stomach and extend upward into the esophagus. Extension submucosally is common and frequently occurs over an extended distance. Due to a lack of serosal layer, invasion of adjacent structures is frequent. Adenocarcinomas may be the result of malignant transformation of the columnar epithelium that has replaced the normal squamous lining of the distal esophagus due to chronic acid reflux. The metaplasia so described has been termed Barrett's esophagus. Approximately 10% of patients with Barrett's esophagus will develop adenocarcinoma.

The symptoms produced by an esophageal malignancy are, unfortunately, frequently insidious at the onset, precluding early diagnosis and thus the opportunity for effective treatment. The rich lymphatic drainage of the esophagus may allow nodal spread of the disease even at this early stage. As the tumor enlarges, progressive dysphagia becomes the predominant symptom. Later weight loss and pain may be present. This ominous scenario mandates immediate and aggressive evaluation of any patient who presents with a complaint of difficulty in swallowing. Even well-informed and highly motivated patients have advanced disease before symptoms are severe enough to bring them to a physician. When weight loss is present, the disease is usually advanced. Benign lesions, in contrast, rarely produce nutritional consequences. It is common for patients with esophageal malignancy to present with an acquired tracheoesophageal fistula due to erosion of the tumor into the trachea or bronchus,

or with frequent episodes of pneumonia due to recurrent aspiration. Patients commonly present with disease so far advanced that they cannot handle their own saliva.

Diagnosis. The diagnosis of esophageal cancer is made by the typical ragged edge, shelf, or apple core that is seen on barium contrast studies of the esophagus (Fig. 15.11). An upper gastrointestinal series is often followed by endoscopy and biopsy of the lesion. Few esophageal cancers remain occult when one has completed a barium and endoscopic study of the esophagus. The extent of tumor involvement is then assessed by CT of the chest and upper abdomen.

Treatment. Squamous or adenocarcinomas of the esophagus carry a very poor prognosis, and generally treatment should be directed toward palliation of the patient, which involves restoration of effective swallowing. Favorable tumors, those without evidence of overt lymph node dissemination, and a small, possibly curable lesion should be aggressively treated based on the location of the tumor. Radiotherapy is the primary mode of treatment for cancer arising in the upper esophagus. Surgical treatment at this level usually requires extirpation of the esophagus en bloc with the larynx, permanent tracheostomy, and restoration of swallowing by a free microsurgically constructed vascular pedicle of jejunum or colon into the neck. Tumors that involve the middle third of the esophagus are usually treated by a staged procedure with total thoracic esophagectomy and bypass. Pulling the stomach into the neck or interposing a segment of colon are reconstructive options. Cancer involving the lower third of the esophagus or proximal stomach is best treated by esophagogastric resection and an end-to-end anastomosis in the midchest.

The cure rate for even very favorable cases seldom exceeds 20% and, in general, the overall cure rate for all esophageal cancers is only 5%. Accordingly, palliation by radiotherapy, laser resection of obstructing tumor, or the placement of an indwelling esophageal tube (stent) can often provide as good palliation with less morbidity than surgery. Even tracheoesophageal fistulas can be tamponaded with these nonsurgical approaches in selected cases.

Traumatic Esophageal Disorders Because of the frequency of occurrence and the morbidity and mortality attendant to the lack of recognition and aggressive management, two traumatic injuries of the esophagus deserve brief mention. These include esophageal disruption or perforation and the ingestion of caustic substances.

Esophageal perforation most frequently is the result of instrumentation, by endoscopic and/or biopsy procedures or the passage of blind nasogastric tubes, instruments designed for dilatation of strictures, or the occasional inflation of devices used to tamponade bleeding varices in the esophagus itself (e.g., Sengstaken-Blakemore tubes, balloon dilatation for achalasia). Spontaneous perforation of the esophagus does occur and follows an episode of forceful vomiting or

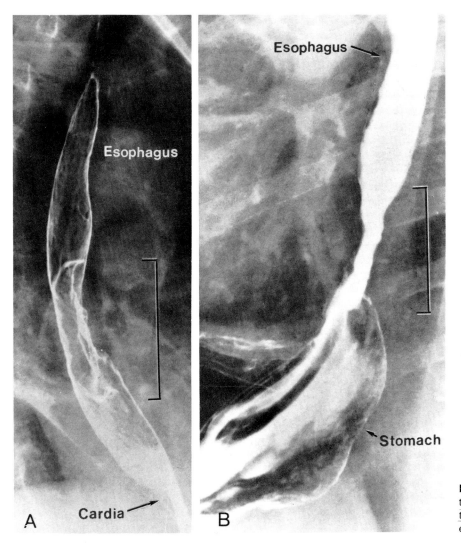

Figure 15.11. **A,** Contrast radiograph showing the typical "apple core" lesion of carcinoma of the middle one-third of esophagus. **B,** Ragged edge seen in carcinoma of the distal esophagus.

wretching, which dramatically increases intraesophageal pressure (Boerhaave's syndrome). The lack of a serosal layer makes perforation more common under this condition than any other place in the alimentary tract. Perforation by external trauma is discussed in Chapter 13.

The symptoms related to esophageal perforation may be dramatic or occult and depend on the location of the perforation and the etiology. Perforation by nasogastric tube may be insidious, and only after several hours will the patient be found in extremus, in profound shock from mediastinal sepsis. At other times the event may be catastrophic from the onset, with severe chest or abdominal pain, hypotension, diaphoresis, nausea, and vomiting to suggest the diagnosis in relationship to the events that preceded the collapse.

Treatment requires aggressive surgical intervention, as mortality is directly related to the interval between the occurrence and intervention. Surgical drainage and repair, if possible, are necessary.

Ingestion of caustic materials, either accidentally (as is seen in children) or intentionally (as is the case in adult suicide attempts) constitutes a medical emergency. The most ominous of these is the ingestion of alkaline-containing products, e.g., Drano, Liquid-Plummer. These solutions can cause destruction of the tissue of varying degrees from the lips well into the small intestine. The most important aspect of treatment involves the early identification of the etiologic agent (acid, alkaline, or specific toxin) as these agent ingestions require different approaches. Secondly, careful physical examination of the oropharyngeal cavity is required to estimate the severity of injury. Invasive endoscopic procedures are usually urgently necessary. Induced vomiting and neutralization of caustic substances are generally not suggested, as they are potentially harmful and ineffective. Airway maintenance is the first priority, followed by maintenance of patency of the esophagus. The use of anti-inflammatory agents is generally recommended for alkaline burns if seen within the first 24 hours. Steroids should not be used when perforation has occurred. Long-term therapy is directed toward the prevention and management of stricture formation. The use of antibiotics as prophylactic, adjuvant agents is controversial.

In summary, diseases that affect the esophagus are

quite common and represent disabling problems for some patients. The diagnosis of virtually all illnesses can be accomplished by a careful barium study of the upper gastrointestinal tract and skilled endoscopic examination and biopsy. An occasional patient not clarified by these studies will require manometric study of the esophagus. Treatment for the benign diseases of the esophagus is generally quite successful, unless one lets progressive distal esophageal inflammation progress to stricture. The treatment of cancer of the esophagus at the time of clinical presentation is usually for palliation. Most recent efforts to improve cure of esophageal cancer have focused on modifying risk factors and earlier diagnosis of the disease. Traumatic injury of the esophagus requires prompt and aggressive management, with surgical consultation from the onset.

SUGGESTED READINGS

Behar J, Biancani P, Sheahan DG: Evaluation of esophageal tests in the diagnosis of reflux esophagitis. *Gastroenterology* 71:9, 1976.

DeMeester TR, Johnson LF, Joseph GJ, et al: Patterns of gastroesophageal reflux in health and disease. *Ann Surg* 184:759, 1976.

Orringer MB: The esophagus. In Sabiston DC (ed): *Textbook of Surgery: The Biological Basis of Modern Surgical Practice*, ed 13. Philadelphia, WB Saunders, 1986, pp 697–748.

Russell COH, Pope CE, Gannan, RM, Allen FD: et al: Does surgery correct esophageal motor dysfunction in gastroesophageal reflux? *Ann Surg* 194:459, 1976.

Sabiston DC, Spencer FC (eds): *Gibbon's Surgery of the Chest*, ed 4. Philadelphia, WB Saunders, 1983.

Shackelford RT: *Surgery of the Alimentary Tract*, ed 2. Philadelphia, WB Saunders, 1978.

Skinner DB: Pathophysiology of gastroesophageal reflux. *Ann Surg* 202:546–556, 1985.

Skinner DB, Belsey RHR, Hendrix TR: et al (eds): *Gastroesophageal Reflux and Hiatal Hernia*. Boston, Little Brown & Co, 1972.

Skills

1. Demonstrate the ability to read a barium swallow in patients with hiatal hernia, esophageal cancer, and achalasia.

2. Interpret manometric results in a patient with achalasia.

3. Develop an algorithm for the management of a patient with dysphagia.

4. Describe a diagnostic evaluation for a patient who presents with dysphagia.

Study Questions

1. Discuss your diagnostic approach to a patient with reflux esophagitis. How can an upper gastrointestinal series, endoscopy, and biopsy contribute to your management of this disease? Discuss the role of manometry.

2. Discuss the medical and surgical treatment of asymptomatic hiatal hernia and symptomatic reflux esophagitis.

3. Describe the clinical presentation of a patient with achalasia. How does this differ from a patient with an esophageal stricture secondary to reflux or a patient with cancer of the esophagus?

4. Discuss the treatment options for a patient with carcinoma of the esophagus.

5. What is Barrett's esophagus? How is it managed? What is the risk of cancer in a patient with Barrett's esophagitis?

6. Find a management plan through additional reading for the management of an 18-year-old man who attempts suicide by the ingestion of a strong alkaline-containing solution. How would this differ if he had, instead, ingested hydrochloric acid?

16

Stomach and Duodenum

J. Patrick O'Leary, M.D., James F. Lind, M.D.,
Raymond J. Joehl, M.D., Edwin C. James, M.D.,
Talmadge A. Bowden, Jr., M.D.,
Mary McCarthy, M.D., Rudy G. Danzinger, M.D.,
Guy Legros, M.D., Gordon Telford, M.D.,
Ajit K. Sachdeva, M.D., F.R.C.S.(C), F.A.C.S.,
Thomas A. Miller, M.D., F.A.C.S., and
Steven T. Ruby, M.D.

ASSUMPTION

The student knows the basic anatomy and physiology of the stomach, including the mechanisms and stimuli for gastric and duodenal secretion.

OBJECTIVES

1. Compare and contrast the common symptoms and pathogenesis of gastric and duodenal ulcer disease, including patterns of acid secretion.
2. Discuss the significance of the anatomical location of either a gastric or duodenal ulcer.
3. List the clinical and laboratory features that differentiate the Zollinger-Ellison syndrome (gastrinoma) from duodenal ulcer disease.
4. Discuss the diagnostic value of upper gastrointestinal roentgenograms, endoscopy with biopsy, gastric analysis, serum gastrin levels, and the secretin stimulation test in patients with suspected peptic ulcer disease.
5. Describe in detail the nonoperative management of patients with peptic ulcer disease.
6. Discuss the complications of peptic ulcer disease, including clinical presentation, diagnostic workup, and appropriate surgical treatment.
7. Compare the risk of carcinoma in patients with gastric ulcer disease with the risk in those with duodenal ulcer disease.
8. Describe and discuss the common operations performed for duodenal and gastric ulcer disease as well as the morbidity associated with each procedure.
9. Discuss the commonly recognized side effects associated with duodenal and gastric ulcer disease surgery, including treatment plans for each.

10. Identify premalignant conditions, epidemiological factors, and clinical features in patients with gastric adenocarcinoma.
11. Describe the common types of neoplasms that occur in the stomach and discuss appropriate diagnostic procedures, therapeutic modalities, and prognosis for each.
12. List the general principles of curative and palliative surgical procedures for patients with gastric neoplasm and discuss the role of adjunctive or alternative therapy.

Anatomy

The stomach is a pliable, saccular organ that is located in the left hypochondrium and epigastrium. It is connected to the rest of gastrointestinal tract by two sphincters. The proximal sphincter is at the junction of the esophagus and stomach. Histologically, a mucosal change from squamous to columnar epithelium can be seen. This area is known as the lower esophageal sphincter (LES) or the esophageal distal high pressure zone (DHPZ). In health, the DHPZ prevents reflux of caustic gastric contents into the esophagus. The distal end of the stomach, or antrum, joins with the duodenum. At this point, a definite epithelial change can be recognized histologically. In this region, there is a well-defined sphincter (pylorus) composed of smooth muscle. The pyloric channel measures from 1–3 cm in length. The pylorus, in association with the antral pump, controls the rate of gastric emptying as well as preventing the reflux of duodenal contents into the stomach. Particles larger than 3–5 mm will not be allowed to leave the stomach until the final "cleansing" wave of peristalsis occurs several hours after the meal.

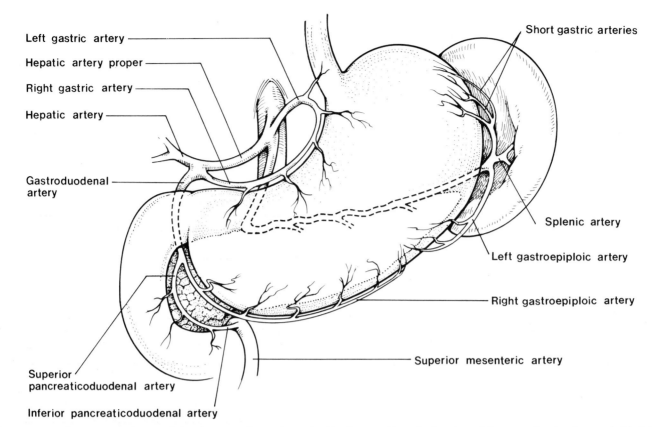

Left gastric artery

Hepatic artery proper

Right gastric artery

Hepatic artery

Gastroduodenal artery

Superior pancreaticoduodenal artery

Inferior pancreaticoduodenal artery

Short gastric arteries

Splenic artery

Left gastroepiploic artery

Right gastroepiploic artery

Superior mesenteric artery

Figure 16.1. The major arteries supplying the stomach are shown in this diagram. Note the location of the gastroduodenal artery behind the duodenum. Posterior penetrating duodenal ulcers may erode into this artery, causing hemorrhage.

The arterial blood supply to the stomach includes the right and left gastric, right and left gastroepiploic, short gastric, and gastroduodenal arteries (Fig. 16.1).

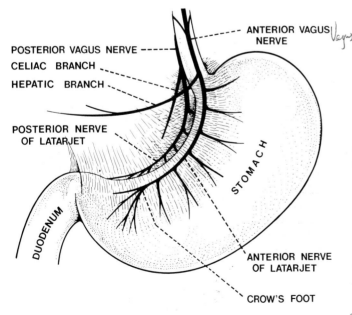

POSTERIOR VAGUS NERVE
CELIAC BRANCH
HEPATIC BRANCH

POSTERIOR NERVE OF LATARJET

ANTERIOR VAGUS NERVE

DUODENUM

STOMACH

ANTERIOR NERVE OF LATARJET

CROW'S FOOT

Figure 16.2. Branches of the vagus nerve innervate the stomach, pylorus, and duodenum. If the distal nerve of Latarjet is denervated, the pylorus will not relax in response to food.

Due to the abundant blood supply, it is quite difficult to devascularize the stomach surgically. Sympathetic innervation parallels arterial flow and parasympathetic innervation comes through the vagus nerve. As the vagus nerves traverse the mediastinum, the left trunk rotates so that it enters the abdomen anterior to the esophagus (Fig. 16.2). The right trunk rotates so that it enters the abdomen posterior to the esophagus. Both innervate the stomach from the lesser curvature. The right vagus gives off a posterior branch that innervates the entire midgut (pancreas, small intestine, and proximal colon), while the left vagus gives off the hepatic branch that innervates the gallbladder, biliary tract, and liver. The vagus nerve stimulates the parietal cell mass to secrete hydrochloric acid; it also controls the motor activity of the stomach.

The wall of the stomach is made up of four layers: the mucosa, submucosa, muscularis, and serosa. The mucosa is separated from the submucosa by the muscularis mucosa. The submucosa contains a rich vascular network that accounts for the abundant blood supply to the mucosa. The mucosa is arranged in a coarse rugal pattern and has a complex glandular structure. Although mucus secreting cells are found throughout the stomach, parietal cells and chief cells are found only in the fundus. The gastrin-producing G cells are found only in the antrum. The simplest way to differentiate antral tissue from fundic tissue is to demonstrate the absence of the brightly eosin-staining parietal cells that are present in the fundus. The pace-making area of the stomach is found in the fundus on the greater curvature near the short gastric vessels.

The duodenum is a metabolically active organ that not only receives the chyme from the stomach, and bile and pancreatic secretion via the ampulla of Vater, but in addition produces a myriad of hormonally active agents. The duodenum is divided into four regions: first part (duodenal bulb), second part (descending), third part (transverse), fourth part (ascending to ligament of Treitz). The descending duodenum is the site of the pacemaker for the entire small intestine.

The blood supply to the duodenum comes primarily from the gastroduodenal artery, although other smaller vessels are contributors. This vessel is the first branch of the proper hepatic artery. It courses immediately posterior to the duodenal bulb and then divides into the pancreaticoduodenal arcades. A duodenal ulcer that penetrates through the posterior wall of the duodenal bulb does so in the vicinity of the gastroduodenal artery. If the vessel wall is exposed to the gastric digestive enzymes and acid, massive bleeding may result.

Mechanisms of Hydrochloric Acid Secretion

Man is the only mammal that secrets hydrochloric acid in the fasting state. This has prompted some investigators to say that duodenal ulcer disease is a disease of civilization.

There are three general phases of stimulation that cause the release of hydrochloric acid from the parietal cell mass. These are the cephalic phase (mediated by the vagus nerve's release of acetylcholine), the gastric phase (mediated by the antral release of gastrin), and the intestinal phase (mediated by the small intestine's release of various gastrointestinal peptides and histamine).

① Cephalic Phase

Central nervous system stimulation by the sight, smell, or thought of food will cause efferent activity in the vagus nerve. Acetylcholine is released in the region of the parietal cell. This is associated with an increase in the metabolic activity of the cell, the consumption of ATP, and the release of hydrochloric acid. Surgical division of the *vagus* nerves supplying the parietal cell mass suppress this response. The response can also be suppressed by anticholinergics.

② Gastric Phase

Alkalinization, distension, or the presence of food in the antrum (particularly amino acids) promotes gastrin release from the G cells. Gastrin is a true hormone that is released into the venous circulation and exerts its effect on the parietal cell. There are at least three species of gastrin. Basal serum gastrin measured in the fasting state is predominantly "big" gastrin containing

a chain of 34 amino acids. The half-life of this molecule is long and its potency is low. In the stimulated state, "small" gastrin is released. This molecule has a 17 amino acid chain and a short half-life. The biological activity of this species of molecule is great. A third moiety, "big, big" gastrin has been identified, but its physiologic function is not well understood.

③ Intestinal Phase

The intestinal phase of gastric acid production occurs when products of digestion reach the small intestine. This phase has been associated with substantial rises in various serum peptides, some of which stimulate gastric acid output while others are thought to be inhibitory. Stimulation of the H_2 receptor may play a role in this phase of acid production.

Physiology of Hydrochloric Acid Secretion

There are at least three types of receptors on the parietal cell membrane, one each for gastrin, acetylcholine, and histamine (Fig. 16.3). Hydrochloric acid is secreted from the cell when any one of these sites is occupied by its appropriate ligand. The effect of any of the ligands is magnified when two receptor sites are occupied simultaneously (synergism). Conversely, when any one of these sites is blocked, the other sites becomes less responsive to stimulation. Thus, when vagal innervation is interrupted, as with vagotomy, the parietal cells become less responsive to stimulation by gastrin, pentagastrin, or by Histalog®.

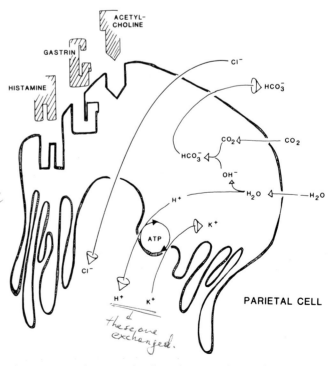

Figure 16.3. The parietal cell in the stomach has three receptors that, when stimulated, result in stimulation of hydrochloric acid.

The parietal cell is capable of secreting hydrogen ion against a 1,000,000:1 gradient. Hydrogen ion is stored within the cytosol of the parietal cell in packets that are surrounded by a membrane. When stimulated, these membranes fuse with the surface membrane and hydrogen is released into the lumen. The secretory process is an active process that exchanges the hydrogen ion for potassium. The chloride ion is transported into the lumen in conjunction with the process. As a by-product of this reaction, water and bicarbonate are produced. These passively diffuse into the plasma and extracellular space.

There are several events that suppress gastric acid production. When acid chyme reaches the duodenum, secretin is released from the duodenal wall. This inhibits gastric acid secretion and gastric emptying. When gastric luminal pH drops below 1.5, antral release of gastrin is inhibited by somatostatin. These are the first autoregulation steps in the control of gastric acid release. Stimulation of the pancreas by secretin causes an increased volume of pancreatic secretion with an increase in bicarbonate concentration and total protein content.

Duodenal sodium bicarbonate production is up to six times greater than that produced by the stomach. The transmucosal electrical gradient is responsible for the transport of the bicarbonate ion into the lumen. Sodium bicarbonate is capable of neutralizing all the hydrogen ion normally presented to the duodenal bulb. The secretin-stimulated pancreatic bicarbonate contributes only a small amount to neutralization of the total acid load. Bicarbonate is also secreted from the gastric glandular epithelium in exchange for chloride ions and is capable of neutralizing a small portion of the maximum acid output. When this effect is added to the protective effect of secreted mucus, the gastric surface epithelium is generally protected from autodigestion. The goblet cells of the stomach produce a mucopolysaccharide that attaches to the luminal surface of the gastric mucosa. Although the luminal pH may drop to as low as 1.0, the pH within the mucus, and therefore at the luminal surface of the mucosal cells, rarely falls below 7.0.

In the acid milieu of the stomach, pepsinogen that is produced by the chief cell is converted to pepsin. Pepsin activity hydrolyzes proteins to peptones and amino acids. This combination of pepsin and hydrochloric acid is potentially damaging to the gastric mucosal cells. Within the mucosa is a sophisticated and highly efficient mechanism (the gastric mucosal barrier) whereby the back diffusion of hydrogen ion can be rapidly neutralized and cleared. If this mechanism is not functioning adequately, damage to the mucosa occurs.

Peptic Ulcer Disease

Stated in its simplest form, peptic ulcers of the upper gastrointestinal tract occur when the mechanisms for defense are inadequate to deal with the phys-

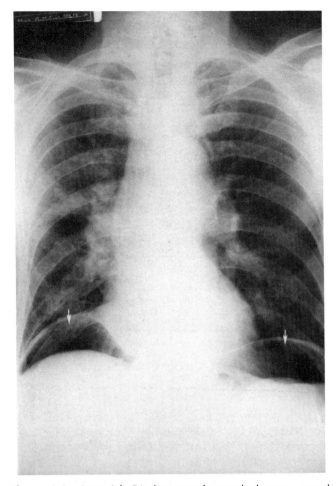

Figure 16.4. An upright PA chest x-ray frequently demonstrates subdiaphragmatic air in patients with a perforated ulcer.

iologic, but hostile, intraluminal milieu. When such an event occurs, autodigestion of the mucosa occurs.

Although grouped together for the purposes of this chapter, there are many differences in the clinical presentation and pathophysiology between ulcers that occur in the stomach and those that occur in the duodenum.

Clinical Presentation of Duodenal Ulcer Disease

It is estimated that 18-20 million patients per year develop acute ulcerations of the duodenum. Although the vast majority of these heal spontaneously, complications are not uncommon. Ulcers most commonly occur in the first part of the duodenum and are associated with the clinical syndrome of burning, epigastric abdominal pain that is accentuated by fasting. The pain frequently awakens patients from sleep and is relieved by antacids or food. Weight gain in this situation is not uncommon. The pain is often characterized as "boring in nature" and may radiate to the back in patients with posterior-penetrating ulcers. Massive upper gastrointestinal hemorrhage may occur when the ulcer erodes into the gastroduodenal artery, producing symptoms of syncope, tachycardia, hypotension, nausea, and hematemesis. An ulcer that perforates through the superior or anterior aspect of the duodenal bulb may spill duodenal contents into the abdominal cavity. In such a circumstance, the patient will have the signs and symptoms of an acute abdomen. These include tachycardia, severe abdominal tenderness and pain, guarding, and rigidity. On an upright chest x-ray, free intraperitoneal air may be seen outlining the diaphragm or liver, confirming the diagnosis of a perforated viscus (Fig. 16.4). Other patients who have repeated bouts of acute ulceration may develop a scarred duodenal bulb. As this cicatrix progresses, gastric outlet obstruction may occur. These patients present with weight loss, persistent vomiting immediately postprandial, and chronic gastric dilatation. Chronic antral dilatation produces sustained release of gastrin, thus initiating a vicious cycle.

A special variant of duodenal ulcer disease is the prepyloric ulcer or the ulcer that occurs in the pyloric channel. These ulcers generally occur at the junction between the antral mucosa and the duodenal mucosa. The gastric acid secretory pattern is that of a duodenal ulcer (as opposed to a gastric ulcer), and the patient should be treated as though the lesion was a duodenal ulcer.

Treatment of Acute Peptic Ulcer Disease

The three complications described above, hemorrhage, perforation, and obstruction, as well as failure of nonoperative management (intractability), are the classic constellation of complications that require surgical intervention.

In patients with free perforation and without other medical diseases that would preclude an operation, an exploratory celiotomy (laparotomy) should be performed immediately. The abrupt onset of severe abdominal pain, findings of a rigid ''surgical abdomen'' and free air under the diaphragm on upright abdominal roentgenograms should lead one to the diagnosis. If perforation is less than 6 hours old, the ulcer is plicated (oversewn) and an acid-reducing procedure is performed. If greater than 6 hours, plication alone is performed.

In patients with an upper gastrointestinal hemorrhage, the stomach should be decompressed with a nasogastric tube. Gastric lavage and antacid therapy should be started. At the initial evaluation, coagulation parameters should also be assessed. An intravenous line should be inserted and blood should be prepared for administration to the patient. Although each case must be judged on its individual merits, if a patient requires six or more units of blood in the initial 12-hour period to maintain hemodynamic stability, then an operation should be performed. Hemodynamically unstable patients and patients who are elderly should be candidates for earlier surgical intervention than younger, stable patients, because hypotension is poorly tolerated in the elderly. The surgical treatment is ligation of the bleeding artery plus an acid-reducing procedure to prevent rebleeding.

In patients with gastric outlet obstruction the stom-

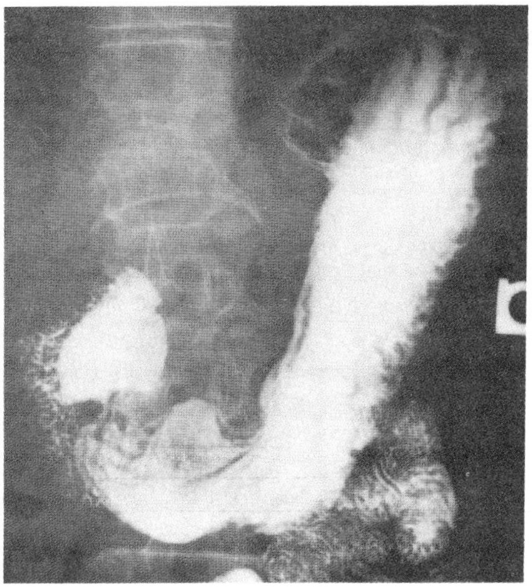

Figure 16.5. An upper GI series showing normal stomach and duodenum. (From Robbins LL (ed): *Golden's Diagnostic Radiology*. Baltimore, Williams & Wilkins, 1969, p 5.187.)

ach should be decompressed with a nasogastric tube for 5 or 6 days or until the stomach has returned to near its normal size. During this time, the patient should be allowed nothing by mouth. Nutrition and fluids should be administered intravenously. In such patients, malnutrition may be ameliorated by total parenteral nutrition (see Chapter 7). An acid-reducing operation as well as a procedure to allow emptying of the stomach are necessary.

A patient should be considered intractable if persistent symptoms interfere with their lifestyle despite adequate medical management. In this situation, surgical intervention may be considered.

Evaluation of Patients with Chronic Ulcer Symptoms

To make the diagnosis of duodenal ulcer disease, the ulcer should be demonstrated *objectively*, rather than relying on vague symptoms.

Upper Gastrointestinal Series. Classically, the diagnosis of duodenal ulcer disease is made by the upper gastrointestinal barium examination (upper GI series) (Fig. 16.5). In this examination, barium and air are swallowed, and the esophagus, stomach, and duodenum are observed fluoroscopically and radiographs are made for permanent documentation. Swallowing, peristaltic and sphincteric function, size, shape, displacement by other organs, distensibility, flexibility, and mucosal pattern are all observed. Ulcers, scars, strictures, cancers, and postoperative changes can all be demonstrated. Because it is widely available, inexpensive, and safe, upper GI series is often the first diagnostic study employed when duodenal ulcer is suspected, especially when symptoms are not clear-cut. Even if an active ulcer is not visualized, ancillary signs of peptic disease, such as duodenal spasm, deformity, and mucosal swelling, usually point to the correct diagnosis.

Endoscopy. To visualize the mucosal surface, upper GI endoscopy is even more reliable than upper GI series. This study involves the passage of a gastroscope from the mouth into the esophagus, stomach, and duodenum. The mucosa can be examined in detail and if an ulcer is present, it can usually be seen. In patients who are bleeding, the exact size of hemorrhage can be determined. Endoscopy can also identify concomitant disease or suggest alternative diagnoses in certain patients. Although adenocarcinoma of the duodenum occurs, it is extremely rare. Only if the ulcer is associated with a mass should a biopsy be performed. This is in contrast to a gastric ulcer where multiple biopsies are mandatory each time an ulcer is identified.

Gastric Acid Analysis. A gastric analysis gives a substantial amount of meaningful information. The test is performed by placing a nasogastric tube into the stomach and collecting the contents from the stomach via constant suction at 15-minute intervals for 2 hours. After a 1-hour basal period, a secretagogue (either Histalog or pentagastrin) is given intravenously and collections are continued at 15-minute intervals for another hour. The gastric analysis in more than one-fourth the patients with duodenal ulcer disease will classically show a high basal acid output (>4.0 mEq/hr) (cephalic phase) and more than one-third will have elevated stimulated acid output. Patients with a gastrinoma (Zollinger-Ellison syndrome) will have a basal acid output that may be 10 times the upper limits of normal; however with stimulation, only a small increase in acid output will occur, since the parietal cell mass is already maximally stimulated by the elevated basal serum gastrin levels.

Medical Treatment

The fundamental problem in patients with duodenal ulcer disease is an accentuation of the cephalic phase of gastric acid output. Therapy is directed at reducing basal acid secretion. The nonoperative treatment of duodenal ulcer disease is aimed at blocking the vagus nerve's stimulation of the parietal cells, or by blocking the parietal cell's response to stimuli. Most dietary regimens are not only ineffective, but actually slow gastric emptying. Presently, diet is only a minor component of nonsurgical treatment. Once the diagnosis of a duodenal ulcer is confirmed, the medical regimen consists of the avoidance of foods that are secretagogues (caffeine, alcohol, chocolates, etc.), intraluminal antacids to neutralize excreted acid, blockade of the H₂ receptor at the parietal cell membrane, the use of surface coating agents, and in certain cases, the administration of systemic anticholinergics. With this regimen, most patients will be asymptomatic within a 7-day treatment period. At this time, the most important modality of treatment is H₂ blockade. The advantages of these medications include: (1) ease of administration, (2) ex-

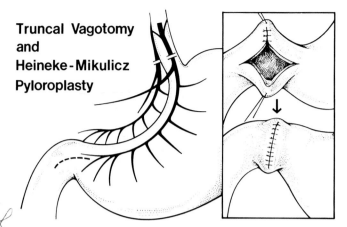

Figure 16.6. When the trunk of the vagus nerve has been divided, a pyloroplasty must also be performed to allow gastric emptying. This pyloroplasty is the most commonly performed.

cellent patient compliance, (3) therapeutic efficacy in excess of 90%, and (4) blocking acid production rather than neutralizing released hydrogen ion. Antacids are also highly effective if taken appropriately. Antacids that contain aluminum hydroxide are frequently associated with constipation, while antacids that contain magnesium salts may produce diarrhea.

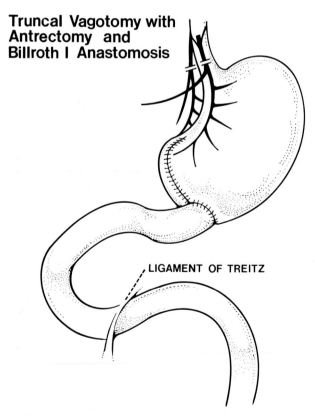

Figure 16.7. An antrectomy removes the distal portion of the stomach, where gastrin is produced. In addition, antrectomy removes the pylorus, thus allowing gastric emptying following vagotomy. In a Billroth I anastomosis, the duodenum is reanastomosed to the stomach in continuity.

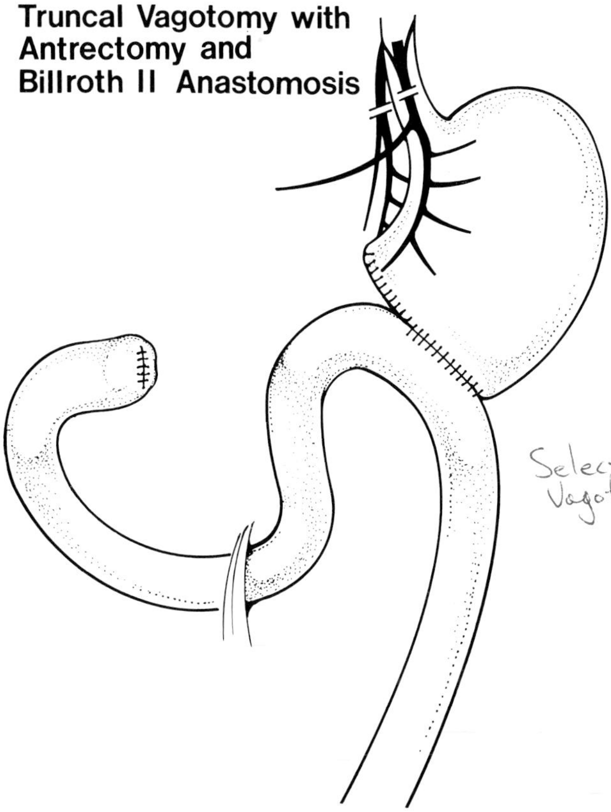

Antrectomy implies removal of the antrum & the pylorus

Truncal Vagotomy with Antrectomy and Billroth II Anastomosis

Figure 16.8. In a Billroth II anastomosis, the duodenum is not reattached to the stomach; rather, the stomach is reanastomosed to a proximal loop of jejunum. This procedure is particularly useful when the duodenum is extensively scarred.

Surgical Treatment

Just as medical therapy is directed at the underlying disease state that predisposes the patient to develop a duodenal ulcer, the surgical approach is also directed at these parameters. Since the most salient feature in the patient with duodenal ulcer disease is a pronounced cephalic phase of gastric acid production, the most critical aspect of surgical intervention is to interrupt the neural pathway responsible for this excess. The vagus nerves can be interrupted in one of three ways: truncal vagotomy, selective vagotomy, or proximal gastric vagotomy (parietal cell vagotomy or highly selective vagotomy). Truncal vagotomy involves the complete transection of all vagal trunks at or above the esophageal hiatus of the diaphragm. This not only denervates the parietal cell mass, but also the antral pump, pyloric sphincter mechanism, and the majority of the abdominal viscera. Because the truncal vagotomy disrupts gastric motility, a gastric drainage procedure is required to facilitate gastric emptying. Otherwise, gastric antral dilation occurs and stimulates gastrin release. The most common complementary procedure is a pyloroplasty, performed by incising the pylorus horizontally and closing it vertically (Fig. 16.6). Various modifications of the pyloroplasty have been proposed and most are known by eponyms. If a pyloroplasty is not possible, a gastroenterostomy is an al-

ternative. Many surgeons add a distal gastrectomy (antrectomy) to the truncal vagotomy (Fig. 16.7) performing an anastomosis between the distal end of the stomach and the end of the duodenum (Billroth I). Gastrointestinal continuity may be reestablished by joining the end of the stomach to a loop of the jejunum (Billroth II), (Fig. 16.8), or a Roux-en-Y gastroenterostomy, (Fig. 16.9). Antrectomy augments the effect of vagotomy by removing the bulk of the gastrin-producing cells. Therefore, these procedures interrupt both the cephalic phase and the gastric phase of acid stimulation. It is not surprising that this combined procedure (vagotomy and antrectomy) is associated with a lower recurrence rate than vagotomy and pyloroplasty (1.5% recurrence rate versus 10% recurrence rate).

The selective vagotomy provides total denervation of the stomach from above the crus of the diaphragm down to and including the pylorus (Fig. 16.11). This procedure spares the parasympathetic innervation of the abdominal viscera, but like the truncal vagotomy, denervates the antral pump and pylorus, necessitating some type of drainage procedure. The most common procedure has been a pyloroplasty. Advocates of this type of vagotomy claim that it gives a more total gastric vagotomy than does a truncal vagotomy, but does not denervate other abdominal organs (liver, gallbladder, pancreas, small intestine, and proximal colon). Postgastrectomy syndromes occur with a frequency equal to a truncal vagotomy and pyloroplasty.

Truncal Vagotomy with Antrectomy and Roux-en-Y Anastomosis

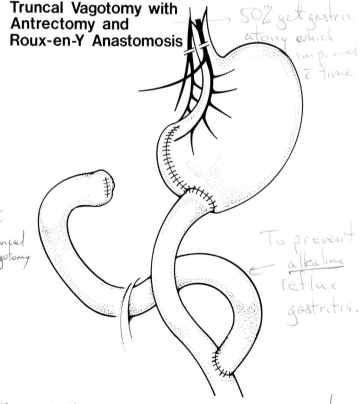

Figure 16.9. The Roux-en-Y anastomosis reduces the reflux of small bowel contents back into the stomach. Peristalsis in the small bowel carries food and fluid away from the stomach. This procedure is particularly used when a patient has a history of alkaline-reflux gastritis.

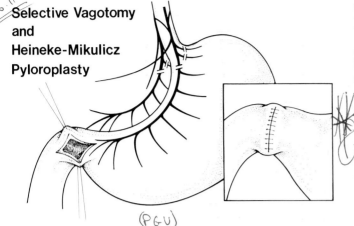

Fig. 16.11

Selective Vagotomy and Heineke-Mikulicz Pyloroplasty

(PGU)

Figure 16.10. A proximal gastric vagotomy (highly selective vagotomy) denervates the acid-producing parietal cells without interfering with the antral pump or pylorus.

Proximal Gastric Vagotomy

The most recent operation to gain popularity is the proximal gastric vagotomy (PGV) (Fig. 16.10). In this procedure, the vagus nerve is identified as it courses along the lesser curvature of the stomach, and only those branches that innervate the parietal cell mass are divided. This allows the antral pump and pyloric sphincter mechanisms to continue to function normally, thus obviating the need for a drainage procedure. Patients with gastric outlet obstruction due to peptic ulcer disease are not candidates for this procedure. This procedure is associated with the lowest incidence of postgastrectomy syndromes. However, the ulcer recurrence rate is in excess of 10%. *(1.5% for vagotomy # antrectomy)*

In some patients, a total gastrectomy (Fig. 16.12) is required to control either the ulcer diathesis or the postgastrectomy sequelae. Although this procedure is associated with the absolute protection of the patient from recurrent ulcer disease, it is associated with significant aberrations in metabolism such as decreased levels of vitamin B_{12}, absent intrinsic factor, pernicious anemia, malnutrition, and weight loss. There is also a

significant operative mortality due to the difficulty of performing an esophageal anastomosis.

The decision about which procedure to perform on an individual patient is complicated, and should be based on the age of the patient, likelihood of ulcer recurrence, severity of symptoms, and the patient's sex and weight. The procedures associated with the highest cure rate (e.g., antrectomy and vagotomy) also have the highest incidence of postgastrectomy side effects, such as dumping syndrome. Likewise, procedures with the lowest cure rate have the lowest incidence of side effects. Therefore, the surgeon's responsibility is to select the procedure for each patient that is likely to be effective in treating the ulcer diathesis without resulting in a high likelihood of side effects. It is possible to predict patients who are at high risk for postgastrectomy complications; young, thin women are particularly vulnerable.

Zollinger-Ellison Syndrome

A special variant of duodenal ulcer disease is the Zollinger-Ellison syndrome (ZES). This syndrome is the direct result of the independent production of gastrin by a tumor arising in the pancreas or paraduodenal area. Approximately 60% of these tumors are malignant. Although long-term survivors are not uncommon, about 50% of patients with the malignant variant of the disease will die within 5 years of the diagnosis. However, a substantial number of people can survive 10 to 15 years. A high degree of suspicion is necessary to identify patients with the ZES. Patients at risk are those with refractory peptic ulcer disease or those with an extremely virulent ulcer diathesis. Many of the latter group will present with multiple ulcers in the duodenum or ulcers in unusual locations (i.e., jejunum and ileum).

The diagnosis should be suspected if fasting serum gastrin levels are high (greater than 300 pg/ml). In addition, a secretin infusion test, performed by injecting secretin intravenously and measuring serum gastrin levels at 2, 5, 10, 15, 30, 45, and 60 minutes after the infusion is frequently confirmatory. In patients with the ZES, there is a profound rise in serum gastrin. This is a safe test with a high specificity and sensitivity.

Therapy for the ZES is controversial. Pharmacological doses of H_2 receptor parietal cell antagonists have been advocated and have proven effective in selected patients (50%). Others have advocated exploratory laparotomy and biopsy or excision of the tumor, if located, to confirm the diagnosis. In a small subset of patients this may be curative. If an isolated tumor is identified, then the tumor should be resected and a proximal gastric vagotomy performed. Even if the tumor cannot be found or totally excised, some have recommended a proximal gastric vagotomy and long-term treatment with an H_2 blocker. These procedures must be compared to the standard of therapy, a total gastrectomy. This procedure removes the end organ, abolishes all acid production, and ablates the majority of symptoms of the disease.

Proximal Gastric Vagotomy

Fig. 16.10

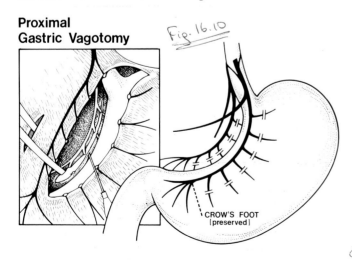

CROW'S FOOT
(preserved)

Figure 16.11. Because a selective vagotomy denervates the pylorus, a pyloroplasty must be performed to allow gastric emptying.

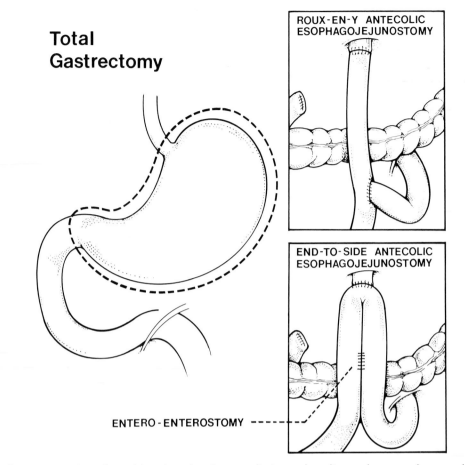

Total Gastrectomy

ROUX-EN-Y ANTECOLIC ESOPHAGOJEJUNOSTOMY

END-TO-SIDE ANTECOLIC ESOPHAGOJEJUNOSTOMY

ENTERO-ENTEROSTOMY ------

Figure 16.12. A total gastrectomy is performed in selected patients to eliminate ulcer disease; however, the procedure is technically more difficult than other procedures and associated with a higher incidence of postgastrectomy complications.

Gastric Ulcer Disease

Gastric ulcers are usually found on the lesser curvature of the stomach within 1 cm of the transition zone between the antrum and body of the stomach. The mechanism producing gastric ulcers is unknown. Suggested mechanisms include a defective mucous barrier, delayed gastric emptying, antecedent gastritis, increased hydrogen ion back diffusion, alkaline reflux, and a defective pyloric sphincter mechanism.

Clinical Presentation

Although both duodenal ulcer disease and gastric ulcer disease commonly present with abdominal pain, the character of the pain is different. Gastric ulcer pain usually occurs in the epigastrium and may radiate through to the back. It is produced by the ingestion of food, while duodenal ulcer pain is relieved by eating. Weight loss is common in patients with gastric ulcers.

Diagnosis

Approximately 80% of patients with gastric ulcers will have a normal or low pattern of gastric acid secretion. Various researchers believe that hydrochloric acid is necessary for mucosal damage to occur, but the un-

derlying cause of the ulcer is probably not acid hypersecretion. Because hydrochloric acid is necessary for a true gastric ulcer, if the patient is found to have achlorhydria, the chances of malignancy are substantially increased. Even with normal hydrochloric acid production, a substantial number of gastric craters will be malignancies mimicking gastric ulcer disease. This is in contrast to the duodenal ulcer, which is seldom malignant.

The diagnosis can be made by upper GI series or by endoscopy. All patients with gastric ulcers should be endoscoped and multiple biopsies taken to establish the presence or absence of carcinoma. Cytology and brushings are also helpful as an adjunct to biopsy. Despite these procedures, false negative results are still common, due to the small sample size.

Nonsurgical Treatment

The treatment regimen proposed in patients with gastric ulcer disease is similar to that for duodenal ulcer disease; however, anticholinergics are generally avoided as they aggravate gastric stasis. With duodenal ulcer disease, greater than 90% of patients will heal their ulcer on a medical regimen; whereas in those with gastric ulcers less than 50% of patients will completely heal. Patients should be taken off all medications that might have contributed to the ulcer's formation or retard healing (aspirin, prostaglandin blockers, steroids, or alcohol). It is imperative in the nonoperative management of patients with gastric ulcer disease that repeat endoscopy be performed after 6 weeks of therapy. If the ulcer has not shown substantial healing, then the patient should be considered for surgical therapy. If the patient is a poor operative candidate, then the medical regimen should be continued and repeat endoscopy scheduled. If after 4 more weeks of therapy the ulcer persists, then it is unlikely that the ulcer will heal without operative intervention. Suspicion that the ulcer harbors a malignancy should be heightened. At each endoscopy where a gastric ulcer is identified, multiple biopsies of the margin of the ulcer should be taken. It is only when these biopsies are reviewed histologically that an ulcer can be said to be nonmalignant.

Despite the best of medical care, the persistence/recurrence rate in the treatment of gastric ulcer disease is extremely high.

Surgical Treatment

The operative approach to benign gastric ulcer disease is in part dependent upon the gastric acid secretory status of the patient. Because the majority of these patients have normal or low total hydrochloric acid production, a distal gastrectomy (approximately 50%) with excision of the ulcer is the appropriate therapy. In gastric ulcer disease, the ulcer must be excised, in contradistinction to the surgical approach to duodenal ulcer disease where the ulcer can be left in situ. Each resected gastric ulcer should be evaluated histologically to make certain that a gastric carcinoma is not hidden in the depths of the crater. If the patient has demonstrated gastric acid hypersecretion, then a truncal vagotomy should be added to the procedure.

The recurrence rate following surgical treatment for gastric ulcer is extremely low. Although postgastrectomy sequelae may occur after such procedures, they appear to be less common than for procedures performed for duodenal ulcer disease.

Postgastrectomy Syndromes

The innervated intact stomach is a careful guardian of the gastrointestinal tract. When the stomach is denervated and especially when the pyloric mechanism is ablated, the exquisite control of gastric emptying is abolished. This fact, in association with the anastomotic characteristics of many of the reconstructions, is at fault in most of the common postgastrectomy syndromes. Several of the reconstructions produce a defunctionalized limb of intestine or place the duodenum or jejunum at risk for obstruction or bacterial overgrowth. Some of the reconstructions provide easy ingress of bile and duodenal secretions into the gastric pouch. These aberrations in normal anatomy produce the various postgastrectomy syndromes.

An UGI series may be useful to document the extent and type of procedure done, to assess gastric emptying and mobility and to determine the cause of vomiting. Gastric emptying can also be defined more physiologically by administering a radionuclide-labelled meal followed by sequential imaging.

Early Dumping

The early dumping syndrome is characterized by a select set of symptoms that occur after the ingestion of food of high osmolarity. Such a meal may be one that contains a large quantity of simple and complex sugars (e.g., milk products). About 15 minutes after the meal has been ingested, the patient will develop anxiety, weakness, tachycardia, diaphoresis, and frequently complain of palpitations. The patient may also describe feelings of extreme weakness and a desire to lie down. Often borborygmi can be heard and diarrhea is not uncommon. Gradually, the symptoms clear and the patient again becomes symptom free.

The patient with early dumping has uncontrolled emptying of hypertonic fluid into the small intestine. There is rapid movement of fluid from the intravascular space to the intraluminal space, producing acute intravascular volume depletion. As the simple sugars are absorbed and as dilution of the hypertonic solution occurs, symptoms gradually abate. Intravascular volume is repleted as fluid moves from the intracellular space and as fluid is absorbed from the intestinal lumen. Fluid shifts, however, fail to explain all the symptoms associated with early dumping. The release of several hormonal substances, including serotonin, histamine, glucagon, vasoactive intestinal peptide, kinins, and others, is thought to contribute to the symptom complex.

This problem is best treated by the avoidance of hypertonic liquid meals and by the ingestion of some fat with each meal to slow gastric emptying. Liquids should be ingested either before the meal or at least 30 minutes after meals. Some authors claim that β blockers (10–20 mg of propranolol hydrochloride) taken 20 minutes before a meal are helpful in about 50% of the cases. Pharmacologic intervention to block hormonal substances may occasionally be of benefit.

In some patients with recalcitrant symptoms, surgical construction of a Roux-en-Y gastrojejunostomy may be necessary. This procedure works by delaying gastric emptying.

Late Dumping

Just as in early dumping, the patient will develop anxiety, diaphoresis, tachycardia, palpitations, weakness, fatigue, and a desire to assume the recumbent position. In late dumping, the symptoms usually begin within 3 hours after the meal. This variant of dumping is not associated with borborygmi or diarrhea. The physiologic explanation for late dumping involves rapid changes in serum glucose and insulin levels. After the meal, a large bolus of glucose containing chyme is presented to the mucosa of the small intestine. The absorption of the glucose occurs much more rapidly than when the intact pylorus is present to meter gastric emptying. Extremely high serum glucose levels may result shortly after the meal. This elicits a profound outpouring of insulin. The insulin response exceeds what is necessary to clear the glucose from the blood and subsequently hypoglycemia results. The symptoms in late dumping are the direct result of rapid fluctuation in serum glucose.

Nonoperative therapy for this syndrome should include the ingestion of a small snack 2 hours after the meals. Crackers and peanut butter make an excellent supplement to abort or ameliorate the symptoms. If symptoms cannot be controlled by nonoperative management, then either conversion of the previous procedure to a Billroth I (if not already present), or the construction of a Roux-en-Y gastrojejunostomy should be considered. Surgical intervention should only be considered in patients refractory to aggressive nonoperative therapy.

Afferent Loop Obstruction

Afferent loop obstruction occurs only after a gastrectomy with a Billroth II reconstruction. It is usually associated with a kink in the afferent limb adjacent to the anastomosis. Pancreatic and biliary secretion are trapped in the afferent limb, producing distention. Symptoms generally consist of severely cramping abdominal pain that occurs immediately after the ingestion of a meal. Patients often characterize the pain as crushing. Within 45 minutes, the patient will feel an abdominal rush that is associated with increased pain followed by nausea and vomiting of a dark brown, bitter-tasting material that has the consistency of engine oil. This results from the spontaneous and forceful decompression of the obstructed limb. Classically, no food is present. With the episode of vomiting, symptoms resolve. Often these patients have profound weight loss because they stop eating to prevent the pain. The best treatment is exploration of the abdomen and conversion of the Billroth II to either a Roux-en-Y gastrojejunostomy or to a Billroth I gastroduodenostomy.

Blind Loop Syndrome

It is more common to develop a blind loop syndrome after a Billroth II procedure than after a Roux-en-Y procedure. It is also seen in patients who have had bypass of the small bowel secondary to radiation injury or morbid obesity. The blind loop syndrome is associated with bacterial overgrowth in the limb of intestine that is excluded from the flow of chyme. This excluded limb of intestine harbors bacteria that proliferate and interfere with folate and vitamin B_{12} metabolism. The patients frequently complain of weakness and are often anemic. A Schilling test is often positive. Treatment consists of orally administered broad spectrum antibiotics that cover both aerobic and anaerobic bacteria. This regimen is often a temporizing step as many patients will require conversion to a Billroth I gastroduodenostomy.

Alkaline Reflux Gastritis

Alkaline reflux gastritis is seen in patients in whom duodenal, pancreatic, and biliary contents are allowed to reflux back into the denervated stomach. These patients complain of weakness, weight loss, persistent nausea, abdominal pain that frequently goes through to the back, and are often anemic. The diagnosis is made by upper gastrointestinal endoscopy, where the gastric mucosa will be edematous, bile stained, atrophic, and erythematous. The visual diagnosis should be confirmed by multiple biopsies taken of the gastric mucosa away from the stoma. The microscopic appearance is often quite characteristic, revealing inflammation and a "corkscrew" appearance of blood vessels in the submucosa.

Although a variety of medical regimens have been proposed to treat alkaline reflux gastritis (the oral ingestion of cholestyramine, antacids, and others), none have proven to be uniformly satisfactory. The surgical correction of this disease consists of diverting the duodenal contents away from the stomach with a long limb Roux-en-Y gastrojejunostomy. The minimum distance between the gastrojejunostomy and the stoma bringing the bile and pancreatic juices into the intestine must be at least 40 cm (18 inches). This procedure has proven effective in most patients.

Recurrent Ulcer Disease

The most common cause of recurrent ulcer disease is an inadequate vagotomy. The vagus nerve most often missed is the right posterior nerve. Each operation is associated with different recurrence rates. The operation associated with the lowest recurrence rate is a total gastrectomy, but it is rarely indicated because of its high early and late morbidity. The next lowest recurrence rate is seen in patients who have had a truncal vagotomy and antrectomy (1–2%). The highest recurrence rate would appear to be in patients who have had a proximal gastric vagotomy (~12%), although results vary substantially among different centers. The average recurrence rates for the different operative procedures as well as the incidence of the various postgastrectomy syndromes are listed in Table 16.1.

Gastric Atony

One of the most difficult problems after any operation that denervates the stomach and ablates the pylorus is aberrations in gastric motility. Rapid emptying, especially of liquids, is common and has been dealt with previously (dumping syndrome). Delayed gastric emptying, especially of solids, is a poorly understood phenomenon that may be the single most common problem after gastric resection. More than 50% of patients with Roux-en-Y gastrojejunostomy have substantial delays in gastric emptying identified by technetium-labeled egg albumin scan. However, only 50% of these patients will have symptoms. The majority will improve with time. If medications are necessary, urecholine or metaclopramide may prove beneficial.

Table 16.1.
Relative Incidence of Recurrence and Operative Mortality Expressed As Percentages[a]

	Recurrence Rate (%)	Operative Mortality (%)	Dumping		Afferent Loop Syndrome	Blind Loop Syndrome	Alkaline Reflux Gastritis	Metabolic Sequelae
			Early	Late				
Vagotomy/pyloroplasty	5–10	1–2	2+	2+	0	0	1+	1+
Vagotomy/antrectomy Billroth I	1–2	1–4	2+	2+	0	0	1+	1+
Vagotomy/antrectomy Billroth II	1–3	1–4	3+	3+	2+	2+	2+	2+
Selective vagotomy	5–10	1–2	2+	2+	0	0	0	1+
Proximal gastric vagotomy	10–15	1	0	0	0	0	0	0
Total gastrectomy	0	2–5	3+	2+	0			2+

[a]These numbers are averages taken from the larger series published in the literature. The relative incidences of the postgastrectomy syndromes are expressed on a scale from 0 to 4+ with 0 implying relative absence of symptoms and 4+ implying frequent profound symptoms.

Nutritional Disturbances

Although a variety of different metabolic abnormalities have been identified following gastric resection, megaloblastic anemia (B_{12} deficiency/folate deficiency) and microcytic anemia (iron deficiency or blood loss) are the most common. Other patients experience steatorrhea and in many instances, weight loss. Diarrhea secondary to vagotomy is extremely rare, although changes in stooling pattern are common. Up to 25% of patients may have loose, frequent stools in the postoperative period.

Gastritis

Diffuse erythema and disruption of the mucosa of the stomach can occur and is frequently associated with a myriad of symptoms including bleeding, nausea, and vomiting. Gastritis is often associated with the intake of caustic agents, such as alcohol, aspirin, steroids, or prostaglandin blockers. Treatment consists of withdrawal of the noxious agents, decompression of the stomach, antacids and H_2 blockers, and nutritional repletion.

Stress Gastritis

In the past, bleeding from stress gastritis was a common cause of morbidity and mortality in burn patients (Curling's ulcer), head trauma patients (Cushing's ulcer), or in patients in intensive care units. With the advent of aggressive neutralization of gastric acidity by titrating intraluminal pH to 3.5 or greater, these syndromes have been virtually eliminated. In a patient at risk, a nasogastric tube should be positioned and the gastric contents aspirated. An antacid should be instilled and left for 1 hour, after which gastric aspiration is again performed. If the pH is below 3.5 the amount of antacid should be increased until the pH is above 3.5. Some authors have recommended using H_2 block-

ers; however, these have not been shown to be substantially better than antacids.

If a patient does experience upper gastrointestinal hemorrhage, the physician should aspirate the stomach and perform endoscopy. If the source of bleeding is from stress gastritis and persists despite aggressive, nonoperative management, then a surgical procedure may have to be performed. A vagotomy and pyloroplasty with oversewing of the bleeding erosions is a quick and conservative procedure that will control bleeding in approximately 50% of patients. If bleeding recurs, a total gastrectomy must be considered.

Gastric Polyp

Gastric polyps are rare, but greater numbers have been diagnosed as more patients have undergone upper gastrointestinal endoscopy. If the polyp measures less than 0.5 cm in size, the risk of malignancy is low, while a polyp greater than 1.5 cm in diameter has considerably greater risk. When a gastric polyp is diagnosed, the physician may wish to evaluate the patient for the presence of other polyps. Multiple benign polyps in the small intestine and melanous spots on the lips and buccal mucosa are known as Peutz-Jegher's syndrome. Peutz-Jegher's syndrome is a Mendelian dominant trait with a high degree of penetrance. In such patients conservative therapy is indicated, as the tumors are hamartomas and are infrequently malignant.

Bezoar

The accumulation of a large mass of undigestible vegetable fiber within the stomach is known as a phytobezoar. If the material is predominantly hair, the mass is known as a trichobezoar. Trichobezoars are more common in children and among inmates of mental institutions. Although most bezoars may be broken up endoscopically, others must be removed surgically.

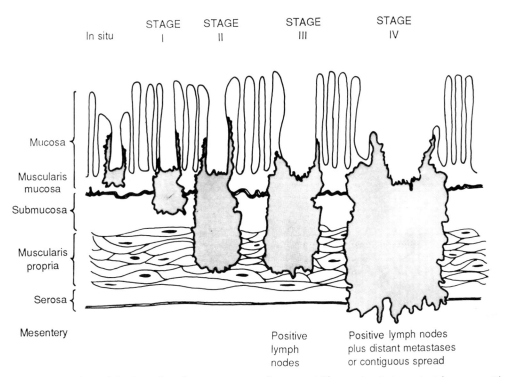

STAGE I   STAGE II   STAGE III   STAGE IV

In situ

Mucosa

Muscularis mucosa

Submucosa

Muscularis propria

Serosa

Mesentery

Positive lymph nodes

Positive lymph nodes plus distant metastases or contiguous spread

Figure 16.13. As tumor penetration of the bowel wall progresses, so does stage. The staging is important because with advanced stages survival is severely limited.

Malignancy of the Stomach

Gastric Carcinoma

The incidence of gastric carcinoma in the population varies greatly. In the United States, the frequency has steadily fallen in the past three decades, while in Japan, China, Chile, Finland, and the Soviet Union, the incidence is considerably higher and has remained essentially unchanged. Immigrants from these countries to the United States seem to have a lower incidence of the disease, suggesting an environmental or dietary factor as a possible etiologic agent.

Conditions that are thought to be premalignant and therefore warrant close observation are the presence in the stomach of adenomatous polyps, chronic gastritis, or a caustic injury secondary to lye ingestion. Also, pernicious anemia, which includes gastric achlorhydria and an extreme atrophic gastritis, is considered premalignant (about 40% will eventually develop a gastric cancer). Therefore, patients with pernicious anemia and without other contraindications should undergo regular endoscopy on a yearly basis.

Clinical Manifestations. Symptoms of gastric carcinoma often occur after the disease is far advanced. The earliest symptom may be weight loss; however, many patients experience epigastric pain as a prodrome that is so vague that a diagnosis cannot be made. Patients may have dysphagia, hematemesis, or melena. Laboratory studies often reveal an iron deficiency anemia or positive stool guaiac.

Diagnosis. The upper gastrointestinal series may show a fixed deformity of the stomach with or without an ulcer. The superficial spreading type of carcinoma, commonly found in Japan, will often show no abnormality on upper gastrointestinal roentgenogram. Endoscopy with biopsy is the best way to establish the diagnosis. The morphologic variants of gastric carcinoma that occur with greatest frequency in the United States include ulcerating, polypoid, and linitis plastica (leather bottle stomach). The prognosis for the disease depends upon the extent of involvement. Resected polypoid lesions have a better 5-year survival than do ulcerating lesions. Patients with linitis plastica have the poorest prognosis.

Sixty percent of gastric carcinomas originate in the distal half of the stomach and the majority of these will occur in the pyloric gland area. Metastatic spread occurs to regional lymph nodes, the omentum, the left supraclavicular area (Virchow's node), the ovary and to the peritoneum. Metastases in the pelvis can often be palpated through the rectum or vagina (Blumer's shelf) or in the ovary (Krukenberg's tumors) or at the umbilicus (Sister Jeane Marie's nodule).

Therapy. The only possible cure for gastric carcinoma is complete surgical resection; however, complete removal of a gastric carcinoma is rarely possible. Because of the lack of early symptoms, patients often present with advanced disease. The best cure rates are reported from Japan where there is a high percentage of the superficial spreading type. Even with this type of tumor, the 5-year survival rate is less than 50%. In a majority of studies from English speaking countries, curative resection is associated with less than a 10% 5-year survival. Pathologic staging of the resected specimen is the best predictor of survival (Fig. 16.13). The case for early diagnosis is made in studies where the 5-year survival has been evaluated in patients who had an incidental carcinoma found in the stomach removed for supposed benign disease. Some studies report that 5-year survival in this highly selected cohort approaches 75%.

Extended total gastrectomy, which is the procedure of choice for cure, removes not only the entire stomach, but also the spleen, distal pancreas, parapyloric nodes, and omentum. The operative morbidity and mortality is acceptable in the hands of experienced surgeons. The 5-year survival, although somewhat improved, is still less than 20%. There is considerable debate about the advantages of this procedure over a subtotal gastrectomy with adequate margins.

Despite these dismal results in the general population, the best palliation is still associated with gastric resection. Surgical resection for palliation should be carried out if possible, even if disease is left behind, to reduce bleeding and improve the patient's ability to eat. The resection should include the lesion with an adequate cephalic margin and the entire stomach distal to the tumor.

Gastric Lymphoma

Gastric lymphoma presents clinically similar to and may be mistaken for gastric carcinoma. The diagnostic evaluation is similar. The treatment of choice consists of exploratory laparotomy and resection. Once the diagnosis is confirmed pathologically, radiation therapy is indicated. The 5-year survival rate for such patients approaches 50%.

Leiomyoma and Leiomyosarcomas (smooth muscle tumors)

Both of these entities present as a submucosal mass. Some observers feel a leiomyoma may degenerate into a leiomyosarcoma. The most common symptom associated with these lesions is vague epigastric gastrointestinal pain. Occasionally, massive bleeding may occur. These lesions appear as a submucosal mass on upper gastrointestinal radiography. At endoscopy, the smooth raised lesion often has a central ulceration. The treatment is surgical resection. The prognosis for the benign lesion is excellent, while the malignant variant may prove very aggressive.

Techniques

Nasogastric Tube Placement

The medical student should be able to pass a nasogastric tube in a patient without abnormalities of the upper respiratory tract. The nasogastric tube should be removed from its package and appropriately straightened. The tube can be lubricated with either a gel or water. A small amount of gel should be placed on the tip of the tube and in the appropriate nasal passage. In some instances, it is necessary to anesthetize the hypopharynx with a small amount of aerosal local anesthetic. The patient is placed in the sitting position and the head bent slightly forward. The nasogastric tube is inserted gently into the nares and gently allowed to pass through the upper nasal passage. When the tip of the nasogastric tube approaches the pharynx, the patient is asked to swallow. As the patient swallows, the tube is advanced. If the patient develops paroxysms of coughing, the tube should be withdrawn slightly, the patient's neck should be fixed, and the tube should be advanced. When the tube has been advanced to such a depth that the aspiration ports should be within the stomach, a small burst of air is delivered into the lumen from a Toomy syringe while auscultation is accomplished over the upper abdomen. If a rushing sound is heard, the tube is in an appropriate position.

Once the tube has been positioned, it should be secured to the patient's integument in such a way as to prevent pressure on the tip of the alae cartilage. This is often best accomplished by securing the tube to the upper lip. The tube should then be positioned on the side of the patient's face and secured to the forehead. This keeps the tube out of the patient's vision and makes it a little easier for the patient to tolerate it.

When the tube is to be removed, the patient should be positioned comfortably in a relaxed position. All of the attachments of the tube to the patient should be disconnected. The tube should be disconnected from suction. At this point, the patient should be given a tissue with which to blow the nose when the tube has been completely removed. The patient should be asked to breathe in and out deeply and then to stare at a fixed object across the room. During exhalation the patient is exhorted to keep his eyes open and the tube is briskly removed. If the patient's eyes remain open, the patient will not gag. Once the tube has been removed, the patient is allowed to blow his nose.

SUGGESTED READINGS

Feldman M: Gastric secretion. In Sleisenger MH, Fordtran J (eds): *Gastrointestinal Disease: Pathophysiology, Diagnosis, Management*, ed 3. Philadelphia, WB Saunders, 1983.

Fink AS, Longmire WT Jr: Stomach. In Schwartz SI (ed): *Principles of Surgery*, ed 3. New York, McGraw-Hill, 1979.

McHardy G: Symposium: Peptic ulcer disease. *South Med J* 72: 251–278, 1979.

Moody FG, McGreevy J: Carcinoma of the stomach. In Sabiston, DC Jr (ed): *Textbook of Surgery*. Philadelphia, WB Saunders, 1986.

Richardson CT: Gastric ulcer. In Sleisenger MH, Fordtran J (eds): *Gastrointestinal Disease: Pathophysiology, Diagnosis, Management*, ed 3. Philadelphia, WB Saunders, 1983.

Soll AH, Eisenberg JI: Duodenal ulcer disease. In Sleisenger MH, Fordtran J (eds): *Gastrointestinal Disease Pathophysiology, Diagnosis, Management*, ed 3. Philadelphia, WB Saunders, 1983.

Thompson JC, Donovan AJ, Karl RC, Walt AJ, Mason GR, Mansberger HR Jr: Stomach and duodenum. In Sabiston DC Jr (ed): *Textbook of Surgery*. Philadelphia, WB Saunders, 1986.

Zollinger RM, Ellison EH: Primary peptic ulcerations of the jejunum associated with islet cell tumors of the pancreas. *Ann Surg* 142:709, 1955.

Skills

1. Given a patient with acute peritonitis from a perforated duodenal ulcer, demonstrate the appropriate maneuvers to demonstrate upper abdominal tenderness and rebound tenderness.

2. Demonstrate the ability to pass a nasogastric tube in a conscious patient. The demonstration should include techniques to lubricate the tube, minimize chances of laryngeal intubation, recognize laryngeal intubation should it occur, and uncoil kinks that might occur in the tube. The final demonstration should be the ability to recognize clearly the presence of the nasogastric tube within the stomach utilizing the techniques of air insufflation.

3. Demonstrate the ability to remove a nasogastric tube.

4. Demonstrate the ability to recognize the presence of a duodenal ulcer in an upper gastrointestinal roentgenogram demonstrating this disorder.

5. Demonstrate the ability to recognize a gastric ulcer in the upper gastrointestinal roentgenogram demonstrating this disorder.

6. Demonstrate the techniques of gastric lavage.

7. Demonstrate the techniques necessary to perform a gastric analysis and an understanding of data gathered from this technique.

Study Questions

1. A 45-year-old hospital administrator complains of severe upper abdominal pain that will often bore "through to his back." The pain is worse when he fasts and is relieved by eating. He is often awakened in the early morning with pain that is relieved by antacids.

   a. How would you approach the clinical evaluation of this patient? This evaluation revealed a duodenal ulcer.
   b. Discuss the pathogenesis of a duodenal ulcer.
   c. Describe the site where such an ulcer is classically found.
   d. Discuss the three phases of gastric acid secretion and state which one plays the most substantial role in patients with duodenal ulcer disease.
   e. Discuss the values that might be obtained if a gastric analysis were performed in this patient.
   f. What should the initial medical management of a patient with these symptoms include?
   g. List the four indications for surgery in a patient with duodenal ulcer disease.
   h. List at least three different operations that might be used in this patient and identify specific indications for each of the procedures listed.
   i. List the pathophysiologic changes that occur in early dumping and contrast those to the physiologic changes that occur in late dumping.
   j. Discuss the nonoperative treatment of patients with early dumping.
   k. Discuss the surgical approach to patients with the dumping syndrome.

2. A 30-year-old high school football coach has been operated upon twice for refractory duodenal ulcer disease. The first time, he had a vagotomy and pyloroplasty. Ulcers were found not only in the duodenum but in the proximal jejunum. When the patient developed recurrent ulcers within the first year, a repeat vagotomy and distal gastrectomy were done. Gastrointestinal continuity was reestablished with a Billroth II anastomosis.

   a. Discuss the difference between a Billroth II anastomosis and a Billroth I anastomosis.
   b. What tests should be performed on this patient at this time?
   c. What conditions should be included in the differential diagnosis in this patient?
   d. What single test would be the most appropriate to establish the diagnosis?

   The patient is believed to have a gastrinoma of the pancreas (Zollinger-Ellison syndrome).

   e. Discuss the sites of origin of a gastrinoma and state the incidence of malignancy.
   f. Discuss the therapeutic options.

3. A 70-year-old woman seeks medical attention because of weakness and dizziness. She reports a 20-pound weight loss and complains bitterly of early satiety. She has upper abdominal pain and rectal exam reveals guaiac positive stools.

   a. Discuss the evaluation of this patient's complaints.

   During the evaluation an ulcer in the stomach is identified.

   b. List the conditions that might be associated with an ulcer of the stomach.
   c. Discuss the pathophysiology of gastric ulcer disease.
   d. What maneuver is most important in this patient's evaluation to establish the diagnosis?
   e. Discuss the gastric secretory pattern found in patients with gastric ulcer disease and contrast this to the gastric acid secretory pattern of patients with duodenal ulcer disease.

   Biopsies of the margin of this ulcer reveal that the patient has gastric carcinoma.

   f. Discuss the appropriate therapeutic modalities that should be considered at this point (surgery, chemotherapy, and radiation therapy).

g. Compare the 5-year survival of patients with gastric carcinoma to those patients who have their stomach removed for gastric ulcer disease and in whom a small occult carcinoma is found in tissue adjacent to the ulcer.

h. Compare the therapeutic modalities used in patients with gastric carcinoma to those utilized in a patient with gastric lymphoma.

i. Compare the 5-year survival for patients with gastric lymphoma to patients with gastric carcinoma.

17

Small Intestine and Appendix

Bruce V. MacFadyen, Jr., M.D.,
Edwin C. James, M.D.,
Gordon L. Telford, M.D., and
James E. Colberg, M.D.

- Littre's hernia - a hernia c̄ a Meckel's diverticulum within it.

ASSUMPTIONS

The student knows the anatomy and embryology of the small intestine and appendix.

The student is familiar with the physiology of the small intestine, with absorption of fluids and nutrients as well as exchange of electrolytes.

The student is familiar with the pathology of small intestinal diseases.

OBJECTIVES

1. List the signs and symptoms of acute appendicitis.
2. Formulate a differential diagnosis of the conditions that commonly mimic acute appendicitis.
3. Outline the diagnostic work up in a patient with suspected appendicitis and list the laboratory findings that would tend to confirm the diagnosis of acute, nonperforated appendicitis.
4. List the common complications following a ruptured appendix and subsequent appendectomy and explain how each can be prevented and/or managed.
5. List three common situations in which acute appendicitis is difficult to diagnose or manage.
6. Describe the incidence and management of appendiceal carcinoid.
7. Discuss the embryologic relationship between umbilical hernias and Meckel's diverticulum.
8. Describe the various clinical presentations of a patient with Meckel's diverticulum.
9. Outline the work up of a child with intermittent right lower quadrant pain.
10. Discuss the treatment of a Meckel's diverticulum.
11. Discuss the relative frequency of the most common malignant and benign small bowel tumors.
12. Describe the carcinoid syndrome.
13. List the features of a carcinoid tumor that suggest it may be malignant. List those features that may cause the carcinoid syndrome.
14. Discuss the clinical presentation and diagnostic approach to the following types of tumors of the small bowel: adenocarcinoma, carcinoid, and lymphoma.
15. Discuss the role of surgery in the management of patients with small bowel tumors.
16. Describe the major etiologies, signs, and symptoms of small intestinal obstruction and contrast them with those of paralytic ileus.
17. Discuss the complications of small intestinal obstruction, including fluid and electrolyte shifts, sepsis, and vascular compromise of the small intestine.
18. Outline the appropriate laboratory tests and x-rays used in the diagnostic evaluation of a patient with suspected small intestinal obstruction.
19. Discuss the clinical manifestation of small bowel strangulation and the potential difficulty of making that diagnosis.
20. Outline a plan of treatment for a patient with small intestinal obstruction, including fluid and electrolyte therapy, intestinal intubation, resuscitation, antibiotic therapy, and indications for operative therapy
21. Describe the various clinical presentations of a patient with Crohn's disease. Differentiate the presentation of Crohn's disease and ulcerative colitis.
22. List the complications of Crohn's disease that may require surgical therapy including extraintestinal manifestations.
23. Discuss the potential nutritional problems in a patient with Crohn's disease and describe treatment methods for each.
24. Outline a diagnostic approach to a patient with Crohn's disease.

Anatomy

From the surgical perspective, the small intestine is composed of three anatomic sections: the duodenum, jejunum, and ileum. The duodenum begins at the pylorus and ends at the ligament of Treitz. The jejunum represents the first 40% of small intestine distal to the ligament of Treitz with the remaining 60% being ileum. Both jejunum and ileum are mobile, in contrast to the duodenum, which is attached to the posterior peritoneal wall beginning in the left upper abdomen and extending across the midline to the right lower abdomen. The arterial supply originates from the superior mesenteric artery, with the major branches consisting of the middle colic artery and the right colic artery. The vascular arcades to the jejunum and ileum terminate in the ileocolic artery and appendiceal artery. Venous drainage from the small intestine is into the superior mesenteric vein that forms the portal vein in conjunction with the splenic and inferior mesenteric veins. The lymphatic drainage is via numerous channels that are parallel to the superior mesenteric vein. They empty into the cisterna chyli, located in the retroperitoneum between the aorta and vena cava, and eventually drain into the thoracic duct and left subclavian vein.

The ileocecal valve is the termination of the small intestine, regulating passage of intestinal contents into the large intestine and preventing reflux of colonic contents into the small bowel. Removal of this valve increases the amount of liquid chyme entering the colon, increases colonic transport time, allows reflux of colon contents into the small intestine, and decreases absorption of bile salts and nutrients from the ileum. The appendix is located at the tip of the cecum at the junction of the three taenia coli, a landmark sometimes used by surgeons to find the appendix.

Physiology

The primary function of the small intestine is efficient absorption of ingested nutrients into the bloodstream. The alkaline intestinal fluid (succus entericus) is composed of mucus and other digestive enzymes, principally enterokinase and amylase. The volume of succus entericus increases during the first 2 hours after a meal. The process of absorption is carried out by simple diffusion and active transport, requiring the expenditure of energy. In the following sections of this chapter, several of the disease processes associated with the small intestine will be discussed, demonstrating the effect of an altered absorptive process.

Intestinal motility is regulated by both sympathetic and parasympathetic stimuli. These nerves follow the blood vessels into the mesentery via the celiac and superior mesenteric ganglia. Parasympathetic supply originates from the vagus nerve, increasing the tone and enhancing motility of the small intestine. Sympathetic nerves have the opposite effect. When both types of autonomic nerves are divided, motility is maintained by intrinsic nerve conduction responding to changes in intraluminal pressure.

Diseases of the Appendix

Acute Appendicitis

Significance and Incidence. Acute appendicitis is the most common cause of the acute surgical abdomen, occurring in the lifetime of approximately 6% of the population. Eighty per cent of the patients are between 5 and 35 years of age. The presentation of the disease in young children and the elderly is frequently atypical, often resulting in a delay in diagnosis and consequently a higher incidence of perforation.

Anatomy. The appendix is usually 9–10 cm long, but reaches 20 cm in some patients. The location is at the base of the cecum on the inferomedial aspect. The tip may be located in any number of positions: retrocecal or retrocolic, pelvic, inferior to the cecum, and superior and anterior to the ileum. The location frequently determines the presentation of the patient. How would a patient with a retrocecal appendix present differently from a patient with an anterior appendix? The appendix is primarily a lymphoid organ with up to 200 follicles throughout its length. The peak number occurs in adolescents and diminishes with age. There is no known adverse effect of appendectomy despite past efforts to demonstrate an association with carcinoma of the colon.

Pathogenesis. The pathophysiology of appendicitis begins with obstruction of the narrow lumen by lymphoid hyperplasia, fecal material, or foreign body. In younger patients lymphoid hyperplasia due to acute viral and bacterial illnesses is the most common cause of obstruction. In older patients, obstruction by fecal material, fecalith, and foreign bodies is more frequently seen. Following luminal obstruction, continued secretion of mucus occurs, producing distention of the distal lumen, ischemia of the appendiceal wall, bacterial proliferation, patchy necrosis, and eventually gangrene with perforation. With distention of the appendix, the visceral peritoneum is stretched and produces an ill-defined and poorly localized pain in the periumbilical region. When there is inflammation of the parietal peritoneum, the pain becomes somatic and localized at the site of parietal peritoneal irritation.

The typical history in acute appendicitis follows the pathophysiologic progression from luminal obstruction and distention to spread of the inflammatory process beyond the appendix. This process causes localized peritonitis progressing to an inflammatory mass or abscess. If the inflammatory process is not controlled or localized, it can spread through the portal system (pylephlebitis), and eventually into the liver and upper abdominal structures. Diffuse peritonitis, general sepsis, and death may occur. As many as 10,000 deaths each year in the United States are attributed to diseases of the appendix, although appendicitis is a much rarer cause of significant morbidity and mortality than it was prior to the development of antibiotics.

Clinical Presentation. The usual progression of signs and symptoms is:

1. Pain in the upper abdomen or periumbilical region;
2. Anorexia, nausea, and/or vomiting;
3. Right lower quadrant pain;
4. Fever; (if ↑↑fever → suspect perforation)
5. Leukocytosis.

Initially the pain is ill-defined, often waking the patient from sleep in the early morning. Nausea with or without vomiting follows the onset of pain. The pain shifts as inflammation spreads beyond the confines of the appendix and involves the parietal peritoneum, typically in the right lower quadrant of the abdomen. Variations of this presentation occur because of the different locations of the distal appendix and its association with other abdominal organs.

Characteristically, the patient with appendicitis prefers not to move and will often have the right knee drawn up to the chest to relieve pressure in the right lower quadrant. Fever is a relatively late sign and tends to be only mildly elevated (37.7–38.3°C). Higher fever increases the suspicion of perforation or some other disease process. The diagnosis is suspected when there are signs of peritoneal inflammation in the right lower abdominal quadrant with direct and rebound tenderness on palpation of the abdomen. Pain may also be elicited by rectal or pelvic examination. Bowel sounds are diminished. A positive psoas sign (pain on extension of the right hip) may be present when the inflamed appendix is retrocolic and adjacent to the iliopsoas muscle. A positive obturator sign (pain on passive internal rotation of the flexed right hip) is observed if the inflammation is adjacent to the obturator internus muscle. All of these signs may be absent when the appendix is anteriorly located or wrapped in an inflammatory mass (phlegmon) of omentum and/or intestine. With progression of the disease past 18 hours, the incidence of perforation and the complications of sepsis and wound infection increase significantly. Occasionally, the inflammation may resolve spontaneously by relief of the obstructive process with discharge of the appendiceal contents into the cecum, before necrosis of the appendiceal wall occurs.

In pregnancy, appendicitis is the most common nonobstetrical acute surgical problem involving the abdomen. With the increased size of the uterus, the appendix is displaced into the right upper quadrant of the abdomen or into the right flank. The normal leukocytosis of pregnancy can be confusing but is rarely greater than 16,000. Diagnosis of acute appendicitis in the pregnant woman must be made early to reduce the incidence of perforation since generalized peritonitis results in fetal loss in 35% of patients.

Diagnosis. Diagnosis is made by history and physical examination and must be considered in any case of abdominal pain, especially in the lower abdomen. To avoid the progression to perforation and possible sepsis, early operative intervention is essential. A 20% rate of negative surgical explorations is acceptable to avoid the risk of perforation; for women of childbearing years this rate approaches 35%. Other gynecologic conditions, such as pelvic inflammatory disease, ruptured ovarian follicle, twisted ovarian cyst, and tubal pregnancy, often require surgical exploration for confirmation; delaying the operation for appendicitis results in an unacceptably high morbidity and mortality.

Other diseases in the differential diagnosis include inflammation of a Meckel's diverticulum, acute ileitis, or other inflammatory bowel diseases, obstructing tumors of the descending colon, sigmoid or cecal diverticulitis, acute cholecystitis, a perforated gastric or duodenal ulcer, early small bowel obstruction, volvulus, and intussusception. Many of these problems also require surgical intervention and should be treated if acute appendicitis is not found. However, it is critical that appendicitis be differentiated from nonoperative conditions such as acute gastroenteritis, mesenteric adenitis, right lower lobe pneumonia, acute hepatitis, acute pyelonephritis, ureteral stones, and cystitis.

Although the diagnosis of acute appendicitis is primarily made on clinical grounds, laboratory and radiologic studies may be confirmatory and help differentiate appendicitis from other problems when the clinical picture is not clear-cut. The white cell count may be normal or only mildly elevated with a slight shift to polymorphonuclear leukocytes and band forms. White cell counts greater than 15,000 raise the concern of perforation or other inflammatory diseases. Urinalysis may demonstrate a few red or white blood cells, but a large number indicates a possible urinary tract etiology rather than appendicitis.

In acute appendicitis prompt treatment is more important than diagnostic certainty, but, when the clinical presentation is confusing, radiologic studies are helpful in differentiating appendicitis from other conditions mentioned above, all of which have their own radiologic findings. Initial studies can be quickly done and should include PA and lateral chest radiographs if right lower lobe pneumonia is suspected, or if a baseline chest radiograph is needed in older patients likely to have postoperative cardiopulmonary problems. At the same time plain and upright or left lateral decubitus (left side down with horizontal beam) abdomen films should be obtained. Plain films are positive although nonspecific in about 65% of cases of appendicitis and in 90% of those with appendiceal perforation. In the clinical setting of acute appendicitis, the finding of an oval calcified appendicolith is pathognomonic, as is a distended gasfilled appendix with a fluid level in it. Supporting signs include localized gas or fluid levels in the cecum and/or terminal ileum, scoliosis from right psoas muscle spasm, and obliteration of the (normally lucent) right properitoneal fat line. If the clinical picture still leaves doubt as to whether surgery is indicated, ultrasound (US) or computed tomography (CT) can be used to show the extent and location of inflammatory disease beyond the appendix and are helpful in surgical planning. Barium enema may show nonfilling of the appendix and mass effect at the base of the cecum, and may be particularly useful in young children.

Treatment. The treatment of acute appendicitis is prompt surgical removal of the inflamed appendix. The treatment of an appendiceal abscess is operative drainage of the abscess with removal of the appendix when feasible. Prior to surgery, initial therapy includes intravenous fluids to correct dehydration and electrolyte imbalances. A nasogastric tube may be necessary to empty the stomach. The preoperative use of antibiotics to decrease wound infection is generally recommended and is continued postoperatively, particularly in cases where the inflammatory process extends beyond the appendix and therefore is not removed. Because early appendicitis is predominantly caused by aerobic bacterial infection, first and second generation cephalosporins may be used. In appendicitis with perforation, antibiotics should be added to provide coverage against anaerobic organisms. When the diagnosis is made and preoperative preparation completed, the patient is taken to the operating room for exploration. Further delay only increases the chance of perforation.

The surgical incision is in the right lower quadrant, crossing McBurney's point (located 1.5–2 inches from the anterior superior iliac spine on a line drawn from the spine to the umbilicus). When perforation is present, the incision should be placed directly over the mass to prevent spillage of purulent material into the peritoneal cavity. When an inflamed appendix is found, the surgical procedure consists of clamping the blood supply to the appendix and amputating the appendix at its junction with the cecum. If the appendix is not inflamed, a search through the abdomen is made for other surgical pathology. The appendix is usually removed, particularly if no other pathology is found. If an abscess is found and a drain is used, it is usually brought through the abdominal wall by a separate stab wound. When possible, in perforation with an abscess, the appendix is removed, since the incidence of recurrent appendicitis in a retained appendix is approximately 20% within 2 months and as high as 50% over the next 5 years.

The mortality following appendectomy for acute appendicitis is less than 0.5% but increases to 15% in the elderly. This is primarily related to uncontrolled sepsis, associated cardiopulmonary complications, and intercurrent diseases. Overall, the incidence of complications in appendicitis is 10–15%, increasing to 25–40% when perforation is present. The most common complication of appendectomy for acute appendicitis is wound infection, ranging from 8% in the uncomplicated case to 17% or higher in cases of perforation. In most clinical series, perioperative antibiotics reduce the rate of wound infection significantly. Minor complications include atelectasis, prolonged ileus, and urinary tract infections. The serious complications that prolong the hospital stay of the patient include uncontrolled sepsis, bleeding, pulmonary embolus, myocardial in-

farction, intestinal fistula, bowel obstruction, hernia, and abscess formation. Two of the most severe complications are spread of infection along the right lateral gutter to form a subphrenic abscess and through the portal venous system into the liver with pylephlebitis and intrahepatic abscess formation. Uncontrolled sepsis is more likely to occur in the diabetic or debilitated patient who has coexisting medical problems. Pelvic abscesses can occur after a perforated appendix and may be first detected by persistent fever, ileus, leukocytosis, and the presence of a palpable mass on rectal examination.

Radionuclide (RN) scans (gallium 67- or indium 111-labeled white blood cells), ultrasonography (US), and computed tomography (CT) are all effective in localizing abdominal abscesses. Sensitivity increases from 60% to 90% when two of the three are used in combination. RN scans are most useful when the patient is not acutely ill (since they require 6–24 hours) or when the patient has no localizing signs. If the patient has localizing signs, it is advisable to begin with US or CT. If the patient is gas distended, obese, has multiple surgical drains, or if retroperitoneal disease is suspected, then diagnosis should begin with CT. Otherwise, US is cheaper and spares radiation. Following detection, radiologically guided fine needle aspiration and percutaneous drainage are both over 90% effective for definitive diagnosis and treatment. Response can be followed clinically and by US, CT, or fistulography (contrast agent visualization of the tract and cavity). Additional drainage may be implemented if needed. If the abscess is located in the pelvis, the abscess can be drained through the rectum or through the vagina in a female.

To reduce the risk of infectious complications, prompt recognition and surgical intervention is necessary when appendicitis is suspected, even though a false positive diagnosis rate of 20% may be the trade-off.

Tumors of the Appendix. The most common tumor of the appendix is a carcinoid tumor, found in 0.5% of all appendices removed. This constitutes approximately one-half of all carcinoids in the gastrointestinal tract. Only 3% of carcinoids are malignant. Patients with carcinoid may be asymptomatic or have signs and symptoms of acute appendicitis. The treatment of choice is an appendectomy when the lesion is less than 2 cm in diameter, has not extended beyond the serosa, and can be removed by appendectomy alone. If the tumor is greater than 2 cm, the incidence of malignancy is higher, and a right hemicolectomy is indicated.

Other tumors of the appendix include adenocarcinoma and malignant mucoid adenocarcinoma, comprising only 0.08% of appendiceal diseases. The treatment of choice in these unusual conditions is a radical right hemicolectomy. A mucocele of the appendix may occur, secondary to luminal obstruction and distention of the appendix with mucus. If it ruptures spontaneously or at the time of removal, pseudomyxoma peritonei may result. Although these appendiceal tumors are rare, aggressive surgical extirpation is indicated.

Meckel's Diverticulum

Significance and Incidence

A Meckel's diverticulum is a remnant of the embryonic vitelline or omphalomesenteric duct and the most common congenital anomaly of the small intestine. Its incidence in the general population is 1–3% with a male/female preponderance of two or three to one in symptomatic patients. Arising from the antimesenteric border of the distal ileum, more than 90% occur within 1 m of the ileocecal valve. Most often, a Meckel's diverticulum is noted as an incidental finding at exploratory celiotomy. Controversy surrounds its management, particularly whether or not resection in asymptomatic patients is indicated. Although it is frequently taught that 25% of patients with a Meckel's diverticulum develop complications, Soltero and Bill suggest the rate is much lower, i.e., 4.2% in infants, 1.5% at age 40, and 0% at the age of 75 years.

Clinical Presentation

In addition to the risk of intussusception, particularly in children, 20–30% of Meckel's diverticula cause problems from the heterotopic gastric, duodenal, pancreatic, or colonic tissue contained within the diverticulum. Diverticulitis, hemorrhage, and perforation may result from acid-producing gastric tissue in the diverticulum, causing peptic ulceration and inflammation in the adjacent normal ileal mucosa. Other common complications include: patent omphalomesenteric duct (congenital umbilical fistula), iron deficiency anemia, malabsorption, neoplastic involvement, impacted foreign bodies with perforation, cutaneous fistulas, and incarceration or strangulation in hernias. A Littre's hernia is a hernia with a Meckel's diverticulum within it; 50% are inguinal, 20% femoral, and 20% umbilical, while the remainder occur in miscellaneous locations.

Diagnosis

The clinical diagnosis is made by a combination of typical symptoms, a high index of suspicion, and carefully selected diagnostic testing. Sudden profuse, painless hemorrhage due to peptic ulceration in a child is a classic but uncommon presentation. In patients with right lower quadrant abdominal pain, the differential diagnosis includes appendicitis, regional enteritis, intussusception, and incarcerated hernia. Volvulus or complications due to Meckel's bands (Fig. 17.1) usually show symptoms and signs of intestinal obstruction, whereas patients with incarcerated Meckel's diverticulum frequently fail to exhibit fever, pain, abdominal distention, or obstipation unless the lumen of the ileum is compromised (Fig. 17.2). However, if the Meckel's diverticulum is incarcerated in a hernia in a palpable location, there may be a tender, nonreducible mass.

If the patient presents with lower gastrointestinal (GI) bleeding, the choice and sequence of radiologic tests depends on the acuteness of bleeding. Patients with massive bleeding and unstable vital signs generally require immediate surgical exploration. A site of active bleeding at 0.5 ml/min or more can be shown by angiography and often stopped by selective infusion of vasopressin into the bleeding artery. RN scans using ^{99m}Tc sulfur colloid can show sites bleeding as slowly as 0.1 ml/min. With ^{99m}Tc-labeled red cells or albumen and repeated scans over a 24-hour period, even intermittently bleeding sites can be found. Even if bleeding has stopped, the ectopic gastric mucosa in the diverticulum responsible for the bleeding can still be demonstrated because it, like the stomach, excretes ^{99m}Tc

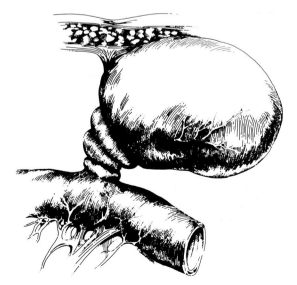

Figure 17.1. Volvulus of intestine around an omphalodiverticular band.

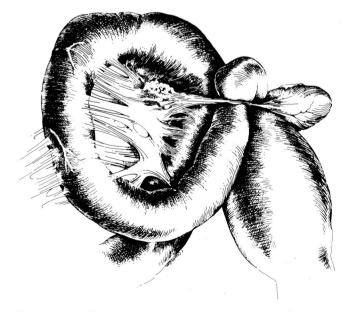

Figure 17.2. Obstruction due to a mesodiverticular band.

pertechnetate. ^{99m}Tc pertechnetate scans are reported to be about 90% accurate in the detection of bleeding Meckel's diverticula.

If the patient presents with acute abdominal pain, radiologic testing begins with plain and upright or lateral decubitus abdomen films and progresses through the same sequences as for suspected appendicitis. In chronic abdominal pain or bleeding, barium studies of the GI tract, including double-contrast barium enema and upper GI series with small bowel follow-up, are indicated. When they are negative and small bowel disease is still strongly suspected, the next radiologic test is enteroclysis (antegrade small bowel enema done by passing a tube through the nose past the stomach and by rapid injection of barium, achieving uniform demonstration of the small bowel). Normal Meckel's diverticula are seldom distinguishable from surrounding small bowel loops, but detection of those causing disease is somewhat more likely.

The treatment of a Meckel's diverticulum is usually simple diverticulectomy. For broad-based diverticula or complications, such as inflammation and perforation, removal of the diverticulum by formal small bowel resection is advocated. For the asymptomatic or incidental Meckel's diverticulum, suggested indications for resection are:

1. Diverticulum 2 inches or greater in length;
2. Age less than 40 years;
3. The detection of palpable heterotopic tissue;
4. The presence of apparent inflammation or irritation;
5. Attached mesodiverticular or omphalodiverticular bands.

Diseases of the Small Bowel

Any histological element of the small bowel is capable of neoplastic transformation, attested to by the wide spectrum of benign and malignant neoplasms found in the intestine. However, in terms of frequency, colon and rectal neoplasms occur 40–60 times more often than small bowel neoplasms. The average age at diagnosis is approximately 60 years with an equal sex distribution. Some studies suggest a male preponderance of 2–3:1 with malignant neoplasms.

Benign Neoplasms

The leiomyoma is the most common benign tumor of the small bowel. Other benign neoplasms include fibroma, lipoma, angioma, hamartoma, lymphangioma, and a variety of adenomas and tumors of neurogenic origin. The majority of gastrointestinal lipomas are found in the small bowel (ileum more frequently than jejunum). Although many benign neoplasms exhibit no symptoms or signs, 50% eventually become symptomatic. Large intraluminal neoplasms may cause intussusception with small bowel obstruction (frequently seen with leiomyomas). Extraluminal leiomyomas may cause small bowel volvulus as a primary clinical presentation. The most frequent tumors to cause bleeding are adenomas, leiomyomas, and hemangiomas.

Malignant Neoplasms

The most common malignant neoplasms of the small bowel are [1]adenocarcinomas, [2]carcinoids, [3]lymphomas, and [4]leiomyosarcomas, usually in that order of occurrence. The most common symptoms are pain, weight loss, and anemia, with other less common symptoms and signs being nausea, emesis, obstruction, bleeding, and the presence of an abdominal mass. Duodenal lesions may also cause ampullary obstruction and jaundice. Pain in the midback region may indicate invasion of the small bowel mesentery and weight loss. Weight loss is particularly common with lymphomas. Approximately 10% of small bowel neoplasms, usually lymphomas or sarcoma, will perforate and produce a localized peritonitis. Massive hemorrhage is rare with adenocarcinomas yet is the most common presenting symptom in leiomyosarcoma.

Adenocarcinomas. Adenocarcinomas of the small intestine constitute only 1% of all GI tract malignancies. However, they represent the most common primary malignancy of the small bowel. Most occur in the duodenum, followed by the jejunum, and then the ileum. Some reports suggest an equal incidence in all three locations. Associated malignancies, both synchronous and metachronous, occur in 25% of patients. Adenocarcinoma often causes intermittent or partial small bowel obstruction due to the slow, constricting encroachment on the intestinal lumen. If bleeding is present, it is frequently insidious and results from direct ulceration of the intestinal mucosa. The diagnosis is difficult in many patients but is aided by testing of the stool for occult blood, fiberoptic endoscopy of the duodenum, and conventional barium-contrast roentgenograms of the duodenum and small bowel. Fifty per cent of patients have a diagnosis made at the time of exploratory celiotomy. Enteroclysis is a useful radiographic diagnostic technique and the wider use of enteroclysis in strongly suspected small bowel disease can be expected to improve this figure.

Surgical treatment includes wide local excision of the involved segment of bowel and mesenteric lymph nodes, preserving the superior mesenteric vessels. Despite an aggressive surgical approach to these lesions, the 5-year survival rate for these patients is 20–30%. The poor survival rate is due to the late clinical presentation of these tumors as well as the difficulty in diagnosis.

Carcinoid Tumors. Carcinoids originate from the APUD (amine, precursor uptake, and decarboxylation) line of cells of neuroectodermal origin. They are found predominantly in the brain and gastrointestinal tract, although these cells have been found in other tissues

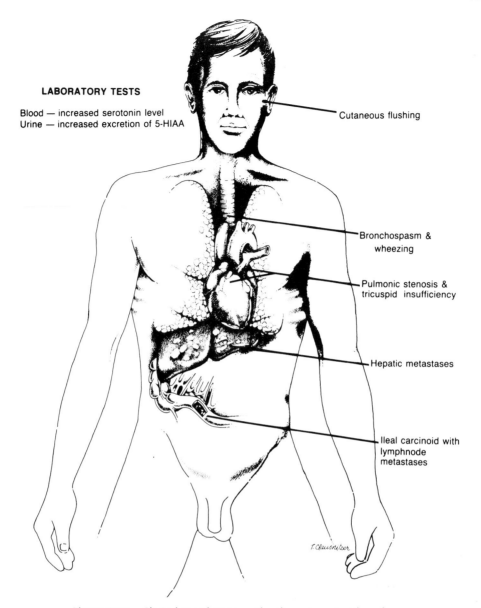

LABORATORY TESTS

Blood — increased serotonin level
Urine — increased excretion of 5-HIAA

Cutaneous flushing

Bronchospasm &
wheezing

Pulmonic stenosis &
tricuspid insufficiency

Hepatic metastases

Ileal carcinoid with
lymphnode
metastases

Figure 17.3. Clinical manifestations of malignant carcinoid syndrome.

as well. They are considered malignant because of the potential to develop metastasis when the tumors are large. Tumors less than 1.0 cm in diameter metastasize with a frequency of approximately 2.0%, compared to a 90% incidence of metastasis when the tumor is larger than 2.0 cm.

Forty to fifty per cent of carcinoids in the gastrointestinal tract occur in the appendix. The second most common location is in the small bowel, where carcinoids occur eight times more frequently in the ileum than in the jejunum. Multicentricity is common, with multiple carcinoids documented in 20–30% of the patients. Although only 3% of carcinoids are malignant, 30% of patients will have another malignancy (histologically different) in the gastrointestinal tract.

The carcinoid syndrome (Fig. 17.3) is most frequently associated with ileal tumors. These tend to metastasize to regional mesenteric lymph nodes and then to the liver through the portal venous system. Clinical mani-

festations include (Fig. 17.3) episodic attacks of cutaneous flushing, hyperperistalsis, bronchospasm and wheezing, pellagra-like skin lesions, vasomotor instability, and valvular heart disease (pulmonic stenosis and tricuspid insufficiency). Chronic watery diarrhea occurs in 85% of patients with cutaneous flushing episodes that are especially prominent over the head and upper trunk. Attacks may occur spontaneously or be stimulated by excitement, physical activity, ingestion of alcohol or foods, or from pressure on the tumor.

Carcinoid tumors cause increased metabolism of dietary tryptophan to 5-hydroxytryptamine (serotonin), a potent neurotransmitter. This peptide is degraded primarily in the liver to 5-hydroxyindole acetic acid (5-HIAA). Other peptides synthesized in this process include 5-hydroxytryptophan, kallikrein, histamine, and adrenocorticotrophic hormone. Serotonin is thought to be the major cause of the diarrheal component of this syndrome. Tumors that drain into the systemic venous circulation (bronchial, ovarian, and testicular) can produce the malignant carcinoid syndrome without liver metastases, as degradation in the liver is bypassed. Carcinoid syndrome has also been reported in the absence of hepatic metastasis. Carcinoid tumors are frequently found at celiotomy for other surgical conditions. Elevated blood serotonin and 5-HIAA urine levels are diagnostic of functioning tumors, although false positive and false negative values are not infrequent with the qualitative 5-HIAA urine test. A more accurate assessment involves the quantitative 5-HIAA urinary determination (normal = 2–10 mg/24 hr, malignant carcinoid syndrome greater than 40 mg/24 hr).

The treatment for carcinoid tumors is surgical resection. When the carcinoid is located in the appendix, appendectomy is adequate when the tumor is less than 2 cm in diameter. For carcinoid tumor in the small intestine, standard resection procedure includes removal of the primary tumor plus metastases in the lymph nodes and liver when technically possible.

The medical therapy of carcinoid syndrome consists of opiates, methylsergide, cyproheptadine, *p*-chorophenylalanine, and somatostatin infusions. They may afford temporary relief for uncontrollable diarrhea. Chemotherapy with doxorubicin, BCNU, methotrexate, 5-fluorouracil, cyclophosphamide, and streptozotocin, alone or in combinations, has been used with varying degrees of success, although the treatment is not specific or predictable.

The overall survival at 5 years following resection of carcinoid tumors of the small bowel is approximately 60%. Ten-year survival falls to 40%. The majority of early deaths following resection occur within the first 3 years following diagnosis. As expected, the presence of hepatic metastases reduces survival to 35% and 15% at 5 and 10 years, respectively. This compares to 72% and 60% for patients without hepatic involvement. Surprisingly, neither the presence of multiple carcinoid tumors nor the size of the primary tumor has any effect upon survival. Patients whose tumors are resected "for cure" have survivals of 76% at 5 years, 60% at 10 years, and 40% at 20 years. Tumors not resected for cure are associated with survival rates similar to those patients with hepatic metastases.

Lymphoma. Lymphomas of the small bowel are rare, comprising 1–3% of all tumors involving the gastrointestinal tract. Although more lymphomas occur in adults, they are the most common small bowel malignancy in children. The majority occur in the ileum, producing symptoms and signs of anorexia and weight loss. An abdominal mass or chronic obstruction may be the only presenting complaints. Histiocytic, lymphocytic, mixed histiocytic-lymphocytic, and Hodgkin's variants are all found. In most patients, involvement of the small bowel is usually part of a systemic disease process.

A small number of patients with long-term malabsorption due to adult celiac sprue will develop intestinal lymphomas. Another variant, the Mediterranean lymphoma, despite its name, occurs worldwide. The most common clinical feature is dysproteinemia and the disease is frequently fatal. Patients with this disease have abnormal alpha heavy chain fragments of immunoglobulin (IgA) in the serum, urine, and intestinal fluid.

The recommended treatment for primary small bowel lymphomas is wide surgical excision of the involved bowel and mesenteric lymph nodes, followed by postoperative irradiation and chemotherapy in selected cases. When resections are performed for cure, the 5-year survival is in the range of 40%.

Small Intestinal Obstruction

Etiology

The most common surgical condition of the small intestine is obstruction. Adhesions, usually the result of previous surgical procedures, are the leading cause of small intestinal obstruction, accounting for greater than 60% of hospital admissions for obstruction. Adhesions produce the obstruction by kinking or angulating the intestine and by compression of the lumen by fibrous adhesive bands. Hernias, both external and internal, are the next most frequently reported cause of obstruction (20%) in patients who have not had previous surgical procedures. Obstruction occurs in external hernias when a loop of small intestine becomes incarcerated in the hernia sac. This can occur at any hernia site and requires surgical reduction of the incarcerated hernia with repair of the abdominal defect before strangulation of the entrapped intestine occurs. Internal hernias occur either as the result of congenital abnormalities or surgically created mesenteric defects. As in external hernias, intestine can become incarcerated in the defect and cause obstruction. Neoplasms, either primary small intestinal tumors or metastatic tumors, are the third most common cause of intestinal obstruction (15%). The remainder of the obstructions (1–5%) are caused by regional enteritis, small intestinal volvulus, gall-stone ileus, and intussusception.

General Considerations

Various complications occur in patients with small intestinal obstruction; the most frequently observed problems are fluid and electrolyte imbalance along with dehydration. Potentially life-threatening dehydration results from the loss of large amounts of isotonic fluid into the small intestinal lumen. Edema of the bowel wall, transudation of fluids into the abdominal cavity, and vomiting also contribute to the acute volume loss. Initially, the accumulation of fluid within the bowel lumen is the result of decreased absorption. With time, there is a gradual increase in secretion in response to the inflammatory process. Six to eight liters of fluid can be sequestered in the bowel lumen and wall of patients with a mechanical small bowel obstruction. Progressive distention causes venous congestion of the bowel wall resulting in edema. In later stages, transudation of fluid into the abdominal cavity also occurs. Decompensation of the bowel function proximal to the obstruction prevents the absorption of secreted fluids. The patient will begin to vomit isotonic, acidic gastric contents and, if allowed to progress, marked dehydration with hypochloremic, hypokalemic metabolic alkalosis, and shock may result. The vomiting is classically described as "feculent," though not to imply colonic content but referring to the foul odor of stagnant small bowel fluid produced by the large numbers of bacteria.

Obstruction with strangulation (death of the bowel wall) occurs when the arterial blood supply to a segment of obstructed intestine becomes compromised. Along with perforation of the obstructed intestine, this is the most serious complication of intestinal obstruction. It occurs most frequently when a loop of intestine is trapped in an internal or external hernia, when an adhesive band occludes the bowel lumen at two points, and with volvulus of the intervening intestinal loop. Such obstructions at two locations separated by a normal interval are termed closed loop obstructions. As in uncomplicated obstructions, the bowel lumen of the closed loop becomes distended, and venous congestion and edema of the bowel wall ensues. However, in closed loop obstructions, the obstructed bowel is entrapped and can not decompress itself by shifting fluid into segments of the intestine proximal to the obstruction. Edema eventually compromises the arterial blood supply, leading to necrosis and gangrene at a much faster rate.

Sepsis is usually seen with perforation, peritonitis, or closed loop obstruction. It can occur in an uncomplicated obstruction if left untreated for more than 24 hours due to bacterial overgrowth in the obstructed segment and bacteremia. The signs and symptoms of progressive sepsis are hypotension, tachycardia, leukocytosis, fever, metabolic acidosis, and mental changes. Unfortunately, clinical signs and symptoms and laboratory tests frequently do not point to strangulation or sepsis until the process is far advanced.

Diagnosis

Symptoms of small intestinal obstruction are intermittent crampy abdominal pain (colic), abdominal distention, nausea, vomiting, obstipation, and failure to pass flatus. When the obstruction is partial, the patient may have the same symptoms but continue to pass flatus. The pain classically occurs in paroxysms several minutes apart early in the course of the obstruction. This is thought to be due to the muscular efforts of the bowel wall to overcome the obstruction, causing a tremendous increase in intraluminal pressure. Later in the course of the disease, the crampy pain may abate, due to progressive distention of the bowel wall and muscular fatigue. Persistent, severe abdominal pain that follows the symptoms described above should lead one to suspect strangulation or perforation with generalized peritonitis. Vomiting may ameliorate the abdominal symptoms temporarily by removing the intraluminal contents and reducing the distention.

The classic physical signs found in uncomplicated small bowel obstruction include abdominal distention, tenderness to palpation, involuntary guarding, and hyperactive bowel sounds with rushes. The bowel sounds may be high pitched and may have an almost tinkling or musical quality. Very early in the process, however, bowel sounds may be normal. Rebound tenderness may not be evident until peritoneal irritation is present secondary to the transudation of fluid from the bowel wall.

Abdominal x-rays are important in confirming the diagnosis of obstruction and in distinguishing large from small bowel, partial from complete, mechanical from paralytic, and simple from strangulated obstruction. Because the diagnosis of suspected bowel obstruction depends mainly on recognizing the distribution of gas and fluid in the bowel, the clinician should begin (before injecting air or fluid through enemas or endoscopy) with plain abdominal radiographs that include a supine abdomen film positioned to include the symphysis pubis, an erect abdomen (which includes the diaphragm), or a left lateral decubitus film if the patient cannot be put upright. At the same time PA and lateral chest x-rays should be obtained to look for free air under the diaphragm if a perforated viscus is suspected. Additional films can be helpful, including right decubitus and prone views to position gas in the descending colon and rectum, and serial films made 10 or more minutes apart to help distinguish fixed from changing gas patterns. In 6% of obstructions the abdomen is gasless; the ultrasound can be used to show the dilated fluid-filled intestine.

If more certainty is still needed, a single-contrast barium enema without bowel preparation can be done to rule out large bowel obstruction and to show the distal small bowel by reflux through the ileocecal valve. Proximal small bowel obstruction can be defined by barium given perorally or through a nasogastric or intestinal decompression tube. There is little or no basis to the traditional beliefs that barium must not be given above an obstruction because it will inspissate and that water-soluble contrast agent is safer. Water-soluble contrast agent instead of barium is only indicated when perforation is suspected. It is hypertonic, draws fluid into the gut, and consequently worsens both the patient's electrolyte balance and his bowel distention. It

Table 17.1.
Characteristics of Paralytic Ileus and Small Intestinal Obstruction

Paralytic Ileus	Small Intestinal Obstruction
1. Minimal abdominal pain	1. Crampy abdominal pain
2. Nausea and vomiting	2. Nausea and vomiting
3. Obstipation and failure to pass flatus	3. Obstipation and failure to pass flatus
4. Abdominal distention	4. Abdominal distention
5. Decreased or absent bowel sounds	5. Normal or increased bowel sounds
6. Gas in the small intestine and colon on x-ray	6. Gas in the small intestine only on x-ray

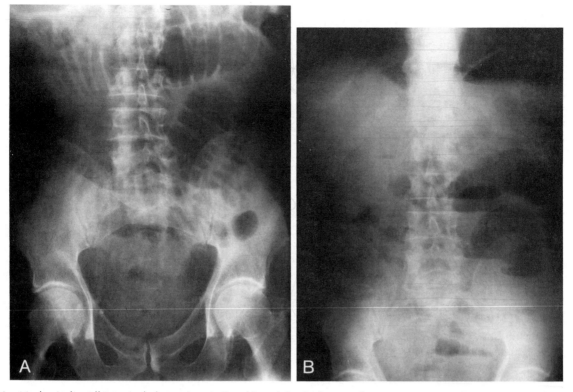

Figure 17.4. Mechanical small intestinal obstruction. **A,** Decubitus abdominal x-ray. There are many, centrally located loops of air-filled small intestine and no gas on the periphery of the abdomen. Valvulae conniventes are clearly depicted. **B,** Upright abdominal x-ray. Multiple air-filled levels are seen.

becomes so dilute that its visibility is inadequate. Furthermore, it is very expensive in the quantities used. It may save time because of its rapid intestinal transit when given perorally; it is also effective as an enema to relieve fecal impaction.

Radiographic interpretation depends on recognizing dilated bowel above and collapsed bowel below an obstruction. Small bowel occupies the center of the abdomen and has mucosal folds (valvulae conniventes) that are smooth, uniform, closely spaced, and cross precisely from one side of the bowel to the other without indenting the wall. The large bowel occupies the periphery of the abdomen and has haustrations that are widely spaced, do not cross the bowel wall, and do indent the bowel margin. The colon is also recognizable when it contains speckled-appearing fecal material mixed with air. Clinical correlation with the duration of illness and serial films are often necessary, because many times plain abdomen films are indeterminate. In intermittent, partial, and early obstruction, the intestine may not show the chararcteristic size discrepancy above and below an obstruction. Finally, plain films should always be used to search for complications, such as perforation with free peritoneal air appearing on upright films; strangulated bowel that is fixed in position, narrowed, rigid, thickened, or has swollen nodular mucosa or crescents of gas in the bowel wall; closed loop obstruction that is immovable and disproportionately distended; inguinal hernia showing gas overlying the pubic rami; gas in the biliary ducts; calculi; or active pulmonary diseases.

Laboratory tests do not help in distinguishing small bowel obstruction from other diagnoses, nor are they helpful in distinguishing uncomplicated obstruction from strangulation. It is essential, however, that determinations of serum electrolytes, blood urea nitrogen (BUN), creatinine, urinalysis, white blood cell count, hemoglobin, and hematocrit be performed. In the early stages of obstruction, all of these tests are usually normal unless there is preexisting disease. With prolonged obstruction and/or continued vomiting, the patient will develop dehydration with a hypochloremic, hypokalemic metabolic alkalosis, elevated BUN and creatinine, and a high urinary specific gravity. The hemoglobin and hematocrit will be elevated secondary to hemoconcentration. The white blood cell count will usually be normal or only slightly elevated. A marked leukocytosis may occur in uncomplicated obstruction as well as in strangulation and is not a distinguishing factor in making the diagnosis of strangulation.

Differential Diagnosis

Differentiation between mechanical small bowel obstruction and paralytic ileus is extremely important. Characteristics of both are listed in Table 17.1. In most cases of paralytic ileus, the cause will be acute pancreatitis, appendicitis, cholecystitis, gastroenteritis, etc. When the cause is not apparent, it may be clinically

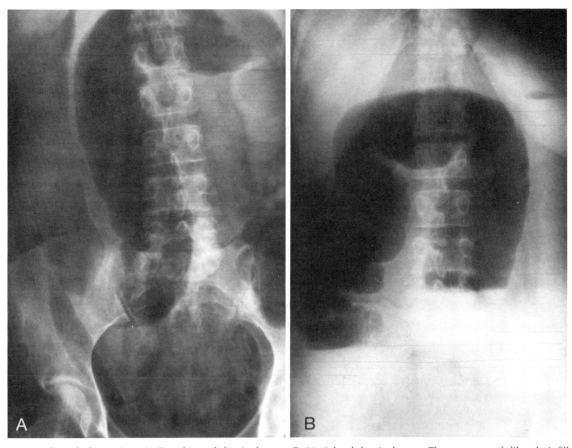

Figure 17.5. Large bowel obstruction. **A,** Decubitus abdominal x-ray. **B,** Upright abdominal x-ray. The presence of dilated air-filled loops of colon on the periphery of the abdomen and centrally located air-filled loops of small intestine with no rectal gas suggests that this patient has a sigmoid obstruction. The patient has carcinoma of the colon.

difficult to differentiate obstruction from paralytic ileus, since both conditions produce the same symptoms and signs. Patients with paralytic ileus frequently have more continuous abdominal pain and have minimal or absent bowel sounds, in contrast to obstructed patients who demonstrate colicky pain and hyperactive bowel sounds. Upright or decubitus abdominal x-rays are the best method to distinguish ileus from intestinal obstruction (Figs. 17.4 and 17.5). In paralytic ileus, large quantities of gas are seen in both the large and small intestine. In small bowel obstruction, air fluid levels are seen mainly in the small bowel. Laboratory tests do not serve to distinguish between diagnoses, since laboratory values can be normal in both. When abnormal in paralytic ileus, they are due to the primary disease causing the ileus.

A major risk in observing patients with a small bowel obstruction is the development of strangulation. The most important factor in strangulated obstruction is the paucity of specific signs and symptoms caused by strangulation. Therefore, patients with complete small bowel obstruction should have an exploratory celiotomy as soon as they have been physiologically stabilized; the physician should not wait for the exact diagnosis. The classic signs of strangulated obstruction are tachycardia, fever, presence of a mass, hypoperis-

talsis, rigidity, and abdominal tenderness. An elevated white blood count is usually seen, although it is not diagnostic of strangulation. Abdominal x-rays do not differentiate strangulation from uncomplicated obstruction since a similar picture is present in both entities.

The signs and symptoms of colonic obstruction are similar to small intestinal obstruction. Because the colon continues to absorb fluids and electrolytes in early uncomplicated colonic obstruction, nausea and vomiting are not often a part of the symptom complex in acute to subacute uncomplicated colonic obstruction. However, with prolonged obstruction, the ileocecal valve may become incompetent and reflux of colonic contents into the ileum can produce signs and symptoms similar to small intestinal obstruction.

As in paralytic ileus, abdominal x-rays are often helpful in distinguishing colonic from small intestinal obstruction. In early colonic obstruction, only colonic gas may be seen with no small intestinal gas or air fluid levels. If there is progression to a point where there is air in both the colon and small bowel, it is usually possible to distinguish colonic gas around the periphery of the abdominal cavity. Paralytic ileus can be differentiated from distal colonic obstruction by the presence of gas in the distal sigmoid and rectum in the former

(Fig. 17.6). If the diagnosis is still in question and the patient is stable, a barium enema will usually distinguish between the two conditions by demonstrating the point of obstruction.

Treatment

The diagnosis of mechanical small bowel obstruction requires prompt surgical intervention. Once a decision has been made to operate, appropriate laboratory tests should be drawn and aggressive fluid resuscitation should be instituted to restore an effective circulating blood volume. A Foley catheter should be inserted to monitor urinary output. Fluid resuscitation is considered adequate when the urine output is greater than 30–50 ml of urine per hour for 2 consecutive hours. Because the fluids that are lost to the vascular space by vomiting or secretion into the bowel lumen are isoosmotic, they should be replaced with a physiologic solution. The best choices are normal saline or lactated Ringer's solution. Once it has been established that the patient has normal renal function, 30–40 mEq of potassium can be added to each liter of intravenous fluid. A nasogastric tube should be inserted into the stomach for decompression and to decrease the possibility of aspiration during the induction of anesthesia. Placement of a long intestinal tube into the jejunum in patients with complete small intestinal obstruction can be used to decompress further the small bowel. Although small bowel tubes have been advocated for definitive treatment, they rarely are successful and increase the

risk of strangulation while determining its effectiveness. Patients should have preoperative broad spectrum intravenous antibiotics with coverage of Gram negative and anaerobic organisms, because of the possibility of strangulated obstruction or perforation and the increased risk of infectious complications.

The objectives of surgery are twofold: removal of the obstruction and resection of any necrotic small intestine. The only therapy necessary for uncomplicated obstruction is to relieve the obstruction, i.e., reduction and repair of an incarcerated hernia, division of an obstructing peritoneal adhesive band, or untwisting of a volvulus. If the intestine has become strangulated and necrotic, resection of the small intestine with reanastomosis is required. Frequently the surgeon must make a clinical decision about the viability of the bowel when it is not clearly infarcted and a large amount of bowel is involved. When the obstructing lesion is unresectable, such as in metastatic carcinoma, it is necessary to bypass the lesion to relieve the obstruction.

The overall mortality from uncomplicated small bowel obstruction is less than 1% when the previously discussed principles of diagnosis and treatment are utilized. However, when delay in diagnosis and therapy with the attendant complications of perforation and infarction occur, the mortality rate rises to 30–50%. Therefore, early diagnosis and treatment are essential.

Crohn's Disease of the Small Intestine

Significance and Incidence

Crohn's disease (granulomatous disease) of the small intestine was described in 1932 by Crohn, Ginsburg, and Oppenheimer, who differentiated it from ileocecal tuberculosis. The incidence varies from 1.5–25 per 100,000 population, with an increase in frequency since 1970, particularly in the colon. The disease is located only in the terminal ileum in 50% of patients and only in the colon in 10% of the patients, with the remaining 40% having combined small and large intestinal disease. There are two peak periods during which Crohn's disease occurs, first in the late teens and early 20's with most disease involving the small intestine and terminal ileum, and the second peak in the 6th and 7th decades of life with most disease involving the colon.

Pathology

The disease may occur anywhere from the mouth to the anus and characteristically has "skip lesions," as opposed to contiguous disease observed in ulcerative colitis (Table 17.2). On gross examination of the bowel, the serosa appears beefy red with a grayish exudate and "creeping" mesenteric fat over the areas of greatest inflammation. In severe cases, single and multiple strictures occur. Perianal complications, such as ulcers, fissures, perirectal fistulas, and abscesses, occur in 30–60% of patients with colonic disease and 8–30% of patients with small bowel disease. The bowel wall and lymph nodes frequently have noncaseating granulomas identified on histologic examination. Microscop-

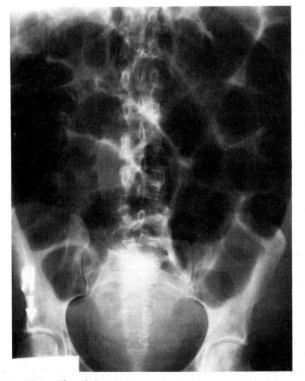

Figure 17.6. This abdominal x-ray shows paralytic ileus of the small bowel. This can be differentiated from mechanical small bowel obstruction and colonic obstruction by air in the distal sigmoid colon and rectum.

Table 17.2.
Characteristics of Ulcerative Colitis and Crohn's Disease

Crohn's Disease	Ulcerative Colitis
Transmural involvement	Mucosal disease
Segmental involvement "skip lesions"	Diffuse involvement of the entire colon
Rectum uninvolved with disease	Rectum involved with disease (90%)
Fistulas common	Fistulas (external, internal, or perianal) are rare
Anal complications common	Anal complications are rare
Toxic megacolon uncommon	Toxic megacolon is common
Bleeding is rare	Bleeding is common
Carcinoma is rare	Carcinoma is common
Surgery is relatively effective	Surgery is curative

ically, the inflammatory process begins in the submucosa and spreads transmurally, frequently producing fistulas and abscesses.

Clinical Presentation

In 65% of patients with Crohn's disease, at initial presentation there will be a 10–20% loss of body weight. These patients appear chronically ill. Hypoproteinemia (decreased serum albumin), edema, muscle weakness, increase of basal metabolic rate, and deficiencies of vitamins A, D, E, and K, are often observed. A rapid intestinal transit time is not uncommon. Protein secretion into the gut may be increased up to 15 times above the normal level of 24 mg of albumin per kilogram body weight per day. In addition 40–50% of patients with Crohn's disease may have malabsorption of carbohydrate, protein, fat, and vitamin B_{12}. Therefore, intensive parenteral and enteral nutrition therapy is necessary to correct these deficiencies, which significantly increase the morbidity and mortality from the disease.

Pain is the most frequent presenting symptom (greater than 90% of patients) and may be intermittent or constant in character. The second most common symptom (85%) is diarrhea that rarely contains blood. This is in contrast to patients with ulcerative colitis, where bloody diarrhea usually occurs. Other symptoms include fever, weight loss, and extraintestinal manifestations, such as ankylosing spondylitis, migratory polyarthritis, erythema nodosum, pyoderma gangrenosum, and uveitis. In general, these extraintestinal manifestations resolve when the disease is in remission or as the result of medical or surgical therapy.

The presenting symptom complex in 10% of patients with Crohn's disease is similar to acute appendicitis, with fever, pain in the midabdomen or right lower quadrant, and possibly a mass. Differentiating acute Crohn's disease from appendicitis may be difficult, requiring an operation to determine the correct diagnosis. Usually the presenting symptoms are primarily related to the complications of the disease, such as bowel obstruction, abscess, fistula, or perianal disease. Carcinoma and significant hemorrhage of the small intestine are rare, but do occur, in Crohn's disease.

Diagnosis

Crohn's disease can mimic other inflammatory and neoplastic lesions of the GI tract radiographically. Radiology is useful in determining not only the diagnosis, but the extent of disease. Intestinal complications, such as fistulas, abscesses, obstructions, or cancers, and the presence of extraintestinal manifestations, including gallstones, sclerosing cholangitis, urinary calculi, retroperitoneal fibrosis, and skeletal diseases, such as osteomyelitis, septic arthritis, and aseptic necrosis resulting from steroid treatment, are all within the diagnostic possibilities of a skilled radiologist.

Radiologic studies to be used depend on the disease presentation. Where the presence of intestinal and extraintestinal complications are suspected and surgery is contemplated, an expeditious and proper sequence of studies should be planned so that one study does not interfere with another. Radiologic consultation for planning can greatly increase the diagnostic yield and minimize radiation and expense. In general barium expulsion is slow and interferes with nuclear scans, ultrasonography, plain films, and intravenous contrast studies. Hence barium studies should be done last and in the following order: barium enema, UGI series, small bowel series, and enteroclysis. Water-soluble contrast agents interfere with the interpretation of ultrasound and plain films; hence the latter should be done first.

Therefore, begin with plain films of the abdomen to search for biliary and urinary calculi, skeletal manifestations, and intestinal complications. Proceed to ultrasonography if biliary calculi or intestinal complications are suspected. This may reveal the thickened walls and narrowed lumens of involved segments and any surrounding abscesses or masses. Nuclear scans are less helpful because they cannot distinguish inflammation in the bowel from that surrounding it. CT may demonstrate complications like abscess or phlegmon in even greater detail. Cost and radiation dose, especially to the female pelvis, must be considered. Excretory urography, if needed, should be done before CT. If extraintestinal (enterocutaneous, enterovesical, or enterovaginal) fistulas are suspected, these should be investigated next using fluoroscopically and endoscopically guided catheter placement and a water-soluble contrast agent.

Thereafter, double-contrast barium enema, double contrast esophagram and upper GI series, and small bowel series should be done (Fig. 17.7). If all segments of small bowel have not been exceptionally well shown, enteroclysis should be used to demonstrate skip lesions and very early lesions, as well as entero-enteric and other fistulous connections. Enteroclysis (small bowel enema) involves passing a tube under fluoroscopic guidance through the nose and GI tract to the proximal small bowel and rapidly injecting a large quantity of barium to fully distend the bowel loops while multiple radiographs are made. After a radiologic overview of the GI tract, endoscopic confirmation and biopsy of Crohn's lesions is needed.

Interpretation depends on finding the earliest, as

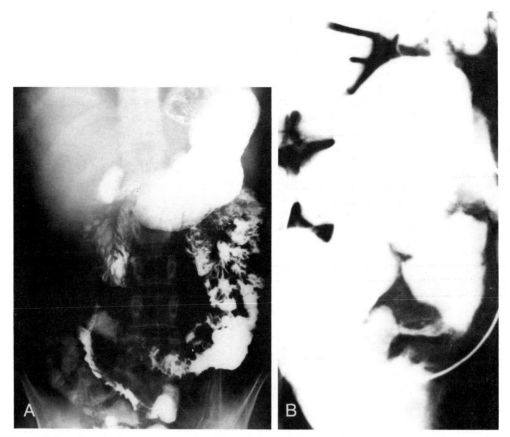

Figure 17.7. **A,** This small bowel study demonstrates a narrowed segment of distal small bowel and a similar change in the antrum of the stomach. The mucosal pattern of the bowel is altered by pseudopolyps and there is absence of the valvulae conniventes. The upper small bowel suggests skip areas of Crohn's involvement whereas the distal bowel is narrowed and contiguously involved with Crohn's disease. **B,** This small bowel study demonstrates the "string sign" in the terminal ileum adjacent to the cecum with proximal dilatation of the ileum.

well as the advanced, Crohn's lesions. The earliest mucosal lesion is an aphthous ulcer, described as a small ulcer crater on top of a mound of edema appearing in a double-contrast barium study as a white fleck on a dark doughnut in an otherwise normal-appearing mucosa. As disease progresses, the mucosa thickens and becomes nodular. The mucosal folds become unrecognizable, cracks representing linear ulcers appear between nodules and the lumen narrows as the bowel wall thickens. Spasm is a frequent finding fluoroscopically. Mesenteric involvement adds to the thickening and the final result is a narrowed "string-like" lumen, fixed in position and size and separated by mass effect from the next adjacent loop. Spasm and edema account for some of the lumen narrowing, but finally irreversible stricturing and partial obstruction occur. Strictures are smooth, without the "shouldering" seen in neoplasms.

Proctocolonoscopy and biopsy are extremely important in differentiating the type of inflammatory bowel disease in the colon. Although Crohn's disease rarely involves the rectum, full thickness rectal biopsy must be performed, even when the mucosa appears normal, to differentiate Crohn's disease from ulcerative colitis. Esophagogastroduodenoscopy is necessary to document the rare involvement of the foregut structures by Crohn's disease.

Treatment

There is no curative therapy for Crohn's disease, and, therefore, treatment is directed toward relieving the symptoms and managing the complications. Diarrhea can be managed using diphenoxylate and codeine. Nutritional deficiencies can be corrected with intensive parenteral therapy and rapidly absorbed enteral diets that are low in fat and free of lactose. The inflammatory response is best treated with broad spectrum antibiotics such as sulfasalazine. Prednisone (60–80 mg/day) and immunosuppression (azathioprine) are occasionally required. Because this disease characteristically has periods of exacerbation and remission, surgery is indicated only when complications develop. Surgical intervention is necessary if there is evidence of obstruction, intractability, perforation, abscess formation, massive bleeding, persistent gastrointestinal fistulas, and the rare finding of carcinoma. In these cases, if the disease is localized, the involved segment of bowel with 7–10 cm of grossly normal proximal and distal bowel should be resected.

Acute terminal ileitis precipitated by the *Yersinia* bacterium, can produce an inflammatory response in the terminal ileum in 20% of patients with Crohn's. Although this problem spontaneously resolves in 90% of the cases, the appendix should be removed if the cecum is normal. This removes the possibility of appendicitis in the differential diagnosis if future attacks of right lower quadrant pain develop. The treatment of gastrointestinal fistulas and abscesses is a particularly complicated problem, because most of these appear in the perianal region. Surgical excision of perianal fistulas and drainage of abscesses is effective in 75% of patients. Additionally, the use of intravenous alimentation and bowel rest can also allow spontaneous closure in 75% of fistulas originating from the small intestine. Colonic fistulas will have a 30% spontaneous closure rate with parenteral nutritional support. Perianal, external, and internal fistulas will rarely heal until there is quiescence of the active disease.

Because of the severity and chronicity of this disease, severe metabolic problems, such as fluid and electrolyte imbalances do occur. Biliary and renal stones occur secondary to chronic ileal disease or from resection of more than 50% of the terminal ileum. Failure of the terminal ileum to absorb bile salts eventually depletes the pool of bile acids and predisposes to the precipitation of cholesterol crystals that can become the nidus for stone formation. Calcium lost in the diarrhea prevents the binding of oxalate produced by gut bacteria and results in increased intestinal absorption of oxalate. Hyperoxaluria is frequently observed in patients with Crohn's disease.

The incidence of recurrence is particularly high in patients who develop this disease during their youth (50–80% over the following 10 years). Early recurrence may be defined as an exacerbation of symptoms that develops within the first 2 years following surgery, or as a late recurrence developing between 5 and 10 years after the operation. Overall, early and late recurrences are greater in the small bowel than in patients with colon involvement. This benign disease produces significant morbidity due to frequent recurrences following bowel resection. The optimal treatment of Crohn's disease requires the highest level of both medical and surgical judgment. Despite excellent medical care, the overall mortality may be as high as 20% over a 20-year period.

SUGGESTED READINGS

Diseases of the Appendix

Berry J Jr, Malt RA: Appendicitis near its centenary. *Ann Surg* 200:567–575, 1984.
Buchman TG, Zuidema GD: Reasons for delay of the diagnosis of acute appendicitis. *Surg Obstet Gynecol* 158:260–266, 1984.
Cooperman, M: Complications of appendicitis. *Surg Clin North Am* 63:1233–1247, 1983.
Kelly, HA, Hardon E: *The Vermiform Appendix and Its Diseases.* Philadelphia, WB Saunders, 1905.
Silen W (ed): *Cope's Early Diagnosis of the Acute Abdomen,* ed 16. New York, Oxford, 1983.

Meckel's Diverticulum and Neoplasms

Davis Z, Moertel CG, McIlrath DC: The malignant carcinoid syndrome. *Surg Gynecol Obstet* 137:637–644, 1973.
Herbsman H, Wetstein L, Rosen Y, et al: Tumors of the small intestine. *Cur Prob Surg* 122–182, 1980.
Perlman JA, Hoover HC, Safer PK: Femoral hernia with strangulated Meckel's diverticulum. *Am J Surg* 139:286–289, 1980.
Soltero MJ, Bill AH: The natural history of Meckel's diverticulum and its relation to incidental removal. *Am J Surg* 132:168–173, 1976.

Small Bowel Obstruction

Bizer LS, Liebling RW, Dlany HM, Gliedman, ML: Small bowel obstruction. *Surgery* 89:407–413, 1981.
Brolin RE: The role of gastrointestinal tube decompression in the treatment of mechanical intestinal obstruction. *Am Surg* 49:131–137, 1983.
Hofstetter SR: Acute adhesive obstruction of the small intestine. *Surg Gynecol Obstet* 152:141–144, 1981.
Stewardson RH, Bombeck CT, Nyhus LM: Critical operative management of small bowel obstruction. *Ann Surg* 187:189–193, 1978.

Crohn's Disease

Kirsner JB, Shorter RG: Recent development in ''nonspecific'' inflammatory bowel disease. *N Engl J Med* 306:775–785, 1982.
Kirsner JB, Shorter RG: Recent developments in nonspecific inflammatory bowel disease. Second of Two Parts. *N Engl J Med* 306:837–848, 1982.
Pillai DK, Flavell Matts SG: Chronic inflammatory bowel disease—a review. *Br J Clin Pract* 37:165–172, 1983.
Weterman, IT, Pena AS, Booth CC (eds): *The Management of Crohn's Disease.* Amsterdam, Excerpta Medica, 1975.

Skills

1. Demonstrate the ability to perform a physical examination of the abdomen.
   a. In patients with diffuse and localized abdominal tenderness;
   b. In patients with abnormal bowel sounds: absent, hypoactive, and borborygmi;
   c. In patients with various abdominal masses;
   d. In patients with abdominal distention.

2. Demonstrate the ability to perform a rectal examination
   a. In a patient with rectal tenderness;
   b. In a patient with rectal mass.

3. Demonstrate the ability to perform a rectal and pelvic examination
   a. In a patient with pelvic inflammatory disease;
   b. In a patient with an ovarian mass;
   c. In a patient with appendicitis.

4. Demonstrate the ability to perform proctosigmoidoscopy.

5. Demonstrate the ability to insert a nasogastric tube.

6. Demonstrate the ability to outline an appropriate radiologic workup and sequencing of studies for the following suspected conditions.
   a. Appendicitis;
   b. Meckel's diverticulum;
   c. Abdominal abscess;
   d. Complicated Crohn's disease;
   e. GI bleeding;
   f. Intestinal obstruction.

7. Demonstrate the ability to interpret roentgenograms.
   a. Plain and upright abdomen;
   b. Differentiate a normal gas pattern from the gas pattern seen with paralytic ileus, small bowel obstruction, and distal colonic obstruction.
8. Given a patient with prolonged small intestinal obstruction with dehydration and vomiting, demonstrate the ability to calculate the estimated fluid deficit and write orders to correct the deficit and provide maintenance fluids. Discuss the clinical and laboratory data that would be used to calculate this deficit.
9. Discuss the indications for placement of a long intestinal tube for bowel obstruction. Demonstrate the ability to pass a long intestinal tube in a patient with a mechanical bowel obstruction.

Study Questions

1. A 22-month-old male infant experiences rectal bleeding for several weeks.
   a. Describe your initial workup of this patient.
   b. What tests would you order?
   c. The workup reveals a hemoglobin of 8.5 gm/100 ml and a nasogastric aspirate negative for gross or occult blood. A technetium [99mTc] pertechnetate scan demonstrates an increased uptake in the distal ileum.
   d. Should contrast x-rays of the upper gastrointestinal tract (a small bowel series) be performed?
   e. Should surgery be performed (elective or emergency)?
   f. Should the technetium scan have been performed after the first episode of rectal bleeding?

2. A 4-year-old boy develops abdominal pain, a temperature of 38.5°C, and moderately severe right lower quadrant tenderness. There is also rectal tenderness on the right side. List your differential diagnosis. How would you workup this problem?

3. An 8-year-old girl has chronic, intermittent, right lower quadrant pain, at times associated with tenderness and mild diarrhea. Her hemoglobin is 9.5 gm/100 ml. What is your differential diagnosis? How would you workup this child?

4. A 40-year-old female has a gastrectomy performed for peptic ulcer disease. The operation is uncomplicated. At the time of surgery, a moderate-sized Meckel's diverticulum is identified in the terminal ileum. How would you manage this diverticulum? List your rationale for resection or nonresection.

5. A 40-year-old man comes to the Emergency Room with a 24-hr history of nausea, vomiting, obstipation, inability to pass flatus, and crampy abdominal pain. He had an appendectomy 5 years ago but otherwise has always been in good health. His abdomen is distended and he has hyperactive bowel sounds.
   a. What is your differential diagnosis?
   b. How would you proceed with this patient's diagnostic workup?
   c. How would you distinguish small intestinal obstruction from paralytic ileus and colonic obstruction?
   d. What are the important elements of the initial therapy in a patient that presents with the signs and symptoms of small intestinal obstruction?
   e. If the patient has a small intestinal obstruction, what would be your definitive therapy?

6. A 35-year-old male presents with a 10-pound weight loss, fever to 101°F orally, three to five diarrhea stools per day, and crampy lower abdominal pain. Physical exam of the abdomen reveals mid to right lower quadrant abdominal pain and a right lower abdominal mass.
   a. How would you initially workup this patient?
   b. The results of the laboratory data show a serum albumin of 2.5 gm/100 ml and hemoglobin 10 gm/100 ml. Upper gastrointestinal and small bowel series show a terminal ileal mass and multiple constricted areas of the small bowel.
   c. What is the diagnosis?
   d. What is your initial treatment?
   e. How would you manage this patient's nutritional problem?
   f. When is surgery indicated?

18

Colon, Rectum, and Anus

Merril T. Dayton, M.D.
James T. Evans, M.D.

ASSUMPTIONS

The student knows the normal anatomy and embryology of the colon, rectum and anus, including blood supply and lymphatic drainage.

The student understands the physiology of the colon.

The student understands the composition of colonic flora.

OBJECTIVES

Diverticular Disease

1. Describe the clinical findings of diverticular disease, differentiating the symptoms and signs of diverticulitis and diverticulosis.
2. Discuss five complications of diverticular disease and their appropriate surgical management.
3. Discuss massive rectal bleeding, including differential diagnosis, initial management, appropriate diagnostic studies, and the preferred treatment for each lesion.
4. List the differential diagnosis, initial management, diagnostic studies, and indications for medical versus surgical treatment in a patient with left lower quadrant pain.

Carcinoma of the Colon, Rectum, and Anus

1. Identify the common symptoms and signs of carcinoma of the colon, rectum, and anus.
2. Discuss the appropriate laboratory, endoscopic, and x-ray studies for the diagnosis of carcinoma of the colon, rectum, and anus.
3. Outline the treatment of carcinoma of the colon, rectum, and anus located at different levels and include a discussion of the role of radiotherapy and chemotherapy.
4. Describe the postoperative follow-up of a patient after colon cancer resection including a discussion of the role of CEA in detecting recurrence.

5. Using Duke's classification, discuss the staging and 5-year survival rate of carcinoma of the colon and rectum.

Ulcerative Colitis and Crohn's Disease of the Colon

1. Differentiate ulcerative colitis and Crohn's disease of the colon in terms of history, pathology, x-ray findings, treatment, and risk of cancer.
2. Discuss the role of surgery in the treatment of patients with ulcerative colitis who have the following complications: intractability, toxic megacolon, cancer, perforation, and bleeding.
3. Discuss the role of surgery in the treatment of patients with Crohn's disease who have the following complications: fistula, bleeding, and stricture.
4. Discuss the nonoperative therapy of ulcerative colitis and Crohn's disease.

Hemorrhoids

1. Discuss the anatomy of hemorrhoids including the four grades encountered clinically; differentiate internal and external hemorrhoids.
2. Discuss the etiological factors and predisposing conditions in the development of hemorrhoidal disease.
3. Describe the symptoms and signs of patients with external hemorrhoids; with internal hemorrhoids.
4. Outline the principles of management of patients with symptomatic external and internal hemorrhoids, including the roles of nonoperative and operative management.

Colonic Obstruction, Volvulus, Intussusception, and Impaction

1. List signs, symptoms, and diagnostic aids for evaluating presumed large bowel obstruction.

2. Discuss at least four causes of colonic obstruction in the adult patient including a discussion of frequency of each cause.
3. Outline a plan for diagnostic studies, preoperative management, and treatment of volvulus; of intussusception; of impaction; of obstructing colon cancer.
4. Given a patient with mechanical large or small bowel obstruction, discuss the potential complications if the treatment is inadequate.

Perianal Infections

1. Discuss the role of anal crypts in perianal infection and describe the various types of perianal infections.
2. Outline the symptoms and physical findings of patients with perianal infections.
3. Outline the principles of management of patients with perianal infections, including the role of antibiotics, incision and drainage and primary fistulectomy.

Fistula-In-Ano

1. Define fissure-in-ano.
2. Describe the symptoms and physical findings of patients with fissure-in-ano.
3. Outline the principles of management of patients with fissure-in-ano.

While the colon and rectum are nonessential organs from the standpoint of biological function, one must understand the physiology, anatomy, and pathophysiology of these structures because of the high incidence of disease originating in them. Conditions, such as diverticulosis coli, colonic polyps, adenocarcinoma of the colon and rectum, and ulcerative colitis, afflict a large number of patients in the United States and the economic, social, and personal costs are enormous. Paradoxically, while the colon is much less vital for nutrition, fluid maintenance, and overall homeostasis than the small intestine, disease conditions are far more common in the colon and rectum.

Anatomy

The large intestine may be divided into several different parts. The cecum is the largest part of the intestine and is found where the small bowel enters the colon. There is an indistinct division between the cecum and ascending colon, which is fixed posteriorly in the right gutter of the posterior abdominal cavity and is therefore considered to be a retroperitoneal structure. The hepatic flexure is the bend in the ascending colon where it becomes the transverse colon, which is suspended freely in the peritoneal cavity by the transverse mesocolon. The transverse colon bends again at the spleen (splenic flexure) and again becomes retro-

peritoneal. The descending colon remains retroperitoneal up to the sigmoid colon, which is a loop of redundant colon in the left lower quadrant. The distal sigmoid colon (which is intraperitoneal) becomes the rectum when it passes the sacrum and becomes a partially retroperitoneal structure. The rectum continues to the sphincters that form the short (3 cm) anal canal.

The rectum is 12–15 cm long and its origins are marked by some anatomic change (compared to colon). The taenia coli disperse at approximately the level of the sacral promontory so that the longitudinal muscle layer becomes a continuous, homogeneous layer. In addition, proximal rectum is covered by peritoneum anteriorly but not posteriorly down to approximately 8–9 cm above the anal verge where rectum becomes an extraperitoneal structure. Because of the latter, rectal biopsy above 8–9 cm is more hazardous on the anterior wall because of the risk of perforation into the peritoneal cavity.

The blood supply (Fig. 18.1) to the colon is more complex than the small bowel. The ascending and proximal one-half of the transverse colon are supplied by branches of the superior mesenteric arteries (same as the small intestine) while the distal one-half of the transverse colon, descending colon, sigmoid colon, and upper one-half of the rectum are supplied by branches of the inferior mesenteric artery. The distal rectum and anus are supplied by branches of the internal iliac artery (middle and inferior hemorrhoidal arteries). The importance of understanding this complex arterial blood supply is that in certain areas of the colon (e.g., splenic flexure), which are at the junction of two separate blood vessel systems, there may be a relatively poor blood supply; anastomoses in this region would carry a higher risk of ischemic complications. The venous drainage of the large bowel is less complex because most branches accompany the arteries and eventually drain into the portal system.

Lymphatic drainage (Fig. 18.2) of the large intestine parallels the arterial blood supply with several different layers of lymph nodes occurring as one moves toward the aorta. In general, tumor metastases move from one layer to another in an orderly progression, with the paracolic lymph nodes being involved first, followed by the middle tier of lymph nodes, and lastly the periaortic lymph nodes.

The bowel wall of colon is divided into the same layers as the small intestine, namely mucosa, submucosa, muscularis, and serosa. The major difference is that the colon has no villi; i.e., the mucosal crypts of Lieberkuhn form a more uniform surface with less absorptive area. Another major difference is the outer longitudinal smooth muscle layer that is separated into three bands (taenia coli) that cause outpouchings of bowel between the taeniae (haustra).

Physiology

The colon and rectum have two primary functions: (1) Water and electrolyte absorption from liquid stool

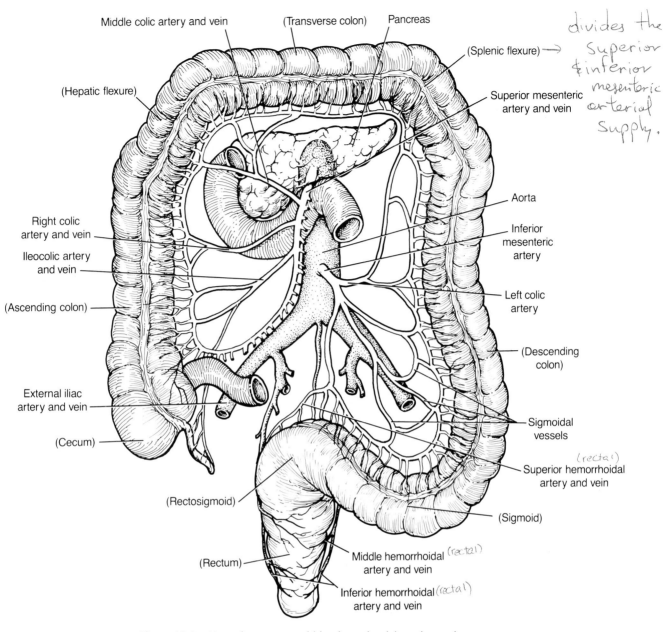

Middle colic artery and vein

(Transverse colon)   Pancreas

(Splenic flexure) →   *divides the superior & inferior mesenteric arterial supply.*

(Hepatic flexure)

Superior mesenteric artery and vein

Right colic artery and vein

Aorta

Ileocolic artery and vein

Inferior mesenteric artery

(Ascending colon)

Left colic artery

(Descending colon)

External iliac artery and vein

Sigmoidal vessels

(Cecum)

(rectal) Superior hemorrhoidal artery and vein

(Rectosigmoid)

(Sigmoid)

(Rectum)

Middle hemorrhoidal *(rectal)* artery and vein

Inferior hemorrhoidal *(rectal)* artery and vein

Figure 18.1.   Normal anatomy and blood supply of the colon and rectum.

and (2) storage of feces. Some 600–700 ml of chyme is presented to the cecum each day. Most of the stool water is absorbed in the right colon, leaving 200 ml of stool evacuated as solids daily. This represents a small fraction of the total water absorbed in the intestinal tract. The left colon and rectum thus function to store solid fecal material and the anorectal apparatus regulates evacuation of solids permitting defecation at a socially acceptable time. Very little digestion and absorption of nutrients occurs in the colon—thus the organ is not essential to life. The composition of colonic gas varies between individuals and is influenced substantially by diet. Some 800–900 ml/day is passed as flatus—70% of which is nitrogen (N_2) derived from swallowing air. Other gases include oxygen, carbon dioxide, hydrogen, methane, indole, and skatole—the

latter two giving colonic gas its characteristic odor.

Colonic motility is unique among organs of the alimentary canal because of the multiple types of contraction patterns including "segmentation" and "mass contractions." The latter are particularly unique to the colon and are characterized by contraction of long segments of colon, resulting in mass movement of stool bulk. Movement of residue through the colon occurs at a much slower rate (18–48 hours) than it does through the small bowel (4 hours). Colonic transit time may be accelerated by emotional states, diet, disease, infection, and bleeding.

Normal frequency of defecation is approximately every 24 hours but may vary from 8–72 hours. Any patient who has a significant change in bowel habit pattern should be evaluated for the possibility of seri-

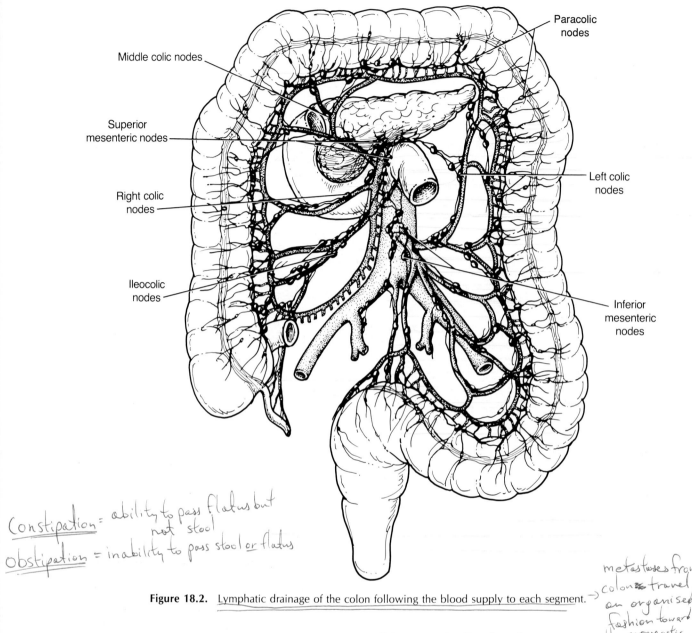

Middle colic nodes

Paracolic nodes

Superior mesenteric nodes

Left colic nodes

Right colic nodes

Ileocolic nodes

Inferior mesenteric nodes

Constipation = ability to pass flatus but not stool

Obstipation = inability to pass stool or flatus

metastases from colon travel in an organised fashion toward the paraaortic nodes.

Figure 18.2.   Lymphatic drainage of the colon following the blood supply to each segment.

ous disease. Severe constipation (ability to pass flatus but not stool) and obstipation (inability to pass stool or flatus) are examples of changes that should be evaluated.

The colon harbors a greater number and variety of bacteria than any other organ in the body. The overwhelming majority of organisms are anaerobes with *Bacteroides fragilis* being the most common. The most common aerobes are *Escherichia coli* and enterococci. While the bacteria perform a number of important functions, such as degradation of bile pigments and production of vitamin K for the host, their high number and variety in the colon make it a hazardous organ to treat surgically because of the risk of infection. Some studies demonstrate postoperative infection rates as high as 25–30% following surgery on colon that has not been "prepared" (cleaned out) prior to operating.

Diagnostic Evaluation

Patients having signs or symptoms referable to the colon or rectum may be evaluated by a host of modalities. The digital exam remains an important means of detecting a number of disease processes including rectal tumors or polyps, rectal abscesses, rectal ulcers, hemorrhoids, and colorectal bleeding. The tendency to defer the digital rectal examination because of patient discomfort or physician inconvenience is an egregious error that the student-physician must avoid.

While rigid sigmoidoscopy was the standard method of visualizing the distal colon and rectum for many years, it has largely been replaced by fiberoptic flexible sigmoidoscopy. The latter provides a higher diagnostic yield and is much less uncomfortable for the patient. This examination allows visualization of the last 30–65

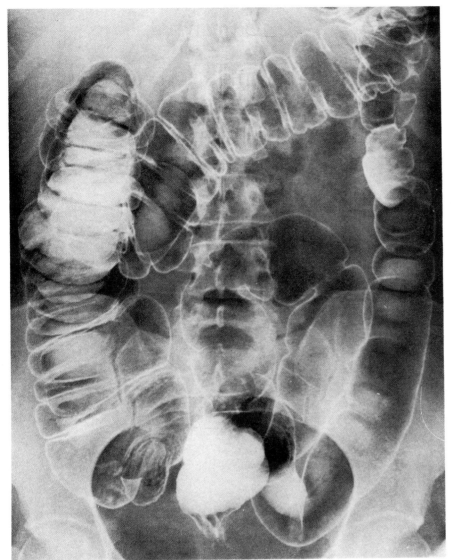

Figure 18.3.   Normal air-contrast barium enema.

cm of the colorectal complex and results in detection of 60% of colorectal neoplasms. In addition to detecting polyps and neoplasms, it can aid in detecting sites of hemorrhage, ascertaining etiology of obstruction, evacuating excessive colonic gas, and removing foreign bodies from the rectum. Because of the frequency of colorectal disease, this exam should be an integral part of the routine examination of patients over age 50.

An abdominal series (flat plate and upright x-ray) should be obtained on any patient presenting with significant abdominal pain. This series continues to be very helpful in detecting pneumoperitoneum, large bowel obstruction (e.g., volvulus or tumor), paralytic ileus, appendicolith, and other less common diseases. It is important to stress that *both* of the x-rays in the series should be obtained and not simply an abdominal flat plate.

Barium enema remains an important diagnostic modality in detecting disease in this region. After properly ''cleaning out'' the colon and rectum, contrast is intro-duced under mild pressure that fills the entire organ. Air insufflation with some intraluminal barium remaining provides for particularly sensitive detection of polyps and small lesions (Fig. 18.3). Barium enema is particularly helpful in diagnosing tumors, diverticulosis, diverticulitis, volvulus, sites of obstruction, and inflammatory bowel disease.

One of the newest and most helpful diagnostic tools is fiberoptic colonoscopy. This instrument allows visualization of the entire colon and rectum as well as the last few centimeters of terminal ileum. It also provides therapeutic options not previously available without surgery such as polyp removal, colonic decompression, stricture dilatation, hemorrhage control, and foreign body removal. After thorough bowel preparation and mild sedation, the device is inserted into the rectum and advanced using a steering mechanism on the handle (Fig. 18.4). Although initially used primarily to evaluate ambiguous findings on barium enema, more physicians are using it for diagnostic purposes and

Proctum = rectum

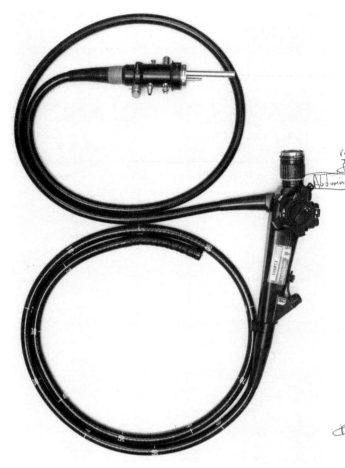

Figure 18.4. Fiberoptic colonoscope used for diagnostic and therapeutic maneuvers in the colon.

postoperation followup. It is indicated to evaluate lower gastrointestinal bleeding of unknown etiology, inflammatory bowel disease, polyps, equivocal barium enema findings, posttumor removal, pseudo-obstruction, and stricture.

Angiography is useful primarily in detecting the source of colonic bleeding when it occurs at a moderate or rapid rate. It is not helpful for low, chronic blood loss.

Miscellaneous Terms

Understanding treatment of colonic diseases requires comprehending a few simple terms that are unique to this organ. The term *colostomy* refers to the surgical procedure in which the colon is divided and the proximal end brought through a surgically created defect in the abdominal wall. The purpose is nearly always to divert stool from a diseased segment distally in the colon or rectum. The distal segment is either oversewn and placed in the peritoneal cavity as a blind limb *(Hartmann's procedure)* or brought out inferiorly to the colostomy through the abdominal wall *(mucous fistula)*. A *loop colostomy* is created by merely bringing a loop of colon through a defect in the abdominal wall, placing a rod underneath, and making a small hole in

ē colostomy bag

the loop to allow stool to exit into a colostomy bag. The term *ileostomy* refers to a similar procedure in which ileum is brought through the abdominal wall to divert its contents from distal disease or, in a proctocolectomy, to serve as a permanent stoma.

Other terms that often confuse medical students include *proctocolectomy*, *abdominoperineal resection*, and *low anterior resection*. "Proctum" is a synonym for "rectum" and thus *proctocolectomy* refers to operative removal of the entire colon and rectum (e.g., for ulcerative colits, polyposis syndromes). *Abdominoperineal resection* refers to operative removal of the lower sigmoid colon and the entire rectum, leaving a permanent proximal sigmoid colostomy (e.g., for low rectal cancer). *Low anterior resection* refers to removal of distal sigmoid colon and approximately one-half of the rectum with primary anastomosis of proximal sigmoid to distal rectum (e.g., for high rectal cancer).

Diverticular Disease

Diverticular disease develops at different rates in different countries with widely varying dietary habits, suggesting the probable influence of diet on the development of this condition. The incidence of diverticular disease is progressive from the fifth to eighth decade of life and it is estimated that 70% of elderly patients have asymptomatic diverticuli. Quite clearly there is some influence of the aging process on the incidence, but whether this is related to general relaxation of colonic tissue or a result of life-long dietary habits is not yet clear. Dietary influences have been implicated based upon comparative geographic epidemiology; these studies implicate the lower fiber content diet found in Western Europe and the United States. It is postulated that lower stool bulk results in higher generated luminal pressures for propulsion. The resultant in-

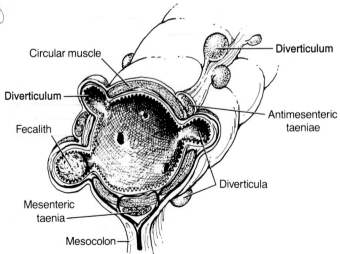

Figure 18.5. Mucosal herniation characteristic of diverticulosis. Most herniations occur at a site where the blood vessel penetrates the bowel wall.

increased work causes hypertrophy that leads to diverticulosis.

There are two types of diverticulae found in the colon. Congenital solitary "true" diverticulae (full bowel wall thickness in the diverticular sac) are uncommonly found in the cecum and ascending colon. Acquired (false) diverticulae are very common in western civilization and 95% of patients with the condition have involvement of the sigmoid colon. These diverticulae consist of mucosal herniations through the muscular wall. The muscles of the colon consist of an inner circular smooth muscle layer and a thinner outer layer organized into three longitudinal bands, the taenia. The most favorable area for herniation occurs where branches of the marginal artery penetrate the wall of the colon (Fig. 18.5). The etiology of herniation is probably related to the colon's exaggerated adaptation for fecal propulsion. One theory suggests that diverticular disease results from the higher than normal segmental contractions of the sigmoid leading to high intraluminal pressure. These high intraluminal pressures were found to be confined to those segments having diverticulae. Specifically, the sigmoid colon developed localized pressure increases because of segmentation between contraction rings. Contraction of the wall generated high pressure zones within the segment that resulted in herniation at the weakest point, near the vascular penetration of the bowel wall.

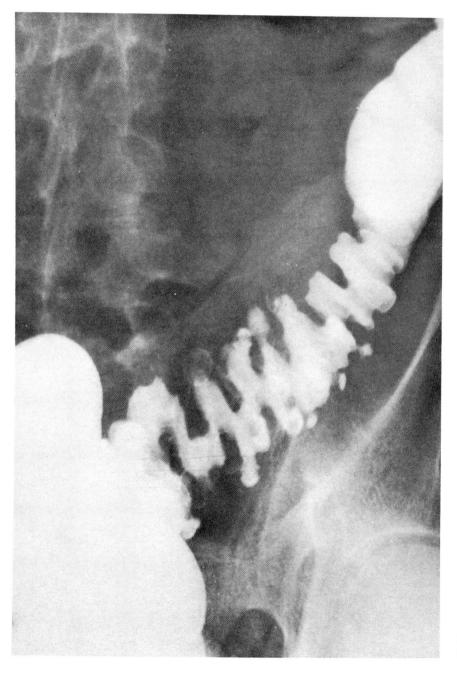

Figure 18.6. Sigmoid diverticulosis shown on barium enema.

Diverticulosis

General use of the term "diverticulosis" has been reserved for the presence of multiple false diverticulae in the colon. This is most often an asymptomatic (80%) radiographic finding when a barium enema is performed for some other diagnostic purpose (Fig. 18.6). Nevertheless, certain symptoms have been attributed to diverticulae in the absence of either inflammation or bleeding. These symptoms include recurrent abdominal pain, often localized to the left lower quadrant, as well as functional changes in bowel habits including constipation, diarrhea, or alternating constipation and diarrhea. The physical examination is most often unremarkable or it reveals mild tenderness in the left lower quadrant. By definition, fever and leukocytosis are absent. The additional roentgenographic findings of segmental spasm and luminal narrowing have been reported. Additional endoscopic evaluation of the lumen generally fails to reveal anything except the openings of the diverticulae. Management of asymptomatic patients with diverticular disease remains controversial. Although certain public health organizations recommend a diet with increased fiber content, no specific definition of fiber dietary content has been given for the normal adult. Patients are generally encouraged to consume fresh fruits and vegetables, whole grain breads, cereals, and bran products. Pharmacologic preparations of fiber, such as psyllium seed products, are more expensive but are more likely to be taken by the patients.

Diverticulitis

Diverticulitis is the term that describes a limited infection of one or more diverticulae including extension into adjacent tissue. The condition is initiated by obstruction of the neck of the diverticulum by a fecolith. The obstruction leads to microperforation that results in swelling in the colon wall or macroperforation that involves the pericolic tissues. The clinical presentation depends on the progression of infection after the perforation. If the perforation is small, it may spontaneously regress. If it is larger, it may be confined to pericolic tissues and abate after treatment with antibiotics. The process may enlarge to form an extensive abscess in the mesenteric fat that remains contained, eventually requiring surgical drainage. It may drain into the peritoneal cavity causing peritonitis or it may burrow into adjacent hollow organs resulting in fistula formation. Occasionally the diverticulum freely ruptures into the peritoneal cavity, causing peritonitis and resulting in urgent exploration.

Approximately one-sixth of all patients with diverticulosis will develop signs and symptoms of diverticulitis. The hallmark symptoms of diverticulitis are left lower quadrant abdominal pain (subacute onset), alteration in bowel habits (constipation or diarrhea), occasionally a palpable mass, and fever. Occasionally free perforation with generalized peritonitis occurs, but the most common picture is one of localized disease. The disease is often referred to as "left lower quadrant ap-

pendicitis." When cicatricial obstruction develops secondary to repeated bouts of inflammation, the patient will present with distention, high-pitched bowel sounds, and severe constipation or obstipation. Fistula formation may be associated with diarrhea, stool per vagina (colovaginal fistula), pneumaturia and recurrent urinary tract infections (colovesical fistula—the most common associated with diverticular disease), or skin erythema and furuncle that ruptures and is associated with stool drainage (colocutaneous fistula). As mentioned above, the clinical spectrum is a function of the complications of the diverticular perforation including abscess formation, fistula development, and partial or total obstruction. Of all life-threatening complications arising from diverticulitis, 44% will be due to perforations or abscess; 8% due to fistula; and 4% to obstruction.

Diagnostic evaluation of diverticulitis or its complications is directed by the clinical presentation of the patient. If acute diverticulitis is suspected, abdominal x-rays are obtained and a barium enema is relatively contraindicated. Barium enema may be obtained 2–3 weeks after the episode to confirm the clinical impression. If the patient has obstructive symptoms or evidence of a fistula (e.g., pneumaturia), a contrast enema is indicated. If free perforation has occurred, abdominal x-rays will reveal pneumoperitoneum.

Treatment

Treatment of the complications of diverticular disease is obviously directed at the specific complication.

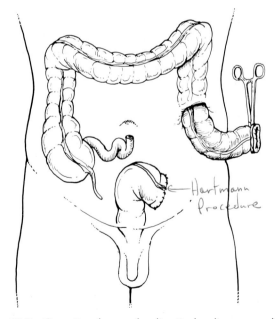

Figure 18.7. Operative therapy for diverticular disease usually involves resection of the sigmoid portion of the colon. If the operation is done for acute perforation or obstruction, the segment may be resected, a diverting colostomy brought to the abdominal wall, and the distal rectal stump oversewn (Hartmann procedure). A second stage of the operation would involve colostomy takedown and anastomosis to the rectal stump.

Treatment of acute diverticulitis is initially conservative in 85% of cases. It usually consists of hospital admission, intravenous hydration, giving the patient nothing by mouth, and giving intravenous antibiotics (usually an aminoglycoside and coverage for *B. fragilis*). The majority of patients will respond to conservative treatment and will not require further therapy. However, a subsegment of this group will have repeated bouts of acute diverticulitis requiring hospitalization. Experience with this disease has shown that the natural history of diverticulitis in those who have repeated bouts is one of gradual progression to one of the serious complications previously discussed. For this reason, most surgeons feel that any patient who has had two severe bouts of diverticulitis requiring hospitalization should be scheduled for elective sigmoid colectomy—the site of the problem in 95% of cases. In the face of perforation, obstruction, or abscess, immediate surgical resection of the diseased sigmoid colon is indicated with a temporary diverting colostomy and a Hartmann pouch (Fig. 18.7). If the disease is refractory or a fistula is present, the patient may undergo a bowel preparation and formal sigmoid colectomy with primary anastomosis.

Colovesical fistula is the most common type of fistula encountered in diverticulitis with a complication occurring in approximately 4% of the cases. The differential diagnosis includes carcinoma of the colon, cancer of other organs, such as the bladder, Crohn's disease, radiation bowel injury, and trauma due to foreign bodies. Some patients will be relatively symptom-free or only mildly symptomatic. However, others may present with refractory urinary tract infections, fecaluria, and pneumoturia. The most common physical finding is a palpable mass and leukocytosis secondary to urinary tract infection is common. The diagnostic triad includes barium enema, cystography, and intravenous pyelogram (IVP); however, in a patient with no demonstrable lesion, the use of dye markers, such as methylene blue, can be instilled into the bladder or rectum. The treatment for colovesical fistula is surgery. Primary closure of the bladder and resection of the sigmoid colon with primary anastomosis is the usual treatment. However, in the presence of severe infection, the colon anastomosis may be delayed and a temporary colostomy may be indicated. Generally, results are successful and recurrence is rare.

Diverticular Bleeding

Diverticulosis is occasionally associated with gastrointestinal hemorrhage, bleeding being the primary symptom in 5–10% of all patients with diverticular disease. Bleeding from diverticulae is occasionally massive (diverticulosis is the most common cause of massive lower gastrointestinal bleeding) and may be lethal. Of all patients with bleeding distal to the ligament of Treitz, approximately 70% have diverticulosis as the source of the bleeding and of this bleeding, approximately 25% is severe bleeding. The patient generally presents with profuse bright red or dark red rectal bleeding and hypotension. Unfortunately the age, sex, and symptoms of patients with bleeding diverticular disease are coincident with those of cancer and other lesions. Patients with cancer are unlikely to bleed as severely as patients with diverticulosis, but carcinomas bleed more frequently. Following the history, physical examination, and resuscitation with volume expanders and blood transfusions, the diagnostic approach to the patient with lower gastrointestinal hemorrhage includes insertion of a nasogastric tube with aspiration to rule out an upper gastrointestinal source, and rectal exam that excludes severe hemorrhoidal bleeding (e.g., due to portal hypertension) or ulcer. The next diagnostic procedure is flexible sigmoidoscopy that extends the examination of the lower portion of the large bowel to rule out other causes of bleeding. If massive bleeding continues, angiography is the diagnostic procedure of choice. If the bleeding is intermittent or angiography is indeterminate, colonoscopy after rapid colonic lavage is the preferred modality. Included in the differential diagnosis (in addition to diverticulosis) are angiodysplasia, solitary ulcers, varices, and rarely, inflammatory bowel disease. If the bleeding does not spontaneously cease, surgical resection of the involved segment is indicated.

Polyps and Carcinoma of the Colon and Rectum

Colorectal Polyps

"Polyp" is a morphologic term used to describe small mucosal excrescences that grow into the lumen of the colon and rectum. A brief discussion of these lesions is warranted because of their clear association with carcinoma of the colon. A variety of polyp types have been described, all with different biological behaviors. Approximately 5% of all barium enemas reveal polyps with about 50% occurring in the rectosigmoid region and 50% being multiple.

Inflammatory polyps (pseudopolyps) are quite common and have no malignant potential. Hamartomas (juvenile polyp and polyps associated with Peutz-Jeghers syndrome) similarly have very low malignant potential and often spontaneously regress. They may be safely observed. However, polyps that fall into the general category of "adenoma" are clearly premalignant and appropriate vigilance is indicated. Three subdivisions of adenomas have been described: (1) tubular (adenomatous) (2) tubulovillous (villoglandular), and (3) villous adenoma. Most polyps occur as either "sessile" (flat and intimately attached to the mucosa) or "pedunculated" (rounded and attached to mucosa by a relatively long, thin neck) (Fig. 18.8). Tubular and tubulovillous adenomas are more commonly pedunculated while villous adenomas are more commonly sessile. Evidence for the malignant potential of these lesions includes: (1) the high incidence of cancer associated with the polyps in familial polyposis and Gardner's syndrome, (2) simultaneous occurrence of cancers

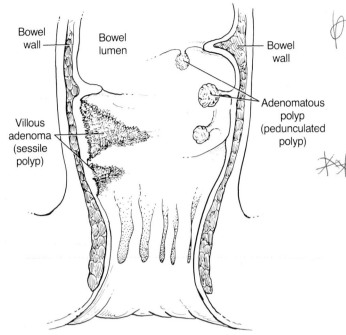

Figure 18.8. Characteristic appearance of villous adenoma (sessile polyp) compared to an adenomatous polyp (pedunculated polyp). Sessile polyps tend to be more difficult to manage because they are difficult to remove endoscopically and because their malignant potential is greater than adenomatous polyps.

and polyps in the same specimen, (3) carcinogens that experimentally produce both adenomas and cancers in the same model, and (4) lower cancer risks associated with those who have polyps removed. Approximately 7% of tubular, 20% of tubulovillous, and 33% of villous adenomas become malignant.

Treatment involves colonoscopic polypectomy of pedunculated polyps where possible. Those that can not be removed colonoscopically should be biopsied and a segmental resection of the colon done if the lesion is a villous adenoma, large, ulcerated, or indurated. For disease conditions characterized by extensive polyposis (familial polyposis, Gardner's syndrome), the treatment of choice is now abdominal colectomy, mucosal proctectomy, and ileoanal pull through.

Epidemiology

Cancer of the colon and rectum remains a major cause of death in the United States as reflected by estimates by the American Cancer Society that approximately 60,000–63,000 people die from this disease annually. Approximately 140,000–145,000 cases are annually identified as new cases. While a large number of factors associated with development of the disease have been elucidated, theories regarding etiology center around the impact of intraluminal chemical carcinogenesis. There are various theories as to whether these carcinogens are ingested or whether they are the result of biochemical processes occurring intraluminally from existing substances that are found normally in the fecal stream. Geographic epidemiologic studies

have revealed that certain populations have a very low incidence of cancer of the colon and rectum apparently as a result of identifiable dietary factors (high fiber, low fat) although social customs and a lack of environmental carcinogens cannot be excluded. Certain health agencies have promoted a low fat, high fiber diet as being protective against cancer of the colon and rectum. Additionally, the question of chemoprevention by ingestion of agents, such as carotenoids and other antioxidants, is as yet not well established.

The majority of large bowel cancers occur in the lower left side of the colon, near the rectum (Fig. 18.9) although recent studies suggest a slow shifting to right side lesions. Synchronous tumors (simultaneously occurring) develop in 5% of patients while 3–5% have metachronous tumors (a second tumor developing at a later time after resection of the first).

Disease conditions, such as familial polyposis and Gardner's syndrome, clearly demonstrate the genetic predisposition to cancer of the colon as does the so-called "cancer family syndrome." Other predisposing diseases include ulcerative colitis, Crohn's colitis, and certain polyps (described previously).

The peak incidence of colon cancer occurs at about 70 years of age, but incidences begin to increase in the fourth decade of life. While rectal cancer is more common in men, colon cancer appears to be more common in women.

Clinical Presentation

The clinical signs and symptoms of colorectal cancer are determined largely by the anatomic location. Cancers that are confined to the right colon are usually exophytic lesions that are associated with occult blood loss and result in iron deficiency anemia (Table 18.1). Advanced stages of the disease may reveal the presence of a palpable right lower abdominal mass. In re-

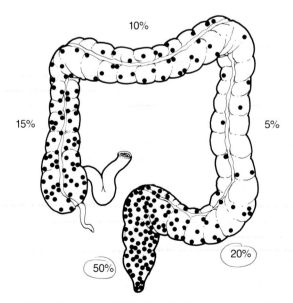

Figure 18.9. Frequency distribution of adenocarcinoma of the colon and rectum.

Table 18.1.
Symptoms of Colon and Rectal Cancers

	Right Colon	Left Colon	Rectum
Weight loss	+	+/0	0
Mass	+	0	0
Rectal bleeding	0	+	+
Tympany	0	0	+
Virchow's node	+	0	0
Blumer's shelf	+	+	0
Anemia	+	0	0
Obstruction	0	+	+

cent years there have been retrospective studies that indicate that the incidence of right colon cancers is increasing at a greater rate than that of left colon cancers. At the present time right-sided lesions may account for as much as one-third of all new cases being seen, with most being diagnosed in a late stage. Cancers arising primarily in the left colon and sigmoid colon are more frequently annular and invasive resulting in obstruction and rectal bleeding of a macroscopic nature (Table 18.1). Cancers confined to the rectum (which is defined as the terminal 12–14 cm of large bowel) also present with a symptom complex of rectal bleeding, obstruction, and occasionally alternating diarrhea and constipation. Tenesmus is frequently associated with far advanced disease.

Diagnosis

Any patient with a change of bowel habits, iron deficiency anemia, or rectal bleeding should undergo the following diagnostic studies: (1) a digital rectal examination with hemoccult testing to rule out occult blood, (2) flexible sigmoidoscopy, (3) barium enema (Fig. 18.10 A, B). If rectal bleeding occurs, workup for a possible malignancy should be initiated even if the "apparent" source is a benign lesion such as hemorrhoids.

If the results of all of these are nonconclusive, a total colon survey by flexible colonoscopy should be considered. Bright red rectal bleeding should always be evaluated by an examination of the perianal region, digital rectal exam, and flexible sigmoidoscopy. The value of preoperative total colonoscopy lies in its ability to detect the 3–5% of patients with synchronous colon cancers, thus allowing one to plan more appropriately the surgical therapy as well as to identify the presence of any associated nonmalignant polyps. Liver scans and computed tomography of the abdomen are not indicated prior to surgery. Preoperative blood tests should be designed to evaluate the patient's overall nutritional status but should include liver function tests and a carcinoembryonic antigen study. The latter test is elevated in many gastrointestinal malignancies and while not specific for colorectal cancer may be useful in following patients after resection to detect recurrence.

Frequently, diagnostic studies will reveal an obstructing lesion in the sigmoid colon that occurs in the presence of diverticulae but is suspicious for malignancy. Because both conditions may coexist and it is occasionally impossible to distinguish between the two, the surgeon should proceed with a "cancer operation" whenever there is any question. Diverticular stricture, polyp, benign tumors, ischemic stricture, and Crohn's colitis should be included in the differential diagnosis.

Treatment

Metastases from colon and rectal cancer can occur in a variety of ways—the most common of which is regional lymph node metastasis. Removal of the lymphatics draining the tumor region should be a part of the operation as nodal involvement will be present in over 50% of specimens. Colorectal cancer may also spread by direct extension, hematogenously, intraluminally, and by peritoneal seeding (Blumer's shelf on rectal exam). The most common organ involved in distal colorectal metastases is the liver.

The surgical treatment employed by the majority of surgeons in the United States includes adequate local excision of the cancer with a length of normal bowel on either side of the tumor and resection of the potentially involved lymph-node draining basin found in the mesentery that is determined by the vascular supply. There may be a certain subset of patients with carcinoma of the colon and rectum with lymph node metastasis at a site fairly distant from the primary lesion who may be rendered disease free by the surgical resection.

Patients whose tumors are no longer confined to the bowel and are adherent to extraperitoneal structures in the pelvis, upper abdomen, or other area should have en bloc resections whenever possible with the area being subsequently marked with metal clips to identify the area of potential recurrence. When the small bowel is involved, it should be included en bloc in the resection because most studies indicate that its involvement does not indicate a difference in the stage-for-stage prognosis. Similarly a partial cystectomy or total hysterectomy should be performed with the resection of the tumor if it is adherent to these organs. Bilateral oophorectomy is recommended by some in menopausal or postmenopausal women due to the high incidence of asymptomatic ovarian metastasis.

Tumors of the cecum and ascending colon are treated by right hemicolectomy that includes resection of the distal portion of the ileum and all of the colon to the midtransverse colon with an ileo-midtransverse colon anastomosis (Fig. 18.11). Lesions that are present in the hepatic flexure are best treated by an extended right colectomy that includes resection to the level of midtransverse colon or beyond. Lesions in the transverse colon or splenic flexure are best treated by a transverse colectomy with complete mobilization and removal of both hepatic and splenic flexures, and anastomosis of ileum to descending colon. Left-sided lesions are treated by a left hemicolectomy that includes resections from the level of the midtransverse colon to the sigmoid. Sigmoid colon lesions are treated by sigmoid re-

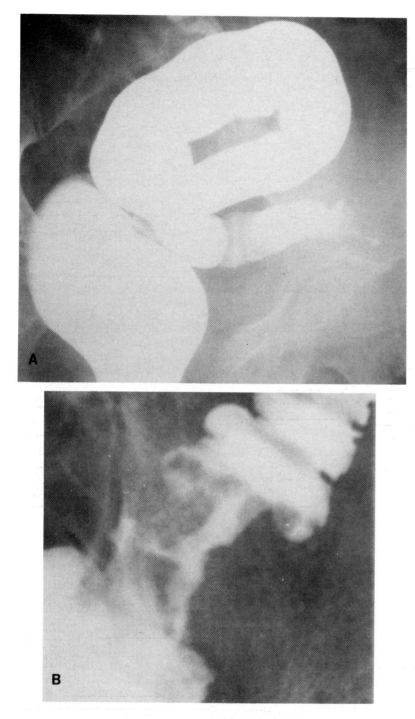

Figure 18.10. A, Carcinoma of the sigmoid colon causing total obstruction. **B,** After administration of antispasmodic agents, barium demonstrates an annular carcinoma.

section. However, sigmoid lesions that are more difficult due to obstruction may require left hemicolectomy and sigmoid colectomy. Obstructive or perforating tumors that prevent bowel preparation and a primary anastomosis should be treated by resection, diverting colostomy, and Hartmann's pouch or mucous fistula.

Tumors in the upper third of the rectum may be treated by a low anterior resection with primary anastomosis. Tumors in the middle and lower third of the rectum require specialized procedures such as a low anterior resection done with a stapled anastomosis or an abdominoperineal resection with permanent end-sigmoid colostomy. In certain selected high-risk patients, when the expertise and the equipment is available, patients with lesions in the rectum that are less than 2 cm and that are exophytic may be treated by local ablation using the laser. There are, in addition, certain surgeons who include fulguration and/or local excision for treatment of these small lesions with very careful follow-up. Following the surgical procedure, the patient's disease stage is defined. A clinical staging system does not exist for colon cancer, and therefore final pathological staging is utilized. A system of stag-

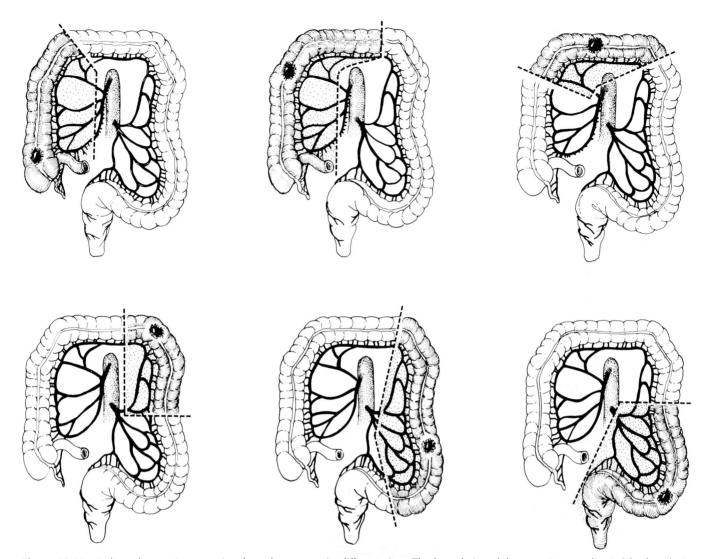

Figure 18.11. Indicated operative resection for colon cancer in different sites. The boundaries of the resection are dictated by lymphatic drainage patterns that parallel the blood supply.

Duke's staging of colon CA.

ing large bowel cancer was first proposed by Dr. Dukes over 50 years ago (Table 18.2). There have been subsequent modifications, particularly those by Astler-Coller, and the subsequent development of the TNM (tumors, nodes, metastases) system by the Joint Committee on End Stage Results. There have been other attempts to look at clusters of prognostic factors (tumor markers and size of lesion) and elements that are not included in Dukes' original classification, which was based on depth of invasion.

The use of adjuvant therapies in the treatment of colon and rectal carcinoma has generated considerable research in the last several decades. The main outcome from the randomized trials with 5-fluorouracil (5-FU) as a single agent in an adjuvant setting was that no improvement occurred in the disease-free interval or increase in cure rate when compared with surgery alone. Thus, one should not recommend adjuvant chemotherapy outside of a clinical trial. → *not helpful*

The utilization of radiation as an adjuvant, particularly for rectal tumors, is a different matter. For rectal tumors that have completely penetrated the rectal wall, with or without lymph node metastases, there is a high risk of recurrence despite the most radical surgical procedure. The risk of recurrence ranges from 30–40%. The question of whether or not to choose preoperative radiation or postoperative radiation would seem to be strictly a matter of choice. However, postoperative radiation seems to be more widely applicable since it permits a selection based on the final pathologic staging and prevents treating patients who are not at risk for local recurrence, as well as eliminating those who are not candidates because of distant disease. The usual tumoricidal doses of approximately 5000 rads can be tolerated in the postoperative period if the surgeon and the radiation oncologist plan the adjuvant radiation therapy prior to surgery even if it is to be given in a postoperative setting. Well-conducted trials have clearly indicated that postoperative radiotherapy prevents recurrence and, thus, increases the disease-free interval and survival rates.

For those patients who have had curative resection

Table 18.2.
Dukes-Astler-Coller System

Stage	Description	5-Year Survival Rate (%)
A	Confined to the mucosa	85–90
B1	Negative nodes; extension into, but not through, the muscularis propria	70–75
B2	Negative nodes; extension through the muscularis propria	60–65
C1	Same level of penetration, but with positive nodes	30–35
C2	Same level of penetration as B2, but with positive nodes	25
D	Distant metastases	<5

and for whom no adjuvant therapy is appropriate, the question of followup surveillance is one of maximal importance to the practitioner. Certain large centers have recommended monthly physical examination, bimonthly carcinoembryonic levels, and either endoscopy or barium enema every 6 months for the first 2 years of followup because the majority of recurrences occur within the first 18–24 months. The use of carcinoembryonic antigen (CEA) is well established with recurrence suggested not by the absolute level of the CEA but, rather, a progressive rise. A progressive rise mandates a complete evaluation of the patient including liver scan, computed tomography, and possible second-look surgical procedure. While there are not a large number of patients who will benefit from this, a sufficient number will benefit to make initiating this thorough survey worthwhile. The prognosis of colon and rectal carcinoma is dependent upon the classification detailed in Table 18.2.

Ulcerative Colitis and Crohn's Disease of the Colon

In addition to the material contained here, the student should refer to Chapter 17 (Small Intestine and Appendix) for discussion of ulcerative colitis and Crohn's disease. Ulcerative colitis is an idiopathic inflammatory bowel disorder involving the mucosa and submucosa of the large bowel and rectum. It occurs in a bimodal distribution with regards to age. The first and largest peak (two-thirds of all cases) includes ages 15–30 while the second, smaller peak (one-third of all cases) occurs around age 55. The disease is slightly more common in Western countries and its annual incidence is 10 per 100,000 population. A family history of ulcerative colitis is positive in 20% of patients, suggesting a genetic predisposition to the disease.

The exact etiology and underlying causative agent are unknown. Infectious, immunologic, genetic, and environmental factors have all been implicated but none have been proven. The female-to-male ratio of occurrence among patients with ulcerative colitis is five to four. There is an increased incidence of the disease among Jews yet it is uncommon among blacks and American Indians.

Pathologic findings include invariable involvement of the rectum (>90%) with variable proximal extension. Occasionally, the rectum alone is involved, a condition referred to as ulcerative proctitis. In contrast to Crohn's disease "skip areas" of normal bowel between diseased segments are not seen in ulcerative colitis. The mucosa is initially involved, with lymphocyte and leukocyte infiltration that then involves the submucosa with microabscess formation. The crypts of Lieberkuhn are commonly affected (crypt abscesses) but muscle layers are rarely involved. The coalescing of these abscesses and erosion of the mucosa leads to pseudopolyp formation, which is identified readily on endoscopic examination. About one-third of the patients affected with ulcerative colitis have pancolitis, where the entire colon is severely involved.

Clinical Course

The clinical presentation of ulcerative colitis is quite variable. The disease may have a sudden onset with a fulminant, life-threatening course or it may be a mild, insidious disease. Patients frequently present with watery diarrhea that contains blood, pus, and mucus accompanied by cramping, abdominal pain, tenesmus, and urgency. There are varying degrees to which the patients are afflicted with weight loss, dehydration, pain, and fever. Fever is usually indicative of multiple microabscesses and/or endotoxemia secondary to transmural bacteremia. About 55% of patients have a mild, indolent course, 30% a moderately severe course requiring large doses of prednisone or azulfidine, and 15% have a fulminant, life-threatening course. The latter presentation is often associated with massive colonic dilatation secondary to transmural progression of the disease and destruction of the myenteric plexus (toxic megacolon). Patients present with severe consti-

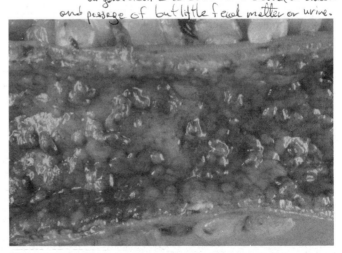

Figure 18.12. Photograph demonstrating the characteristic mucosal pattern in advanced ulcerative colitis. Ulceration, friability, and pseudopolyps are seen in this photograph.

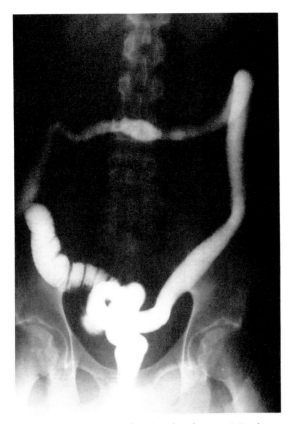

Figure 18.13. Barium enema showing the characteristic changes associated with chronic ulcerative colitis. One sees loss of the haustral pattern, ulcerations, and foreshortening. Because of these changes, the colon is said to resemble a "lead pipe."

"String sign" for Chrone's.

tutional symptoms related to sepsis, malnutrition, anemia, acid-base disturbances, and electrolyte abnormalities.

Extraintestinal manifestations occur in a smaller percentage of patients, including ankylosing spondylitis, peripheral arthritis, uveitis, pyoderma gangrenosa, sclerosing cholangitis, pericholangitis, and pericarditis. The amount of information obtained on physical examination is directly dependent upon the acuteness and severity of the disease process at the time of examination. If the patient is seen in a quiescent phase, there may be few or no findings; if the patient is seen in an acute phase, an acute abdominal condition may be present.

Diagnosis

The mainstay of diagnosis is endoscopy with biopsy. The typical endoscopic findings are those of friable, reddish mucosa with no normal intervening areas, mucosal exudates, and pseudopolyposis (Fig. 18.12). A secondary diagnostic study is barium enema (Fig. 18.13) in which mucosal irregularity may be demonstrated; frequently shortening of the colon, loss of normal haustral markings, and a "lead pipe" appearance may also be demonstrated. No specific laboratory tests are diagnostic for ulcerative colitis; however, leukocytosis

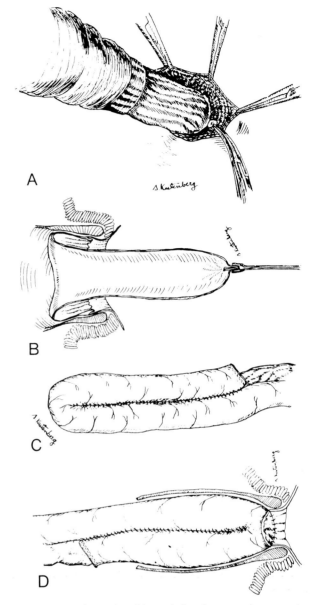

Figure 18.14. Ileoanal pullthrough has become the operation of choice for definitive treatment of ulcerative colitis and familial polyposis. **A,** After removal of the entire colon, the mucosa is stripped away from the muscular layers of the rectum. **B,** This dissection is continued down to the dentate line and the mucosa everted out through the anus and resected. **C,** A small reservoir is constructed from terminal ileum using a J-shaped configuration. **D,** This J-shaped pouch is then pulled through the muscular cuff and anastomosed to the dentate line, thus creating a neorectum.

with the presence of toxic granules and anemia may be present.

Differential diagnosis includes other inflammatory or infectious disorders, including Crohn's disease, bacterial colitis, and pseudomembranous colitis. The disease most commonly confused with ulcerative colitis is Crohn's disease involving the colon. Table 18.3 reveals distinguishing characteristics of both disease processes.

Table 18.3.
Comparison of Ulcerative Colitis and Crohn's Colitis

	Ulcerative Colitis	Crohn's Colitis
Symptoms/Signs		
Diarrhea	Severe, bloody	Less severe, bleeding infrequent
Perianal fistulas	Rare	Common
Strictures/obstruction	Uncommon	Common
Perforation	Free, uncommon	Localized, common
Pattern of Development		
Rectum	Virtually always involved (90%)	Often normal
Terminal ileum	Normal	Diseased in majority
Distribution	Continuous	Segmented, "skip lesions"
Megacolon	Frequent	Less common
Appearance		
Gross	Friable, bleeding granular exudates, pseudopolyps, isolated ulcers	Linear ulcers, transverse fissures, cobblestoning, thickening, strictures
Microscopic	Submucosa and mucosa inflamed, "crypt abscesses"; fibrosis uncommon	Transmural inflammation, granulomas, fibrosis
Radiologic	"Lead pipe," foreshortening, continuous, concentric	"String sign" in small bowel; segmental, asymmetric, internal fistulae
Course		
Natural history	Exacerbations, remissions, dramatic flareups	Exacerbations, remissions, chronic, indolent
Medical treatment	Initial response high (>80%)	Response less predictable
Surgical treatment	Curative	Palliative
Recurrence after	No	Common

Treatment

Medical therapy is usually the initial treatment and is successful in about 80% of cases. In mild disease, the treatment is primarily symptomatic with the use of antidiarrheal agents that slow gut transit (e.g. loperamide) and bulking agents (psyllium seed products) that result in semiformed, less watery stools. In more severe disease, sulfasalazine which is the antiinflammatory agent of choice, should be tried in all patients, as it is successful in inducing remission in about half of all patients initially. Steroids remain a mainstay of therapy and most patients respond dramatically to steroid administration. Unfortunately, because of severe side effects, the dose must be tapered and minimized whenever possible. Elimination of milk from the diet is occasionally helpful and supportive therapy, including physical and emotional support is important.

Major complications of ulcerative colitis are toxic megacolon, colonic perforation, massive hemorrhage, serious anorectal complications, and carcinoma development after years of disease. Initial therapy for toxic megacolon is aggressive medical care including gastric decompression, antibiotics, intravenous administration of fluids, hyperalimentation, and elimination of all other medications, specifically anticholinergics. Surgical therapy is indicated whenever medical therapy fails or surgically treatable complications ensue, such as hemorrhage, perforation, obstruction, or carcinoma. Long-standing ulcerative colitis, because of the increased risk of carcinoma, is also an indication for surgical intervention. The risk is calculated to go up 2% per year after the initial 10 years of disease. In years past, the definitive operative procedure for cure of ulcerative colitis has been total proctocolectomy with permanent ileostomy. Recently, other procedures have been devised in an attempt to maintain fecal continence, including the development of an operation that involves construction of a reservoir with a nipple valve out of the small intestine (Kock's continent ileostomy); this operation has met with only limited success. Subtotal colectomy with ileoproctostomy is attempted in some patients who have less severe rectal involvement and absolutely no perianal problems. Unfortunately, this operation does not represent a cure for the disease and subjects the patient to the risks of recurrent disease or the development of a malignancy in the remaining remnant. The operation of choice for this disease is a relatively new operation that cures the disease and yet maintains fecal continence. The operation, total colectomy with mucosal proctectomy and ileoanal anastomosis (Fig. 18.14 A–D), is usually done with an ileal reservoir and spares the patient a permanent abdominal ileostomy. Those patients with toxic megacolon, perforation, or other complications have a much higher morbidity and mortality and, thus, early surgery may be indicated.

Colonic Obstruction and Volvulus

Obstruction of the Large Intestine

Only 10–15% of intestinal obstruction in adults is the result of obstruction of the large bowel. The most frequent anatomic site of obstruction is the sigmoid colon

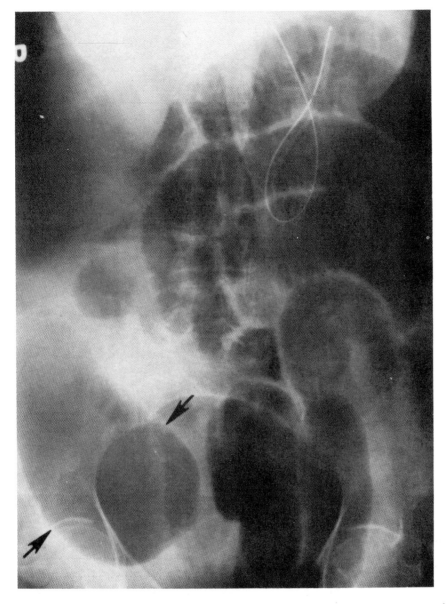

Small Bowel Obstruction:
1) Adhesions   60%
2) Hernias   20%
3) Cancer   15%

Large Bowel Obstruction:
1) adenocarcinoma   65%
2) scarring 2° to
      diverticulitis   20%
3) volvulus   5%

Figure 18.15. Carcinoma of the transverse colon (arrows) causing cecal and small bowel distention.

N.B.: "closed-loop" obstruction

and the three most common causes of complete colonic obstruction are adenocarcinoma (65%), scarring associated with diverticulitis (20%), and volvulus (5%). Inflammatory disorders, benign tumors, foreign bodies, and other miscellaneous problems account for the remainder. Obstructive adhesive bands, as seen in the small bowel, are extremely uncommon in the colon.

Signs and symptoms include abdominal distension with or without tenderness, cramping abdominal pain, usually manifesting in the hypogastrium, and nausea and vomiting. Radiologic findings demonstrate distended proximal colon, air-fluid levels, and no distal rectal air (Fig. 18.15).

An important element that affects the clinical expression of large bowel obstruction is whether or not the ileocecal valve is competent. If the valve is incompetent, the signs and symptoms produced are indistinguishable from those of routine small bowel obstruction. If the colon has a competent ileocecal valve, as is the case with approximately 75% of the patients, a so-called "closed loop" obstruction results between the ileocecal valve and the obstructing point distally. Massive colonic distention results and the cecum may reach a diameter of 12 cm, thus increasing the possibility of perforation with or without gangrene. Physical examination usually reveals abdominal distention, tympany, high-pitched metallic rushes, and gurgles. On palpation, a localized, tender, palpable mass may indicate a strangulated closed loop or an area of inflamed diverticular disease. All patients with large bowel obstructions should be treated with intravenous fluids, nasogastric suction, sigmoidoscopy, and continuous observation, preferably in an intensive care unit, until the diagnosis is established and definitive therapy is undertaken. Potentially lethal complications of large bowel obstruction are perforation and abdominal peritonitis and sepsis. The major causes of severe colonic obstruction leading to these complications include car-

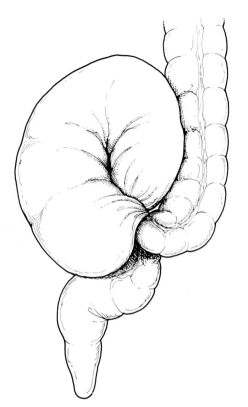

Figure 18.16.   Volvulus of the sigmoid colon.

cinoma of the colon, with or without perforation, diverticulitis, sigmoid volvulus, or cecal volvulus. The appropriate diagnostic techniques include plain films of the abdomen; in those patients in whom the cecum measures more than 12 cm and a definitive lesion cannot be delineated, laparotomy is undertaken. Use of barium enema will confirm the diagnosis of colonic obstruction and identify the exact location. If the obstruction is delineated on plain abdominal films, barium enema is not necessary. Barium should never be given orally in the presence of suspected colonic obstruction. Colonoscopic examination has a major role to play in Ogilvie's syndrome; otherwise, it is reserved for the occasional case of volvulus for decompression. Emergency laparotomy is undertaken for acute large bowel obstruction with cecal distention beyond 12 cm, severe tenderness, evidence of peritonitis, or generalized sepsis. Perforation due to volvulus, obstructing cancers, or diverticular strictures usually results in laparotomy with the appropriate surgical procedures; these usually include resection and diverting colostomy.

For the occasional case of Ogilvie's syndrome where there is enormous dilatation of the right colon without mechanical obstruction (pseudo-obstruction), the currently recommended therapy is fiberoptic colonoscopy, with decompression and placement of a long rectal decompression tube. Cecostomy may be necessary in cases of recurrence.

The various conditions leading to large bowel obstruction result in differing prognoses, most of which are dependent upon the age and the comorbidity of existing diseases in the patient, particularly with regard to cardiovascular disease. The major predictive feature is the presence or absence of perforation, regardless of the cause of obstruction and the promptness of surgical management. Unfortunately, the overall death rate of patients who have a cecal perforation approaches 30%. Thus, prompt laparotomy is the mainstay in treatment of large bowel obstruction.

Volvulus of the Large Intestine

Volvulus may be defined as rotation of a segment of the intestine on the axis formed by the mesentery (Fig. 18.16). The most frequent sites of occurrence in the large bowel are the sigmoid (70%) and cecum (30%). They account for almost 5–10% of all cases of large bowel obstruction and are the second most common cause of complete colonic obstruction. Stretching and elongation of the sigmoid with age is a predisposing factor, as witnessed by the fact that over 50% of the patients are 65 years of age or older at the time of their first occurrence. For unknown reasons, patients who are confined to mental institutions or nursing homes have an increased risk of this disease. Volvulus also occurs in those patients who have hypermobile cecums, owning to incomplete fixation of the ascending colon at the time of intrauterine development. This allows the cecum to twist about the mesentery, forming a closed loop obstruction at the entry and exit points with major pressure at the sites of the twist. The vessels are partially occluded and circulatory impairment leads to prompt gangrene and perforation. The patient presents with abdominal distention, often massive, as well as vomiting, abdominal pain, obstipation, and tachypnea. Physical examination reveals distention, tympany, high-pitched tinkling sounds, and rushes. Diagnostic studies involve abdominal x-ray films and barium enemas. Abdominal x-rays reveal a massively dilated cecum or sigmoid without haustra that often assumes a kidney-bean appearance. Barium enema reveals the exact site of obstruction with a characteristic funnel-like narrowing often resembling a "bird's beak" or "ace of spades." Sigmoidoscopy with rectal tube insertion in order to decompress sigmoid volvulus is the recommended initial treatment for that location. Emergency operation, however, is performed promptly if strangulation or perforation is suspected or if attempts to decompress the bowel are unsuccessful. Surgical therapy involves resection without anastomosis and the creation of a temporary colostomy. Most patients with sigmoid volvulus are easily decompressed conservatively and subsequently require elective resection, except in very poor risk elderly patients. Cecal volvulus is virtually always treated surgically either by cecopexy (suturing the cecum to parietal peritoneum) or right hemicolectomy with ileotransverse colostomy if cecum is gangrenous.

Anorectum

The anorectum is the site of a number of disease conditions that cause great discomfort and consterna-

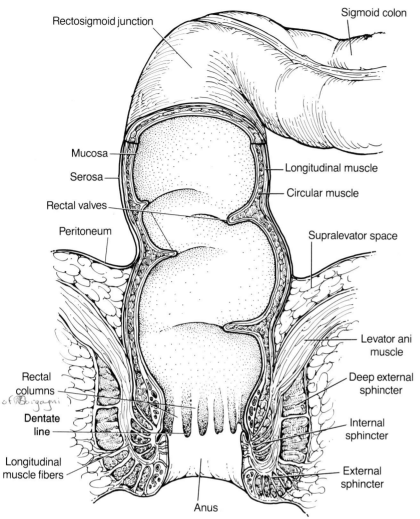

Figure 18.17. Normal anatomy of the anorectal canal.

tion to the patient due to lumps, bleeding, and pain that occur in this area with some frequency. An understanding of this important alimentary junction is necessary because the anal canal and rectum have different epithelia, different nerve supplies and lymphatics, and different venous drainage patterns. All of these differences affect the expression of disease in this area.

Anatomy and Physiology

The anal canal is approximately 3 cm long and comprises the distance from the anal verge to the dentate or pectinate line (Fig. 18.17). The lining of the canal is squamous cell epithelium that contains somatic sensory nerves and responds to painful stimuli. The junction between the columnar epithelium of the rectum and the anoderm is marked by the dentate line. Immediately proximal to the dentate line are longitudinal folds called the columns of Morgagni. At the distal base of these columns are blind sacs called anal crypts into which the anal glands secrete. Perirectal abscesses usually originate in this area. The anoderm venous system drains into the caval system whereas the rectum generally drains into the portal system. A plexus of small veins (hemorrhoidal plexus) connecting the two systems often becomes distended and enlarged leading to hemorrhoidal disease.

The anorectal sphincteric apparatus is composed of an outer external sphincter, which is striated, voluntary muscle, and an inner, smooth involuntary muscle. Also important in this mechanism are the puborectalis sling and the levator ani muscles.

Arterial perfusion of the area is derived from a branch of the inferior mesenteric artery (superior hemorrhoidal) for upper rectum and branches of the hypogastric artery (internal pudendal) via the middle and inferior hemorrhoidal arteries for middle and lower rectum.

When a bolus of stool distends the upper rectum, autonomic nerve stimulation results in proximal colon contraction and internal sphincter relaxation distally, thus facilitating defecation.

Examination of this area should be a routine part of every physical examination. Inspection reveals fissures, hemorrhoids, fistulae, excoriation, and tumors. Digital examination reveals tumors, polyps, fluctuance, *internal hemorrhoids* { 1°, 2° & 3° hemorrhoids → banding → excellent results ; 4° hemorrhoids → surgical excision

bogginess, weak sphincters, and nodal disease. Anoscopy allows detection of more subtle lesions such as ulcers, villous adenomas, and infectious disorders.

Hemorrhoids

The most important system relative to the development of hemorrhoids is the venous drainage system including the inferior hemorrhoidal veins that connect directly to the systemic circulation. The venous drainage system also includes the superior hemorrhoidal system that drains the upper rectum into the portal system via the inferior mesenteric vein.

The rectum derives its nerve supply from both the sympathetic and parasympathetic systems via complex plexes. The rectum is relatively insensitive to touch but quite sensitive to stretching and distention. Below the dentate line, the somatic nerves make the anal canal sensitive to touch because of increased frequency of receptors. While surgical manipulation above the dentate line causes no discomfort, anesthesia of some type must be used when procedures are done below the dentate line. Hemorrhoids are associated with a number of variables that may be causal. Excessive straining at stool, a low-residue diet, pregnancy, and excessive exercise are frequently associated factors, but others include increased anal sphincter tone, musculoskeletal disease, and systemic abnormalities such as portal hypertension. Hemorrhoids are not simply varicose veins but represent a complex of the vascular cushion that contains venous and arterial components.

Treatment of hemorrhoids depends upon their designation as either internal or external. Internal hemorrhoids, by definition, arise above the dentate line and are covered by the insensitive rectal mucosa, whereas external hemorrhoids originate below the dentate line and are covered by the generously innervated epithelial component of the anoderm. The hemorrhoidal plexes are most commonly described as being in the left lateral, right anterior, and right posterior anal canal. The symptoms of external hemorrhoids usually include severe pain that develops when they undergo thrombosis. Conversely, internal hemorrhoids often present with discomfort, bleeding, and prolapse. Physicians are now able to direct their therapy based upon classification of internal hemorrhoids. First degree hemorrhoids may be defined as those that do not prolapse. Second degree hemorrhoids occasionally prolapse into the anal canal and spontaneously reduce after defecation. Third degree hemorrhoids prolapse with straining and coughing and frequently require manual reduction. Fourth degree hemorrhoids remain partially prolapsed at all times and cannot be reduced. A finding of hemorrhoids requires examination and inspection using the anoscope. However, the rectal and perineal exam should be sufficiently thorough to rule out other concomitant disease such as rectal prolapse, prurituis, anorectal inflammation, cancers, and inflammatory bowel disease. There are advocates for all of the following modalities of therapy for hemorrhoids: (1) sclerotherapy; (2) cryosurgery; (3) dietary manipu-

lation; (4) banding; and (5) surgical hemorrhoidectomy. It is the author's experience that banding techniques for first, second, and occasionally third degree hemorrhoids has met with excellent results in most patients. Surgical excision is required in most patients with fourth degree hemorrhoids.

Evaluation of patients with hemorrhoids always includes a careful history. Review of the patient's general health history in addition to his or her colon and rectal complaints should always be investigated. A distended anal canal in the absence of local pathologic changes, for example, may indicate a neurologic disease or may merely be a variation of the normal. The checklist below may be helpful to the investigator in obtaining a quick proctologic profile of patients presenting with hemorrhoids and may help differentiate hemorrhoids from other diseases. For instance, a decrease in the diameter of stools may suggest an anal stricture, benign or malignant. Ribbon-shaped stools have frequently been associated with malignant anorectal tumors. The examining physician should inquire about the following signs and symptoms, their duration, and rapidity of onset:

1. *Bleeding:* What is the amount? Is it unmixed or mixed with stool? Is it bright red or dark red blood?
2. *Constipation:* Are laxatives, enemas, or suppositories used?
3. *Diarrhea:* What is the frequency of bowel movements during a 24-hour period?
4. *Discharge:* What is the type, color, and consistency?
5. *Itching:* How severe? Is it limited to anus only? Does it worsen at night?
6. *Mucus:* What color? Is it bloody? Is it coagulated?
7. *Pain of the anorectal area:* Is it constant or only after bowel movement? What is the nature of the pain (throbbing, burning, etc.)? Is it worse on coughing or straining?
8. *Protrusion:* What is the extent? Is it constant or at bowel movement only?
9. *Stools:* Are they of unusual diameter or uneven formation? Are they soft or hard?
10. *Tenesmus:* Is there a frequent or constant urge for bowel movement?

After examination of the abdomen, complete evaluation of the perianal region is carried out. First, one should begin with an inspection of the anal area. The patient may lie on his side or in the knee-chest position. The buttocks are slowly and carefully separated in order not to aggravate any existing pain. The anus should be inspected under brightly lighted conditions. Fissures may be detected by spreading the skin of the anal area or by observing the small tag of skin in the posterior anal margin. One should be careful to examine for masses, perianal disease, protruding external hemorrhoids, skin irritation, lichenification, or hyperemia of the skin. A peeling white or crusting area is suggestive of fungus infection; the physician should also note sphincter spasm, ulceration, fistulas, draining sinuses, cysts, warts, and discharges.

The examination should then proceed with a gentle digital examination. The tension and force of contraction of the internal and external sphincters can be evaluated with the examining finger, as well as sites and origin of pain secondary to abscesses, fissures, and in males, evaluation of various prostate conditions. Benign polyps can occasionally be differentiated from the solid masses associated with adenocarcinoma. Stenosis and tumors can be detected, as well as characteristics of the coccyx, prostrate, and cervix uteri. Occasionally, masses involving the cul-de-sac may be found including Blumer's shelf, which is a firm mass in the cul-de-sac secondary to metastasis, usually from a gastrointestinal malignancy. Fluctuant masses due to pelvic abscess may be palpated and digital examination may help with the differential diagnosis of diverticulitis, appendicitis with or without perforation, and adnexal female disease. One must always differentiate the normal tenderness associated with the exam in patients with a low pain threshold.

The examining physician is now ready to progress to instrumentation and examination of the anorectal canal. The instruments available are the anoscope, the rigid sigmoidoscope, and the flexible sigmoidoscope. The usual preparation includes administration of an enema just prior to sigmoidoscopic examination. The inverted knee-chest position on a power table is frequently used; however, the patient may be examined adequately in the lateral position. Preparation should consist of physician reassurance and an explanation of the procedure in order to minimize any anxiety. The anoscope is gently inserted and complete inspection of the entire anoderm and the anal canal is carried out. The patient is asked to bear down in order to recreate conditions occuring at bowel movement. When symptoms are detected in the anal canal and visible rectum, no further examination should be carried out until these conditions are successfully treated.

Most hemorrhoids can be successfully treated conservatively with stool softeners, stool bulking agents, sitz baths, and topical anesthetics. The preferred method of treatment for refractory symptomatic internal hemorrhoids is rubber band ligation (Fig. 18.18). Local anesthesia is usually required to obtain sphincter relaxation and insertion of the operating anoscope. The operation consists of the following steps: The apex of the internal hemorrhoid is grasped and drawn through the double-sleeve cylinder of the pistol with the loaded elastic band. The hemorrhoid is completely drawn into the inner cylinder, the trigger is pulled, and the elastic band is attached around the base of the hemorrhoid. The hemorrhoid undergoes eventual degeneration and sloughs over variable lengths of time. The great advantage of this particular treatment is that it can be repeated, usually at intervals not more frequently than every 3 weeks. For large stage III prolapsing hemorrhoids that cannot be treated using the banding method, actual excision of the hemorrhoids must be carried out. The preferred technique is the closed technique of hemorrhoidectomy where the wound created by excision is closed completely to the level of the anoderm.

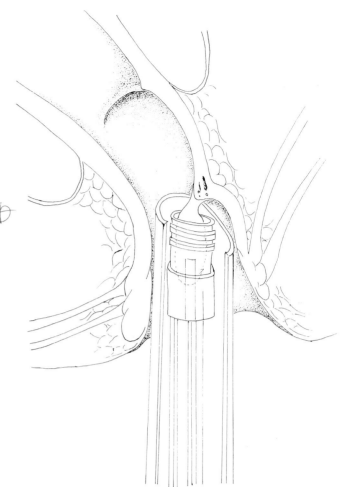

Figure 18.18. Illustration demonstrating the "banding technique" for hemorrhoidal treatment.

The amount of therapy offered for external hemorrhoids is a function of degree of pain. The application of anesthetic ointments and sitz baths, as well as application of 1% hydrocortisone foam may suffice in many instances. If a single, well-delineated external thrombotic hemorrhoid is present, a small amount of local anesthesia may be introduced, a simple eliptical incision made, and the clot evacuated. The wound margins fall together and only pressure is needed to control bleeding. When there is bleeding, it can be controlled by fulguration, ligation, or closure of the skin. Multiple confluent external hemorrhoids require hemorrhoidectomy. This requires multiple incisions as described above through which the venous plexes are dissected and excised. Multiple skin incisions often heal better than incisions used in radical excision to remove the hemorrhoids. Postoperative care includes meticulous anal hygiene, warm water soaks, soaked pads, and stool softeners. Long-term management of patients who have had either internal or external hemorrhoids should also include the uses of stool bulking agents.

Anorectal Abscesses and Fistula-In-Ano

The major types of abscesses found in the perianal area can be classified as follows: (1) infralevator (common), including perianal, ischiorectal, and postanal abscesses, and (2) supralevator (rare), including postrectal and pelvirectal abscesses. Most of these abscesses develop from crypts that are present at the dentate line and become infected. The infecting organisms burrow into the anal glands, producing circumscribed areas of microabscesses in the subcutaneous, submucosal, and intramuscular perirectal regions of the rectum. They present with perianal cellulitis and diffuse inflammation, characterized by generalized edema, swelling, and redness that is not yet localized.

Other abscesses begin at sites other than crypts, as in Crohn's disease and, rarely, in tuberculosis. While they may begin anywhere in the anal canal or the rectum, the etiology of noncryptitic abscesses is not clearly understood. The signs and symptoms of patients presenting with perirectal abscesses include pain as the overwhelmingly most common presenting symptom. A few patients may present with systemic symptoms such as fever, chills, generalized malaise, nausea, and vomiting. The physician should be most suspicious of a supralevator abscess in patients who present with rectal pain and systemic symptoms. If a diagnosis cannot be made by inspection and palpation, with clear delineation of the swelling and induration, a digital examination may reveal the diagnosis, locating the presence of the abscess higher in the anal canal or the perianal tissue. The preferred technique for confirming the diagnostic impression is needle aspiration of the pus under local anesthesia. For those abscesses that are clearly delineated externally and have a "pointing" area, dermal injection of local anesthesia over the area of maximum flucuation followed by adequate incision and drainage, including excision of a portion of the skin, is clearly the surgical procedure of choice. The incision should be as wide as the fluctuating area. There are some proponents of packing the wound with gauze for several days; however, the preferred technique is inserting a drain, suturing the drain in place, and beginning prompt local therapy. Perirectal abscesses in children require general anesthesia; this may be performed on an outpatient basis. Additionally, all patients should be educated with regard to the necessity for followup. Following an acute abscess, patients will require additional observation and therapy. Patients may subsequently develop a fistula that is an abnormal passage between the interior of the anal canal or rectum and the skin surface. Nearly all fistulas begin with anorectal abscess formation. The hallmark of a fistula is a history of a previous abscess followed by purulent discharge and drainage of pus or stool from the perianal area. Localized skin irritation with associated symptoms of itching and swelling are present. Occasional recurring obstruction of fistulas produce pain and recurrent abscesses; obstruction may also present with inability to control flatus that escapes spontane-

ously by the fistulous tract. Major definitive diagnostic procedures include complete inspection, palpation, digital examination, and insertion of a probe through the skin opening. The margin of the fistula is most likely delineated at a crypt, which is easily visualized using an operating anoscope. Anal fistulas will rarely heal spontaneously and thus are treated almost exclusively by surgery. The fistulous tract must be opened up along with the source of infection (usually a crypt). After the crypt is opened and complete hemostasis is accomplished using electrocautery, rapid healing usually occurs. In a patient with a very long anal canal and a very deep fistula that extends into the rectum or has numerous openings, the fistula needs to be completely excised. In those instances in which the sphincter is transected, prompt repair of the sphincter is required in order to prevent incontinence.

Fissure-In-Ano

painful linear ulcer at the margin of the anus.

Fissure-in-ano is a painful linear ulcer at the margin of the anus. Constipation or diarrhea are the most likely historical antecedents, usually combined with anxiety over prolonged periods of time, producing anal abrasions and acute ulcers at the anal verge. The ulcer is frequently associated with infections in the crypts, an enlarged papilla, associated skin tags, and a narrow anal canal. Anal fissures may also develop secondary to anal surgery, proctitis, or basal cell carcinoma of the anus. A fissure may be one of the most painful conditions encountered by a surgeon. The pain is clearly disproportionate to the size of the lesion, occurs at defecation, and persists for several hours. The patient may never be pain free. Small amounts of bright red blood, which are not mixed with stool, are a common association. Inspection reveals an external skin tag. Frequently, simple gentle separation of the skin of the anal verge reveals the ulcer posteriorly. The internal sphincter muscle may be seen at the base of the punched-out ulcer; another cardinal sign is an enlarged papilla.

Diagnosis is made by inspection. The fissure can be distinguished from lesions caused by Crohn's disease, leukemia, or malignancy in that it is usually clear, punched out, and not large or indolent. Fissures are rarely multiple. The use of topical anesthetic lubricant upon digital inspection and palpation, plus insertion of a stricture anoscope, are helpful in diagnosis. Treatment of fissure usually depends on the duration of the existence of the condition. Fissures that are acute and have been present for less than two weeks may respond to nonoperative therapy consisting of good anal hygiene, cleansing with sponges, and the application of hydrocortisone foam or suppositories. The patient should also be placed on a high residue diet. For severe pain, an anesthetic ointment can be applied with finger cots. Conditions that have been present longer than two weeks will generally require surgical therapy. Associated conditions, such as skin tags and papillae, need to be excised and any associated internal or external hemorrhoids should be removed. Many surgeons currently employ a partial internal spincterotomy, which releases the thickened spasmed sphincter and has given good results in simple fissures. Most of these surgical procedures can be carried out in the outpatient clinic or single-day surgery.

Anal Malignancy
→ epidermoid carcinoma
→ malignant melanoma

The student should also be familiar with the neoplasms arising in the area of the anus. There are essentially two major types: epidermoid carcinoma and malignant melanoma. Epidermoid carcinoma constitutes less than 2% of all anorectal carcinomas. Squamous cell carcinoma occurs with equal frequency above and below the dentate line and has had a relatively poor prognosis. Delay in diagnosis is frequently a function of both patient and physician neglect. The primary symptoms are rectal pain and bleeding. Therapy of squamous cell carcinoma has been primarily surgical in the past but there is an emerging role for radiotherapy combined with adjuvant chemotherapy. The treatment of choice in the past has been abdominoperineal resection with wide excision of perineal node-bearing tissues. However, excellent results have been obtained with combined radiation therapy and chemotherapy; this regimen spares the sphincter and provides comparable survival rates.

One of the major areas of controversy centers around the surgery for lymph nodes. The final resolution of whether or not prophylactic lymph node dissection should be carried out is as yet still unclear; however, most practitioners feel that patients benefit from excision of palpable nodes and close follow-up with subsequent inguinal node dissections when clinically apparent disease is present. The overall incidence of inguinal node involvement in these patients is 35–40%. The appropriate type of groin dissection is radical groin dissection with complete evacuation of both the superficial and deep inguinal node basins.

Malignant melanoma, a relatively rare disorder of the anal canal, requires diligence in early detection and therapy. The tumors can be generally considered treatable in the same category as melanomas in other parts of the body; however, this requires accurate staging and treatment. Students should consult Chapter 27 for information on staging and thickness of melanomas. The tumors arise from the epidermal lining of the anal canal and present with rectal bleeding, although pruritus may be a component. The major difficulty in diagnosis is the lack of pigmentation in a fairly high percentage of these tumors. Treatment should be early radical surgery. Once again, the management of the lymph node basins is important, although less so in melanoma than in the epidermoid carcinomas, primarily due to the high rate of hematogenous spread and the poor prognosis that these patients have with lung and liver involvement.

SUGGESTED READINGS

Adams D, Kovalcik PJ: Fistula in ano. *Surg Gynecol Obstet* 151:731, 1981.

Anuras S, Shirazi SS: Colonic pseudo-obstruction. *Am J Gastroenterol* 79:525, 1984.

August L, Wise L: Surgical management of perforated diverticulitis. *Am J Surg* 141:122, 1981.

Boyd JB, Bradford B Jr, Watne A: Operative risk factors of colon resection in the elderly. *Ann Surg* 192:742, 1980.

Chrabot CM, Prasad ML, Abcarian H: Recurrent anorectal abscesses. *Dis Colon Rectum* 265:105, 1983.

Classen JN: Surgical treatment of acute diverticulitis by stage procedures. *Ann Surg* 184:582, 1976.

Deveney KE, Way LW: Follow-up of patients with colorectal cancer. *Am J Surg* 148:717, 1984.

Evans JT, Vana J, Aronoff BL, Baker HW, Murphy GP: Management and survival of carcinoma of the colon: results of a national survey by the American College of Surgeons. *Ann Surg* 188:716, 1978.

Goldenberg HS: Supralevator abscess. *Surgery* 91:164, 1982.

Hass PA, Fox TA, Hass GP: The pathogenesis of hemorrhoids. *Dis Colon Rectum* 27:442, 1984.

Khubchandani IT: A randomized comparison of single and multiple rubber band ligations. *Dis Colon Rectum* 26:705, 1983.

Lavery IC, Jagelman DG: Cancer in the excluded rectum following surgery for inflammatory bowel disease. *Dis Colon Rectum* 25:522, 1982.

Maxfield RG: Colonoscopy as a routine preoperative procedure for carcinoma of the colon. *Am J Surg* 147:477, 1984.

Murrie JA, Sim AJ, Mackenzie I: Rubber band ligation vs. hemorrhoidectomy for prolapsing hemorrhoids: a long-term prospective clinical trial. *Br J Surg* 69:536, 1982.

Ray JE, Penfold JC, Gathright JB Jr: Lateral subcutaneous internal anal sphincterotomy for anal fissure. *Dis Colon Rectum* 17:139, 1974.

Reid JDS, Robins RE, Atkinson KG: Pelvic recurrence after anterior resection EEA stapling anastomosis for potentially curable carcinoma of the rectum. *Am J Surg* 147:629, 1984.

Riddell RH, et al: Dysplasia in inflammatory bowel disease: standardized classification and the provisional clinical applications. *Hum Pathol* 14:931, 1983.

Sanfey H, Bayless TM, Cameron JL: Crohn's disease of the colon: is there a role for limited resection? *Am J Surg* 147:38, 1984.

Umpleby HC, Williamson RCN: Survival in acute obstructing colorectal carcinoma. *Dis Colon Rectum* 27:299, 1984.

Skills

1. The student should demonstrate the ability to perform a thorough digital rectal exam including use of the guaiac test for stool blood.

2. The student should be familiar with the flexible sigmoidoscope and indications for its use.

3. The student should demonstrate competence in reading a barium enema.

4. The student should demonstrate the ability to perform anoscopy.

5. The student should be able to write orders for a preoperative bowel prep.

6. The student should be able to point out the dentate line in a patient undergoing anorectal surgery.

Study Questions _____

1. How does the blood supply of the right colon differ from that of the left colon? What is the marginal artery of Drummond?

2. What are the indications for surgery in patients with diverticular disease? With ulcerative colitis?

3. Describe six ways in which ulcerative colitis differs from Crohn's colitis.

4. What constitutes appropriate management of a patient with his first attack of uncomplicated acute diverticulitis?

5. Describe the Duke's system of prognosticating survival in colorectal cancer.

6. What is the appropriate operative procedure for a patient with a malignant tumor in the low rectum? in the high rectum? in the ascending colon? in a patient with familial polyposis?

7. Describe appropriate management of a patient who presents with large bowel obstruction secondary to sigmoid volvulus.

8. What is the most common complication of the treatment for perirectal abscess? How is that complication treated?

9. Define first, second, third, and forth degree hemorrhoids and tell how their respective forms of treatment differ.

10. What type of colonic polyps has the greatest malignant potential? Describe appropriate management for that polyp.

11. What is the most common cause of chronic, severe anal pain? How is it treated?

12. Describe the appropriate treatment for a 2-cm squamous cell carcinoma of the anus.

The Biliary Tract

Merril T. Dayton, M.D.
Jeffrey E. Doty, M.D.
Ajit K. Sachdeva, M.D.
James B. Peoples, M.D.

(handwritten margin note: usually pancreatic CA)

(handwritten notes at top of right column:)
* — Courvoisier's sign → non-gallstone obstruction of bile duct.
* — Murphy's Sign → acute cholecystitis
* — Charcot's triad (fever [high], pain [RUQ], jaundice)
  └→ "acute ascending cholangitis"

ASSUMPTIONS

The student knows the physiochemical characteristics of normal bile, its production, and the physiologic mechanism of bile salt resorption.

The student knows the mechanism for the stimulation of bile secretion and the hormonal mediators of this response.

The student knows the normal anatomy of the biliary tree and its common variations.

T tube, including purpose and circumstances of use,
Gallstone ileus.
12. Contrast carcinomas of the gallbladder, bile duct, and ampulla of Vater with regard to survival and presenting symptoms.

(handwritten notes:)
— Reynold's pentad (fever, pain, jaundice, hypotension, mental confusion)
  └→ "acute suppurative cholangitis" (pus under pressure)
  = a surgical emergency

Anatomy

The anatomy of the extrahepatic biliary system varies considerably from individual to individual and innumerable anomalies have been reported. To prevent inadvertent and frequently irreparable injury to the extrahepatic bile ducts during cholecystectomy, anticipation of anomalous anatomy and careful, bloodless dissection in this region are vitally important.

The gallbladder is a thin-walled, contractile storage bag attached to the undersurface of the liver at the anatomic division of the right and left lobes of the liver. It is usually tubular in shape, measuring about 10 cm long and 5 cm in diameter. Most commonly, 75% of the gallbladder is covered by peritoneum and the remainder is intimately attached to the liver. In some patients, the gallbladder is completely covered by peritoneum and suspended by a mesentery, or it can be almost completely embedded in the liver. In general, the less the gallbladder is attached to the liver, the easier is its surgical removal. The gallbladder itself consists of the fundus, the body, Hartmann's pouch, and the cystic duct, which is lined by the spiral valves of Heister (Fig. 19.1).

The cystic duct, which drains the gallbladder, joins the common hepatic duct, which drains the liver, to form the common bile duct. The common bile duct enters the head of the pancreas, joins the pancreatic duct of Wirsung usually within 1 cm of the wall of the duodenum, and then empties into the second portion of the duodenum through the ampulla of Vater (Fig. 19.1).

OBJECTIVES

1. List the common types of gallstones and describe the pathophysiology involved in their formation.
2. List several diseases known to predispose to gallstones.
3. Describe the signs and symptoms in a patient with biliary colic. Contrast these symptoms with those of acute cholecystitis.
4. List the tests commonly used in the diagnosis of calculus biliary tract disease and describe the indications for, limitations, and potential complications of each.
5. Describe the likely natural history of a young patient with asymptomatic gallstones.
6. List the possible complications of biliary calculi and describe the history, physical examinations, and laboratory findings for each.
7. Outline the medical and surgical management of a patient with acute cholecystitis.
8. Describe the signs, symptoms and management of choledocholithiasis.
9. Outline a diagnostic and management plan for a patient with acute right upper quadrant pain.
10. Describe the diagnostic evaluation and management of a patient with fever, chills, and jaundice.
11. Define the following:
    Murphy's sign,
    Courvoisier's sign,

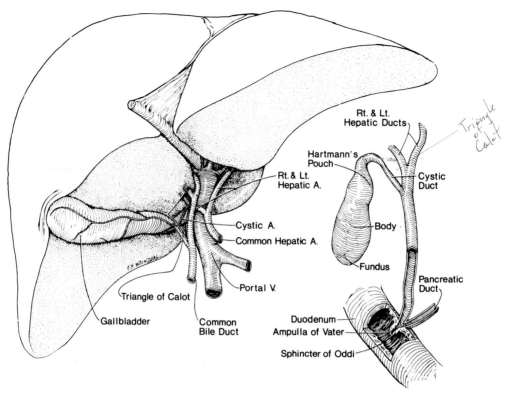

Triangle of Calot

Pringle maneuver

Figure 19.1. Gallbladder, extrahepatic bile duct, and porta hepatis anatomy.

Bile flow into the duodenum is, in part, regulated by the sphincter of Oddi, which encircles the distal bile duct. The bile ducts can be obstructed at different levels by neoplasms, strictures, or gallstones.

The common bile duct lies anterior and to the right of the portal vein and adjacent to the more medial hepatic artery in the porta hepatis (hepatoduodenal ligament). Excessive hepatic or biliary bleeding during surgery can be controlled by compressing this structure (the Pringle maneuver), temporarily occluding the hepatic artery and the portal vein. Most commonly the cystic artery branches from the right hepatic artery just distal to the cystic duct and enters the gallbladder after traversing the triangle of Calot, an anatomic space bordered inferiorly and to the left by the cystic duct, medially by the common hepatic duct, and superiorly by the undersurface of the liver.

Physiology

Man is fundamentally an aqueous solution separated from the environment by lipid membranes. Bile permits the exchange of lipids with the environment. Numerous chemicals metabolized by the liver are excreted in the bile. It facilitates the emulsification, digestion, and absorption of cholesterol and fatty acids; the fat-soluble vitamins A, D, K, and E; and minerals, such as calcium and magnesium. Along with pancreatic bicarbonate and protein secretion, bile also neutralizes gastric acid in the duodenum.

The liver secretes between 500 and 1200 ml of bile a day. The electrolyte composition of hepatic bile is quite similar to that of serum, and hepatic bile generally can be replaced with lactated Ringer's solution in patients with external biliary drainage. Cholesterol, bile salts, and phospholipids (primarily lecithin) are the major biliary lipids; they are solubilized in aqueous bile in a complex emulsion called a micelle. Cholesterol, the least soluble of the three, is solubilized by the more polar bile salts and lecithin. These two lipids have both a water-soluble component that interacts with the aqueous phase of bile and a fat-soluble component that interacts with the other phospholipid and bile salt molecules in the lipid micelle to "shield" the cholesterol from the surrounding polar, aqueous environment. Small amounts of cholesterol can be solubilized in this manner. The relative concentrations of cholesterol, bile salts, and lecithin in bile must be maintained within a fairly limited range or bile falls outside of the "zone of solubility" and becomes supersaturated; this increases the likelihood of cholesterol precipitation (Fig. 19.2). Bile from a normal patient contains approximately 75% bile salts, 20% lecithin, and 5% cholesterol. Reduced cholesterol solubility could result from either increased hepatic bile cholesterol secretion or diminished cholesterol-emulsifying capability (i.e., reduction in bile salt pool). The small area under the *curved line* in Figure 19.2 demonstrates how little tolerance for change in concentrations of the biliary lipids exists before the emulsion falls out of the "zone of solubility."

In addition to solubilizing cholesterol, bile salts and phospholipids solubilize ingested lipids and facilitate their absorption by the intestine. More than 95% of the

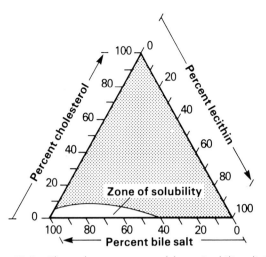

Figure 19.2. The molar percentages of the major biliary lipids (cholesterol, lecithin, and bile salts) in bile plotted on triangular coordinates. The small area under the curved line is called the "zone of solubility" and represents the percentage of each biliary lipid required for micellar formation and thus cholesterol solubilization. If the relative concentrations of the biliary lipids change so as to fall outside this small zone, the cholesterol-solubilizing capacity is diminished and gallstone formation is likely.

bile salts are resorbed by the distal ileum into the portal blood, extracted by the liver, and excreted again in the bile. Only the bile salts are recirculated by this "enterohepatic circulation." This bile salt pool circulates six to eight times a day during fasting and even more rapidly during meals. Bile salts lost in the stool are replenished by hepatic synthesis of bile salts from cholesterol. Bilirubin, which is constantly being produced by the breakdown of red blood cells, is extracted from the blood by the liver and conjugated with glucuronic acid to form bilirubin diglucuronide, the water-soluble, direct bilirubin, which is then actively excreted into the bile.

In the fasting state, hepatic bile is stored and concentrated in the gallbladder by absorbing Na^+, Cl^-, HCO_3^-, and water. After a meal, fat and, to a lesser degree, protein release cholecystokinin (CCK) from the duodenum, which stimulates gallbladder contraction and relaxation of the sphincter of Oddi, thus releasing concentrated bile into the duodenum. Hepatic bile flow is also increased during eating by the release of secretin, which is stimulated by acidification of the duodenum. In the intestine, the bile emulsifies ingested fat and facilitates absorption. The bile salts are resorbed in the distal ileum and reexcreted in the bile.

Gallbladder Disease

Diseases of the biliary system can be divided into three groups: (1) gallstone disease, (2) neoplastic disease, and (3) uncommon inflammatory diseases and anatomic anomalies, such as sclerosing cholangitis and choledochal cysts. The vast majority of clinical problems are related to gallstones, which result in clinical disease by obstructing the biliary system. The anatomic

site and duration of obstruction by a gallstone, the presence of infection and the body's response to this insult, and the medical management instituted determine the course of benign biliary tract stone disease. Once formed, the precise chemical composition of the gallstones is less important.

Gallstone Formation

Approximately 75% of people in the United States with gallstones have stones composed primarily of cholesterol (this includes both pure and mixed stones). As previously discussed, cholesterol is insoluble in an aqueous medium and is solubilized in bile by the detergent action of bile salts and phospholipid. If hepatic cholesterol secretion is greater than the solubilizing capacity of the bile salt and phospholipid micelles, the bile is supersaturated and cholesterol precipitates into crystals in the bile. Cholesterol supersaturation of bile may occur because of increased hepatic cholesterol secretion or decreased bile salt secretion. These crystals agglomerate in the gallbladder and grow into gallstones. Not all individuals with cholesterol-supersaturated bile form gallstones. Gallbladder stasis and nucleating or solubilizing factors may account for this discrepancy, but this is as yet unproven.

Twenty-five per cent of gallstones in the United States and 60% in Japan are composed of bile pigments that are primarily calcium bilirubinate. Pigment gallstones are associated with hemolytic disorders, cirrhosis, and bile stasis. Pure and mixed cholesterol gallstones are usually radiolucent, but pigmented stones are frequently visible on plain abdominal radiographs.

Epidemiology

Approximately 10% of the population of the United States (25 million people) has gallstones. Nearly 500,000 cholecystectomies are performed annually in this country, which accounts for a sizable portion of our health care costs. Gallstones are rare in children and infrequent in young adults but steadily increase in incidence with age. They are more common in females and in certain ethnic groups, such as Pima Indians and Mexican-Americans. Gallbladder disease clusters in some families and is increased in certain disorders, such as alcoholic cirrhosis, chronic hemolytic anemia, terminal ileal disease, and obesity. Multiparity, in and of itself, is not a strong risk factor for developing gallstones, whereas oral contraceptives and estrogen seem to increase the risk of forming gallstones. Patients on long-term total parenteral nutrition also have an increased incidence of gallstone formation.

Diagnostic Evaluation

Patients with biliary tract disease generally present with right upper quadrant pain, jaundice, or sepsis. In evaluating these patients, several laboratory tests are valuable. An elevated white blood cell count and differential suggest acute inflammation and infection. An

[handwritten margin notes at top: 1) direct bilirubin → conjugated bilirubin (eg. extrahepatic biliary obstruction or cholestasis) 2) indirect bilirubin → unconjugated bilirubin (eg. ↑ in hemolysis) eg. hepatocellular disease → conjugated & unconjugated bili is ↑ed.]

increased serum amylase indicates pancreatitis. Liver function tests are helpful in detecting jaundice and determining its cause. Unconjugated bilirubin or indirect bilirubin increases in the serum with increased hemolysis. With hepatocellular disease, both indirect and direct (unconjugated and conjugated) bilirubin are increased in the serum. With extrahepatic biliary obstruction or cholestasis, primarily the direct, conjugated fraction is elevated. The serum alkaline phosphatase is released by the bile canalicular cells and, therefore, provides a sensitive test for bile stasis, either from extrahepatic biliary obstruction or, less commonly, cholestasis caused by a drug reaction or primary biliary cirrhosis. Frequently this enzyme is moderately elevated in hepatitis, and it can also be released from bone. Elevated alkaline phosphatase due to biliary disease may be differentiated from that of other sources by virtue of the fact that biliary alkaline phosphatase is heat stable on heat fractionation. The test for 5'-nucleotidase is also helpful in cases in which the source of elevated alkaline phosphatase is uncertain. If the results are elevated, they confirm that the disease is of biliary origin. The serum glutamic oxaloacetic transaminase (SGOT) and serum glutamic pyruvic transaminase (SGPT) are released from the hepatocyte and are increased significantly in hepatitis of various etiologies. These enzymes are frequently elevated with biliary obstruction, particularly when it is acute. As a rule, however, the increase in alkaline phosphatase is relatively greater than the increase in the transaminases in biliary obstruction and vice versa in hepatitis.

If only part of the biliary ductal system is obstructed, for example by a primary or metastatic tumor, the serum alkaline phosphatase will be released into the serum from the obstructed ducts, but the bilirubin will be normal as it is cleared by the unaffected liver.

Radiographic Evaluation

Numerous tests are available to aid the clinician in evaluating the patient who presents with either right upper quadrant pain or jaundice. Determining which tests will yield the diagnosis most expediently with the least risk and expense to the patient requires an understanding of both the pathophysiology of biliary tract disease and the specificity, sensitivity, risk, and cost of each test. Some are highly operator dependent; hence, their value will vary between institutions.

A plain film of the abdomen is easily and safely obtained. Approximately 15% of the time it will reveal gallstones if they are radiopaque (Fig. 19.3). Air in the biliary system indicates communication of the biliary system with the intestines either secondary to prior biliary-enteric bypass surgery or a pathologic fistula.

Ultrasonography has become the initial study in the evaluation of many patients with suspected biliary tract disease. Ultrasound is 95% accurate in detecting gallstones in the gallbladder and rarely is falsely positive; therefore, it is quite valuable in the initial evaluation of the patient with right upper quadrant pain that is suggestive of either biliary colic or acute cholecystitis (Fig. 19.4). In the jaundiced patient, ultrasonography can demonstrate dilated intrahepatic ducts if the jaundice is secondary to extrahepatic obstruction. If the gallbladder is distended as well, the obstruction is probably distal to the cystic duct junction with the hepatic duct. A mass in the head of the pancreas would sug-

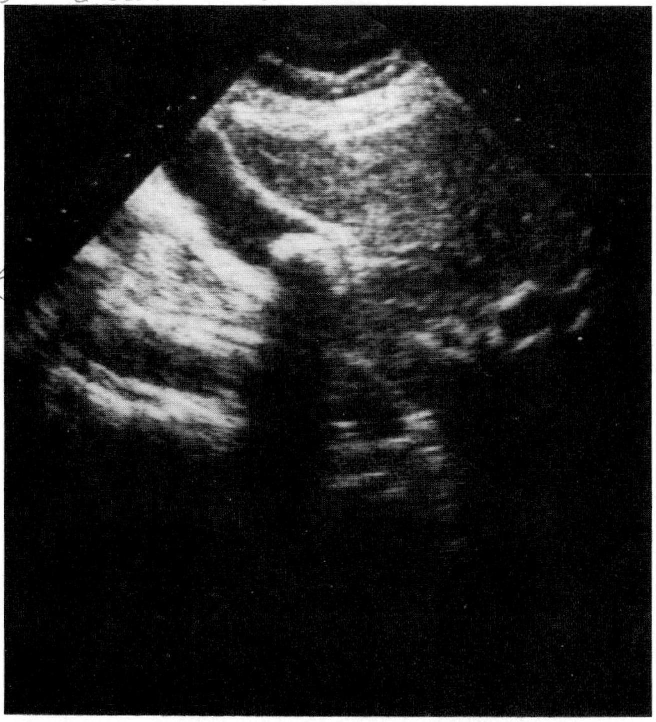

Figure 19.4. Ultrasound of gallbladder with gallstones.

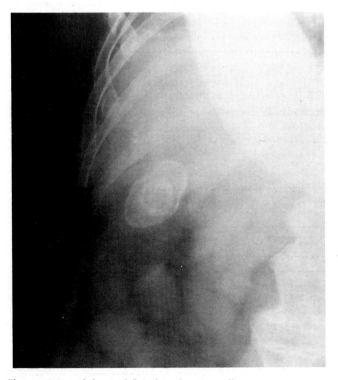

Figure 19.3. Abdominal flat plate showing gallstones.

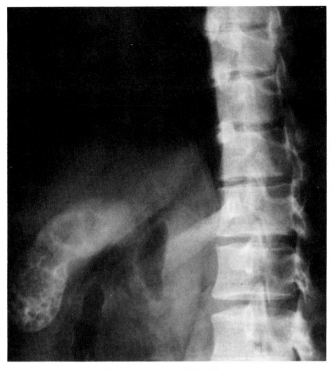

Figure 19.5. Oral cholecystogram with gallstones.

gest that pancreatic cancer is responsible for the patient's biliary obstruction and jaundice. Ultrasonography is painless, relatively inexpensive, and does not entail the use of radiation nor require any specific preparation of the patient.

The oral cholecystogram (OCG) has essentially been replaced by ultrasonography. To obtain an adequate sonogram, the patient need only fast overnight. To visualize the gallbladder with an oral cholecystogram, the patient takes an oral contrast agent (Telepaque or Bilopaque) the night before the examination. This agent must then be absorbed by the intestine, and absorption can be impaired by many acute abdominal illnesses. After absorption, the compound is taken up by the liver, excreted into the bile, and then concentrated by the gallbladder. Radiographs of the right upper quadrant are taken the following morning (Fig. 19.5). If the serum bilirubin is greater than 3 mg/dl, the contrast agent is not adequately taken up by the liver. If gallbladder absorption is impaired, the contrast agent will not be sufficiently concentrated by the gallbladder for it to be visualized radiographically. If a second dose is given and the gallbladder still cannot be visualized (a nonvisualization on a double-dose OCG), there is a 95% chance that the gallbladder is diseased. However, the presence of gallstones can be as reliably and more readily obtained with a single ultrasonographic examination.

By definition, acute cholecystitis is caused by acute and persistent obstruction of the cystic duct. In the past this was primarily a clinical diagnosis, but radionuclide biliary scans (HIDA) are now a rapid and reliable (95% accurate) means to determine whether the cystic duct

is patent. In this test, a technetium-99m-labeled derivative of iminodiacetic acid (IDA) is injected intravenously and rapidly excreted in high concentrations into the bile ducts even in the presence of significant jaundice. Visualization of the common bile duct without filling of the gallbladder indicates cystic duct obstruction and strongly supports the diagnosis of acute cholecystitis (Fig. 19.6). Other inflammation at the site of the gallbladder may produce the same picture.

In patients with jaundice, particularly with evidence of extrahepatic obstruction and dilated intrahepatic ducts on ultrasonography, radiographic visualization of the biliary ductal anatomy is often valuable in making the diagnosis and planning therapy. Although this is at times done initially at surgery, preoperative cholangiograms can facilitate a safe and expedient operation. Two methods are available whose relative merits are still being determined. The percutaneous transhepatic cholangiogram (PTC) is obtained by percutaneously sticking a thin needle through the liver and injecting contrast medium directly into an intrahepatic bile duct. Dilated bile ducts facilitate this procedure (95% success rate). If the ducts are of normal caliber, the test is successful only 60–70% of the time. Transhepatic cholangiography is particularly valuable in demonstrating the proximal ductal system. It also has therapeutic capabilities in aiding placement of a biliary drainage catheter into the obstructed bile ducts. It is contraindicated in patients with ascites, clotting abnormalities, or a small, shrunken liver. The endoscopic retrograde cholangiopancreatogram (ERCP) requires a skilled endoscopist, who endoscopically cannulates the sphincter of Oddi and injects contrast agent to obtain a radiograph of the pancreatic and biliary ductal anatomy. This study is particularly valuable in patients with normal-sized bile ductules and in those with suspected ampullary lesions when a biopsy can be obtained for diagnosis. This procedure also has valuable therapeutic capabilities that are in the process of development and refinement. HIDA scanning is not indicated in the evaluation of jaundice because of its poor specificity under these conditions.

Clinical Presentation

Asymptomatic Gallstones

Initially, gallstones do not cause clinical symptoms. Many individuals with gallstones have been followed for decades without developing complications. Although controversy persists as to whether asymptomatic gallstones are an indication for cholecystectomy, most data suggest that many individuals will never develop symptoms and, if they do, a cholecystectomy can then be safely performed. Certainly, the cost burden of removing nearly 25 million gallbladders in the United States would be prohibitive. Patients with asymptomatic gallstones have a 20% chance of developing symptoms from their stones at some time during their lifetime. There are, however, certain high-risk patients,

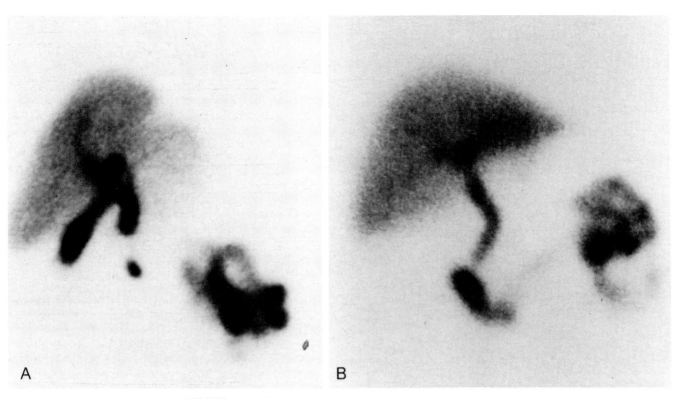

Figure 19.6.   HIDA scans, with (**A**) and without (**B**) gallbladder visualization.

such as diabetics, who should have elective cholecystectomies since the clinical course is generally more severe once they develop inflammation of the gallbladder.

Biliary Colic

Approximately three-quarters of the patients requiring surgery for gallstones have biliary colic, or chronic cholecystitis, caused by obstruction of the cystic duct by a gallstone. This visceral pain is similar to the colic of early acute appendicitis, small intestinal obstruction, or ureteral obstruction, although the pain cycle is less frequent. Because the peritoneum is not inflamed, the patient frequently writhes about as compared to the patient with acute cholecystitis and localized peritonitis, who lies completely still. The pain usually follows a meal, begins abruptly, and is constant until it abates in minutes to several hours. The pain of biliary colic is usually upper abdominal and may be greatest in the right upper quadrant with radiation through to the back. It may mimic or be confused with angina, pneumonia, pyelonephritis, duodenal ulcer, or pancreatitis. Nausea and vomiting frequently occur during an attack.

Indigestion, fatty food intolerance, flatulence, belching, heartburn, and other nonspecific symptoms that have been blanketed under the term "dyspepsia" are frequently relieved by cholecystectomy. However, these symptoms are so frequent in the general population that they may be unrelated to a given individual's gallstones. The surgeon must be certain that the patient understands that these symptoms may well persist after the gallbladder has been removed.

Physical examination during an episode of biliary colic is often unremarkable because there is no peritoneal inflammation. Palpation in the right upper quadrant may elicit tenderness by compressing the distended gallbladder.

Patients presenting with biliary colic can be managed with parenteral analgesics and observation. Once the acute episode has resolved, further elective evaluation can be undertaken. A sonogram or oral cholecystogram is frequently used to demonstrate gallstones. If the right upper quadrant pain persists or if the physical examination or white blood cell count suggests more severe inflammation, the patient should be hospitalized and further evaluation initiated.

Efforts to develop an oral medication to dissolve gallstones continue. Chenodeoxycholic acid (Chenodiol), a bile acid, is the only agent presently available. It is effective in approximately 10–20% of cases and usually requires 1–2 years to dissolve gallstones completely. The gallstones will frequently recur within 5 years after discontinuation of the medication. Because of its poor long-term success rate, Chenodiol should be reserved for the elderly patient with associated medical illnesses that preclude a safe operation.

Most patients with symptoms believed secondary to documented gallstones should undergo an elective cholecystectomy for symptomatic relief and to prevent the development of acute cholecystitis or choledocholithiasis. The individual with symptomatic gallstones has a 70% chance of developing a complication from the disease at some time during his life. During a cholecystectomy, the cystic duct is initially isolated and controlled to prevent gallstones from migrating into the common bile duct. The cystic artery is then sought in the triangle of Calot and ligated to decrease blood loss during dissection of the gallbladder from the liver. The artery at greatest risk for injury during this maneuver is the right hepatic artery. In the face of unusual anatomy or significant inflammation, great care is taken not to divide any structures until they are clearly identified. When confused during biliary surgery, the careful surgeon obtains a cholangiogram, a "roadmap," early during the operation to demonstrate the ductal anatomy, thereby avoiding injury to the vital bile ducts. An intraoperative cholangiogram should be obtained in every patient undergoing a cholecystectomy to look for occult common bile duct stones. The operative mortality rate of an elective cholecystectomy is 0.3% and approaches 1 in 1000 in young, healthy patients. Surgery for infrequent biliary colic should be deferred in patients with severe chronic illness or advanced hepatic cirrhosis unless more significant complications develop.

Acute Cholecystitis

In terms of their pathogenesis, acute cholecystitis and biliary colic are quite similar. A gallstone impacted in Hartmann's pouch or the cystic duct causes obstruction with its attendant morbidity. In biliary colic, the obstruction is temporary and the biliary colic spontaneously abates. In acute cholecystitis, the obstruction persists and the gallbladder becomes progressively more distended, inflamed, and tender. Although most episodes of acute cholecystitis resolve spontaneously, some attacks may progress to gangrene, empyema, or perforation of the gallbladder. Usually acute cholecystitis is associated with gallstones, but, particularly in the diabetic, immunosuppressed, or postoperative patient, acute cholecystitis may occur without gallstones.

The majority of patients presenting with acute cholecystitis have had previous episodes of biliary colic. However, unlike previous attacks, this one persists. The pain usually becomes more localized to the right upper quadrant and is exacerbated by movement and palpation. Accentuated tenderness and inspiratory arrest during palpation in the right upper quadrant are often present; this pattern is called Murphy's sign.

Low grade fever, leukocytosis, and a slight increase in liver function tests are frequently present. The mild rise in bilirubin is secondary to edema obstructing the common hepatic duct adjacent to the inflamed gallbladder. The differential diagnosis includes pancreatitis, perforated duodenal ulcer, right lower lobe pneumonia, acute appendicitis, and hepatitis. Careful evaluation of an upright chest x-ray for free subdiaphragmatic air or pneumonia and of the serum amylase and liver enzymes will help to exclude these diagnoses.

Ultrasonography can usually be easily obtained and will demonstrate gallstones and often thickening of the gallbladder wall. If doubt still persists as to the diagnosis, a radionuclide excretion scan (HIDA, PIPIDA) can demonstrate obstruction of the cystic duct and, essentially, confirm the diagnosis.

Patients with acute cholecystitis should be admitted to the hospital, fluid resuscitated intravenously, and treated with antibiotics. The incidence of positive bile cultures increases with the duration of symptoms prior to surgery. The most common organisms are *Escherichia coli, Klebsiella pneumoniae, Clostridium welchii* or *Clostridium perfringens*, and *Streptococcus faecalis*. As a rule, early cholecystectomy is the preferred method of managing acute cholecystitis. It shortens overall hospital stay and ensures exploration of individuals with occult complications of cholecystitis, such as empyema or perforation, in whom an expectant approach would be catastrophic. Because two-thirds of cases of acute cholecystitis will resolve spontaneously, an expectant approach can be taken in patients with significant acute medical problems to allow time for these to be treated optimally. However, if a patient's condition deteriorates during observation or has not improved within 24–48 hours, surgery should not be delayed.

Cholecystectomy with an operative cholangiogram is the preferred surgical procedure for the treatment of acute cholecystitis. If the patient is severely unstable for reasons unrelated to the inflamed gallbladder, the gallbladder may be opened, the gallstones evacuated, and an external drainage catheter secured in the fundus of the gallbladder—a cholecystostomy. The mortality and morbidity rates for cholecystectomy done for acute cholecystitis are approximately 5% and 15%, respectively. Postoperative complications most commonly seen include wound infection, intraabdominal abscess, atelectasis, pneumonia, and retained common duct stone.

Complications of Cholelithiasis

The majority of operations for gallbladder disease are for chronic and acute cholecystitis. In approximately 15% of these cases choledocholithiasis, or gallstones in the common bile duct, will be encountered. Although in about one-half of the cases these are asymptomatic and are detected only by intraoperative cystic duct cholangiography, common duct stones can present quite dramatically with jaundice and cholangitis. These complications will be discussed in detail in the section on choledocholithiasis. Passage of a common bile duct stone through the ampulla of Vater can also induce acute pancreatitis. Therefore, all patients with acute pancreatitis should be carefully evaluated for gallstones. If stones are present, an elective cholecystectomy should be performed after the acute pancreatitis has resolved.

As with other organs of the gastrointestinal tract, obstruction of the biliary tree can lead to perforation. In the gallbladder, the gallstone obstructs the cystic duct and the perforation is most commonly located in the fundus of the gallbladder. Usually the perforation is localized to the right upper quadrant because chronic inflammation of the gallbladder induces adhesions to form between the gallbladder and surrounding organs, such as the colon, duodenum, and omentum, that may lead to erosion into one of these organs or form a pericholecystic fistula. Infrequently, the gallbladder perforates freely into the abdomen, causing a diffuse peritonitis with abdominal tenderness and rebound, so-called "bile peritonitis." Because of the rapid shift of fluid into the peritoneal cavity, these patients require a significant amount of volume resuscitation. Once this has been accomplished, emergent laparotomy and cholecystectomy should be performed. This condition is associated with a 50% mortality.

Empyema of the gallbladder is defined as a gallbladder filled with pus. It represents an advanced stage of acute cholecystitis similar to gangrenous cholecystitis where part or all of the wall of the gallbladder has necrosed secondary to ischemia. The latter condition is frequently associated with a localized perforation. Both of these complications are seldom diagnosed preoperatively and occur more frequently in the elderly, diabetic, or immunocompromised patient. Most likely, these patients fail to manifest the outward signs of a severe intraabdominal infection. This, coupled with the physician's reluctance to operate on a "high-risk" patient, often results in procrastination, where early intervention would prevent the development of gangrene and empyema with their associated high morbidity and mortality. A corollary to this observation is that occult sepsis in the debilitated patient is not infrequently secondary to cholecystitis or cholangitis, which will be overlooked unless aggressively sought.

Biliary-enteric fistulae are seen more frequently in patients with chronic rather than acute cholecystitis and are often, themselves, asymptomatic. They develop secondary to adherence of the adjacent duodenum or colon to the chronically inflamed gallbladder with gradual erosion of a gallstone from the gallbladder into the adjacent organ. Gallstone ileus develops when a gallstone erodes into the duodenum and then obstructs the intestine, usually at the ileocecal valve. The classic radiographic appearance of gallstone ileus is air in the biliary tree associated with small bowel obstruction.

Gallbladder Cancer

Gallbladder cancer is an uncommon malignancy, accounting for less than 2% of malignant tumors in the United States. Because the gallbladder is a blind sac, obstruction by tumor does not cause jaundice, and presenting symptoms are usually secondary to local spread causing vague right upper quadrant pain or systemic complaints such as malaise and weight loss due to widespread metastases. Therefore, gallbladder cancer, similar to cancer of the tail of the pancreas, is seldom detected early. The prognosis is equally poor in both of these malignancies—less than 5% survival at 5 years. Gallbladder cancer is frequently not diagnosed preoperatively, has often metastasized by the time it is detected, and responds poorly to any therapy. If encountered in a localized state, which happens most commonly during an elective cholecystectomy, wedge resection of the gallbladder fossa and liver bed and regional lymphadenectomy of the porta hepatitis have been advocated. Therefore, every gallbladder removed should be opened and carefully examined for cancer prior to completing the operation.

Gallstones are present in nearly 80% of cases of gallbladder cancer. Although this might argue for prophylactic cholecystectomy for asymptomatic gallstones, the relative rarity of gallbladder cancer compared to the prevalence of gallstones, and the risks and expense of surgery render this approach both medically and economically impractical. On the contrary, if porcelain gallbladder (calcification of the gallbladder wall) is seen on an abdominal film, the incidence of carcinoma in this unusual condition is up to 60%. Elective cholecystectomy is indicated for porcelain gallbladder.

Common Bile Duct Disease

The common bile duct is a 6-mm tubular, collagen-rich structure with minimal elastin. Because of its narrowness, its lack of distensibility, and its position in an important alimentary intersection, it may be occluded by a variety of disease conditions, including biliary calculi, stricture, primary malignancy, metastatic malignancy, and various inflammatory conditions. Understanding common bile duct disease mandates understanding the pathophysiology of biliary obstruction, which is clinically manifested by jaundice. An algorithm for evaluation of the jaundiced patient is seen in Figure 19.7.

Most jaundiced patients of concern to the surgeon are those with extrahepatic biliary obstruction. They present with a conjugated (direct) hyperbilirubinemia with predominant alkaline phosphatase elevation and lesser SGPT increases. These patients often have bile in the urine, which has diagnostic implications. Since conjugated bile is water soluble, it is excreted in urine; unconjugated bile is water insoluble and, therefore, not excreted. If urine urobilinogen is present, complete biliary obstruction is not present since urobilinogen is formed in the gut by the action of bacteria on conjugated bilirubin. The remainder of this chapter will focus on the most common causes of common bile duct obstruction and their diagnosis and treatment.

Choledocholithiasis

Approximately 15% of all patients with gallbladder stones will have, as a complication of their disease, passage of stones from the gallbladder into the common bile duct (choledochus). While a sizable percentage of stones entering the common bile duct may pass into the duodenum without causing symptoms, significant morbidity and mortality result each year from the sequelae of stones occluding the biliary and pancreatic ducts. If 15% of the 500,000 cholecystectomies performed in the United States each year require common bile duct exploration (75,000), the magnitude of this disease becomes evident.

Clinically, the patient often gives a history of multiple previous episodes of biliary colic that resolved spontaneously. Commonly, the patient presents with

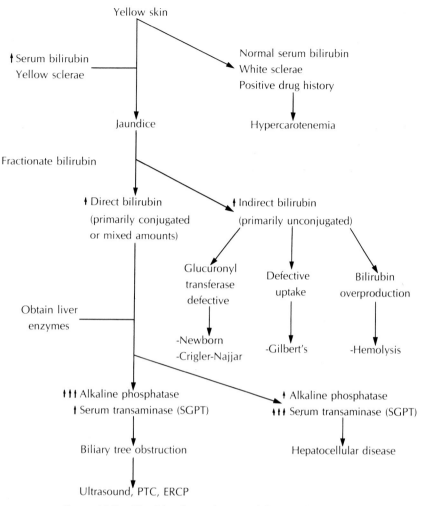

Figure 19.7. Algorithm for evaluation of the jaundiced patient.

jaundice, acholic stools, or biliuria as the initial manifestation of his disease. A characteristic feature of the jaundice associated with common bile duct calculi is its "fluctuating" nature as opposed to a continuous "nonfluctuating" jaundice seen in biliary obstruction caused by malignant disease. The patient may describe either midepigastric (gallstone pancreatitis) or right upper quadrant (biliary colic) pain associated with the jaundice. In more serious cases, the patient will have jaundice, right upper quadrant pain, and chills and high fever (Charcot's triad), which are associated with acute ascending cholangitis. If the patient has hypotension and mental confusion in addition to Charcot's triad (Reynold's pentad), he almost certainly has acute suppurative cholangitis ("pus under pressure"), a surgical emergency. Physical examination usually reveals jaundice that is first detected in the sclerae and mucous membranes, right upper quadrant pain, and, in cholangitis, hepatic tenderness to percussion. Additional findings may include grey-colored stool on rectal examination and brown urine. The gallbladder is usually not palpable in chronic gallstone-related disease.

The diagnostic workup of jaundice associated with probable choledocholithiasis starts with bilirubin fractionation and the liver function tests mentioned above. Ultrasonography is believed by most to be the diagnostic screening procedure indicated initially. Multiple studies confirm its efficacy as a screening procedure in common duct stone-related disease; it demonstrates dilated intra- and extrahepatic ducts 80% of the time. It also detects gallbladder stones with 95% accuracy, often suggesting the likely source of the common duct obstruction. Its disadvantages include its 20% false-negative rate in detecting dilated bile ducts and its inability to determine the site or cause of the obstruction in many patients. The computed tomography scan may also be used as a screening test. It detects dilated ducts when present with 90% accuracy, but it is expensive and, like ultrasound, often misses the site and cause of obstruction. Percutaneous transhepatic cholangiography (PTC) and endoscopic retrograde cholangiopancreatography (ERCP) are the two most accurate and definitive tests available for diagnosing bile duct obstruction. Because PTC is technically easier and visualizes the entire biliary ductal system proximal to the obstruction, most authorities consider it to be the definitive diagnostic test in common duct obstruction. In Figure 19.8, PTC reveals the "meniscus sign" in the

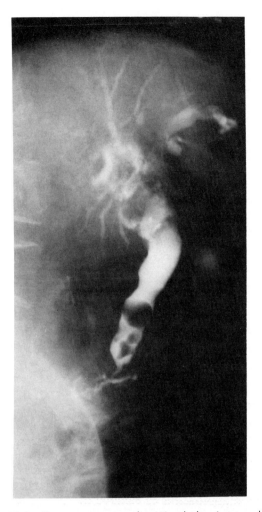

Figure 19.8. Percutaneous transhepatic cholangiogram demonstrates common bile duct obstruction secondary to a gallstone.

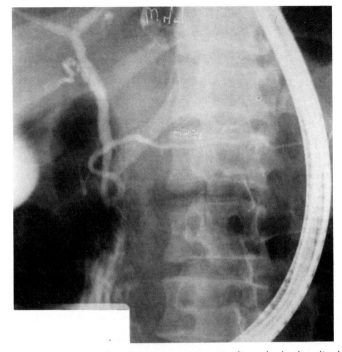

Figure 19.9. Cholangiopancreatogram visualizes both the distal common bile duct and the pancreatic duct.

distal common duct, indicating a diagnosis of obstruction secondary to calculi. PTC is invasive, however, and is associated with 5% morbidity (bleeding, sepsis, bile leak). ERCP visualizes the distal bile duct and pancreatic duct (Fig. 19.9) and is indicated when coagulopathy makes PTC prohibitive or when an ampullary or duodenal lesion is suspected and biopsy is desired. Oral cholecystography, intravenous cholangiography (IVC), and HIDA scan are not useful in the diagnosis of common bile duct obstruction.

After the diagnosis is made, preparation for operative therapy depends on the clinical condition of the patient. In the absence of sepsis, the patient may be completely worked up and hydrated, clotting abnormalities may be corrected with vitamin K, and the patient may be scheduled for surgery without a sense of urgency. In a patient with Charcot's triad, the approach must differ. Cholangitis, by definition, is obstruction of the biliary ducts with infected, nondraining bile behind the obstruction. Again, the most commonly cultured organisms include *E. coli, K. pneumoniae,* and *S. faecalis.* Before a diagnostic workup can be considered, treatment of the cholangitis is imperative. The

patient is given nothing by mouth and IV hydration is initiated with monitoring of urine output via a Foley catheter. Nasogastric decompression is helpful if the patient has been vomiting. However, the keystone of treatment involves immediate aggressive antibiotic treatment with an aminoglycoside and a penicillin (usually ampicillin or a semisynthetic penicillin). Clotting abnormalities may be corrected by giving vitamin K. Over 70% of patients with cholangitis will defervesce and improve clinically on the above regimen, thus allowing a diagnostic workup prior to operative therapy. In the small percentage of patients who do not respond to therapy, urgent or emergency exploration may be required to open the common duct, evacuate the pus, and thus decompress the biliary tree—a lifesaving procedure.

The operative procedure for common duct stone obstruction includes cholecystectomy (the source of stones 97% of the time), and intraoperative cholangiography via the cystic duct prior to opening the common bile duct. "Absolute" indications to explore the duct include a palpable common duct stone, common duct stones visualized on intraoperative cholangiogram, the presence of cholangitis, and a serum bilirubin of greater than 7 mg/100 ml. "Relative" indications for common duct exploration include duct dilatation, gallstone pancreatitis, recurrent jaundice, small gallbladder stones, a biliary-enteric fistula, and a single-faceted gallbladder stone. A small vertical incision is then made in the common duct (choledochotomy) and the lumen explored using a variety of instruments, including forceps, scoops, inflatable balloon catheters, and collapsible wire "baskets." A small endoscope (choledochoscope) is then advanced through the open-

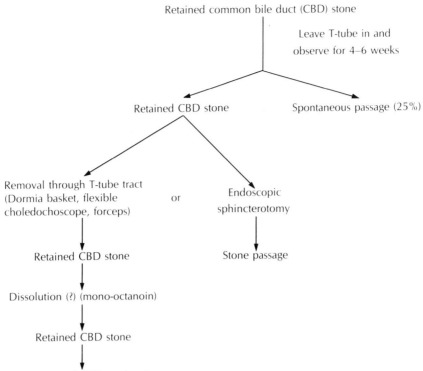

Figure 19.10. Algorithm for management of retained common duct stones.

ing and the proximal and distal duct is carefully visualized. All stones, mucus, and debris are removed and the duct is irrigated with saline. A T-tube is then placed in the lumen of the duct and the choledochotomy is closed around the T-tube. Its function is to decompress the common bile duct while the duct heals. A "completion cholangiogram" is obtained to assure that no further defects remain in the duct before the abdomen is closed.

The postoperative management involves placing the T-tube to gravity drainage for 1 week at which time a "T-tube cholangiogram" is obtained. If no residual filling defects are seen, the patient is sent home for about 2 weeks with the T-tube clamped. If no jaundice develops, the T-tube is pulled out through the fibrous tract that developed around it postoperatively. The operative mortality for cholecystectomy and common bile duct exploration of 8–10% increases to 20% if cholangitis is present.

Postoperative complications could include bleeding, recurrent cholangitis, a bile leak, duodenal leak, pancreatitis, and subphrenic abscess. One of the most frustrating complications seen by biliary surgeons in spite of thorough and compulsive duct exploration is a "missed" or retained stone. This occurs in about 7% of common duct explorations. The stone places the patient at risk to develop the same complications that brought him to the hospital, and so it must be removed. Management of retained common duct stones is suggested in Figure 19.10. In the presence of a retained common duct stone, the T-tube is left in place for 4–6 weeks to allow maturation of the tract around

the T-tube and to allow spontaneous passage of the stone, which occurs in a small number of patients. At the end of the 4- to 6-week period, one of two approaches may be utilized to remove the stone. The most common approach is to remove the T-tube, advance a maneuverable, collapsible basket under fluoroscopy through the T-tube tract and into the duct, and retrieve the stone (Fig. 19.11). This can be done successfully in 80–90% of cases, depending on the skill of the retriever and the size of the stone. A flexible choledochoscope may also be advanced down the tract to assist with stone retrieval, under direct vision using the basket. Special forceps have also been designed to remove stones under fluoroscopy. The other approach involves ERCP with intubation of the ampulla from the duodenum. An electrocautery wire is used to divide the sphincter of Oddi, thus allowing the stone to pass spontaneously. If none of the above methods is successful, operative reexploration of the duct may be necessary. Chemical dissolution of cholesterol stones has been described by some investigators using an organic solvent, mono-octanoin (Capmul). Preliminary studies appear promising and suggest another possible weapon in the armamentarium against retained common duct stones.

Common Duct Stricture

Because of a low elastin content, little redundancy, and poor blood supply, the common bile duct is an unforgiving organ when injured. Over 90% of common duct strictures occur as the direct result of an inadvertent injury during an operative procedure. Approxi-

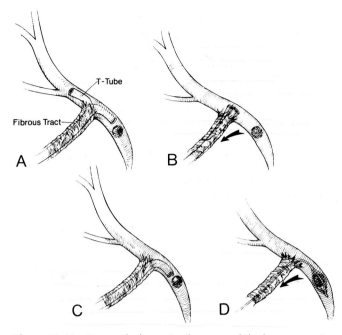

Figure 19.11. Removal of a retained common bile duct stone using a Dormia basket.

"U-tube"

mately 75% of injuries occur during a simple cholecystectomy, underscoring the importance of recognizing the anatomic variations of the biliary tree and the importance of proceeding in a cautious, systematic fashion even during a "routine" cholecystectomy. If injury occurs and is immediately recognized, primary repair may be done over a T-tube stent brought out elsewhere on the common duct. Stricture rates are low under these circumstances. However, many injuries occur when the duct is ligated (while tying off bleeders), clamped with a hemostat, or divided with a scalpel and a section of the duct is removed. Under these circumstances, the injury may not be recognized immediately and the complication may be recognized in one of two fashions: as a life-threatening bile peritonitis that requires immediate reexploration, and as postoperative jaundice, sometimes occurring in the immediate perioperative period and sometimes weeks or even months later. Under the latter circumstances, cholangitis is often present and may be life threatening.

Diagnostic workup of the delayed postoperative jaundice associated with stricture is conducted in a similar fashion to that with common duct stones. A history of recent gallbladder surgery, nonfluctuating jaundice (often) with cholangitis, conjugated hyperbilirubinemia, and predominant alkaline phosphatase elevation suggests the diagnosis. The diagnostic procedure of choice in this disease is PTC, although ERCP is occasionally helpful. Before either of these procedures is done, the patient should be given prophylactic antibiotics because of the relatively high incidence of cholangitis and septicemia that occurs after they are obtained. PTC usually reveals narrowing of the common duct in one of three sites: (1) at or near the common hepatic duct bifurcation, the most common site;

(2) cystic duct-common hepatic duct junction; and (3) in the distal duct near the ampulla.

Long experience has demonstrated the futility of attempting to resect a strictured segment of this rigid, already foreshortened structure and doing an end-to-end, duct-to-duct anastomosis, because restricturing is inevitable. Operative therapy nearly always involves anastomosis of the dilated proximal biliary ductal system to a segment of small bowel, most commonly a Roux-en-Y loop of jejunum. A mucosa-to-mucosa anastomosis is usually done in an end-to-side fashion using a small needle and meticulous technique. A Silastic stent is usually passed through the anastomosis and left in place for prolonged periods of time to prevent restricturing from occurring. If the injury is in the distal duct, a T-tube may be used as the stent. However, very proximal lesions near the hilum of the liver nearly always require a transhepatic stent. This involves placement of a Silastic tube through the abdominal wall, through hepatic parenchyma, into a major bile duct, through the biliary-enteric anastomosis, down the limb of jejunum, and back out through the abdominal wall (the so-called "U-tube"). Patients who have a meticulously constructed biliary-enteric anastomosis with proper stenting have an excellent result in 80% of cases. Restricturing occurs in a minority of patients under the above circumstances.

Common Duct Malignancies (uncommon 0.1-0.9%)

Malignancy of the extrahepatic bile ducts is uncommon, the incidence ranging from 0.1–0.9%. The etiology of bile duct cancers is unknown, but as many as 57% are associated with gallstones. Other diseases with an increased incidence of bile duct cancers include choledochal cysts, Caroli's disease, and ulcerative colitis. Histologically, the lesions are usually adenocarcinoma (cholangiocarcinoma) and are frequently firm, well-circumscribed tumors that occlude the biliary ductal system. In general, these are slow-growing, locally invasive tumors that rarely metastasize. Unfortunately, because of the intimate association of the extrahepatic bile ducts with the portal vein and common hepatic artery, curative resection of these lesions is the exception rather than the rule.

The two most common presenting symptoms are jaundice (50%) and right upper quadrant pain (30%). Pruritus, chills and fever, and weight loss are occasionally seen. In contrast to the fluctuating jaundice often seen in patients with common duct stones, the jaundice associated with bile duct cancers is nonfluctuating. A small percentage of patients with biliary obstruction secondary to malignancy (most commonly pancreatic) will present with a palpable, nontender mass in the right upper quadrant. On exploration, a tense, noninflamed, distended gallbladder is seen to be the source of the palpable mass. This clinical finding of a palpable, nontender gallbladder is called Courvoisier's sign and is frequently a harbinger of unresectable pancreatic malignancy. Courvoisier's sign rarely occurs with gallstone disease. Laboratory tests will reveal total bilirubin

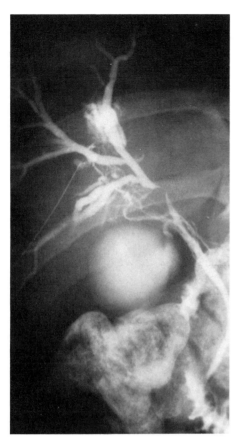

Figure 19.12. Bile duct carcinoma at the bifurcation of the common hepatic duct (Klatskin tumor).

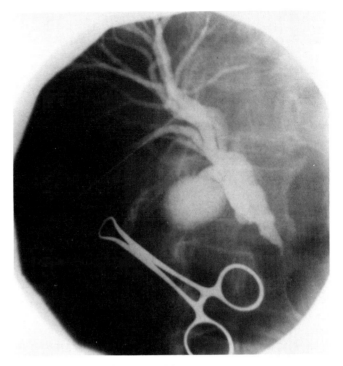

Figure 19.13. Distal common bile tumor seen on PTC.

elevation that averages 20 mg/dl with the direct fraction predominating. Similarly, alkaline phosphatase is usually more than three times normal. Ultrasound may function as a good screening test, but it rarely suggests a diagnosis in this disease. PTC and ERCP are the diagnostic procedures of choice in evaluating jaundice not associated with calculi. PTC is particularly accurate and sensitive in demonstrating the lesion and the proximal biliary tree. Most authorities consider it to be the premier diagnostic modality in this disease.

Treatment and prognosis of adenocarcinoma of the extrahepatic bile ducts are particularly dependent on the level of the tumor in the bile duct. For this reason, the extrahepatic ductal system is divided into three regions when discussing its clinical behavior—the upper, middle, and lower thirds. The most common site of bile duct cancer is at the bifurcation of the common hepatic ducts in the upper third (>50%). Tumors located here are called ''Klatskin tumors'' and have a particular clinical behavior characterized by slow growth and late metastases (Fig. 19.12). While resection of these lesions may be technically possible in up to 47% of cases, the resection is rarely curative and 5-year survival in most series is 0–5%. The treatment of choice is complete surgical excision of the lesion whenever possible; however, in the majority of patients, in whom that is not possible, excellent palliative treatment may be rendered by opening the bile duct, pass-

ing dilators through the tumor-narrowed bile duct, inserting a U-tube stent through the narrowed area, and bringing it out in two places as previously described. Should the U-tube become occluded with biliary debris, a new tube may be attached to the upper end of the occluded one and pulled into position as the occluded one is pulled out. Patients often live 2–3 years with excellent quality of life following this procedure. Biliary drainage catheters can also be placed by interventional radiologic methods, as primary therapy or in conjunction with surgery. Rapid advances in equipment and techniques are being made in this field.

Tumors of the middle and distal thirds are less common but have a better prognosis than Klatskin tumors. Middle-third tumors are usually treated by resection with choledochoenterostomy or simple bypass choledochoenterostomy in which the tumor is not resected but merely bypassed. The 5-year survival rate for middle-third lesions averages 10%. Distal-third lesions have a significantly higher resection rate and 5-year survival rate than lesions elsewhere in the biliary tree. Lesions here cause jaundice at an early stage but must be distinguished from ampullary, duodenal, and pancreatic malignancies—all of which cause distal duct obstruction, but all of which have a poorer prognosis than distal common duct tumors (Fig. 19.13). The operation of choice for distal common duct tumors is a Whipple procedure. This procedure, one of the most difficult and technically demanding in gastrointestinal surgery, involves resecting distal stomach, distal common duct (with the tumor), the pancreatic head, and the entire duodenum. Three anastomoses—pancreaticojejunostomy, choledochojejunostomy, and gastrojejunostomy—must be completed after the resection is accomplished. The 5-year survival rate after a Whipple

30%. Whipple procedure

procedure for a lesion in the distal third of the common duct is 30%.

SUGGESTED READINGS

Acosta, JM, Pellegrini CA, Skinner DB: Etiology and pathogenesis of acute biliary pancreatitis. *Surgery* 88:118–125, 1980.

Elias E, Hamlyn AN, Jain S, et al: A randomized trial of percutaneous transhepatic cholangiography with the Chiba needle versus endoscopic retrograde pancreatography for bile duct visualization in jaundice. *Gastroenterology* 71:439–443, 1976.

Girard RM, Legros G: Retained and recurrent bile duct stones. Surgical or nonsurgical removal. *Ann Surg* 193:150–154, 1981.

Glenn F: Acute cholecystitis. *Surg Gynecol Obstet* 143:56–60, 1976.

Glenn F: Biliary tract disease. *Surg Gynecol Obstet* 153:401–402, 1981.

Ralls PW, Colletti PM, Halls JM, et al: Prospective evaluation of ^{99m}Tc-IDA cholescintigraphy and grey-scale ultrasound in the diagnosis of acute cholecystitis. *Radiology* 144:369–371, 1982.

Thompson JE, Tompkins RK, Longmire WP: Factors in management of acute cholangitis. *Ann Surg* 195:137–145, 1982.

Tompkins RK, Thomas D, Wile A, et al: Prognostic factors in bile duct carcinoma: analysis of 96 cases. *Ann Surg* 194:447–452, 1981.

Way LW, Admirand WH, Dunphy JE: Management of choledocholithiasis. *Ann Surg* 176:347–359, 1972.

Way LW, Bernhoft RA, Thomas JM: Biliary stricture. *Surg Clin North Am* 61:963–972, 1981.

Wenckert A, Robertson B: The national course of gallstone disease. Eleven-year review of 781 nonoperated cases. *Gastroenterology* 50:376–381, 1966.

Skills

1. Given a patient with acute cholecystitis, demonstrate the right upper quadrant physical findings that indicate this diagnosis.
2. Demonstrate an understanding of drains by advancing and/or removing subhepatic drains and a T-tube.
3. Discuss when an intraoperative cholangiogram and a T-tube cholangiogram are indicated. Demonstrate ability to read the above radiologic studies, pointing out pertinent anatomy and pitfalls leading to misdiagnosis.
4. Demonstrate ability to read a percutaneous transhepatic cholangiogram and an endoscopic retrograde cholangiopancreatography (ERCP) study. Tell when each is indicated.

Study Questions

1. What is the difference between biliary colic and acute cholecystitis clinically and what is the difference in their management?
2. Describe five complications of gallstone disease.
3. What two conditions must be present for cholangitis to develop? What does optimal management of cholangitis entail? How can uncomplicated acute ascending cholangitis be differentiated from acute suppurative cholangitis?
4. As the physician of someone with asymptomatic gallstones, what recommendations would you make? With symptomatic gallstones?
5. When is a cholangiopancreatogram (ERCP) preferred over a percutaneous transhepatic cholangiogram (PTC)?
6. What is the diagnostic procedure of choice for someone with acute cholecystitis? With chronic cholecystitis? With jaundice and guaiac positive stools? With deep jaundice, weight loss, and anorexia?
7. A cholangiocarcinoma in what part of the biliary tree has the best prognosis? The worst?
8. What is the most common cause of biliary stricture? How can biliary strictures be avoided?
9. What is the most common cause of air in the biliary tree (pneumobilia) in the patient with a virgin abdomen? How do patients with this problem present clinically?
10. What kind of antibiotic(s) should be administered to the patient with acute cholecystitis? With cholangitis?

20

Pancreas → retroperitoneal

Royce Laycock, M.D., L. Beaty Pemberton, M.D.,
Philip J. Huber, Jr., M.D., Steven T. Ruby, M.D.,
Ajit K. Sachdeva, M.D., and
Jeffrey T. Schouten, M.D.

Cullen's sign → bluish discoloration of the periumbilical area
Grey-Turner's sign → bluish discoloration of the flank   *→ Severe hemorrhagic pancreatitis*

ASSUMPTIONS

The student is familiar with the anatomy of the pancreas and understands its relationship to the biliary tree.

The student understands the physiology of the pancreas, including endocrine and exocrine function.

OBJECTIVES

1. Classify pancreatitis on the basis of the severity of injury to the organ.
2. List four etiologies of pancreatitis.
3. Describe the clinical presentation of a patient with acute pancreatitis, including indications for surgical intervention.
4. Discuss at least five potential early complications of acute pancreatitis.
5. Discuss four potential adverse outcomes of chronic pancreatitis as well as surgical diagnostic approach, treatment options, and management.
6. Discuss the criteria used to predict the prognosis for acute pancreatitis.
7. Discuss the mechanism of pseudocyst formation with respect to the role of the duct and list five symptoms and physical signs of pseudocysts.
8. Describe the diagnostic approach to a patient with a suspected pseudocyst, including indications for and sequence of tests.
9. Discuss the natural history of an untreated pancreatic pseudocyst as well as the medical and surgical treatment.
10. List four pancreatic neoplasms and describe the pathology of each with reference to cell type and function.
11. Describe the symptoms, physical signs, laboratory findings, and diagnostic workup of a pancreatic mass on the basis of the location of the tumor in the pancreas.
12. Describe the surgical treatment of pancreatic neoplasms.
13. Discuss the long-term prognosis for pancreatic cancers on the basis of pathology and cell type.

Diseases of the pancreas are common and often require surgical intervention as treatment. The pancreas is subject to congenital, inflammatory, infectious, post-traumatic, and neoplastic diseases. The gland was named by Galen and it was originally believed that its only function was to protect blood vessels. Its exocrine role in digestion was not known until the 1800s, and its ability to modulate glucose metabolism was demonstrated in 1921 by Banting and Best. Inflammatory diseases of the pancreas were described in the late 1800s by Fitz and surgery for pancreatic neoplasms was popularized by the work of Whipple et al. in the 1930s. As a result of our greater understanding of pancreatic anatomy, physiology, and pathophysiology, we are now able to better identify patients with pancreatic disease who will benefit from surgical intervention.

Anatomy

The pancreas is a gland that lies in a transverse orientation in the retroperitoneum at the level of the second lumbar vertebra. Its length is generally between 12–18 cm and it weighs between 70 and 110 gm.

The gland itself is divided into four distinct parts: head, neck, body, and tail (Fig. 20.1). The head of the pancreas accounts for approximately 30% of the gland and is surrounded by the ''C-loop'' of the duodenum. Its lower portion is referred to as the uncinate process. The neck of the gland is the portion to the left of the head, directly anterior to the superior mesenteric vessels. The body of the pancreas extends to the left and slightly cephalad. The tail enters the splenorenal ligament and often makes contact with the inferior aspect of the splenic hilum.

The anterior surface of the gland is in contact with the transverse mesocolon as well as the posterior wall of the stomach. Its posterior surface is devoid of peritoneum and is bounded by the common bile duct, the superior mesenteric vessels, the inferior vena cava, and the aorta.

245

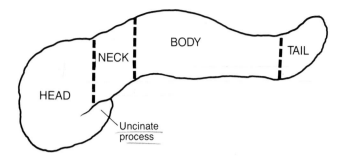

Figure 20.1.   Regional anatomy of the pancreas.

Ductal Anatomy

The duct of Wirsung is the main pancreatic duct and its position within the gland is relatively constant (Fig. 20.2). It begins in the tail and courses toward the head with smaller subsidiary ducts joining it along its length. It will eventually join the common bile duct within the head of the pancreas. These structures will then pass through the medial wall of the second part of the duodenum in an oblique course to form an ampulla within the papilla of Vater. This nipple-like protrusion (papilla) is referred to as the major papilla. The pancreas will usually (>95%) have an accessory duct known as the duct of Santorini. Its anatomic configuration is quite variable but most commonly it enters the duodenum separately through the lesser papilla usually located 2 cm proximal to the papilla of Vater. The accessory duct has a tributary that joins the main duct within the head of the gland in the majority of cases and in a small percentage of cases (2%) may fail to enter the duodenum. The duct of Santorini may be the main pancreatic duct in 5–10% of people because of a congenital anomaly that is referred to as pancreas divisum.

The common bile duct passes behind the first portion of the duodenum and descends directly posterior to the head of the pancreas. It will generally enter the

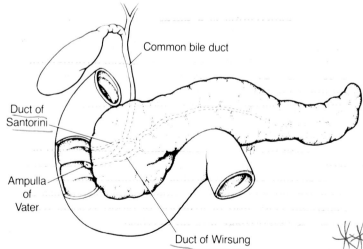

Figure 20.2.   Anatomy of the pancreatic ductal system demonstrating the ducts of Wirsung (major duct) and Santorini (minor duct) and their relationship to the common bile duct.

substance of the gland just prior to entering the duodenum, either as a common channel with the duct of Wirsung (38%) or as a separate opening adjacent to the pancreatic duct (42%).

The sphincter of Oddi is a complex series of circumferential smooth muscle sphincters surrounding the ampulla. Constriction of this sphincter mechanism will result in a cessation of bile flow. The pancreatic duct may have its own sphincter mechanism within the ampulla of Vater.

Arterial Blood Supply

The pancreas receives its arterial blood supply from branches of the celiac axis and the superior mesenteric artery (Fig. 20.3). The head of the pancreas is nourished by a set of paired, matched vessels known as the anterior and posterior arcades. The gastroduodenal artery is a branch of the hepatic artery and gives rise to the anterior superior pancreaticoduodenal artery, which is a major component of the anterior arcade. The other component of the anterior arcade is the anterior inferior pancreaticoduodenal artery, which is a branch of the superior mesenteric artery. The gastroduodenal artery also gives rise to the posterior superior pancreaticoduodenal artery, a component of the posterior arcade. The other component of the posterior arcade is the posterior inferior pancreaticoduodenal artery, a branch of the superior mesenteric artery. Of note is that the arcades also provide a major source of blood supply to the duodenum.

The dorsal pancreatic artery is present in 90% of people but has a variable origin. In most cases, it arises from the proximal splenic artery but may be a branch of the celiac axis or superior mesenteric artery. It will divide into a right branch, which passes along the upper margin of the uncinate process and joins the anterior arcade, as well as a left branch, which becomes the inferior pancreatic artery and supplies the body and tail of the gland. The splenic artery is the source of multiple superior pancreatic branches that supply the body of the pancreas. The largest of these branches is known as the pancreatic magna (great pancreatic artery).

Venous Drainage

The venous drainage of the pancreas and duodenum corresponds to the arterial supply. The veins, in general, are immediately superficial to the arteries. The anterior venous arcade drains into the superior mesenteric vein while the posterior venous arcade generally drains into the portal vein.

Innervation

Inflammatory as well as neoplastic diseases of the pancreas often manifest with pain that is mediated via the abundant supply of afferent sensory nerve fibers. The pancreas is also innervated by motor fibers of both the sympathetic (greater splanchnic nerve) and parasympathetic (vagus nerve) autonomic nervous systems. All fibers pass through the celiac or superior

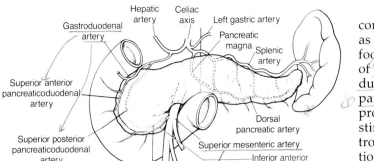

Figure 20.3. Blood supply of the pancreas.

mesenteric plexus. Pain fibers accompany the sympathetic fibers and follow the blood vessels to the gland.

Anomalies

Anomalies of the pancreas are well known to surgeons. Heterotopic pancreas occurs in up to 6% of autopsy cases. These accessory nodules of pancreatic tissue, also known as pancreatic rests, occur most commonly in the submucosae of the stomach, duodenum, or the jejunum. The rests may or may not contain islet tissue. Annular pancreas is a congenital anomaly resulting in a ring of pancreatic tissue encircling the duodenum. Another anomaly occurs when faulty rotation of the ventral primordium results in lack of fusion with the dorsal primordium. This condition is referred to as pancreas divisum, and it occurs in 5–10% of the population.

Physiology

Exocrine → pancreatic juice

The main function of the exocrine pancreas is to secrete 1000–5000 ml/day of isosmotic, alkaline (pH-8.00) pancreatic juice through the pancreatic duct into the second portion of the duodenum. The components of pancreatic juice are electrolytes, protein, and digestive enzymes. The concentration of sodium and potassium is similar to plasma. The pH of pancreatic juice is 8.0 because of a high concentration of HCO_3^- which is secreted by an active mechanism under the catalytic influence of carbonic anhydrase. Pancreatic enzymes necessary for digestion include chymotrypsin, trypsin, carboxypeptidase, amylase, and lipase. Proteins that are ingested are broken down to peptides by the digestive enzymes trypsin and chymotrypsin. The latter are formed by the activation of trypsinogen and chymotrypsinogen, which are precursors synthesized within the pancreatic cell. Amylase is the enzyme most commonly associated with the pancreas because its measurement in clinical medicine is used as a marker for inflammatory disease of the gland. Its function is to split starch into dextrins and disaccharides. Lipase splits fats into glycerol and fatty acids, but requires the presence of bile acids.

Pancreatic secretions are controlled by a number of complex mechanisms. Stimulation of the vagus nerve as well as distention of the antrum of the stomach by food will increase pancreatic secretions. The presence of amino acids, sodium oleate, or an acidic pH in the duodenum will lead to the release of cholecystokinin-pancreozymin (CCK-PZ) and secretin, two hormones produced by the mucosae of the duodenum. Secretin stimulates the flow of bicarbonate-rich water and electrolytes from the pancreas. CCK-PZ potentiates the action of secretin and increases the enzyme concentration of pancreatic juice. The major effect of surgical removal of the pancreas is the loss of all pancreatic secretions, which leads to severe impairment of digestion and absorption.

Endocrine → Islets of Langerhans

The islets of Langerhans make up 1.5% of the pancreas by weight and are responsible for the endocrine functions of the gland. Islets measure 75–150 μm and are more abundant in the tail of the gland. The major function of the islets is the control of glucose homeostasis. The α cells secrete glucagon, which is a peptide made of 20 amino acids. Its release is stimulated by a low serum glucose and it results in glycogenolysis and the release of glucose into the blood stream. The β cells constitute 60% of the islets and secrete insulin, a peptide with a molecular weight of 6000. Insulin is released in response to increases in serum glucose and promotes the transfer of glucose across cell membranes. The inability of the β cells to produce insulin results in hyperglycemia (high serum glucose), which leads to the clinical syndrome known as juvenile onset diabetes mellitus. The complications of this disease are well known and include blindness, kidney failure, and accelerated atherosclerosis.

Acute Pancreatitis → 85% < alcohol ingestion / biliary calculi

Acute pancreatitis is a diffuse inflammation of the pancreas often associated with complications that occasionally lead to death. A number of well known factors are associated with acute pancreatitis, although the precise etiology is not well understood. The two most common causes of pancreatitis are alcohol ingestion and biliary calculi. These two factors account for 85% of cases.

Acute pancreatitis is characterized by enzymatic destruction of the pancreatic substance by release and activation of pancreatic enzymes into the glandular parenchyma. The microscopic (histologic) changes include the presence of acute inflammatory cells, loss of pancreatic cells, and destruction of blood vessels with resulting hemorrhage and fat necrosis.

Etiology

All causes of acute pancreatitis can be categorized into the following groups: metabolic, mechanical, vascular, and infectious. The most common etiology within the metabolic group is alcohol, which accounts for up to 40% of cases. Generally, the first episode is preceded by 6–8 years of significant alcohol ingestion and is often followed by recurring acute attacks. After multiple attacks of acute pancreatitis, the pancreas becomes permanently damaged and the result is the clinical syndrome known as chronic pancreatitis. Exactly how alcohol causes pancreatitis is not known. A common theory is that alcohol induces changes in the secretory response of the pancreas resulting in higher protein content in the secretions. This leads to the precipitation of protein and the blockage of small pancreatic ductules. Other metabolic causes of pancreatitis include types I, IV, and V hyperlipoproteinemia, hyperparathyroidism, adrenocorticosteroids, thiazide diuretics, estrogens, and furosemide.

The most common mechanical etiology of acute pancreatitis is gallstones and it is estimated that up to 60% of nonalcoholic patients with pancreatitis have gallstones. Like alcohol, the etiology of gallstone-induced pancreatitis is not completely understood. In 1901, Opie proposed the common channel theory based on his observation of a common channel within the ampullae made up of the common bile duct and the pancreatic duct. He proposed that a gallstone could block the pancreatic duct within the ampulla leading to a reflux of bile into the pancreatic duct resulting in acute pancreatitis. This theory has been disputed by some who have shown experimentally that bile in the pancreatic duct at physiological pressures does not cause pancreatitis. It has been suggested that transient obstruction of a common channel might lead to reflux of pancreatic juice into the common bile duct. The mixing of bile and pancreatic juice may lead to the formation of a substance highly toxic to the pancreas. Other mechanical causes of pancreatitis include blunt and penetrating trauma to the pancreas and malignant obstruction of the pancreatic duct by tumors of the distal common duct, pancreas, ampulla of Vater, and duodenum.

Ischemic injuries to the pancreas, either secondary to hypotension or devascularization during upper abdominal surgery, may initiate pancreatitis or may play a role in the progression of pancreatic edema to pancreatic necrosis. Postoperative pancreatitis may be seen following gastric surgery in up to 15% of cases and following biliary surgery in 10% of cases. Acute pancreatitis is a complication in 1% of patients undergoing an endoscopic radiographic evaluation of their pancreaticobiliary ductal anatomy known as endoscopic retrograde cholangiopancreatography (ERCP). This is thought to be due to an acute increase in intraductal pressure. Mumps, coxsackie virus, chlorthiazide, and steroids may cause pancreatitis as well. Approximately 8–10% of cases of pancreatitis have no recognizable etiology and these are generally termed idiopathic pancreatitis.

Diagnosis

Patients with acute pancreatitis will complain of noncrampy, epigastric abdominal pain. The character of the pain is variable and frequently radiates to the left or right upper quadrant and/or the back. The pain may be relieved by sitting or standing. It is associated with nausea and often a significant amount of vomiting. There will usually be a history of alcohol ingestion or gallstones. Physical examination is characterized by fever, tachycardia, and upper abdominal tenderness with guarding. Bowel sounds are generally absent because of the presence of an adynamic ileus. Physical signs of severe hemorrhagic pancreatitis are a bluish discoloration of the periumbilical area (Cullen's sign) or the flank (Grey-Turner's sign). In addition, generalized abdominal and rebound tenderness may occur in severe pancreatitis. Laboratory evaluation reveals leukocytosis and elevated serum amylase. Urinary levels of amylase are elevated, which is reflected in an increased ratio of amylase clearance/creatinine clearance. In severe cases of pancreatitis there may also be abnormalities in liver chemistries, hyperglycemia, hypocalcemia, and elevated blood urea nitrogen (BUN) and creatinine levels, as well as hypoxemia. The differential diagnosis of acute pancreatitis includes acute cholecystitis, perforated peptic ulcer, mesenteric ischemia, ruptured esophagus, and myocardial infarction. Patients with suspected acute pancreatitis should be evaluated radiologically including (1) chest x-ray, which may show left pleural effusion, plate atelectasis, or hemidiaphragm elevation; (2) plain and upright abdomen x-rays, which may show calcifications indicating chronic pancreatitis, gallstones, or local adynamic ileus; and (3) ultrasonography to detect gallstones, pancreatic enlargements, and pseudocysts. If complicated acute pancreatitis is suspected, CT is preferred over ultrasound because of its greater sensitivity. Ultrasound is preferred for following the course of pseudocysts.

Prognostic Factors

Acute pancreatitis may vary from a mild episode to a rapidly lethal illness. Ranson et al. have devised a system to estimate the risk of major complications or death depending on the number of prognostic signs

Table 20.1.
Prognostic Factors: Risk of Major Complications or Death

At admission	mortality	signs
Age > 55 years	20%	3–4
WBC > 16,000		
Glucose > 200 mg/100 ml	40%	5–6
LDH > 350		
SGOT > 250	100%	≥7
During 48 hr after admission		
HCT > 10 point decrease		
BUN > 5 mg/100 ml increase		
Ca²⁺ < 8.0		
pO₂ < 60 mm Hg on room air		
Base excess > 4 mEq/liter		
Estimated fluid sequestration > 6,000 ml		

present at the time of admission or within 48 hr after admission (Table 20.1). The risk of mortality is 20% if there are three to four signs, 40% for five to six signs, and virtually 100% if the patient has seven or more signs. Acute hemorrhagic pancreatitis has a much higher mortality than the edematous pancreatitis most frequently seen in alcoholics.

Treatment

The medical therapy of acute pancreatitis can be divided into general supportive therapy and specific treatment of pancreatic inflammation. In patients with pancreatitis, it is important to maintain adequate tissue perfusion by monitoring cardiovascular parameters and maintaining adequate intravascular volume. A massive amount of fluid can be sequestered in the retroperitoneal tissues because of the presence of activated enzymes and inflammation. In severe cases, this may require several liters of isotonic solution to be given rapidly through large bore intravenous tubes during resuscitation. Fluid management may be aided by the use of a central venous line or Swan-Ganz catheter to monitor cardiac function and a Foley catheter to evaluate urine output. Electrolytes must be carefully monitored and respiratory, as well as nutritional, support must be instituted when appropriate.

Respiratory function, particularly arterial blood gases, must be monitored carefully as respiratory failure is insidious and is the most common cause of death. Specific inhibition of pancreatic secretions in an effort to decrease peripancreatic inflammation has been attempted with the use of nasogastric suction. Studies in patients with mild alcoholic pancreatitis have not shown a benefit with this mode of therapy; however, nasogastric suction may be useful in patients with more severe forms of pancreatitis. Anticholinergics, somatostatin, specific enzyme inhibitors, such as aprotinin, and snake antivenom, and antacids have all been used in an attempt to decrease the degree of pancreatic inflammation, but none have been shown to be of any significant benefit. Antibiotics similarly have not been shown to decrease morbidity or mortality in patients with mild pancreatitis; however, they are used quite liberally by surgeons in the treatment of gallstone pancreatitis. H$_2$ blockers have been used when there is associated gastritis or ulcer disease.

The surgical management of patients with pancreatitis is controversial. Diagnostic laparotomy is recommended by some when the diagnosis is not clear. This is meant not only to establish the diagnosis of pancreatitis but also to rule out other nonpancreatic lesions that may mimic pancreatitis such as perforated ulcer, gangrenous cholecystitis, and mesenteric infarction. In patients with gallstone pancreatitis it has been suggested by some that early surgical evaluation of the biliary tree may lessen the severity of the pancreatitis. This is based on the belief that persistent obstruction of the ampulla of Vater may be a major factor in determining the progression of acute pancreatic inflammation. Depending on the findings at surgery, inter-

vention may consist of tube cholecystostomy, cholecystectomy, or common duct exploration. This is a controversial issue, and many surgeons report a higher mortality associated with early surgical intervention. Other forms of surgical therapy used on occasion include pancreatic resection and open pancreatic drainage with large sump drains.

Peritoneal lavage was first introduced in 1965 as a form of therapy for patients with acute pancreatitis. The bathing of the peritoneal cavity with an isotonic balanced salt solution infused via catheters has proven to be safe, and seems to be an effective adjunct in management of early cardiovascular and respiratory complications. However, it does not seem to influence the incidence or severity of late septic complications of acute pancreatitis.

Complications of acute pancreatitis

There are many minor and major complications of acute pancreatitis. The metabolic complications include hyperglycemia, hypocalcemia, and renal failure. Varying degrees of respiratory insufficiency and hypoxemia may be present. They develop secondary to a combination of factors including diaphragmatic elevation resulting in decreased ventilation, fluid overload during resuscitation, pulmonary thromboemboli, and the release of an antisurfactant factor. Severe cases may require mechanical ventilation with positive end-expiratory pressure (PEEP). In extremely severe cases, patients may go on to cardiovascular collapse not only because of intravascular fluid depletion but also because of the presence of a probable myocardial depressant factor. Coagulopathy and hemorrhage may also be seen due to depletion of coagulation factors or erosion into a major vessel. The most common local complications seen are paralytic ileus and sterile peripancreatic fluid collections. Patients may develop obstruction of the biliary tree or duodenum as well as thrombosis of the nearby splenic vein, which can lead to the formation of esophageal varices. One of the most serious complications of acute pancreatitis is the formation of a pancreatic abscess that may result from infection of a pseudocyst or the development of infection in peripancreatic devitalized tissue. This complication is associated with a very high mortality and demands prompt surgical intervention.

Chronic Pancreatitis

Inflammation of the pancreas can progress to a chronic stage for a variety of reasons. If the initial inflammatory insult is severe enough to cause permanent ductal damage, recurring pancreatitis can develop, usually because of ductal obstruction or stasis (Table 20.2). Possible causes of such a significant injury include trauma and cholelithiasis. The most important cause of chronic pancreatitis is persistent alcohol ingestion. Infrequently metabolic disturbances precipitate acute or chronic pancreatitis; these include

Table 20.2.
Marseilles Classification of Pancreatitis

I. Acute pancreatitis—a single episode of pancreatitis in a previously normal gland.
II. Acute relapsing pancreatitis—recurrent attacks that do not lead to permanent functional damage; clinical and biological normalcy in interval between attacks.
III. Chronic relapsing pancreatitis—progressive functional damage persisting between attacks; frequent pain-free intervals.
IV. Chronic pancreatitis—inexorable and irreversible destruction of pancreatic function; constant pain.

hypercalcemia, hyperlipidemia, and hemachromatosis. Congenital causes include cystic fibrosis, familial pancreatitis, and pancreatic divisum. The last entity occurs when the dorsal and ventral segments of fetal pancreas fail to meet and fuse. This results in most of the pancreas being drained by the smaller duct of Santorini with consequent stasis and increased likelihood of inflammation.

Repeated episodes of pancreatitis result in disruption and obstruction of large and small pancreatic ducts with subsequent autodigestion. With the edema and tissue destruction, the pancreas undergoes scarring and fibrosis with loss of functional substance. The result of this process is pancreatic insufficiency manifesting as exocrine and endocrine failure. Loss of exocrine function leads to malabsorption. When pancreatic secretion of enzymes drops below 10% of normal, protein and fat cannot be adequately absorbed. The resulting steatorrhea can be quantitated by measuring stool fat in a patient who is on a prescribed fat diet. Pancreatic endocrine dysfunction produces diabetes. Generally these patients respond to insulin treatment and do not seem to be as vulnerable to small vessel disease as other diabetic patients. Nonetheless, insulin administration is hazardous in this chronic pancreatitis population, since most continue their heavy alcohol intake.

Pain is the most frequent symptom of chronic pancreatitis. The pain is usually intermittent but, with the development of subsequent attacks of pancreatitis and more scarring and fibrosis of the gland, the pain may become inexorable and unrelenting. Eating may become impossible because of pain production. Patients often resort to increased alcohol intake and use of pain-killing drugs to obtain relief. Drug dependency, malnutrition, vitamin B_{12} deficiency, and severe pain are usual in the group with chronic pancreatitis. Pseudocysts are not uncommon in this group.

Patients with chronic pancreatitis should be managed conservatively with the intention of reducing trauma to the pancreas and, when necessary, considering surgery to deal with appropriate complications such as pseudocysts. Because alcoholism is the leading cause of pancreatitis, abstinence should be strongly advised. If other specific causes are identified, these too should be corrected to minimize further pancreas difficulties.

Patients with suspected chronic pancreatitis or those with known chronic pancreatitis presenting with new symptoms should be assessed by computed tomography (CT) to search for surgically correctable causes or complications of pancreatitis. CT has the greatest sensitivity for showing gland enlargement or atrophy, duct enlargement, calcifications, masses, pseudocysts, inflammation, and extensions beyond the pancreas. Liver, gall bladder, and bile ducts are also visualized. Ultrasonography is cheaper than CT but less successful in showing the pancreas, especially in obese patients and in patients with gas-filled intestines. However, ultrasonography is the preferred diagnostic study for following changes in pseudocysts if the latter are clearly visualized. It is also the preferred method for initial study of the jaundiced patient even with a pancreatic cause of his jaundice.

Prior to surgery, ductal anatomy should be defined by pancreatic ductography, usually using ERCP. In this procedure endoscopy and fluoroscopy are used in combination to facilitate cannulation and opacification of the pancreatic and biliary ducts with contrast agent. Radiographs are made during the filling and emptying phases to map ductal anatomy as well as to delineate obstructions, strictures, calculi, duct ectasia, and pseudocysts. ERCP is invasive and carries a small but definite risk of causing exacerbation of pancreatitis, biliary or pancreatic sepsis, or infection of a pseudocyst.

Segmental ductal obstruction with dilatation or altering areas of stricture and ectasia in the pancreatic duct, the "chain of lakes" picture, are amenable to surgical intervention. Both problems can be overcome by opening the pancreatic duct throughout its length and performing a side-to-side Roux-en-Y pancreaticojejunostomy. This side-to-side pancreaticojejunostomy seems to control the obstruction and usually alleviates the pain associated with chronic pancreatitis. Progression of the exocrine and endocrine dysfunction is, however, usually not reversed. If no definable ductal abnormality is delineated during diagnostic workup, the patient with chronic pancreatitis should be carefully monitored for pancreatic function and nutritional status. Medication for pain is of limited efficacy and 95% pancreatic resection may be considered for pain relief. This operative procedure is followed by an extremely high complication rate in alcoholics. In general, pain relief may be obtained in 70–80% of patients managed by one of the surgical therapies, and treatment should be tailored to the individual.

Pseudocysts

Another complication of pancreatitis is the development of a pancreatic pseudocyst. A pseudocyst is a cavity lined by nonepithelial elements. This cavity is formed during the process of pancreatitis and is caused by ductal disruption and gland autolysis. Enzymatic fluid collects in or around the pancreas and is "walled off" by surrounding adjacent structures to form a pseudocyst. Pseudocyst development can occur anywhere from the stomach to the pelvis and may include any tissues in this broad area. Pancreatic ductal structure includes many minute ducts through which digestive enzymes and bicarbonate-rich fluid are secreted into the main and accessory pancreatic ducts. For a variety of reasons, disruption in the system—involving either small or large ducts—creates extravasation of highly irritating enzymes. This extravasation can flow into the peritoneal cavity, or it can be localized in the form of a pseudocyst.

The most frequent symptoms associated with pseudocysts relate to the inflammation that created the pseudocyst. Epigastric pain is the most common symptom, but nausea and vomiting may also occur with both pancreatitis and/or pseudocysts. On occasion, pseudocysts can create mechanical obstruction of either the stomach or duodenum, but this is unusual. Jaundice secondary to biliary obstruction can occur due to pseudocyst formation, but this is also unusual. Unexplained fever raises the possibility of an infected pseudocyst. A palpable upper abdominal mass is frequently found with pseudocysts. The mass may or may not be tender and can present without a definite attack of pancreatitis.

To initiate workup of a pancreatic pseudocyst, a thorough history and physical is mandatory. Obviously, obtaining a history of alcoholism and previous pancreatitis is important. Fever, weight loss, and a history of jaundice are other salient clinical features. Appropriate lab data include complete blood chemistry (CBC), liver function studies, serum amylase, and serum lipase. These last two tests are noteworthy in that the serum amylase level in chronic pancreatitis patients may not be as sensitive a marker as the serum lipase level.

In the past, a barium upper gastrointestinal series was the most useful radiologic technique; presently sonography and CT scans have become the first line noninvasive studies to assess an abdominal mass. Sonography has been a marvelous technical advance because it is relatively inexpensive and is quite accurate in distinguishing solid from cystic masses. Further delineation of the mass and surrounding tissue structures is obtained with a CT scan (Fig. 20.4). Not only can the mass and its relationship to surrounding structures be neatly outlined, but serial examinations can show growth or shrinkage of the mass over time. Furthermore, CT and sonography can be utilized in more invasive techniques in which direct needle or catheter aspiration/drainage of the fluid collection may be accomplished. Thus, they may be diagnostic or they may actually be primary treatment of the patient. More and more literature is appearing that supports radiologically directed biopsies, aspirations, or drainage procedures. This modality has clearly had a major impact on diagnosis and treatment of many lesions. A pseudocyst that lies adjacent to the abdominal wall is easily accessible to catheter drainage under local anesthesia. Moreover, a septic patient with a pseudocyst that is the possible origin of the infection can undergo aspiration to determine if the pseudocyst contains pus. Generally, sonography and CT are the two primary studies that permit the diagnosis of a pancreatic pseudocyst.

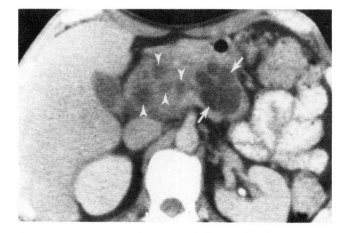

Figure 20.4. A CT scan showing multiple pseudocysts (arrows) in a patient with chronic pancreatitis.

Approximately 30% of pseudocysts resolve spontaneously with conservative medical management. The conservative approach consists of resting the pancreas by maintaining the patient on total parenteral nutrition. During observation of the patient over a period of weeks, one should see progressive decrease in size if the pseudocyst is going to resolve. Simple palpation on daily exam will show reduced tenderness and diminished size. Ultrasound, and, if necessary, CT can document disappearance of the pseudocyst very accurately. Clearly, patients with acute pancreatitis and a sudden onset of a pseudocyst are much more likely to resolve than patients with a history of chronic pancreatitis and a long-standing mass. The initial management of all pseudocysts consists of hospitalization and restricted activity. This mandatory precaution is indicated because pseudocysts in their initial phase are poorly walled off collections that can leak and/or rupture with very severe consequences. By restricting the patient's activity and stopping food intake, the pseudocyst will stabilize its size, and the walls will firm up over time to provide a thickened "rind" or shell that is unlikely to leak or burst. Complications from pseudocysts can be catastrophic and may occur in 30–50% of patients. The pseudocyst is susceptible to infection and abscess formation. Patients with a pseudocyst who develop a fever have an infected pseudocyst until proven otherwise. These infected cysts require drainage.

Hemorrhage from a pseudocyst can be life-threatening. As the definition implies, the lining of the pseudocyst is made from surrounding peripancreatic tissues that abound with major blood vessels. Erosion into an artery can occur with rapid onset of hypotension and exsanguination. Immediate operative intervention is obligatory and the prognosis is poor even when control of bleeding is prompt.

The initial treatment of a pseudocyst consists of intensive medical management until a "mature" cyst wall is formed or the cyst resolves. Maturation of the cyst wall generally requires in excess of 4 weeks. Maturation is the process of developing enough fibrosis in the

external drainage → ↑ recurrence rates

∴ internal drainage → Roux-en-Y cyst-jejunostomy if cyst has resolved or cyst-gastrostomy

cyst wall to support suturing to stomach or jejunum for internal drainage. Following a course of restricted activity and relative bowel rest, drainage is carried out if the cyst has not resolved within 4–6 weeks. If the pseudocyst is approachable by CT-directed drainage technique, aspiration may be attempted, but recurrence rates are high. This decision is best made jointly by the radiologist and surgeon. When the pseudocyst cannot be easily drained percutaneously, surgical exploration is indicated. Two basic techniques are used to drain pseudocysts surgically. Internal drainage of the pseudocyst is accomplished by opening the pseudocyst in a Roux-en-Y cyst-jejunostomy or in some cases where the cyst is fixed to the stomach, performing a cyst-gastrostomy. Internal drainage is preferred, but if this cannot be done because of technical problems, immature cyst wall, or infection, then external drainage is done. Internal drainage is acceptable over 90% of the time while external drainage requires a second operation at least 25% of the time. Biopsy of the cyst wall is recommended at the time of surgical drainage to confirm that the process is benign. Rarely, cystadenocarcinoma of the pancreas can mimic a pseudocyst. Pseudocysts that develop as a complication of pancreatitis need not create life-threatening situations for the patient. An orderly diagnostic approach to determine the extent and anatomic location of the cyst is a significant first step. Conservative management of the patient until the cyst either matures or disappears is most important. A persistent pseudocyst needs surgical intervention to avoid significant complications and to treat the patient effectively.

Pancreatic Neoplasms

Incidence and Significance

Pancreatic adenocarcinoma is the fourth most common cause of cancer deaths in the United States, accounting for over 20,000 deaths per year. The ratio of males to females in most series is approximately 2:1 while the annual incidence is between 9 and 10 cases per 100,000 population. The principle risk factors for the development of pancreatic carcinoma appear to be increasing age and cigarette smoking. While controversy exists over the etiologic role of diabetes and alcohol, cigarette smoking appears to double the risk of developing pancreatic carcinoma. MacMahon published an epidemiological review reporting a threefold increased risk of developing pancreatic cancer for nonsmokers who ingested three or more cups of coffee a day. However, other studies are needed to collaborate these findings. The most common location for pancreatic carcinoma is in the head of the gland, accounting for approximately two-thirds of all cases. The most common malignancy of the pancreas is a poorly differentiated adenocarcinoma originating from the ductal epithelium. Several studies have documented a high incidence of multicentricity. The remainder of neoplasms arising in the pancreas are islet cell tumors and cystadenocarcinomas.

Clinical Presentation

The signs and symptoms of pancreatic carcinoma relate to the anatomy of the region. Tumors originating in the periampullary region may present relatively early with asymptomatic jaundice. However, most patients present with a combination of weight loss, jaundice, and pain due to regional infiltration in the peripancreatic region. Pain tends to be in the posterior epigastric region with radiation to the back. The pain of pancreatic disease can be differentiated from biliary colic based on the *constant* posterior radiating nature of the pain associated with pancreatic disease versus the intermittent *colic* usually associated with biliary tract disease. A palpable nontender gallbladder has been suggested to be associated more commonly with malignancy than with cholelithiasis (Courvoisier's Law). This is due to the ready distensibility of the nonfibrotic gallbladder associated with carcinoma. The existence of a palpable mass at the time of presentation argues against resectability and represents advanced disease. Often patients with pancreatic cancer give a history of phlebitis.

Evaluation and Diagnosis

The most common abnormal laboratory findings are those associated with biliary obstruction. The alkaline phosphatase and direct bilirubin increase proportionally higher than the indirect bilirubin and the serum transaminase levels. Occult blood is present in the stools in one-half of all patients. Hyperamylasemia is infrequently detected (5% of cases). — *amylase is (N) as opposed to pancreatitis.*

Radiologic Findings

The standard plain film of the abdomen is unremarkable in most patients with pancreatic carcinoma. Calcifications, when present, are associated with chronic pancreatitis and not with pancreatic carcinoma. Sonography should be done when the initial history, physical, and laboratory assessment indicate that obstructive jaundice or a pancreatic mass is present. The sonogram is useful in demonstrating dilated ducts, the presence of cholelithiasis and/or choledocholithiasis, the presence of a mass in the head of the pancreas, and the presence of liver metastasis. Following the sonogram, the radiographic workup is individualized. The following additional tests may be useful in evaluating patients with pancreatic carcinoma. Computed tomography (CT) of the pancreas has become a very useful test to evaluate both the local extent of lesions as well as the presence or absence of metastatic lesions. CT may demonstrate local vascular invasion indicating unresectability (i.e., portal vein and superior mesenteric vessels). Additional procedures that may be useful include CT-directed percutaneous fine-needle biopsy of pancreatic lesions and endoscopic retrograde cholangiopancreatography (ERCP). ERCP provides information regarding the anatomy of the pancreatic duct and assesses whether or not a tumor has occluded the duct. Additionally, biopsy specimens may be obtained and a periampullary lesion may be diagnosed based on the endoscopic biopsy results. Similarly, ERCP allows one to perform endoscopy to rule out any other associated lesions relative to the gastroduodenal intestinal tract. Injection of the common duct allows one to delineate anatomically the site and extent of obstruction of the common duct as well as demonstrating the anatomy of the pancreatic duct. Early results evaluating CEA levels and cytology of pancreatic fluid appear encouraging in establishing a diagnosis of pancreatic carcinoma.

Percutaneous transhepatic cholangiography (PTHC) is a useful test, particularly for delineation of the proximal extent of disease. The test can usually be performed with minimal morbidity in a patient with dilated biliary radicals if a percutaneous catheter is left in to decompress the obstructed system following the procedure. In addition, a catheter may be passed through the obstruction to allow for internal biliary drainage. The issue of preoperative decompression of the biliary tree remains controversial relative to its effect upon operative morbidity and mortality. However, in a patient undergoing an extensive preoperative workup, percutaneous transhepatic cholangiographic drainage is useful to prevent any further damage to the liver from the obstructive process.

Angiography allows further delineation of the extent of tumor invasion into the local vascular anatomy of the pancreatic region as well as delineating the vascular supply of the tumor itself. The utilization of angiography has decreased with the widespread availability of CT and other diagnostic procedures mentioned above but may be of value in selected patients.

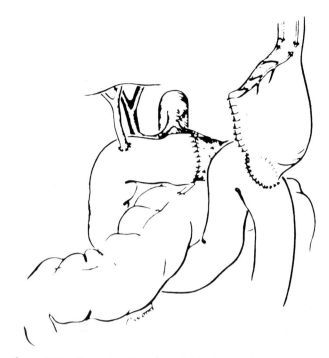

Figure 20.6. Reconstruction after a Whipple resection showing pancreaticojejunostomy, choledochojejunostomy, and gastroenterostomy.

Preoperative Management

Patients undergoing major surgical procedures with obstructive jaundice should receive nutritional supplementation as well as correction of vitamin K-related coagulopathies that may be present because of biliary obstruction and liver injury. Baseline studies are recommended to evaluate hepatic function and nutritional status, including albumin, transferrin, and prothrombin time. Nutritional support preoperatively as well as preoperative biliary tract decompression remain controversial; however, they may lower operative morbidity and mortality in selected patients.

Operative Management

In the operating room, resectability of pancreatic carcinomas is assessed by a thorough examination for any evidence of peritoneal or hepatic metastasis; evaluation of retroperitoneal, mesocolic, periaortic, and periduodenal lymph nodes; evaluation of major blood vessels, including the superior mesenteric artery and vein and the portal vein; and evaluation of the posterior extent of the tumor relative to the vena cava. Lesions in the periampullary region may originate from the duodenum, ampulla of Vater, distal common bile duct, or the head of the pancreas. The first three sites are associated with a reasonable chance of cure following a complete removal of the tumor. The details of a pancreaticoduodenectomy (Whipple procedure) are shown diagrammatically in Figures 20.5 and 20.6. The antrum, duodenum, proximal jejunum, head of pancreas, gallbladder, and distal common bile duct are removed en bloc and a vagotomy is performed. Conti-

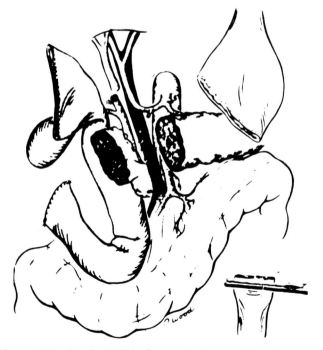

Figure 20.5. Details of Whipple resection (pancreaticojejunostomy) showing antrectomy, duodenectomy, cholecystectomy, distal common bile duct resection and partial pancreatectomy. A vagotomy is also performed.

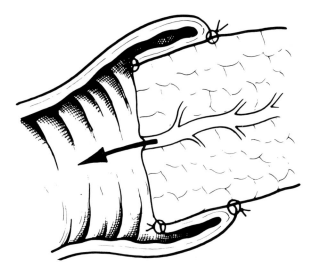

Figure 20.7. Detailed view of pancreaticojejunostomy, emphasizing inversion of pancreas into jejunum.

nuity is reestablished by anastomosing the distal pancreas to the proximal jejunum (Fig. 20.7). Sequentially then the transected common bile duct is reimplanted into the jejunal limb and a gastroenterostomy is performed distal to the other two anastomoses.

All patients should be monitored with adequate arterial and venous access lines as well as a nasogastric tube, Foley catheter, and a Swan-Ganz catheter in selected patients.

The majority of pancreatic cancers are unresectable, and a palliative operative procedure is performed in most patients. The three areas of palliation addressed intraoperatively include relief of biliary obstruction, duodenal obstruction, and chemical splanchnicectomy. The standard palliative operation would include a cholecystojejunostomy or choledochojejunostomy, a gastroenterostomy, and a chemical splanchnicectomy for pain relief (phenol or alcohol).

Controversy centers on the selection of patients for radical resection as well as the possible role of total pancreatectomy in combination with the Whipple procedure. Several studies have shown that pancreatic carcinoma is multicentric in at least one-half of the patients, and there is a significant incidence of intraductal and perineural spread within the gland. Total pancreatectomy also eliminates the potential morbidity of a leak occurring at the site of the pancreaticojejunostomy. However, most surgeons feel that the added morbidity outweighs the benefit. Patients require insulin replacement following total pancreatectomy, and a potentially increased risk of devascularization of proximal stomach is associated with this procedure due to removal of the spleen. Approximately 25% of patients will develop duodenal obstruction prior to their death if a *routine* prophylactic gastroenterostomy is not performed.

Operative Morbidity

The operative procedures outlined above are all associated with significant morbidity and mortality due to the advanced nature of the disease in most patients undergoing surgical treatment. Routine preoperative improvements in liver function and nutritional support have lowered the operative mortality associated with these procedures. Major complications in the postoperative period include leakage from the pancreaticojejunal and choledochojejunal anastomoses as well as sepsis and cardiovascular complications. All patients should be monitored closely in the pre- and postoperative period to assure maximal recovery. Antibiotics are recommended in the perioperative period due to the increased risk of biliary sepsis associated with obstruction.

Prognosis

The prognosis for patients with pancreatic carcinoma remains dismal. This is due to the aggressive biologic nature of the neoplasm as well as the inability to identify a high risk subgroup of patients for early detection via routine screening. Computerized tomography has not made a significant impact on earlier diagnosis. Currently, lesions originating at the ampulla of Vater have a 25–45% chance of cure after a curative resection. However, lesions originating in the pancreatic gland itself are associated with a 0–2% 5-year survival after a curative resection. Only 10–20% of patients presenting with obstructive jaundice are resectable at the time of exploration. The median survival following palliative bypass procedures is 6 months. Radiotherapy and chemotherapy have not proved to have a major impact on the natural history of pancreatic carcinoma. Reports of a 40% response to the chemotherapy regimen of 5-fluorouracil, adriamycin, and mitomycin-C (FAM) have not been reproduced. Body and tail lesions usually are unresectable at the time of diagnosis and are associated with a very poor prognosis. Intraoperative radiotherapy may be of benefit.

Cystadenoma and Cystadenocarcinoma

Cystadenocarcinoma of the pancreas occurs infrequently (1–2%). These lesions originate in the body or tail of the gland and present as a cystic lesion lined by epithelial cells. These are in distinction to pseudocysts that have no true epithelial lining. Cystadenomas and cystadenocarcinomas of the pancreas typically occur in middle-aged women and are associated with malignancy in the mucosal lining approximately 60% of the time. Because these tumors usually arise in the body and tail of the pancreas, a distal pancreatectomy is usually adequate treatment. The prognosis for cystadenocarcinoma of the pancreas is much better than adenocarcinoma originating in the body or tail of the pancreas. Cystadenocarcinoma is usually diagnosed incidentally on a CT scan or sonogram performed for another indication. Aggressive treatment of cystic lesions in the body and tail of the pancreas is recommended because of the favorable prognosis associated with resection. All cystic lesions of the pancreas should be biopsied to look for the presence of epithelial cells in the cyst wall. All epithelial-lined cysts of the pancreas should be excised and not drained internally.

Islet Cell Tumors of Pancreas

The two most common islet cell neoplasms of the pancreas arise from the beta cells (insulinoma) and the delta cells (gastrinoma). Other islet cell neoplasms of the pancreas have been reported to secrete serotonin, ACTH, MSH, glucagon, and somatostatin.

The classic symptoms of insulin-producing neoplasms are described by Whipple's triad consisting of attacks precipitated by fasting, fasting blood sugars less than 50 mg/100 ml, and the relief of symptoms associated with the prolonged fast. Reactive hypoglycemia and spontaneous hypoglycemia always occur following eating. Simultaneous measurement of the serum insulin and blood glucose levels are diagnostic in revealing an inappropriately high serum insulin level relative to the blood glucose. Patients classically have been treated for psychiatric illnesses due to the abnormal behavior associated with prolonged and recurrent hypoglycemia.

Localization of the tumor remains the goal of the preoperative evaluation. The majority of insulinomas are solitary and benign. Angiography demonstrates hypervascular lesions in approximately one-half of the patients. Percutaneous transhepatic sampling of the portal and splenic vein blood for measurement of insulin levels and intraoperative sonography may also be helpful in the detection of insulinoma.

Treatment

Surgical resection is the preferred management for patients with insulinoma. Delay in treatment is associated with neurologic damage due to recurrent episodes of hypoglycemia. The surgical treatment is resection of the tumor if it can be found. Usually the tumor can be simply enucleated.

Medical treatment is reserved for patients with unresectable malignant lesions or lesions that are not managed adequately by an 80% pancreatectomy. Streptozotocin is an effective drug in the treatment of patients with malignant insulinomas. Diazoxide has been useful in the suppression of insulin release from islet cells.

Zollinger-Ellison Syndrome

Islet cell tumors originating from the delta cells are associated with high levels of gastrin production. This has been associated with complications of peptic ulcer disease. The goal of surgery in patients with Zollinger-Ellison syndrome is two-fold. First, the surgeon makes a careful attempt to identify the infrequent single, resectable gastrin-producing tumor. Second, the surgeon may also operate to prevent complications of ulcer diathesis. Total gastrectomy is performed in patients who do not have an identifiable tumor or who have a tumor that is not resectable. Lesser ulcer operations have been associated with a high rate of recurrence in patients who do not undergo complete removal of a gastrin-producing tumor. A minority of patients with Zollinger-Ellison syndrome have a benign neoplasm of the islet cells that may be removed. The differentiation between benign and malignant islet cell tumors of the pancreas is based on the evidence of clinical metastasis. Histologically, differentiation between benign and malignant islet cell tumors, like most neuroendocrine tumors, is difficult.

SUGGESTED READINGS

Acosta JM, Rossi R, Galli OMR, et al: Early surgery for acute gallstone pancreatitis. Evaluation of a systemic approach. *Surgery* 83:367, 1978.

Banting FG, Best CH: The internal secretion of the pancreas. *J Lab Clin Med* 7:251, 1922.

Camer SJ, Tan EGC, Warren KW, Braasch, JW: Pancreatic abscess—a critical analysis of 113 cases. *Am J Surg* 129:426, 1975.

Grieco MB, Braasch JW, Rossi RL: Mass in the head of the pancreas: a practical approach. *Surg Clin North Am* 60:333–347, 1980.

Hodgkinson DJ, ReMine WH, Weiland LH: Pancreatic cyst-adenoma: a clinicopathologic study of 45 cases. *Arch Surg* 113:512–519, 1978.

Kelly TR: Gallstone pancreatitis: pathophysiology. *Surgery* 80:488, 1976.

MacMahon B, Yen S, Trichopoulos D, Warren K, Nardi G: Coffee and Cancer of the pancreas. *N Engl J Med* 11:630–633, 1981.

Modlin IM, Brennan MF: The diagnosis and management of gastrinoma. *Surg Gynec Obstet* 158:97–104, 1984.

Moossa AR, Altorki N: Pancreatic biopsy. *Surg Clin North Am* 63:1205–1214, 1983.

Moossa AR: Pancreatic cancer: approach to diagnosis, selection for surgery and choice of operation. *Cancer* 50:2689–2698, 1982.

Opie EL: The etiology of acute hemorrhagic pancreatitis. *Bull Johns Hopkins Hosp* 12:182, 1901.

Ranson JHC, Rifkind KM, Roses DF, et al: Prognostic signs and the role of operative management in acute pancreatitis. *Surg Gynec Obstet* 139:69, 1974.

Ranson JHC, Spencer FC: The role of peritoneal lavage in severe acute pancreatitis. *Ann Surg* 187:565, 1978.

Sabiston C Jr: *Davis-Christopher Textbook of Surgery.* Philadelphia, WB Saunders, 1981, p 1288.

Sarr MG, Cameron JL: Surgical management of unresectable carcinoma of the pancreas. *Surgery* 91:123–133, 1982.

Silen W: *Principles of Surgery.* New York, McGraw-Hill, 1979, pp 1353–1380.

Warshaw AL, Richter JM: A practical guide to pancreatitis. In *Current Problems in Surgery.* Chicago, Year Book Medical Publishers, 1984, vol 21, pp 57–67.

Whipple AO, Parson W, Mullins S: Treatment of carcinoma of the ampulla of Vater. *Ann Surg* 102:763–779, 1935.

Skills

1. Demonstrate the ability to perform a complete abdominal examination of a patient with an upper abdominal mass.

2. Given a patient with suspected pancreatitis, interpret a plain abdominal x-ray and identify pertinent positive and negative findings.

Study Questions _____

1. What are the two most common causes of pancreatitis?

2. Discuss why an elevated white blood cell count (above 16,000), an elevated glucose (above 200 mgm%), and a falling hematocrit increase the risk of major complications or death in a patient with acute pancreatitis.

3. Name four causes for an elevated serum amylase.

4. What is thought to be the pathophysiology of the formation of pancreatic pseudocysts?

5. What are the chances for a cure in a patient with carcinoma of the ampulla of Vater?

6. Discuss five complications of acute pancreatitis.

7. Discuss the classic symptoms of a patient with a neoplasm of the β cells of the pancreatic islets.

21 Breast and Adrenals

Adel Al-Jurf, M.D., *Nicholas Lang, M.D.,*
Martin Max, M.D., Roger Christian, M.D.,
and Frank Clingan, M.D.

ASSUMPTIONS

BREAST

The student understands the topographic and structural anatomy of the breast.

The student understands the hormonal changes that affect the breast during the menstrual cycle.

ADRENALS

The student understands the anatomy and physiology of the adrenal gland including the role of the pituitary gland in hormonal control.

The student understands the "dual organ" nature of the adrenal gland including its production of both catecholamines and steroid-type hormones.

The student understands the role the adrenal plays in homeostasis and fluid and electrolyte balance.

OBJECTIVES

BREAST

1. Identify and describe the major types of breast lumps.
2. List common risk factors for benign breast disease and five risk factors for breast cancer.
3. List diagnostic modalities and their sequence in the workup of a patient with a breast mass and a patient with nipple discharge.
4. Describe the natural history of benign and malignant breast neoplasms.
5. Describe the treatment for a fibroadenoma and fibrocystic disease.
6. List and discuss the types of breast cancer and their clinical staging.
7. Define the anatomic limits of surgical treatments of breast cancer.
8. List and discuss the treatment options for regional and systemic breast cancer (surgical, nonsurgical, and combined).
9. Describe the rationale for adjuvant chemotherapy, radiation, and hormonal therapy in the treatment of breast cancer.
10. List the current survival and recurrence rates of treated breast cancer, according to clinical stage.
11. Define a treatment plan for local recurrence and metastatic breast cancer.

ADRENALS

12. List and discuss three major adrenal dysfunctions, their clinical presentation, etiology, diagnostic procedures, and treatment options.
13. Describe the clinical features of Cushing's syndrome and tell how causal lesions in the pituitary, adrenal cortex, and extra-adrenal sites may be distinguished from a diagnostic standpoint.
14. Discuss medical and surgical management of Cushing's syndrome in patients with adrenal adenoma; with pituitary adenoma causing adrenal hyperplasia; with an ACTH-producing neoplasm.
15. Discuss the clinical and laboratory findings associated with adrenal insufficiency as well as the most common cause of its occurrence.
16. Describe the likely pathology, clinical features and laboratory findings of a patient with hyperaldosteronism.
17. Discuss the diagnostic workup of a patient with suspected hyperaldosteronism as well as the preferred operative treatment.
18. Discuss the most common tumor of the adrenal medulla including its associated signs and symptoms, an appropriate diagnostic workup and treatment.
19. Describe the features of the multiple endocrine neoplasia syndrome associated with pheochromocytoma.
20. Discuss the possible causes of virilization in a patient, including the clinical presentation and diagnostic workup that distinguish gonadal from adrenal lesions.

Breast

Topographic and Structural Breast Anatomy

During the reproductive years, the female breast is a heterogenous structure. It is made of glandular, ductal, connective, and fatty tissue. The breast tissue located on the anterior chest wall may extend to the clavicle superiorly, midsternal line medially, sixth rib inferiorly, and anterior axillary line and axilla laterally (Fig. 21.1). It is composed of lobules that may reach 12–24 in number. The lobules are supported by fibrous tissue, interconnected by ducts, and interspersed in variable amounts of fatty tissue. The ductal system extends from the lobules to the nipple.

The connective tissue extends from the pectoralis fascia to the skin (Cooper's ligaments). Fibrosis and shortening of the ligaments by benign (more often) or malignant disease causes "dimpling" of the skin.

The lymphatic drainage of the breast is primarily to the axilla, while a minor portion of it courses to the internal mammary nodes (Fig. 21.2). Because of the predominance of the former route, axillary lymph node metastases remain the most useful and reliable indicator of prognosis in breast cancer. Less frequently, drainage from medially located cancers may be to the mediastinal nodes without evidence of axillary metastases. Supraclavicular, interpectoral, and contralateral axillary nodes are not within the primary drainage pathways of the breast, and involvement of such nodes with tumor is a sign of widespread disease.

Physiology and Function

The breast is an apocrine gland modified for the formation of milk under normal physiologic circumstances. It varies considerably in gland structure during the menstrual cycle and lifetime of the organ. The infant breast consists primarily of ducts with few, if any, acini present. At puberty, increased estrogen and progesterone produced by the ovary along with trophic pituitary hormones result in ductal budding and initial acinar formation. Thereafter, the mature breast undergoes cyclic changes during each menstrual cycle. In the postmenstrual phase, the pituitary gland produces the follicle stimulating hormone (FSH), which causes ovarian follicle ripening. The latter leads to increased estrogen production, which leads to proliferation of the breast ductal system. After ovulation, estrogen and progesterone levels from the ovary diminish and breast ducts begin to diminish in size. Variations of this cycle often occur leading to a number of benign breast diseases—usually related to duct hypertrophy and subsequent sloughing of duct epithelial cells. In pregnancy, estrogen and progesterone levels remain relatively high. This results in further hypertrophy and budding of the ductal system with associated acinar development. At the time of parturition, the sudden decrease in hormonal levels plus prolactin secretion from the pi-

tuitary gland results in the onset of lactation. At menopause there is loss of breast parenchyma and increased fibrous tissues.

Benign Breast Masses

Benign masses of the breast are either benign tumors or benign tissue changes that have been errantly labelled "masses." This includes the fibrous and cystic components of "fibrocystic disease" (or "condition"). The following is a description of some of the most frequently encountered benign breast masses.

Fibroadenomas (benign)

Fibroadenomas are the easiest to recognize of all breast masses because of their specific character on physical exam. They are quite common, usually occurring in younger women (late teens to early thirties), but they may be found at any age. Most of the time they are discovered at the 1–3 cm size, but occasionally they may grow to larger sizes. In a few patients (10–15%) fibroadenomas are multiple in one or both breasts.

Fibroadenomas are firm, smooth, round, well defined, and extremely movable (formerly described as a "breast mouse"). Histologically, they are encapsulated, homogenous fibromas characterized by fibrous whorls. Rapid growth of fibroadenomas often occurs with high levels of estrogen (pregnancy, lactation, and premenopause), suggesting the hormonal responsiveness of this benign tumor. Some cysts may feel like fibroadenomas, but they generally lack the same firmness and mobility. In addition, cysts of the breast generally occur at an older age (late twenties to early forties).

The treatment of fibroadenomas is complete surgical excision because (1) they do not disappear spontaneously, although they may regress with age (postmenopause); (2) a very small percentage may harbor a sarcoma (usually large fibroadenomas or cystosarcoma phyllodes); and (3) because the diagnosis of a breast mass is never a certainty without histologic confirmation.

Fibrocystic Disease (benign)

Fibrocystic disease is the most common lesion affection the female breast. This condition may be a manifestation of physiologic changes in the breast that are caused by the menstrual hormonal cycle. Indeed, the majority of women are likely to have some manifestation of the condition in their lifetime. Areas afflicted with these changes are composed of fibrous elements and cysts that may be in close proximity or at a distance from each other. It may affect a single area or multiple areas in one or both breasts. Monthly cyclic tenderness is common with this condition. Recognition of this condition may be easy because of the irregular fibrous "rubbery" tissue of some areas and the distinct "cystic" feeling of some other areas. However, on occasion, areas of fibrosis may form a hard, well demar-

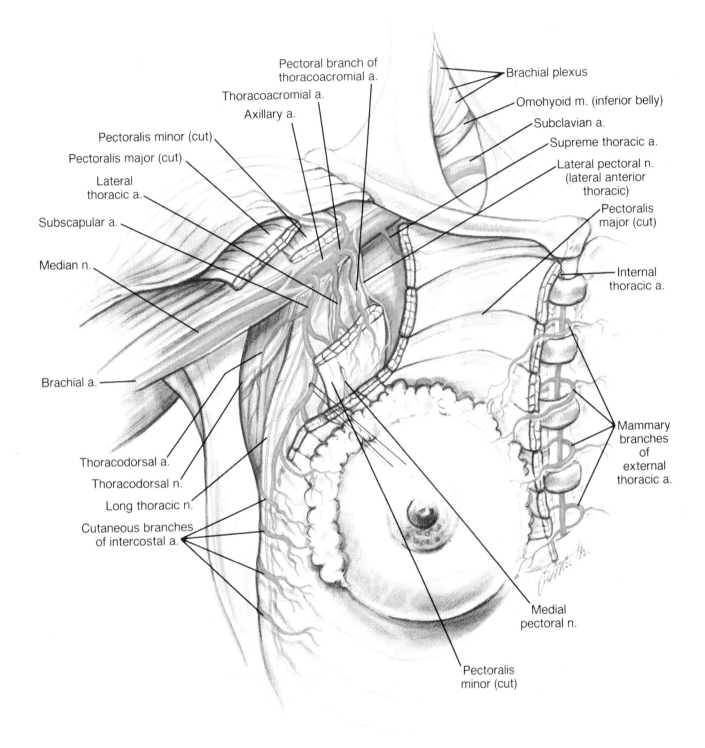

Figure 21.1. Normal breast anatomy demonstrating vascular and neural origins.

cated mass with ill-defined margins that may feel suspiciously like cancer. Fibrocystic disease occurs most commonly in women 30–50 years of age. Although histologically it is demonstrable in postmenopausal women, it rarely produces masses or tenderness in that age group.

If a cyst is suspected, it can be simply aspirated with a needle and syringe. The cystic fluid is usually straw colored and occasionally turbid or green. Smears of cyst fluid may be obtained but rarely help with the diagnosis. A mass suspected to be a cyst that cannot be aspirated (usually a fibroadenoma) should be excised.

Aspiration should be attempted when cysts are suspected and/or prior to planned biopsy. If no fluid is

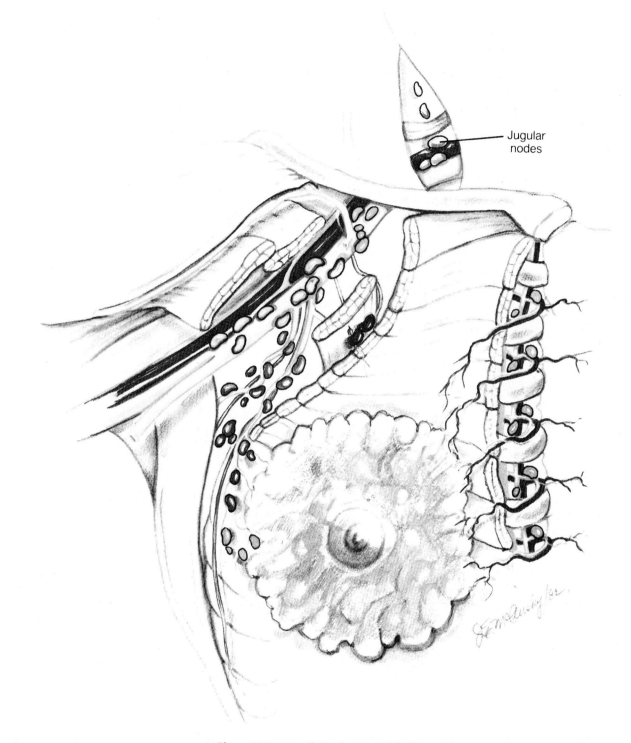

Jugular
nodes

Figure 21.2. Lymphatic drainage of the breast.

retrieved, an excisional biopsy should be done. Histologically one sees glandular hyperplasia, connective tissue hyperplasia, apocrine epithelium, cyst formation, lymphatic infiltration, and, occasionally, sclerosing adenosis. The latter lesion is benign but is commonly confused with carcinoma. Biopsy is also indicated for cysts with particulate matter in the aspirate, residual masses after aspiration, cysts with bloody aspirate, and cysts that recur after repeated aspiration.

Fibrocystic disease fluctuates with the menstrual cycles and most of the tenderness and engorgement of the breast occurs 1 week prior to the menstrual period and subsides 1 week later. However, particular areas of tenderness, cysts, or fibrosis may persist for weeks, months, or years. Therefore, needle aspiration should be done in midcycle if the cyst persists for at least a month.

Fibrocystic disease requires no specific treatment; indeed, there is no consistently effective treatment. Explanation and reassurance are usually effective in reducing anxiety. Limiting caffeine intake may reduce the symptoms of pain and tenderness. Vitamin E ingestion or tobacco abstinence are less helpful in alleviating symptoms. The androgenic hormone danocrine is effective, but it can result in significant and prohibitive side effects and should not be recommended routinely in the therapy of fibrocystic disease.

Most women tolerate symptoms of fibrocystic disease with little or no need for analgesics. An occasional patient will require treatment of extremely severe symptoms. Fibrocystic disease often leads to biopsy because of the uncertainty about the diagnosis. Subcutaneous mastectomy and prosthetic implant is a last resort in the treatment of fibrocystic disease and should be reserved for the very occasional woman with severe fibrocystic disease.

Rare Benign Masses

Other benign masses of the breast occur infrequently. These include lipomas, papillomas, galactocele, fat necrosis, breast abscess, and cystosarcoma phyllodes. The latter tumor is a very rare one and may be confused with fibroadenomas on physical exam; however, it is usually much larger (historically referred to as giant fibroadenoma). It may occur at any age but is most common in young girls or middle-aged women. Cystosarcoma phyllodes rarely metastasizes but have a high tendency to recur locally. The treatment is wide, local excision (segmental mastectomy) to reduce the incidence of local recurrence.

Nipple Discharge

Nipple discharge can be categorized as spontaneous or induced, unilateral or bilateral, and bloody or nonbloody.

Women can occasionally express a small amount of nipple discharge with digital manipulation. Clear, straw-colored, and greenish drainage suggest fibrocystic disease. Spontaneous, bloody unilateral nipple discharge is most commonly caused by intraductal papillomas; however, it should be investigated primarily to rule out cancer (10–15% of all cases). Cytologic exam of nipple drainage (and cyst aspirates) produces

Table 21.1.
Some Facts and Statistics About Breast Cancer in the United States

The leading cause of cancer deaths in women. (The recent increase in lung cancer may soon make it the leading cause of death.)

The leading cause of death, from all causes, in women 40–44 years of age.

114,000 new cases are expected to be diagnosed per year.

About 35,000–40,000 deaths from breast cancer are also expected per year.

One of every 11 women is expected to develop breast cancer in her lifetime.

such a low yield in diagnosing cancer that it has no practical value.

Breast Cancer

In addition to the very specific and distinct character of a cancer on physical exam, increasing age is another factor that suggests a breast mass could be malignant. Breast cancer usually presents as an irregular mass with ill-defined margins that "invades" adjacent tissues, is not movable, and is inseparable from adjacent tissues. Fat necrosis of the breast, which is a very rare condition, may be hard to distinguish from breast cancer on physical exam.

Some facts about breast cancer in the United States are shown in Table 21.1.

Risk Factors

Some of the known risk factors for developing breast cancer are:

1. Sex—99% of breast cancers occur in women. (1% in men)
2. Age—80% of breast cancers occur after age 40.
3. Family history—A mother and sister with breast cancer increase a woman's risk significantly.
4. Nulliparity, late pregnancy, early menarche, and late menopause all increase the risk of breast cancer.
5. Previous or current use of estrogens or birth control pills does not increase the risk of breast cancer.
6. Contrary to popular belief, a history of fibrocystic disease (except for certain types) may not increase the risk significantly.

Diagnosis

Three axioms in the recognition of breast cancer are important in its management: (1) A firm diagnosis of cancer is made only by the pathologist; nevertheless, clinical suspicion leads to biopsy by the clinician. (2) Mammograms are only radiologic images that increase or decrease the suspicion of cancer. They are not conclusive diagnostic tools and have a high false-negative rate in young women. (3) A distinct breast mass should be biopsied or the patient referred to a surgeon with experience in breast disease. No breast mass should be followed for a period of more than 2 months without histologic confirmation that it is benign. (Screening mammography for asymptomatic women is valuable and is discussed elsewhere in this chapter.)

In symptomatic women (presenting to the physician with a breast complaint), the symptoms and physical exam are the two most valuable aids to the diagnosis. If the symptom or complaint is a breast mass, then its character on physical exam should be the major indicator for advising and/or performing a biopsy for definitive diagnosis (Fig. 21.3). Some items in the medical history (Table 21.2) or signs (Table 21.3) observed by the patient or detected by the physician may increase

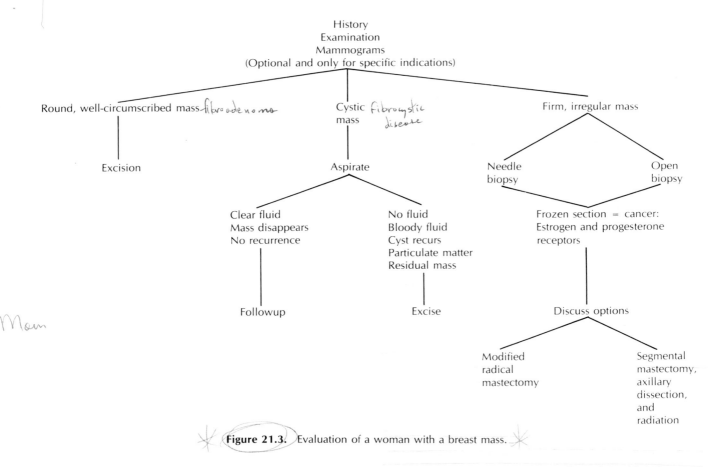

History
Examination
Mammograms
(Optional and only for specific indications)

Round, well-circumscribed mass—fibroadenoma

Cystic fibrocystic mass disease

Firm, irregular mass

Excision

Aspirate

Needle biopsy

Open biopsy

Clear fluid
Mass disappears
No recurrence

No fluid
Bloody fluid
Cyst recurs
Particulate matter
Residual mass

Frozen section = cancer:
Estrogen and progesterone receptors

Followup

Excise

Discuss options

Modified radical mastectomy

Segmental mastectomy, axillary dissection, and radiation

Mam

Figure 21.3. Evaluation of a woman with a breast mass.

the suspicion of cancer. It is critical that the history and physical findings be documented in detail, including location of the mass, for future reference.

Mammography (Fig. 21.4) in symptomatic women is used to evaluate the opposite breast and to evaluate other areas in the ipsilateral breast. The false-negative rate of mammography (up to 15% especially in younger women) reduces the reliability of mammography in the diagnosis of palpable masses. In other symptomatic women, mammography may be useful in evaluating:

1. Nipple drainage, especially when bloody, without palpable masses. If mammography also shows no mass, mammary ductography, by demonstrating the bleeding duct with contrast medium, can appropriately direct surgical biopsy.
2. Suspected Paget's disease of the nipple without palpable masses.
3. Women with any complaint who request a mammogram. This is done for reassurance of the patient and because of the possibility that an occult

Table 21.2.
Pertinent Items in the Medical History of Patients with Breast Complaints

1. Age
2. Noted changes in size of a mass (cyclic changes or progressive increase)
3. Pain and tenderness in the breast
4. Family history of breast cancer (mother or sister)
5. History of fibrocystic disease (by biopsy or cyst aspiration)
6. History of other (benign or malignant) breast lesions
7. Age at first menses and menopause
8. Age of first pregnancy and number of pregnancies
9. History of breast feeding
10. History of previous mammograms and results of those mammograms
11. History of nipple drainage and its character

Table 21.3.
Physical Signs To Be Looked for During Breast Examination

1. Asymmetry (most women have slightly asymmetrical breasts)
2. Skin discoloration
3. Skin edema or thickening
4. Skin dimpling or retraction
5. Skin redness
6. Skin ulceration
7. Nipple discharge
8. Nipple crusting or ulceration
9. Nipple retraction
10. Prominent or palpable veins
11. Breast mass without tenderness
12. Breast mass with tenderness
13. Pain and tenderness without mass
14. Lymph nodes
15. Arm edema

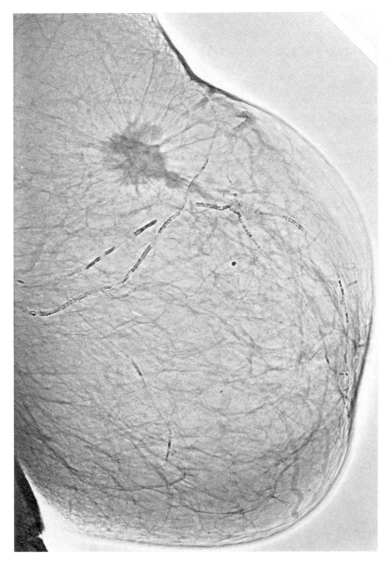

Figure 21.4. A xeromammogram, lateral view, shows a large stellate carcinoma of the breast with associated skin thickening. Calcification in the vascular system is noted incidentally.

cancer (not palpable on physical exam) may coexist and would be detectable by mammography (e.g., minimal cancers and areas of calcifications).
4. Women in high risk categories. →mammography
5. Mammography also serves several adjuvant roles: to place a localizing needle prior to surgical biopsy of a nonpalpable, mammographically discovered mass; to confirm that a mammographically suspicious lesion has indeed been included in the biopsy specimen and to localize the lesion in the tissue for the pathologist.

①from ductal system → 90%

Types of Breast Cancer

② from lobules → 10%

Breast cancers can arise from the ductal system (90%) or breast lobules (10%) and are consequently termed "ductal" or "lobular." Other malignancies occur in the breast that are not considered "breast cancers" such as fibrosarcoma; these are rare, however. The firmness

of breast cancer is due to the considerable amounts of fibrous tissue seen on histologic examination in a majority of the tumors and has given rise to the term "scirrhous." Histologic types in order of their prognosis are listed in Table 21.4.

Distinction should be made between in situ intraductal (noninvasive) and infiltrating ductal carcinoma (invasive). Similarly, distinction should be made between in situ and invasive lobular cancers.

Clinical Staging of Breast Cancer

The TNM system (tumors, nodes, metastases) is gaining wider use in the staging of breast cancer. Its major advantage is the attention given to tumor size. This factor has been neglected in other classifications and has proven to be of prognostic value. Definitions and staging are listed below.

T = Tumor itself
  T_1 Tumor < 2 cm

TNM system:
(tumors, nodes, metastases)

Table 21.4.
Types of Breast Cancer in Order of Prognosis

1. In situ intraductal or lobular cancer
2. Comedo carcinoma or papillary carcinoma confined within the ducts
3. Paget's disease of the nipple associated with intraductal carcinoma
4. Well differentiated adenocarcinoma
5. Medullary carcinoma
6. Colloid or mucinous carcinoma
7. Tubular carcinoma
8. Infiltrating ductal (scirrhous) carcinoma and infiltrating lobular carcinoma
9. Undifferentiated carcinoma with obvious blood vessel invasion
10. Inflammatory carcinoma *→ worst prognosis*

---

    a. Not fixed to pectoralis fascia
    b. Fixed to pectoralis fascia
T_2 Tumor > 2 cm, < 5 cm
    a and b similar to above
T_3 Tumor > 5 cm
    a and b similar to above
T_4 Tumor invading chest wall (beyond pectoralis muscle)
    a. Fixation to chest wall
    b. Edema (peau d'orange) or skin ulceration, satellite nodules of cancer on skin of same breast
    c. Both of above
    d. Inflammatory cancer

N = *Node involvement*
N_0 = No palpable axillary nodes
N_1 = Movable palpable nodes
    a. Not suspicious for metastases
    b. Suspicious for metastases
N_2 = Nodes containing metastases and fixed to one another
N_3 = Supraclavicular or infraclavicular nodes with metastases or edema of the arm

M = *Metastases*
M_0 = No evidence of distant metastases
M_1 = Distant metastases or skin recurrence beyond breast area

After the TNM classification has been completed, the stage is determined as follows:

Stage I	$T_{1a \text{ or } b}$	N_0 or N_{1a}	M_0
Stage II	T_0, $T_{1a \text{ or } b}$	N_{1b}	M_0
	$T_{2a \text{ or } b}$	N_0, $N_{1a \text{ or } b}$	M_0
Stage III	$T_{1a \text{ or } b}$	N_0, N_1, N_2	M_0
	$T_{2a \text{ or } b}$	N_2	M_0
	$T_{3a \text{ or } b}$	N_2	M_0
Stage IV	T_4	any N	any M
	any T	N_3	any M

The conventional classifications use similar guidelines, but differ in the respect that they disregard tumor size. The most commonly used classification is the Columbia Clinical Classification (the clinical classification is dependent upon clinical rather than histological verification). Using this system a clinical stage may change after surgery and histological examination of the tissue.

Stage A: Tumor in the breast. Axillary nodes not clinically involved. No "grave" signs.
Stage B: Tumor in the breast. Axillary nodes clinically involved but less than 2.5 cm in diameter. No "grave" signs.
Stage C: Tumor in the breast, associated with one of the five "grave" signs.
    1. Edema of less than one-third of the skin of the breast;
    2. Skin ulceration;
    3. Tumor fixed to the chest wall;
    4. Massive involvement and enlargement of axillary lymph nodes (greater than 2.5 cm);
    5. Fixation of axillary nodes to adjacent structures.
Stage D: Signs of more advanced disease than above:
    1. Two or more of the "grave" signs;
    2. Edema of more than one-third of the skin of the breast;
    3. Satellite skin nodules;
    4. Involved supraclavicular nodes;
    5. Edema of the arm;
    6. Inflammatory carcinoma (so termed because of rapid enlargement of the breast with warmth, erythema, and tenderness suggesting inflammation but caused by early lymphatic invasion and skin lymphatic blockage);
    7. Distant metastases.

Treatment of Breast Cancer

Surgical Treatment

In the vast majority of cases surgical treatment is indicated for earlier clinical stages (I and II, A and B), where there is potential for cure. When the potential for cure is small or nonexistent (stage III and IV, C and D), surgical therapy alone is not recommended and mastectomy is performed in addition to other modalities, for palliation only (Fig. 21.5).

The philosophy regarding surgical treatment has evolved over the years because of changing hypotheses regarding the method of progression of breast cancer and the desire of some patients to preserve the breast. One theory proposes a progression in an orderly, local-regional-systemic fashion. Such theory argues for aggressive local therapy. Aggressive local therapy has ranged from the removal of all breast tissue, underlying pectoral muscles, axillary contents, and sometimes mediastinal lymph nodes (radical and extended radical mastectomies, Fig. 21.6A) to removal of all the breast tissue and axillary contents but with preservation of the pectoralis major muscle and either leaving or removing the pectoralis minor muscle (modified radical mastectomy, Fig. 21.6B). An opposing theory suggests that breast cancer has a potential for early nonorderly

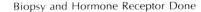

Biopsy and Hormone Receptor Done

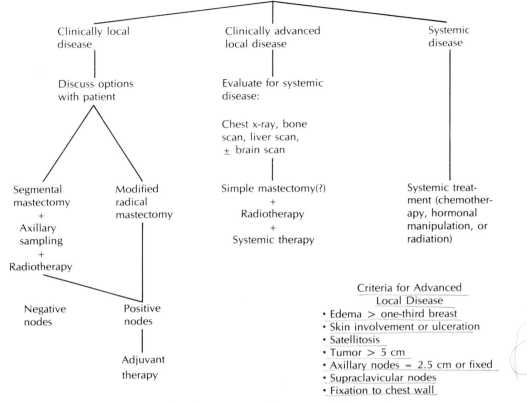

Figure 21.5. Approach to the treatment of a woman with known breast cancer.

systemic spread from inception. Such theory minimizes the role of local therapy. Now with evidence supporting the early systemic nature of breast cancer and with increasing pressure on the part of some women to preserve the breast, simple mastectomy (Fig. 21.6C), segmental or quadrant mastectomy (Fig. 21.6D), and "lump" removal (lumpectomy) with axillary dissection (Fig. 21.6E) followed by radiation to the breast are being applied more often.

The anatomical limits of surgical resection for breast cancer may include:

A. Breast tissue extending from
   1. midsternal line medially to,
   2. clavicle superiorly to,
   3. sixth rib inferiorly to,
   4. margin of pectoralis minor (axillary fascia) laterally.
B. Axillary contents extending from
   1. lateral margin of pectoralis minor muscle anteromedially,
   2. the long thoracic nerve—posteromedially,
   3. axillary vein superiorly,
   4. margin of latissimus dorsi muscle posterolaterally.

Segmental mastectomy (or quadrantectomy) removes the tumor and a segment of normal breast to assure complete removal of the cancer.

Treatment Options for Local-Regional Breast Cancer

The terms local, regional, and systemic disease are often used in describing the extent of breast cancer. Treatment is dependent on the clinical extent of the disease. Treatment of local-regional disease (stages I and II or A and B) is essentially surgical. Options of treatment are:

A. Radical mastectomy, removing all breast, pectoralis muscles and axillary contents. This treatment is now almost completely abandoned because of significant morbidity without significant improvement in survival.

B. Modified radical mastectomy, removing all breast tissue, axillary contents, with or without removal of the pectoralis minor muscle (now the most commonly applied treatment).

C. Simple mastectomy without axillary dissection (or with "sampling" of the axillary nodes for staging and prognostic reasons; used in special circumstances).

D. Segmental mastectomy (as well as "lumpectomy") with axillary dissection and radiation of the residual breast tissue (now meeting growing acceptance and application).

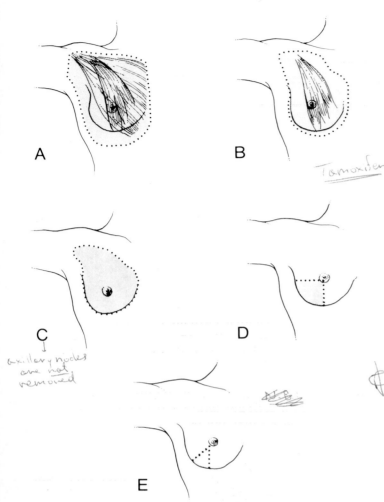

Tamoxifen

axillary nodes are not removed

Figure 21.6. Surgical procedures for carcinoma of the breast. **A,** Standard radical mastectomy. In this procedure both pectoral muscles and axillary nodes are removed. **B,** Modified radical mastectomy. The pectoralis major is preserved and the pectoralis minor may or may not be preserved. Axillary lymph nodes are removed. **C,** Simple mastectomy. Axillary nodes are not be removed. **D,** Quadrantectomy. Nodes are removed or sampled. **E,** "Lumpectomy." Nodes are removed or sampled.

Adjuvant Chemotherapy, Radiation Therapy, and Hormonal Therapy

The rationale behind employing additional (adjuvant) therapy in breast cancer treated (and potentially cured) by surgery is dependent upon three factors: (*1*) The evidence supporting the "early systemic" nature of breast cancer; (*2*) The high recurrence rate despite what appears to be adequate local surgical therapy at the time of diagnosis; and (*3*) The hypothesis that a small tumor load (clinically undetectable disease immediately after surgery) may respond better to chemotherapy, radiation, or hormonal therapy.

The earliest trials with adjuvant chemotherapy began in the late 1950s. Initial results were encouraging and somewhat confirmatory of the hypothesis. Subsequently, radiation therapy and hormonal therapy (in premenopausal women) were used but no improve-

ment in survival was demonstrated. Many chemotherapeutic agents have been used (L-Pam, 5-FU, cytoxan, methotrexate, adriamycin, etc.) in different combinations. The place and role of adjuvant therapy in breast cancer was recently addressed in a statement of a Consensus Development Conference from the National Institutes of Health. The statement indicates that adjuvant combination chemotherapy should become standard care in premenopausal women with positive axillary nodes, regardless of hormone receptor status. Adjuvant therapy with tamoxifen (an antiestrogen agent) should be given to postmenopausal women with positive nodes and positive receptor levels. There is no justification for the routine use of adjuvant chemotherapy in other patients. Until more data become available, other treatment modalities should continue, but only within the constraints of study protocols.

Treatment of Advanced and Systemic Disease

Once there is evidence that the tumor is beyond stages I and II (A and B), surgical therapy alone is rarely utilized. Locally advanced disease can be treated with combined modalities. Mastectomy preceded or followed by chemotherapy and radiation therapy to reduce the local problems of ulceration and infection is an acceptable management option.

There are many modalities for treatment of local and systemic breast cancer. These include:

(*1*) Radiation therapy. Radiation therapy is most effectively used for local chest wall and regional lymph node recurrences, bony metastases and brain metastases.

(*2*) Hormonal manipulation. The word "manipulation" is often used because alteration of hormonal influences is used in these therapies. In premenopausal women, oophorectomy would be the procedure of choice to remove the source of endogenous estrogen. In postmenopausal women, exogenous estrogens, progesterones, androgens, or antiestrogens (tamoxifen) are given. Tamoxifen has been used recently in premenopausal women in place of oophorectomy. Andrenalectomy is used less frequently now. Hypophysectomy is used occasionally and appears to reduce, temporarily, the bone pain from metastatic breast cancer regardless of its effect on the disease progression. The median duration of response to the first effective hormonal maneuver is over 11 months, but each subsequent treatment may add additional prolongation of response. The response rate to hormonal manipulation is dependent on the steroid receptor status of the tumor (estrogen or progesterone positive) and thus hormone dependency of the tumor. Hormone-dependent tumors may show response rates in excess of 50%. Hormone-independent tumors will show response below 8%.

(*3*) Chemotherapy. Combination chemotherapy has shown a high response rate in breast cancer (in excess of 50–60%, exceeding single agent therapies). Single agents produce a 20–40% response rate. The median duration of response is about 8–13 months.

The choices of radiation, hormonal manipulation,

and chemotherapy are dependent on many factors, including site of recurrence of metastases, number of metastatic sites, estrogen and progesterone receptor status, and general status of the patient. Obviously, the least noxious modality should be chosen since all treatments are palliative and none of them is curative. It is unlikely that treatment of metastatic breast cancer will prolong overall survival of patients. It may prolong the survival of some patients with a good response. The most effective chemotherapeutic agents are the same used in adjuvant therapies (5-FU, cytoxan, adriamycin, methotrexate, and L-PAM).

(4) Immunotherapy has not been, so far, proven effective in breast cancer.

Hormonal Receptors

It is now known that the growth of some breast cancers may be dependent upon the presence of estrogen or progesterone receptors in the cytoplasm of the cancer cell. It is also known that the presence or absence of those receptors in cancer cells can be used to predict the response of metastatic disease to hormonal manipulation. Two receptors are now useable, the estrogen and progesterone receptors. Tumors with positive receptors respond well to hormonal manipulation, while tumors with negative receptors have very low response rates. Because of that important therapeutic implication, all tumors should have measurement of these receptors at the time of biopsy. The measurements can only be done on fresh tissue (not imbedded in formalin) and, thus, should be done at the time of frozen section. The receptors are expressed in fmol/mg cytosol. Positive values are usually considered greater than 10 fmol/mg cytosol.

Results of Treatment of Breast Cancer

The cure of breast cancer by any treatment is obviously dependent on the stage of disease at the time of treatment and, in surgically curable disease, it is dependent on the presence or absence of metastases in the axillary lymph nodes and the number of nodes involved. Tumor size appears also to influence survival. Some types of breast cancer are associated with a better prognosis than others (Table 21.4). Survival by stage is shown in Table 21.5.

Table 21.5.
Survival in Breast Cancer According to Stage of Disease and Number of Lymph Nodes Involved[a]

Axillary Nodes	10-Year Survival (%)
Nodes negative	72–76
Nodes positive (overall)	25–48
1–3 nodes involved	34–68
4 or more nodes involved	14–27
Metastatic disease	0

[a]Range of results from six reported series.

Table 21.6.
Sites of Breast Cancer Metastases[a]

Organ	Incidence (%)
Lymph nodes	75
Lungs ± pleura	70
Liver	60
Bone	60
Brain	15
Other organs	10

[a]In most patients more than one site is involved.

Treatment of Local Recurrence and Metastatic Breast Cancer

The treatment of local recurrence, as well as metastatic breast cancer, is dependent upon the site of recurrence of metastases (Table 21.6), the symptoms produced by the recurrence, the estrogen and progesterone receptor status, and the potential side effects of the treatment. There is virtually no cure from recurrent or metastatic disease, though treatment may alleviate symptoms or prolong survival in some patients whose disease responds to treatment.

Local chest wall recurrence can be treated by radiation therapy or by hormonal manipulation (if the tumor is positive for estrogen and/or progesterone receptors). Bony metastases may not be amenable to extensive radiation and can be treated by hormonal manipulation or chemotherapy.

For almost all metastases (except liver metastases), hormonal therapy should probably be tried before chemotherapy is used if estrogen and progesterone receptors are positive. Although the response rate in certain sites is not as good with hormonal therapy as it is with chemotherapy, the low potential for side effects or toxicity of hormonal therapy makes that treatment more acceptable. If, after a period of 6 weeks to 3 months, there is no obvious response to the hormonal manipulation and/or there is progression of the disease, then chemotherapy can be tried. There are some physicians who consider lung, pleural, and liver metastases an indication for initiation of chemotherapy without any attempts at hormonal manipulations.

Treatment of Complications of Breast Cancer

Bone pain from metastases usually responds to radiation to localized areas. For widespread disease and pain, hormonal therapy, chemotherapy, or hypophysectomy may help.

Pleural effusion from pleural metastases may be treated by aspiration (repeated if needed), or chest tube drainage with injection of sclerosing agents (e.g., chemotherapeutic agents or tetracycline). Response is variable and temporary.

Hypercalcemia may occur from bony metastases or from the production of a humoral substance by the tumor. Hypercalcemia temporarily responds to hydration, diuresis, phosphate by mouth and mithramycin.

Role of Mammography in Breast Disease Evaluation

For screening of asymptomatic women, there is now substantial proof that mammography can detect occult (nonpalpable) breast cancers and can reduce mortality from breast cancer because of early detection of minimal cancers. → even though 15% false negatives in younger ♀.

Recommendations for screening (mainly by mammography and physical examination in otherwise asymptomatic women) as outlined by the American Cancer Society are shown below. These recommendations have continued to evolve as new information becomes available.

Women 20 years of age and older should perform breast self-examination every month.

Women 20–40 years of age should have a physical examination of the breast every 3 years, and women over age 40 should have a physical examination of the breast every year.

Women between the ages of 35 and 40 should have a baseline mammogram.

Women between the ages of 40 and 50 should have a mammogram every other year and should consult their personal physicians about the need for mammography.

Women over 50 years of age should have a mammogram every year when feasible.

Women with personal or family histories of breast cancer should consult their physicians about the need for more frequent examinations or about beginning periodic mammography before age 50.

The pros and cons of mammography in symptomatic women (breast mass, pain, tenderness, and/or nipple discharge) are discussed elsewhere in the chapter. Periodic screening mammography should continue following biopsy or surgery for breast cancer. A comparison mammogram prior to biopsy or mastectomy is helpful because interpretation of screening mammograms is heavily dependent on detecting asymmetry and change over time. Mammography following biopsy is technically much more difficult because compression views are painful postoperatively and scarring hinders interpretation.

The physician should be warned not to allow negative results of mammography to override clinical judgment. A biopsy of a dominant and palpable breast mass should be performed despite a ''negative'' mammogram.

Adrenal Glands

Anatomy

The adrenal glands are located superior and medial to the upper pole of each kidney (Fig. 21.7). The anatomical relationships of each adrenal are different. The right adrenal is in close proximity to the inferior vena cava and, when the liver in enlarged, it may be located behind it in the retroperitoneum. The left adrenal is in closer proximity to the aorta, pancreas, and spleen. The arterial supply to the adrenal glands is from multiple, small, and inconsistent arteries. The venous drainage is more consistent. The right adrenal venous drainage

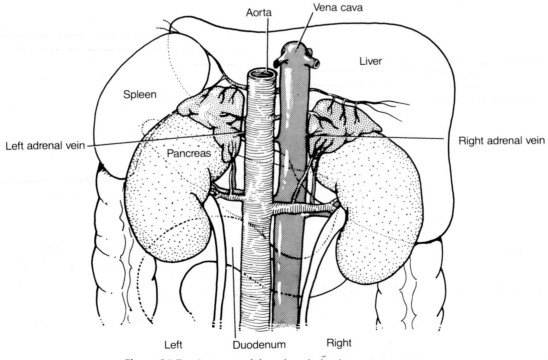

Figure 21.7. Anatomy of the adrenal glands (posterior view).

is to the inferior vena cava via a short but relatively large vein. The left adrenal vein drains into the left renal vein.

Adrenal Function

The adrenal glands produce a large number of hormones, primarily by the adrenal cortex. Understanding the function of the adrenal gland, the hormones produced, and their metabolism and degradation is essential; such understanding makes possible appreciation of the clinical presentations and manifestations of the diseases associated with adrenal malfunction and hormone-producing tumors, and facilitates directing the diagnostic workup in these conditions. The adrenal medulla primarily produces catecholamines. The cortex produces a number of hormones which may be divided into three major categories, according to their function.

1. *Glucocorticoids (cortisone and hydrocortisone).* These are essentially involved with protein and carbohydrate metabolism and their presence is essential for survival. Corticoids are secreted in the zona fasciculata.
2. *Minerocorticoids.* They exert predominant action on electrolyte metabolism, aldosterone being the chief example. Aldosterone is secreted in the zona glomerulosa.
3. *Progesterone, androgens, and estrogens.* Though adrenal progesterone is not secreted in the blood stream, it acts as a precursor for other hormones. Adrenal androgens and estrogens both circulate in the blood. These hormones are secreted in the zona reticularis.

Steroids have a tetracyclic carbon skeleton, consisting of three six-sided rings and one five-sided ring containing 17 carbon atoms (the cyclopentanoperhydrophenomthrene nucleus is derived from and similar to that of cholesterol). The conversion, derivation, and degradation of all steroidal hormones concerned can be found in more detailed textbooks, but some of the degradation products or pathways will be discussed with individual diseases.

Dysfunction of the adrenal may be primary or it may be secondary to other organ dysfunction (e.g., pituitary). Each hormonal disturbance produces a disease state with special characteristics that may be specific and obvious in some cases or nonspecific and subtle in others.

The following is a brief review of the major dysfunctions that can manifest clinically from abnormal hormonal production.

Cushing's Disease and Cushing's Syndrome

Characterized by excessive glucocorticoid secretion, this condition may be produced by dysfunction of the adrenal cortex secondary to tumors, by excessive secretion of ACTH by the anterior pituitary gland, or by an ectopic source of ACTH such as oat cell carcinoma of the lung. Cushing's syndrome refers to patients having the constellation of certain clinical findings because of excessive circulating of glucocorticoids. The term Cushing's disease is applied when the excessive glucocorticoids are secondary to excess ACTH produced by the pituitary gland.

Clinical Manifestations

Clinical manifestations include the symptoms of fatigue and weakness, truncal obesity with the typical "buffalo hump," hypertension, amenorrhea or irregularity of the menstrual periods, easy bruising, nervousness, irritability, back and bone pain, osteoporosis, hirsutism, headache, ankle and hand edema, diminished libido in females and feminization in males. It is unlikely that a single patient will display all of these characteristics simultaneously.

Etiology

Diffuse adrenal cortical hyperplasia secondary to a functioning pituitary adenoma (Cushing's disease) is the most frequent adrenal finding (60%); however, benign adenomas and carcinomas of the adrenals are seen in 15% of the cases. Occasionally, the excess hormone secretion is secondary to a malignant tumor (e.g., lung cancer) producing ectopic ACTH. Exogenous steroid intake and diseases interfering with the normal metabolism of steroids may produce signs and symptoms of the syndrome.

Diagnosis

The physical findings may be prominent or subtle. It is rare to palpate a tumor on physical examination. The best way to make the diagnosis is to measure glucocorticoid hormones or their breakdown products (Fig. 21.8). The urinary excretion of cortisol is raised and plasma cortisol values are generally elevated. There is loss of the diurnal variation in corticoid secretion as well as loss of the ability of the adrenal gland to increase its cortisol secretion in response to ACTH stimulation.

The dexamethasone suppression test is often used to confirm the presence of Cushing's syndrome and to discriminate between Cushing's syndrome and Cushing's disease. Dexamethasone, in small (2 mg) doses, will suppress cortisol secretion in normal subjects. In Cushing's syndrome, there will be no suppression by this small dose of dexamethasone. In Cushing's disease, dexamethasone in large doses (8 mg) will suppress plasma cortisol levels by more than 50% and will be associated with normal or mildly elevated ACTH. When Cushing's syndrome is caused by ectopic ACTH production, cortisol levels will not be suppressed by large doses of dexamethasone and plasma ACTH will be very high. When Cushing's syndrome is caused by an autonomous adrenal tumor, cortisol levels will not be suppressed by large doses of dexamethasone and plasma ACTH will be low.

EXCELLENT

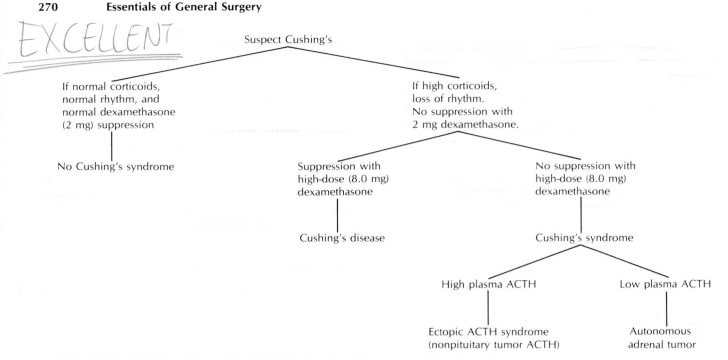

Figure 21.8. Workup of patients with suspected Cushing's disease or syndrome.

There are other biochemical laboratory changes in Cushing's disease such as mild hyperglycemia, glycosuria, low-serum potassium, and elevated carbon dioxide content. These, however, may be normal in many cases and cannot be used for diagnosis. Radiologic examinations may be helpful in identifying adrenal lesions, if present. These include plain abdominal films, intravenous pyelograms with nephrotomography, computed tomography (CT), selective arteriography, and selective retrograde adrenal venography. Not every patient needs to be subjected to all procedures and a few may be sufficient to establish the diagnosis. Recent use of adrenal photoscanning with $^{131}I^-$ labeled cholesterol has been helpful in demonstrating the adrenal lesion in Cushing's syndrome. The CT scan has become one of the most important diagnostic techniques today for identifying the presence and lateralization of an adrenal tumor (Fig. 21.9). This has resulted in decreased use of invasive techniques, such as arteriography and venography.

Treatment

There is a difference of opinion over whether the primary treatment of Cushing's disease should be ablation of the pituitary gland or the adrenal glands. Surgical ablation of the pituitary is advisable if a pituitary mass is identifiable on CT scan of the head and if there is a clear-cut positive dexamethasone suppression test. However, this approach is associated with a relatively high failure rate. Alternatively, adrenalectomy is an assured successful treatment and is used if the syndrome reappears after hypophysectomy. Some surgeons believe that adrenalectomy should be the first treatment of choice. In 90% of cases, adrenal gland exploration will disclose pathologic changes in either one or both adrenal glands. Obviously, bilateral simultaneous exposure of both glands must be carried out because of the possibility of multiple adenomas, nodular hyperplasia, or diffuse hyperplasia of both glands. This can be done either transabdominally or by a combined bilateral posterior approach. In solitary adenomas and carcinomas, total adrenalectomy on the involved side is the treatment of choice. If there are multiple adenomas, they should be incised intact with a rim of uninvolved adrenal gland leaving some adrenal tissue to maintain endogenous endocrine function. In bilateral cortical hyperplasia, total adrenalectomy is the procedure of choice since it prevents recurrence. In such cases, daily maintenance doses of cortisone (equivalent to 37.5 mg cortisone) should be given to provide the functional requirements in these patients.

Following adrenalectomy, enlargement of the pituitary may occur causing visual field loss and hyperpigmentation (Nelson's syndrome).

One should use perioperative cortisone therapy when total adrenalectomy is planned. Gradual reduction of the dose is carried out postoperatively, until the daily maintenance dose of cortisone is reached within a period of 2–3 weeks. *Nelson's Syndrome*
— visual field loss & hyperpigmentation following adrenalectomy due to pituitary enlargement.

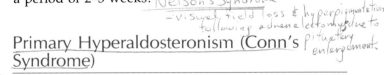

Primary Hyperaldosteronism (Conn's Syndrome)

Patients with hyperaldosteronism have an excessive production of aldosterone that is caused by a benign adenoma of the zona glomerulosa of the adrenal cortex. Hyperplasia and adenomatous hyperplasia may cause hyperaldosteronism. Rarely do malignant tumors cause this condition. Aldosterone is normally secreted in response to sodium and volume restriction or potassium loading in the absence of pituitary influence. In secondary hyperaldosteronism, aldosterone secretion is increased in response to elevated renin and angiotensin levels.

Clinical Manifestations

Findings include mild hypertension, polyuria, polydypsia, muscular weakness, excessive renal potassium loss with resulting hypokalemia and alkalosis, and moderate hypernatremia. Occasionally, hypomagnesemia, tetany, and periodic paralysis may be noted. There are no characteristic somatic abnormalities in hyperaldosteronism.

Diagnosis

Diagnosis can be made by measuring urinary aldosterone levels (and excluding secondary hyperaldosteronism). To do this, low or normal plasma renin levels must be demonstrated as well as an absence of other causes of secondary hyperaldosteronism (Fig. 21.10). Demonstration of excessive aldosterone production after 3 days of saline loading (saline loading test) provides the most sensitive and specific test to exclude secondary hyperaldosteronism. Following this test, elevation of serum aldosterone will be demonstrated, with reduction of plasma renin activity. Many patients with essential hypertension may have an early prehypokalemic phase of hyperaldosteronism. Localization of the dysfunctional adrenal gland (tumor) preoperatively is possible by analysis for aldosterone of adrenal vein blood obtained from each side. The standard radiologic techniques, such as selective arteriography and retrograde venography, may be very helpful. Retrograde venography must be done with great care because rupture of the adrenal veins may occur, making exploration difficult. The scanning technique using [131I]iodocholesterol has also been helpful; the adeno-

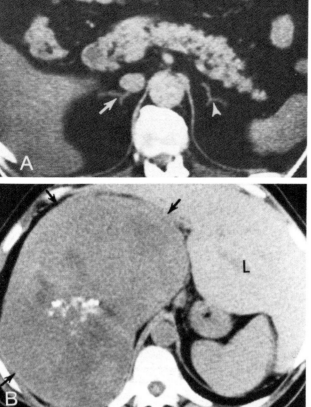

Figure 21.9. **A,** CT scan showing normal adrenal glands (arrows). **B,** A different patient with adrenal carcinoma. CT scan shows a large unhomogeneous mass (arrows) containing calcification and displacing the liver (L). (From Lee JT, Sagel SS, Stanley RJ (eds): *Computed Body Tomography.* New York, Raven Press, 1982, pp 381 and 386.)

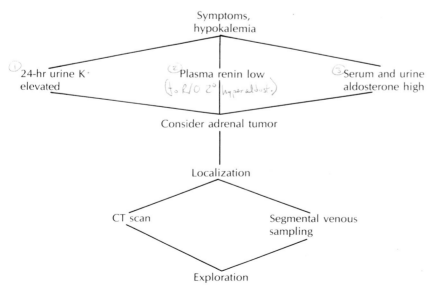

Figure 21.10. Workup of possible hyperaldosteronism.

i.e: Conn's Syndrome

adenomas appear as localized hot spots of increased uptake. In addition, this uptake of hyperplastic glands in aldosteronism can be suppressed by dexamethasone. Currently CT scanning is becoming one of the most useful tests for the diagnosis of this disease and is used as the first test for diagnosis. Adrenal venous sampling approaches a 100% accuracy rate in the diagnosis. The tumors are usually small and more commonly located in the left adrenal.

Treatment

Operative approaches to removal of the adenoma in hyperaldosteronism include abdominal and flank (or back) incision. If the lesion is thought to be bilateral or there is uncertainty, an abdominal approach is preferred. If unilateral, it may be removed through the less morbid back approach. The procedure consists of removing the entire adrenal on the affected side. The right adrenal is usually more treacherous to remove because of the short, large right adrenal vein that immediately enters the vena cava after leaving the adrenal gland.

If an adenoma is excised, prompt and definite improvement in the hypertension occurs. However, in patients diagnosed to have adrenal hyperplasia as the cause of hypertension (idiopathic and secondary hyperaldosteronism), treatment by total adrenalectomy may not result in significant improvement in the hypertension and it is now believed that such patients should be treated medically with aldosterone antagonists.

Pheochromocytoma

Pheochromocytoma is a disease of the adrenal medulla manifesting as hypertension. In a small number of patients, it is produced by tumors in other locations arising from the extraadrenal paraganglionic system alongside the vertebral axis and extending from the pelvis to the base of the skull. The cell of origin is part of the APUD system. Pheochromocytoma may be part of the multiple endocrine neoplasia syndrome, type II. Pheochromocytomas may occur in adults and children.

Clinical Manifestations

The clinical hallmark of pheochromocytoma is hypertension. The high blood pressure is sustained in about one-half of the patients but in the rest it is paroxysmal with normotensive periods in between the hypertensive episodes. Headaches, palpitations, diaphoresis, weight loss and hypermetabolism, nausea and vomiting, nervousness, tachycardia, bradycardia, arrhythmias, fever, dilated pupils, pallor, Raynaud's phenomenon, flushing, and other manifestations of catecholamine excess are the most common symptoms, occurring in 30–85% of all patients. Asymptomatic pheochromocytomas may be discovered incidentally or accidentally.

Pathology

Single adrenal pheochromocytomas are the most common cause of the disease (50–70% of the tumors), but occasionally the two adrenal glands are involved by tumors (5–10%). In the rest of the cases, a tumor outside the adrenal gland is the cause (usually originating in the sympathetic nervous system in the abdomen and rarely in the chest). Patients with pheochromocytomas have contracted vascular volume with hemoconcentration. High catecholamine levels produce hyperglycemia, glucosuria, and an abnormal glucose tolerance test. The symptoms (tachycardia, nervousness, weight loss, etc.) may suggest hyperthyroidism, and this possibility can be excluded by measuring serum thyroxine levels.

The tumor in the adrenal is usually encapsulated, and differentiation between benign and malignant tumors is very difficult histologically unless there is extension of the tumor outside the capsule or there is metastasis.

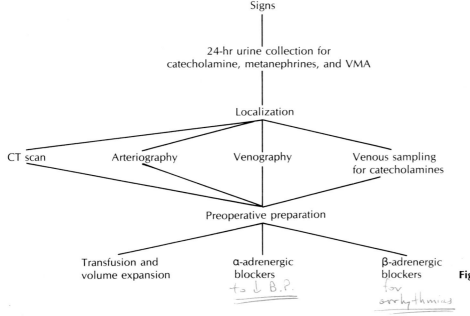

Figure 21.11. Workup of pheochromocytoma.

Diagnosis

Because of paroxysmal hypertension in many patients with pheochromocytoma, the presence of other symptoms should indicate further workup, especially in young patients with no other explanation for hypertension (Fig. 21.11). The symptoms may be brought on by exercise, emotional stress, coughing or straining, alcohol, smoking, drugs (histamine), or hormones (glucagon). The method of diagnosis involves collection of urine for a 24-hr period for measurement of catecholamines and their products (metanephrines, normetanephrines, and vanillylmandelic acid) (Fig. 21.12). If all values are normal (Table 21.7), the presence of pheochromocytoma is unlikely. Plasma catecholamines can be measured if the above urine tests are not diagnostic. Epinephrine-producing pheochromocytomas are always adrenal or are located in the organs of Zuckerkandl. If both tests are negative but suspicion persists, tests may be repeated in a few months. A therapeutic trial with phenoxybenzamine (20–60 mg/day) to lower blood pressure may be helpful.

If tests are positive, localization becomes the second important step in diagnosis. Extraadrenal tumors (in the chest) can be diagnosed by chest x-ray or CT scan of the chest. Tumors in the abdomen can be seen on CT scan in 80–90% of the cases. Vena cava catheterization and epinephrine and norepinephrine assays are diagnostic in 80% of cases. Arteriogram may be helpful in identifying the tumor in 60–85% of the cases.

Some drugs (e.g., theophylline, clonidine, levodopa, methyldopa, etc.) elevate epinephrine and norepinephrine and their products in the urine, and this possibility should be considered in patients with hypertension.

Treatment

Preoperative preparation of patients with pheochromocytoma is of significant importance to reduce

Table 21.7.
Normal Values of Catecholamines and Their By-products Under Normal Conditions

Plasma catecholamines (supine resting)	0.0 mg/ml
Urine norepinephrine	7–150 mg/24 hr
Epinephrine	0.1–2.4 mg/24 hr
Normetanephrine and metanephrine	0.02–1.7 mg/24 hr
Vanillymandelic acid	1–13 mg/24 hr
Homovanillic acid	1–8.5 mg/24 hr

mortality and morbidity. Volume expansion with one or two units of blood 12–18 hr before surgery, generous replacement of operative blood loss and α-adrenergic blocking agents, such as phenoxybenzamine (10–20 mg two or four times a day) for 7–10 days preoperatively will all tend to prevent fluctuations of blood pressure during operation. Pretreatment with a β-blocking agent is not routinely necessary in the absence of arrhythmias. Propranolol (1–2 mg) intraoperatively will control arrhythmias, if needed. Nitroprusside can be used for hypertensive crises. Preoperative localization (and treatment of metastatic pheochromocytomas) with [131I]metaiodobenzylguanidine has been reported.

Surgical removal of the offending tumor by complete adrenalectomy is the treatment of choice for this lesion. Because manipulation of the tumor during surgery may release large amounts of catecholamines into the bloodstream, one should monitor carefully for evidence of paroxysmal hypertension. Nitroprusside is effective for treatment of such crises. An abdominal approach is usually used for this lesion.

Adrenogenital and Masculinization Syndrome

This syndrome is caused by excessive secretion of androgens by the zona reticularis causing masculini-

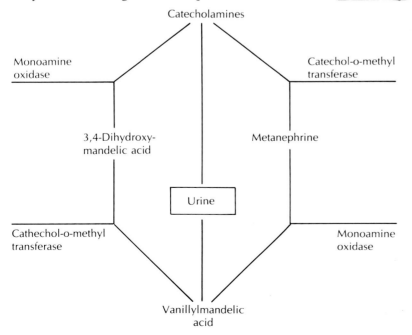

Figure 21.12. Metabolism of catecholamines.

Signs
|
Urine 17-ketosteroids elevated
|
Suppression with dexamethasone positive
|
Localization
|
Operation

Figure 21.13.   Workup for adrenogenital syndrome.

zation. In adults who develop virilization, a malignant functioning adrenocortical tumor is the usual cause. This excessive production of androgens by the adrenal is the most common situation for such condition. Rarely an adrenal rest tumor in the ovary or a true ovarian tumor may be the cause.

Feminizing tumors in males are quite rare and the most common presenting symptom or sign is gynecomastia. Urinary estrogen levels are usually markedly elevated and tumors may be benign, although most are malignant; by the time the diagnosis is established, distant metastases are common.

In evaluating adrenocortical conditions, a high degree of suspicion and a logical sequential approach to diagnosis before undertaking therapy must be carried out so as to achieve the optimal result with a minimum of side effects.

Clinical Manifestations

This usually occurs in children, chiefly females, who will develop deepening of the voice, hair growth of male distribution, muscular development, and growth of the clitoris. In males, the syndrome will present as precocious puberty.

Diagnosis

CT scan is the most important radiologic investigative method. Measurement of urinary 17-ketosteroids and a positive dexamethasone test are important aids to the diagnosis (Fig. 21.13).

Adrenalectomy is the treatment of choice. Postoperatively, most of the masculinizing features will regress except for the deep voice, if it has been well established. Assurance must be made that the tumor responsible is not in the ovary.

In some patients, treatment with cortisone or its derivatives will suppress the secretion of androgens and it is important to begin this treatment early in the course of the disease to avoid premature arrest of bone growth.

SUGGESTED READINGS

Auda SP, et al: Evaluation of the surgical management of primary aldosteronism. *Ann Surg* 191:1, 1980.
Bravo EL, Gifford RW Jr: Current concepts; Pheochromocytoma: Diagnosis, localization, and management. *N Engl J Med* 311:1298, 1984.
Bravo EL, Gifford RW: Pheochromocytoma: diagnosis, localization and management. *N Engl J Med* 311:1298, 1984.
Ferris JB, et al: Primary hyperaldosteronism. *Clin Endocrinol Metab* 10:419, 1981.
Delaney JP, Solomkin, JS, Jacobson ME, Doe RP: Surgical management of Cushing's syndrome. *Surgery* 84:465–470, 1978.
Dluhy RG, Williams GH: Cushing's syndrome and the changing times. *Ann Intern Med* 97:131, 1982.
Grant CS, et al: Primary aldosteronism: Clinical management. *Arch Surg* 119:585, 1984.
Herwig KR: Primary aldosteronism: experience with thirty-eight patients. *Surgery* 86:470–474, 1979.
Howanitz PJ, Howanitz JH: Hypercortisolism. *Clin Lab Med* 289:1519, 1984.
Irvin GL, et al: Familial pheochromocytoma. *Surgery* 94:938, 1983.
Migeon CJ: Diagnosis and management of congenital adrenal hyperplasia. *Hosp Pract* 12:75–82, 1977.
New MI, Levine LS: Congenital adrenal hyperplasia. *Adv Human Genet* 4:251, 1973.
Orth DN, Liddle GW: Results of treatment in 108 patients with Cushing's syndrome. *N Engl J Med* 285:243, 1971.
Skalkeas G et al: Cushing's syndrome; Analysis of 18 cases. *Am J Surg* 143:363, 1982.
Streeten DH, Tomycz N, Anderson GH Jr: Reliability of screening methods for the diagnosis of primary aldosteronism. *Am J Med* 67:403–413, 1979.
Van Heerden JA, et al: Pheochromocytoma: Current status and changing trends. *Surgery* 91:367, 1984.
Weinberger MH, Grim CE, Hollifield JW, Kem DC, Ganguly A, Kramer NJ, Yune HY, Wellman H, Donohue JP: Primary aldosteronism: diagnosis, localization and treatment. *Ann Intern Med* 90:386–395, 1979.

Skills

BREAST

1. Demonstrate the ability to predict whether a breast mass is benign or malignant on the basis of physical examination findings.
2. Given a patient with a breast mass, perform or assist in the aspiration of the mass.
3. Given a patient with a breast mass, clinically stage the patient.
4. Accurately interpret a mammogram of a patient with a large breast cyst.
5. Accurately interpret a mammogram of a patient with carcinoma of the breast.
6. Demonstrate the ability to perform an exam
   a. In patients with a breast mass,
   b. In patients with nipple drainage,
   c. In patients with axillary mass,
   d. In patients with breast tenderness.
7. Demonstrate the ability to outline a workup for women with palpable breast masses.

8. Demonstrate the ability to outline a workup of patients with recurrent (metastatic) breast cancer.
9. Demonstrate ability to interpret
   a. Roentgenograms of the chest showing metastases,
   b. Bone survey showing bony metastases,
   c. Bone scan showing bony metastases,
   d. Nucleotide liver scan or CT scan of the liver showing liver metastases,
   e. CT scan of the head showing brain metastases.
10. Outline appropriate use of screening mammography according to American Cancer Society guidelines.

ADRENALS

1. Demonstrate the ability to outline a workup of patients with hypertension, who are suspected of having:

   a. Cushing's syndrome,
   b. Hyperaldosteronism,
   c. Pheochromocytoma.
2. Demonstrate the ability to interpret
   a. CT scan of the abdomen showing an adrenal mass,
   b. CT scan of the head showing a pituitary tumor.
3. Explain the method and interpretation of
   a. Dexamethasone suppression test,
   b. Salt-loading test,
   c. α- and β-Blocker use in pheochromocytoma.

Study Questions

BREAST

1. In a 22-year-old female presenting with a discrete breast mass:
   a. Outline pertinent points in history taking.
   b. Outline specific features to be looked for on physical exam.
   c. What other workup should be done?
   d. What is the proper diagnostic/therapeutic approach in this patient?
2. In a 55-year-old female presenting with a discrete breast mass:
   a. Outline workup and plan.
   b. If a mammogram is negative, what would the plan be?
   c. If a biopsy proves malignancy, what further workup is needed?
   d. If operative therapy is indicated, what methods of therapy are acceptable?
3. Discuss the place and indication for adjuvant therapy for potentially curable breast cancer.
4. Discuss the rationales for and against screening for breast cancer.
5. Discuss one method of classification of the stages of breast cancer.
6. Discuss the therapeutic options for metastatic breast cancer to various organs, e.g. lymph nodes and skin, bone, lungs, liver, and brain.
7. A 45-year-old large breasted woman with negative physical examination of the breasts has a screening mammogram that shows a 3-mm discrete, highly suspicious lesion visible on only one view. Discuss the appropriate use of repeat mammography, needle localization, and specimen radiography.

ADRENALS

1. In a 52-year-old woman with hypertension who also complains of fatigue, recent weight gain (60 pounds), easy bruisability, and facial acne:

   a. What tests should you order to confirm the diagnosis?
   b. What specific tests and studies can be used to localize the lesion?
   c. What specific measures should be used in preparing the patient for surgery?
2. In a 45-year-old woman with long-standing hypertension who also complains of fatigue, headaches, polyuria, and polydipsia and whose serum Na^+ is 147 mEq/liter, serum K^+ is 2.9 mEq/liter, and serum Cl^- is 110 mEq/liter:
   a. What other tests would you order to reach the diagnosis?
   b. What other specific tests do you order to localize the abnormal gland?
   c. What specific measures can be taken in preparing the patient for operation?
3. In a 67-year-old woman with long-standing hypertension who also complains of fatigue, headaches, sweating, palpitations, facial pallor, tremor, and weight loss:
   a. What tests should you order to confirm the suspected diagnosis?
   b. What specific studies can be used to localize the tumor?
   c. What specific measures should be used in preparing the patient for surgery?
4. In patients with suspected adrenal disease, what tests can be done to localize the abnormal gland(s)?
5. In patients with Cushing's syndrome, outline the workup to differentiate Cushing's disease from Cushing's syndrome secondary to ectopic ACTH or adrenal carcinoma.
6. Outline the histologic "zones" in the adrenal gland and the hormones secreted by each.
7. Discuss the basis and mechanism behind the saline-loading test in the diagnosis of hyperaldosteronism.
8. Discuss the basis and mechanism behind the dexamethasone suppression tests in hypercortisolism.

22 Thyroid and Parathyroid

Martin Max, M.D., Jay Jeffrey Brown, M.D.,
Arlie R. Mansberger, Jr., M.D.,
Roger S. Foster, Jr., M.D., Nicholas P. Lang, M.D.,
and Enrique Vazquez-Quintana, M.D.

ASSUMPTIONS

The student understands the anatomy and embryology of the thyroid and parathyroid glands.

The student understands the physiology of the thyroid and parathyroid glands.

The student is familiar with the pathology of the common diseases of the thyroid and parathyroid glands.

OBJECTIVES

1. List the risk factors for carcinoma of the thyroid gland.
2. Discuss the common presenting symptoms and physical findings in a patient with a thyroid carcinoma.
3. Discuss the differential diagnosis and workup of a patient with a thyroid nodule.
4. Discuss the different types of cancer of the thyroid, including treatment and prognosis differences.
5. Discuss the role of surgery in treating patients with hyperthyroidism and patients with carcinoma of the thyroid, including surgical risks.
6. Discuss the multiple endocrine adenoma syndromes that involve the thyroid gland and discuss their clinical significance.
7. Differentiate between primary, secondary, and tertiary hyperparathyroidism.
8. List the diseases, signs, and symptoms associated with hypercalcemia.
9. Discuss the workup of a patient with hypercalcemia.
10. Discuss the role of surgery in primary, secondary and tertiary hyperparathyroidism.
11. Contrast the pathologic findings of parathyroid adenoma and hyperplasia and discuss associated clinical implications.
12. Discuss the multiple endocrine adenoma syndromes that involve the parathyroid and discuss their clinical significance.

The Thyroid

Anatomy

Because of their close embryologic and anatomic association, the thyroid gland and parathyroid glands will be discussed together. The main precursors of the thyroid gland start as a downgrowth from the first and second pharyngeal pouches. The thyroid descends to just below the cricoid cartilage, at which point it divides into two lobes. The site of origin persists as the foramen cecum at the base of the tongue, and anywhere along the path of descent, ectopic thyroid tissue can be found (lingual thyroid or thyroglossal remnant cysts). The parathyroid glands develop from the third and fourth branchial pouches and descend to lie adjacent to the posterior capsule of the thyroid gland. There are four glands present in over 90% of the population, and occasionally one or more may be incorporated into the thyroid or thymus gland.

In the adult, the normal thyroid weighs 15–25 gm and is composed of two lobes, connected by an isthmus lying over the second tracheal ring (Fig. 22.1). The highly vascularized thyroid derives its blood supply principally from the superior and inferior thyroid arteries. Each thyroid lobe is drained by three sets of veins, the superior, middle, and inferior thyroid veins, which empty into the jugular and innominate veins bilaterally. The parathyroid glands are paired organs, two on each side, found on the posterior surface of each thyroid lobe. The inferior parathyroid (arising from the third branchial pouch) gland location is less predictable than the upper parathyroid, and may be found overlying or alongside the trachea as low as the anterior mediastinum. The upper parathyroids (from the fourth branchial pouch) usually remain in close association with the upper portion of the lateral thyroid lobes but can migrate posteriorly along the esophagus into the posterior mediastinum. The normal parathyroid has a distinct yellowish-brown color, averages 2 × 3 × 7 mm

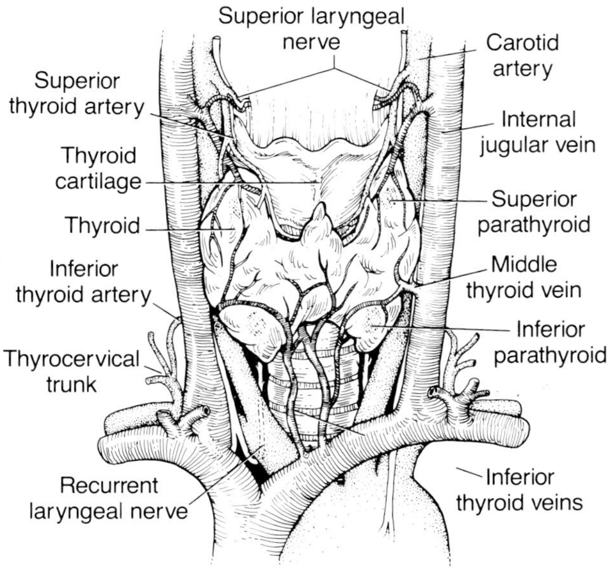

Figure 22.1.   Anatomy of thyroid and parathyroid glands.

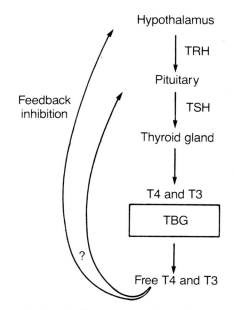

Figure 22.2.   The hypothalamic-pituitary-thyroid axis.

in size, and the total mean weight of four normal parathyroids is about 140 mg. Their blood supply is primarily from the inferior thyroid artery but may also have some component from the superior thyroid vessels.

Physiology

The function of the thyroid gland is to synthesize, store and secrete the hormones thyroxine (T4) and triiodothyroxine (T3). This is performed by the follicular cells of the thyroid, which have the unique ability to trap and to concentrate iodide from the serum. The iodide is then oxidized to iodine and the iodine is incorporated into the amino acid tyrosine to form either monoiodotyrosine (MIT) or diiodotyrosine (DIT). These are coupled to form the active hormones T4 and T3. After initial storage in the colloid of the gland, the thyroglobulin is hydrolyzed and T4 and T3 are secreted into the plasma, binding to plasma proteins. Most T3 is produced by extrathyroidal conversion of T4 to T3.

Thyroid gland function is controlled by a hypothalamic-pituitary-thyroid feedback system (Fig. 22.2). Thyrotropine-releasing factor (TRF) is formed in the hypothalamus and stimulates the release of thyrotropine (TSH) from the pituitary. The thyrotropine then binds to TSH receptors on the thyroid plasma membrane, which increases cyclic AMP production through the production of adenylate cyclase, stimulating thyroid cellular function. If excessive concentrations of T3 or T4 are present in the serum, a negative feedback system shuts off the secretion of TSH, and thus decreases the rate of synthesis and release of T3 and T4 from the thyroid gland. Thyroid hormones control metabolic rate, influence a wide variety of enzyme systems, and stimulate oxidative phyosphorylation.

The parathyroid glands, through the release of parathyroid hormone (PTH), play a vital role in calcium and phosphorus metabolism in bone, kidney, and gut, with interrelationships with vitamin D and calcium. The control mechanism for calcium homeostasis is primarily through the parathyroid glands. In the normal individual, as serum ionized-calcium level diminishes, the parathyroid glands secrete more PTH. This increased level of circulating PTH then acts upon the gut, kidney, and bone to raise serum calcium concentration to normal. Conversely, when there are elevated serum calcium levels, PTH secretion is lessened and the serum ionized-calcium level returns to normal.

Serum calcitonin, though a regulator of serum calcium levels, is not a major component of this system. While the parafollicular cells of the thyroid do secrete calcitonin, its role is primarily that of gross modulation and not a major control of serum calcium homeostasis.

Diseases of the Thyroid

The Thyroid Nodule

The physician confronted by a patient with a thyroid nodule faces the problem of distinguishing whether the lesion is symptomatic and whether it is benign or malignant. Since thyroid cancer frequently presents as a palpable abnormality in the thyroid gland, it must be separated from all other conditions that cause thyroid deformities. Abnormalities of the thyroid gland usually appear as thyroid enlargements that can be either diffuse or nodular. Diffuse enlargement is seen with colloid goiter, hyperplasia of Grave's disease, subacute thyroiditis, and the early stages of Hashimoto's thyroiditis. Only an occasional patient with these conditions is suspected of having thyroid cancer. Although thyroid cancer usually appears as a nodule, some forms may produce diffuse enlargement, for example, lymphoma, sarcoma, or undifferentiated carcinoma. Because most thyroid cancers present as a nodule, all clinically solitary nodules are suspect. Many nodules that appear to be single clinically prove to be multiple on histologic examination and are simple focal manifestations of an adenomatous goiter (diffuse colloid goiter). True single nodules are usually either a nodule of an adenomatous goiter, a follicular adenoma, or a thyroid malignancy.

Single benign nodules in the thyroid are categorized as either an adenomatous goiter or an adenoma. Single nodules of adenomatous goiter show poor encapsulation, variable histologic structure, a growth pattern similar to that of the normal gland, and no significant compression of the adjacent gland. True adenomas, on the other hand, demonstrate good encapsulation, uniform structure, a growth pattern different from that of the normal gland, and compression of abutting normal follicles. Nevertheless, the histologic criteria that separate nodules and adenomas are not always easily recognized in a surgical specimen. Adenomas are considered to be true neoplasms, whereas nodules are not. Clinically, nodules and adenomas should be evaluated and managed in a similar fashion.

Grossly, single thyroid lumps, whether nodules or adenomas, are well circumscribed lesions that vary from 1–10 cm in diameter. They are soft and bulge from the cut surface of the gland. Hemorrhage occurs frequently in these lesions and may produce cysts, intralesional fibrous septae, and calcification. Nodules may be seen as single lesions (uninodular), or several nodules may coalesce and remain segregated in one lobe of the thyroid gland (plurinodular), or several nodules may be found scattered irregularly throughout the thyroid gland, assuming different sizes (multinodular) and deforming the outline of the gland. Multiple adenomas are infrequent.

Based on their microscopic appearance, adenomas have been subdivided into embryonal, fetal, microfollicular, follicular, Hürthle cell, papillary, and atypical. All should be carefully examined by the pathologist. The occurrence of vascular, lymphatic, and/or capsular invasion is considered a sign of malignancy in spite of the benign cytologic appearance of the intralesional cell population.

Evaluation of the Thyroid Nodule

The goal of patient evaluation is to determine which patients with thyroid nodules should undergo surgery and which can be managed medically. During the history, questions should be asked regarding previous irradiation of the head and neck, a family history of multiple endocrine adenomatosis (MEA type II), the patient's age, the patient's sex, and the symptoms. Since 85% of pediatric and 30% of adult thyroid cancer occurs in patients with a history of head and neck irradiation, a history of x-ray exposure is critical. A family history of MEA type II suggests medullary carcinoma of the thyroid (see "Multiple Endocrine Neoplasms" later in this chapter). Nodules in the glands of the young or old are more likely to be cancer than in the middle-aged. Fifty percent of thyroid nod-

ules in patients under 15 years of age are malignant. Solitary nodules in elderly patients have a high incidence of malignancy. Solitary thyroid nodules in men are more likely to be cancer than in women. The symptoms may also help differentiate various thyroid conditions (See clinical evaluation of thyroid cancer).

Physical evaluation of the thyroid gland may be crucial in selecting therapy. Diffuse enlargement suggests benign conditions, such as diffuse colloid goiter, thyroiditis, or hyperplasia. The consistency of the gland and systemic signs may help differentiate these conditions. A single nodule within the thyroid gland, on the other hand, is suspicious of cancer. A single, hard nodule adherent to adjacent tissue or growing rapidly suggests malignancy. Conversely, a smooth, relatively soft nodule of long duration is probably a benign process. Indirect laryngoscopy should be done on all patients with thyroid abnormalities. Hoarseness or the presence of a paralyzed vocal cord indicates recurrent nerve involvement. Enlarged lateral neck nodes or a midline prethyroid (delphian) node suggests metastatic disease.

Imaging of the thyroid gland can be accomplished by radionuclide scanning, ultrasound, or computed tomography (CT) scanning. Classic thyroid scanning is done with ^{131}I. With ^{131}I scanning, most cancers show decreased uptake, but so do the majority of benign lesions. Follicular cancer has been detected in some hot nodules. In one series of thyroid cancers, the nodule was cold in 60%, normal in 34%, and hot in 6%.

Although ^{131}I is the radionuclide commonly used for thyroid scanning, ^{123}I has several characteristics (except cost) that make it attractive (Table 22.1). ^{99m}Tc, the most readily available radionuclide, may also be used initially in nodule evaluation. Technetium is trapped by the thyroid gland in the same manner as iodine. It provides excellent delineation of the gland, particularly on oblique views. Currently, ^{99m}Tc is used in many centers for the initial thyroid scan and is followed with iodine scanning for functional nodules.

Evaluation of a single nodule is a difficult and complicated subject. One method of approach is given in Figure 22.3. The primary decisions are made in differentiating cystic lesions and ascertaining the functional characteristics of solid lesions. Ultrasound scanning of the thyroid is a useful tool for thyroid examination. Improved techniques now allow detection of nodules

Table 22.1.
Isotopes Used in Thyroid Evaluation

Isotope	Half-life	Thyroid Dose (rads)	Cost	Test Performed
^{131}I	8 days	5.50 (5 µCi)	Low	24-hr after injection
^{123}I	13 hr	1.00 (100 µCi)	High	4-hr after injection
^{99m}Tc	6 hr	0.27 (1 mCi)	Very low	Study done immediately

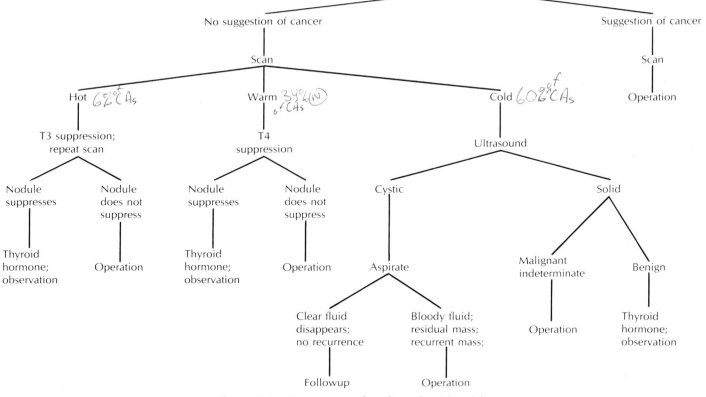

Figure 22.3. Management of a solitary thyroid nodule.

or cysts down to 3 mm in diameter and can differentiate cysts with 95% accuracy. Additionally, the evaluation of change in the size of thyroid lesions is now more reliable.

Thyroid function tests currently used in the evaluation of thyromegaly include examination of circulating thyroid hormones (T3 and T4), thyroglobulin (TG), thyroid antibodies (TAB), and TSH. These test findings are not usually critical in determining whether or not to operate on a nodular lesion. They are important to determine the functional status of the gland; that is, when it is hyperfunctional, hypofunctional, or normally functioning.

Plasma calcitonin levels above the normal maximum of 200 pg/ml may be seen in patients with extensive medullary carcinoma. Patients with a family history of MEA and no clinically evident disease require a stimulation test. The test may be done with a calcium infusion (14 mg/kg over 4 hours) or with an intravenous pentagastrin bolus (0.5 mg/kg).

Both core-needle biopsy and aspiration techniques have been used in thyroid evaluation. Core-needle biopsy of the thyroid gland has been used in several large medical centers but has not gained general acceptance. Its greatest use is the diagnosis of Hashimoto's thyroiditis. A normal needle biopsy finding cannot rule out malignancy, and it is therefore of less value in the evaluation of nodular thyroid problems. Aspiration of nodules suspicious for thyroid cancer with a fine nee-

dle is a very safe technique and appears reliable in centers that use it extensively. Many pathologists, however, are not prepared to provide a definitive thyroid diagnosis from a cytologic specimen.

Thyroid Carcinoma

Pathology. Thyroid cancer may originate from the follicular, parafollicular, or supporting cells of the thyroid gland. Various classifications have been developed but, for clinical purposes, division into the basic histologic types is adequate. These types include papillary, follicular, medullary, undifferentiated, and miscellaneous tumors. Most thyroid carcinomas present as moderately firm, unifocal, nontender enlargements of the thyroid, so-called solitary nodules. In a minority of thyroid carcinomas, there can be multiple nodules or even no detectable abnormality of the thyroid whatsoever. Rarely, the initial presentation of thyroid carcinoma may be related to metastases to regional lymph nodes or to a distant metastasis.

Clinical Evaluation. The patient should be questioned about the known duration of the thyroid nodule, whether the enlargement has been gradual or sudden, and whether there are local symptoms of discomfort. In patients under the age of 50, rapid enlargement of a nodule is almost always associated with conditions other than malignancy, such as thyroid cysts or a subacute thyroiditis. Most thyroid malignancies grow very slowly and actually appear to remain unchanged for many years. Only in elderly patients with anaplastic carcinoma will thyroid malignancies enlarge rapidly and cause significant symptoms of local discomfort. The patient should be questioned about a family history of goiter, thyroid malignancy, or a history suggestive of multiple endocrine neoplasia (MEN-II). The patient should be questioned about any history of therapeutic irradiation to the head and neck area, and about any medications that may have an effect on goiter formation. It is appropriate to determine whether there is any voice change, but almost all thyroid malignancies causing hoarseness are advanced malignancies with relatively obvious gross physical findings.

The main goals on physical examination of the patient with a possible thyroid malignancy are to document carefully the size and consistency of the abnormality in the thyroid gland and whether there are additional abnormalities of the thyroid, such as other nodules, enlargement of the opposite lobe, the pyramidal lobe, or the isthmus. Thyroid carcinomas most commonly metastasize to the nodes of the central neck, the tracheoesophageal grooves, superior mediastinum, and the prelaryngeal nodes (delphian nodes). The neck must be carefully palpated for any abnormalities of the cervical lymph nodes. Except for the delphian node area, central neck nodes are relatively difficult to palpate on physical examination. The most commonly palpable nodes in thyroid carcinoma are in the area of secondary lymphatic drainage; that is, the anterior cervical chain and the supraclavicular area. Most thyroid carcinomas are relatively firm. In general, the firmer the nodule, the greater the suspicion for malignancy. Extremely firm nodules, however, may be related to calcification of a long-standing benign nodule or development of the fibrous variant of lymphocytic thyroiditis. Large papillary carcinomas of the thyroid may undergo an area of cystic degeneration. It is possible for either the primary or the cervical node metastases to be cystic. A minority of thyroid malignancies will have fixation to the surrounding tissue secondary to extracapsular invasion. In all other cases, however, the thyroid and the tumor within it will move on swallowing.

Indirect laryngoscopy should be carried out in all patients preoperatively to detect the function of the vocal cords. Except in the case of patients with obvious advanced thyroid malignancy, most of the abnormalities of vocal cord function detected preoperatively will be related to idiopathic laryngeal nerve dysfunction. It is important to recognize preoperatively the presence of any dysfunction so that postoperative dysfunction is not inappropriately attributed to operative injury.

Treatment. Surgery plays a crucial role in the diagnosis and treatment of thyroid cancer. In recent years, there has been a decrease in the total number of thyroid procedures done, whereas the incidence of malignancy found in such procedures has increased. This finding indicates better selection of patients for thyroid exploration. Thyroid surgery is an anatomic exercise best performed only when armed with a thorough knowledge of neck anatomy. In general, the thyroid gland should be explored when there is significant risk of malignancy. Specifically, surgery is recommended in the following circumstances:

1. Any thyroid abnormality in a patient with previous irradiation of the neck.
2. A solitary nodule in a patient under 20 years of age.
3. A solitary nodule in a male patient.
4. A nodule associated with signs suggestive of malignancy, including recurrent nerve paralysis, palpable nodes in the neck, extreme hardness, or extension into adjacent tissues.
5. A solitary thyroid nodule in a patient over 60 years of age.
6. Most solitary cold nodules.
7. A normal thyroid gland in a patient with proven metastatic thyroid cancer.
8. A patient with an abnormal calcitonin stimulation test.

These indications include most cases involving solitary nodules, except middle-aged women with functional nodules. These patients are usually treated with suppressive doses of T4 for 6 months. If the nodule shrinks, thyroid suppression is continued. If the nodule does not shrink, the thyroid is explored. Nodules that appear cystic on ultrasound may be aspirated. If the aspiration is clear, and the nodule resolves and does not recur, this is adequate treatment.

When operating upon a nodule in the thyroid, the minimum procedure is a lobectomy on the side of the lesion. Incisional biopsy or nodulectomy plays little role in the operative management of these lesions. Once a frozen section is performed with histologic confirmation of a benign or malignant lesion, further surgical excision will depend upon the nature of the histologic diagnosis. Various surgical resections for thyroid disease are illustrated in Figure 22.4.

The methods of management of medullary and anaplastic carcinoma of the thyroid are generally agreed upon by most thyroid oncologists. Medullary carcinoma is usually approached by total thyroidectomy and nodal dissection of the neck on the ipsilateral side of tumor presentation. Anaplastic carcinoma carries a poor prognosis regardless of the mode of treatment or combinations of therapies employed. The treatment of well differentiated thyroid carcinomas is controversial. The debate not only involves medical versus surgical therapy, but whether total or subtotal thyroidectomy is most appropriate. Strong arguments can be made for either approach. There are those who favor subtotal thyroidectomy with or without postoperative ablation of residual thyroid tissue by radioactive iodine, and those who favor total thyroidectomy and reserving radioactive iodine treatment for recurrence or metastasis. Part of the problem concerns the relatively indolent nature of most well differentiated thyroid neoplasms, with mortality from these tumors accounting for a little more than 1000 cases per year.

Most well differentiated thyroid tumors are respon-

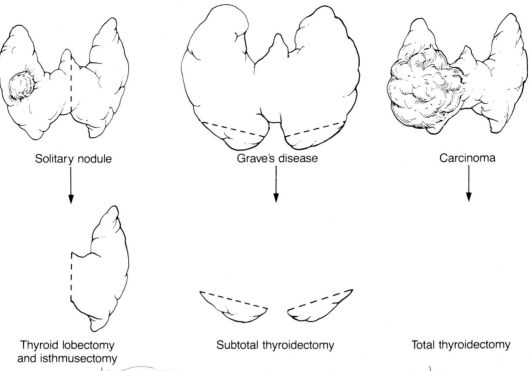

Solitary nodule   Grave's disease   Carcinoma

Thyroid lobectomy and isthmusectomy   Subtotal thyroidectomy   Total thyroidectomy

Figure 22.4. Various surgical resections for thyroid disease.

sive to thyroid-stimulating hormone. Postoperative thyroid evaluations have demonstrated supressed TSH production and therefore TSH has become standard adjuvant therapy. However, careful neck examination is the mainstay. Serum thyroglobulin following total thyroidectomy may be a useful tumor marker for recurrence.

Thyrotoxicosis

Thyrotoxicosis is a syndrome that is due to an oversecretion of thyroid hormone. The most common cause of thyrotoxicosis today is Grave's disease or diffuse toxic goiter. More rarely this may occur as a result of a toxic nodular goiter or a hyperfunctioning adenoma. The signs and symptoms of Grave's disease relate to the hypermetabolic state and can take many forms. These are seen in Table 22.2. Most cases of Grave's disease are found in women. In addition to the symptoms and signs as listed, these patients may also have exophthalmos, a diffuse goiter, and pretibial myxedema. Laboratory findings demonstrate the elevated levels of serum T4 and T3. Serum TSH levels are uniformly low.

There are three forms of treatment available: antithyroid drugs, radioactive iodine, and surgery. Most individuals are initially treated with antithyroid drugs, but this is permanently successful in only about 25% of patients. Also, approximately 5–10% of individuals develop a side effect to these antithyroid drugs. Noncompliance to these drugs, which need to be taken regularly, is also high. Radioactive iodine therapy is an attractive form of treatment because no operation is

necessary and the cost is low. However, radioactive iodine cannot be given to pregnant women since it could destroy the fetal thyroid. Long term risks of infertility and genetic abnormalities and increased incidence of thyroid cancer or leukemia have been disproved; however, there are still some patients afraid of the potential effects of radiation. In addition, greater than 50% of individuals treated with radioactive iodine develop hypothyroidism 10 years after treatment and require thyroid replacement therapy. Thus, radioactive iodine should usually not be given to children or young adults, women who are pregnant, or people who are concerned about the effects of radiation.

Surgery is the third treatment modality for patients with Grave's disease. It provides rapid control of the disease and shows a lower incidence of hypothyroidism than radioactive iodine treatment. It is often the preferred treatment (1) in the presence of a very large goiter or a multinodular goiter with relatively low radioactive iodine uptake; (2) in the presence of a suspicious thyroid nodule; (3) in the treatment of pregnant patients or children; (4) for the treatment of patients who wish to become pregnant within a year of treatment; and (5) for the treatment of psychologically or mentally incompetent patients who may not be able to maintain adequate long-term followup. The risk of thyroidectomy in this setting has become negligible since the introduction of drugs that can adequately prepare the patient for the operation. Giving iodine therapy preoperatively blocks the output of thyroid hormone and decreases the vascularity of the toxic thyroid gland. The β adrenergic blocker, propranolol, may be used. This slows the heart rate to normal and eliminates the

Table 22.2.
Clinical Manifestations of Thyrotoxicosis

Tachycardia, palpitation
CNS manifestations
  Restlessness
  Excitability
  Emotional lability
  Nervousness
  Insomnia
Increased sweating
Tremor
Menstrual irregularity
Increased appetite
Weight loss
Hypersensitivity to heat
Fatigue
Weakness
Bowel changes (diarrhea)
Mammary changes
Dyspnea
Skin changes
Clubbing

tremor. The operative treatment is usually subtotal thyroidectomy, sparing approximately 5–10 gm of thyroid tissue and protecting the recurrent laryngeal nerves and the integrity of the parathyroid glands. The mortality and morbidity is extremely low, with mortality less than 0.1% and major morbidity in less than 2% of the cases.

Complications of Thyroid Surgery

Major complications of thyroid surgery include hypoparathyroidism, nerve injury (recurrent laryngeal or superior laryngeal), and excessive bleeding (Table 22.3). The incidence of hypoparathyroidism is related to the extent of the thyroidectomy. It never occurs with a lobectomy and occurs in up to 29% of patients undergoing total thyroidectomy. It can usually be prevented by identification of the parathyroid glands and preservation of their blood supply. If all parathyroids are unintentionally removed and this problem is recognized, the excised parathyroid tissue should be cut into 1-mm cubes and placed into pockets within the sternocleidomastoid muscle. Return of function can be anticipated. In most cases, hypocalcemia that develops in the postoperative period is temporary, often due to edema or ischemia of the remaining parathyroid gland. During the early postoperative period, calcium is administered for either symptoms or for a serum calcium level of less than 7.5 mg/100 ml. Calcium chloride in a 10% solution is given intravenously, if a rapid increase

Table 22.3
Complications of Thyroid Surgery

Hypoparathyroidism
Recurrent Laryngeal Nerve Injury
Superior Laryngeal Nerve Injury
Excessive Bleeding

in serum calcium is required. Otherwise, a calcium gluconate infusion of 1–2 gm every 8 hours may be administered. Hypocalcemia that persists beyond 1 week is treated with oral calcium in sufficient amounts to provide 2 gm of calcium per day. Vitamin D (1.25–2.25 mg/day) is begun only if permanent hypoparathyroidism is suspected.

Recurrent nerve injury should be practically nonexistent in patients undergoing thyroid lobectomy and should be rare in all patients except those with massive cancers. Although some surgeons do not expose the nerves, injury to the recurrent laryngeal nerve is best prevented by direct visualization of the nerve before sharp dissection or clamping of any adjacent tissue. Demonstration of the recurrent laryngeal nerve is made possible by complete mobilization of the thyroid gland. Once the nerve is located, it should be handled gently and dissected minimally. All dissection should be limited to its medial border. The most dangerous site is the point of entry into the cricothyroid membrane. Here, small vessels are common and are divided medial into the nerve. If the nerve is divided and recognized, it should be repaired, since there is experimental work indicating that function may return. Even with anatomically intact nerves, temporary vocal cord weakness may be detected in a significant number of patients if they are checked carefully. Function usually returns within a few weeks to months. Permanent injury results in a paralyzed cord, but the voice improves considerably with time. If persistent problems occur (poor voice or aspiration), injection of the cord with synthetic material to narrow the glottis may be indicated. Bilateral cord paralysis requires a tracheostomy in most patients.

The external branch of the superior laryngeal nerve accompanies the vascular bundle toward the superior pole of thyroid before it turns toward the midline, terminating in the cricothyroid muscle. The nerve is protected by retracting the superior pole vessels downward and laterally before dividing them. The nerve is frequently seen medial to these vessels, which should be divided very low on the superior aspect of the gland. Damage to this nerve results in a weak voice and significant alteration in the ability to shout or sing. Although in most patients such an injury is not a major disability, it should be avoided.

Excessive bleeding may occur during the procedure or postoperatively and may arise from the gland or its blood supply. Glandular bleeding may develop either from the capsule or from the cut surface. Capsular bleeding results from tears in small vessels and should be controlled with suture ligatures. When thyroid tissue itself is to be divided, it should be clamped, divided, and ligated. Bleeding from the vessels is usually arterial and may develop from branches of either the superior or the inferior thyroid artery. Bleeding from the superior vessels is more dangerous, since these vessels may retract high in the neck, and frantic attempts to gain control may produce injuries to significant structures. Bleeding from the inferior thyroid artery usually occurs from its terminal branches located near the point where the recurrent laryngeal nerve enters the larynx. Usually, firm pressure for a few minutes will provide hemostasis from small vessels. Careful ligation may be needed for larger ones.

Postoperative bleeding may result in respiratory distress. Drains or pressure dressings will not prevent bleeding or hematoma formation. If a significant hematoma develops, the patient should be returned immediately to the operating room, the hematoma evacuated, hemostasis accomplished, and the neck wound reapproximated. Acute respiratory distress may necessitate opening the wound in the patient's room, but this procedure should rarely be indicated.

Multiple Endocrine Neoplasms

The multiple endocrine neoplasia (MEN) syndrome is a genetically transmitted disorder with protean manifestations. Awareness of this entity was stimulated by the description in 1955 of the Zollinger-Ellison syndrome (ZES), in which the association of pancreatic non-β-cell lesions and recurring peptic ulcer disease was established. Eventually, two distinct syndromes were described, depending on the glands involved and known as MEN-I and MEN-II, the latter further subdivided into A and B (Table 22.4).

Multiple Endrocrine Neoplasm—I. In 1903 J. Erdhemin published a treatise on the histology of the thyroid, parathyroid, and pituitary glands. He also described a patient with multiglandular involvement. The familial incidence was recognized in various sporadic reports, and in 1954 Wermer proposed a genetic mechanism, a dominant autosomal gene with high penetrance.

The glands most frequently affected are the parathyroid (85%), pancreas (65%), and pituitary (38%). Less frequently the adrenal and thyroid glands are involved. In the parathyroids the most common finding is chief cell hyperplasia, although an adenoma may also occur. The former finding implies secondary hyperparathyroidism (hypergastrinemia and hyperinsulinism) and the latter autonomous primary hyperparathyoidism. The recommended treatment for hyperplasia is removal of 3½ glands; for solitary adenoma, removal of

the only affected gland is needed but all the glands must be identified and their size ascertained. Ideally, PTH hormone levels should be obtained preoperatively.

The pancreas is the next most commonly affected gland in MEN-I. Non-β-cell pancreatic lesions, ZES, WDHA (watery diarrhea, hypokalemia, achlorhydria), and β-cell pancreatic lesions (insulinomas) have been described.

Over 55% of MEN-I patients present with pituitary tumors. Chromophobe adenomas predominate, but functioning lesions in the pituitary producing acromegaly may occur. Nonfunctioning tumors, if large, might produce pressure on the optic nerve requiring surgery or radiation therapy.

Miscellaneous lesions, such as adrenal adenomas, may also occur in MEN-I syndrome. Generally, the lesions are nonfunctional. Thyroid adenomas also rarely occur.

Multiple Endocrine Neoplasm—IIA. Medullary carcinoma of the thyroid (MCT) was described in 1959 by Hazard et al. Sipple in 1961 described a patient with bilateral pheochromocytomas, multiple thyroid carcinomas, and an enlarged parathyroid gland. The thyroid carcinoma was interpreted as poorly differentiated follicular adenocarcinoma but later proved to be medullary carcinoma. Subsequently it was observed that medullary carcinoma cells were similar to the parafollicular cells (C cells) of the normal mammalian thyroid gland and that this tumor produces thyrocalcitonin. Since 1970 serum thyrocalcitonin has been used as a marker to detect medullary carcinoma, even before symptoms or signs of the disease are present; it is also useful to detect metastatic disease activity. Calcium infusion and pentagastrin injection are provocative tests for calcitonin and are used for screening.

Medullary carcinoma accounts for 4–12% of all thyroid tumors. There is no sex or race predilection. The familial incidence varies from 10–25%; it is inherited as an autosomal dominant trait with high genetic penetrance. It is multicentric, with bilateral thyroid tumors seen in over 50% of the patients at the time of operation.

The most common clinical presentation of patients with MCT is an asymptomatic thyroid nodule or cervical lymphadenopathy. Approximately 10% of patients may have hoarseness secondary to recurrent laryngeal nerve involvement as part of their initial symptom complex.

Involvement of the parathyroid glands in MEN-II syndrome is believed to be secondary to the hypocalcemic effect of calcitonin, although this is not entirely clear. Genetically directed factors and increased production of prostaglandin E$_2$ (PGE$_2$) in patients with medullary carcinoma of thyroid are other possible explanations for the hypercalcemia. The most frequently described pathologic finding is hyperplasia of the parathyroid gland.

Once the diagnosis of MCT has been made or seriously considered, a diligent search for occult pheochromocytoma

Table 22.4
Men Syndromes

MEN 1: Parathyroid, Pancreas, and Pituitary (Adrenal and Thyroid-Rarely)	
MEN-II A	**MEN-II B**
Bilateral Medullary Ca of Thyroid	Same
Pheochromocytoma(s)	Same
Parathyroid Hyperplasia	Rare
None	Specific Phenotype
Autosomal dominant	Sometimes–usually non-familial
Indolent Progression of MCT	Rapid Progression of MCT

chromocytoma should be undertaken because of the risks of general anesthesia in patients with pheochromocytoma. If a pheochromocytoma is discovered, bilateral adrenalectomy should be the initial operative procedure because of the high incidence of bilateral adrenal involvement (70%).

The treatment of MCT is total thyroidectomy. In patients with familial and MEN-associated MCT the disease process is usually multicentric and bilateral, while patients with sporadic MCT are at significant risk for recurrence of tumor in the thyroid remnant if less than total thyroidectomy is performed. Metastases of MCT to cervical lymph nodes should be treated by radical neck dissection if there is no evidence of distant disease. MCT responds poorly to irradiation therapy, ^{131}I, and chemotherapy. The 5-year survival rate after resection ranges from 55–80%, and the presence of nodal metastases affects survival. Surgical treatment of the parathyroid disease, when necessary, will usually require subtotal parathyroidectomy.

Multiple Endocrine Neoplasm—IIB. Medullary carcinoma and pheochromocytomas have been associated with multiple neuromas in the conjunctiva, lips, and buccal mucosa. Megacolon, diverticulosis, and marfanoid habitus without cardiovascular defects have been described. However, the parathyroid glands are normal.

The Parathyroids

Primary Hyperparathyroidism

Primary hyperparathyroidism is due to excess PTH secretion from a single parathyroid adenoma, multiple adenomas, hyperplasia, or carcinoma. This results in hypercalcemia. The prevalence of primary hyperparathyroidism has been recognized more regularly in patients in recent years, and it is estimated that this is diagnosed in about 1 in every 500 patients who enter a hospital. The gross findings pathologically in patients with primary hyperparathyroidism demonstrates a single adenoma in 80–85% of patients, multiple parathyroid adenomas in 2–4% of patients, primary parathyroid hyperplasia in 5–10% of patients, and parathyroid carcinoma in less than 1% of patients. In patients with adenomas, the size usually parallels the degree of hypercalcemia. Microscopically, these tumors may be chief-cell, water-cell, or, rarely, oxyphil-cell type. In patients with primary parathyroid hyperplasia, all of the glands are usually involved, and microscopically there are two types, either chief-cell hyperplasia or water-clear-cell hyperplasia. Parathyroid cell carcinoma is rare and only if invasion of surrounding structures is present, can one be sure of the diagnosis of carcinoma.

Causes of Hypercalcemia

The release of PTH resulting from the stimulation of intracellular cylic AMP (cAMP) is produced by a vari-

Table 22.5.
Causes of Hypercalcemia

A. Malignancies
 1. Bone metastasis from breast, thyroid, kidney, or GI tract.
 2. Producing PTH-like polypeptides: lung, kidney, or bladder.
 3. Hematologic malignancies: multiple myeloma, lymphoma, or leukemia.
B. Diseases that produce increased PTH via stimulation of intracellular cAMP: primary hyperparathyroidism, hyperthyroidism, or pheochromocytoma.
C. Diseases associated with increased calcium absorption or resorption: sarcoidosis, milk-alkali syndrome, vitamin D intoxication, vitamin A intoxication, prolonged bed rest, or thiazide diuretics.
D. Congenital diseases: familial benign (hypocalciuric) hypercalcemia, congenital hypophosphatemia, or idiopathic hypercalcemia of infancy.
E. Diseases associated with hyperproteinemia: Addison's disease, multiple myeloma.

ety of stimuli (Table 22.5). In *primary hyperparathyroidism* a negative feedback mechanism exists by which a lowered serum calcium stimulates the release of PTH through the generation of intracellular cAMP. This feedback "cycle" is so sensitive that a decrease of 0.4 mg/100 ml in serum calcium will double the PTH under physiologic circumstances. The exact reason for interference with this cycle in primary hyperparathyroidism is not well understood.

Cancer, in a variety of forms and for a variety of reasons, may result in elevated serum calcium levels. Solid tumors with osteolytic metastatic bone destruction and excess calcium in the extracellular space is the most common cause of hypercalcemia. Those malignancies with a predilection for osseous metastases are carcinoma of the breast, thyroid, lung, kidney, and the gastrointestinal tract.

Bone destruction, however, is not the exclusive reason for calcium elevations in solid tumor metastases. Certain malignancies of this group have the capacity to produce humoral substances that may act alone or in concert with osteolysis to promote hypercalcemia. Carcinoma of the lung, kidney, pancreas, and bladder are capable of producing PTH-like polypeptides that may result in serum calcium elevations. Certain breast cancers may create hypercalcemia via the production of prostaglandins.

Hematologic malignancies, notably multiple myeloma, leukemia, and lymphoma, are examples of calcium-elevating hematologic malignancies. Multiple myeloma, in addition to its capacity for bone destruction, may produce a lymphokine osteoclast-activating factor that further stimulates calcium liberation.

In *hyperthyroidism*, certain amines, notably epinephrine, dopamine, and histamine, may liberate PTH via the cAMP mechanism cited previously. Thus, because of increased cellular sensitivity to catecholamines in hyperthyroidism, mild hypercalcemia may be present prior to definitive therapy with antithyroid drugs or β-adrenergic receptor blockers.

With *pheochromocytoma* there is always the possibility

that hyperparathyroidism coexists as part of the MEN-IIA syndrome. However, pheochromocytoma without coexistent hyperparathyroidism can result in elevated calcium levels secondary to β-adrenergic receptor site activation and generation of cAMP with liberation of PTH. β-Adrenergic receptor blockade (but only following α blockade) will cause return to normocalcemia.

There are also diseases associated with increased calcium absorption and/or resorption. The hypercalcemia associated with granulomatous diseases (including tuberculosis rarely, as well as sarcoidosis) is probably due to increased sensitivity to vitamin D. Elevation of calcium levels will be seen in approximately one-fifth of the patients with sarcoidosis at some time in the course of their disease. PTH levels in these patients will be low to nonmeasurable and steroid therapy results in return to normocalcemia.

The milk-alkali syndrome is far less common as a cause of hypercalcemia since the advent of nonabsorbable antacid medication. However, it is still seen occasionally in patients with peptic ulcers who ingest large volumes of milk and antacids containing calcium carbonate (commercially available, nonprescription items). Cessation of milk-alkali intake restores calcium homeostasis in these patients.

Hypercalcemia will occur in patients who take large doses of vitamin D daily for weeks or months. Increased amounts of calcium are absorbed from the gastrointestinal tract and accompanied by increased bone resorption. Similarly, large doses of vitamin A taken daily over an extended period will result in hypercalcemia. These vitamins are fat soluble, and cessation of vitamin intake does not result in rapid return to normocalcemia. Steroid therapy effects prompt reversal of hypercalcemia.

In patients, particularly the young, who have a high rate of turnover of bone, forced inactivity may result in significant hypercalcemia from bone resorption. The hypercalcemia will disappear rapidly with ambulation.

With thiazide therapy, there is an initial contraction of extracellular volume. In addition, thiazides have an effect on both kidney and bone. The renal excretion of calcium is decreased with thiazide therapy and bone turnover rates increased. This combination of drug-induced activity results in temporary mild hypercalcemia.

There are several congenital diseases that may cause hypercalcemia, and there is the hypercalcemia associated with hyperproteinemia. These conditions and all of the aforementioned causes of hypercalcemia are listed in Table 22.4.

Diagnosis of Patients with Hypercalcemia

The classic paraphrase for symptoms in primary hyperparathyroidism is "stones, bones, and abdominal groans." While it is true that there is an increase in the incidence of renal calculi and peptic ulcer disease associated with primary hyperparathyroidism, classic von Recklinghausen's disease of bone is seldom seen. The symptom complex of the modern disease is usually subtle, nonspecific, and related to a variety of organ systems, particularly musculoskeletal, renal, neurological, and gastrointestinal. Therefore, the historian must seek information relating to not only the obvious (renal colic, hematuria, gout, pancreatitis, pathologic fracture, etc.) but must ask for data concerning a variety of musculoskeletal aches and pains, constipation, lethargy, mental aberrations (especially depression), polyuria, polydipsia, and hypertension.

Physical examination will, likewise, generally be nonspecific and positive findings will relate to the organ system or systems involved. Benign parathyroid disease can rarely be identified in the neck. However, examination of the eye by slit lamp may reveal band keratopathy, which suggests hyperparathyroidism. The relatively early onset of symptoms related to subaortic stenosis may rarely be the initial clue to steer one toward a concomitant diagnosis of primary hyperparathyroidism.

Bone roentgenograms show a wide variety of findings in this disease from giant-cell tumors [Brown tumors (osteoclastomas)] and diffuse osteopenia to an absence of bony abnormalities (Fig. 22.5). Subperiosteal resorption is the disease's hallmark, best seen on the radial side of the middle phalanges, the skull, and the lateral one-third of the clavicles. Magnification radiographs of the hands are particularly helpful in detecting subperiosteal resorption. Nephrocalcinosis and renal calculi may be seen on plain abdominal films or an intravenous pyelogram (IVP), but rarely coexist in the same patient.

The relationship between serum calcium and parathormone levels is shown in Table 22.6. When evaluating biochemical abnormalities, it must be understood that the effect of PTH on renal tubules results in increased tubular resorption of calcium, and decreased tubular resorption of phosphorous and, to a lesser extent, bicarbonate. Therefore, the patient with primary hyperparathyroidism is expected to have hypercalcemia and hypophosphatemia with hyperphosphaturia. Because of the bicarbonaturia, the patient may have a mild metabolic acidosis with an elevated serum chloride. A chloride/phosphorus ratio that exceeds 33 enhances the diagnostic possibility of primary hyperparathyroidism. Hypercalcemia is frequently intermittent,

Table 22.6
Relationship between Serum Calcium and Parathormone Level

	Calcium	Parathormone
Normal	⟷	⟷
1° HPT	↑	↑↑
2° HPT (renal failure)	↓	↓↓↓
3° HPT	⟷ ↑	↑↑↑
Ectopic HPT	↑↑	↑
Hypo-PT	↓↓	↓
Pseudohypo-PT	↓↓	⟷

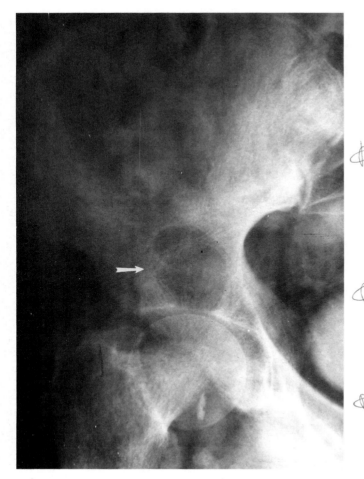

Figure 22.5. Right hip x-ray demonstrating Brown's tumor of acetabulum (arrow).

↳osteoclastoma
of 1° hyperparathyroid

and at least three serum samples should be analyzed if primary hyperparathyroidism is suspected. Most patients will have hypercalciuria, but it will be relatively mild. Severe hypercalciuria should alert one's suspicion relative to some other abnormality of calcium metabolism.

If available, the determination of ionized calcium levels is preferable to calcium levels determined by automation (total serum calcium). Roughly one-half of the circulating calcium (46%) is bound to protein (almost all to albumin). Thus, when total calcium levels are obtained, the reported calcium levels are obviously influenced by the level of protein (particularly albumin). Ionized calcium is elevated in some patients with primary hyperparathyroidism who have normal calcium levels when determined by other methods. Ionized calcium levels are unaffected by changes in serum protein.

Hyperparathormonemia is not necessarily diagnostic of hyperparathyroidism, because some patients on thiazide diuretics or with idiopathic hypercalciuria may have an elevated PTH. Similarly, patients with tumors producing PTH-like polypeptides may have mild elevations of PTH. Conversely, a mid- to high-normal PTH level is often seen in patients with hyperparathyroid-

ism. When a patient has a normal calcium level and the PTH is elevated or within a high normal range and primary hyperparathyroidism is suspected, measurement of the serum magnesium level is indicated. Correction of a low magnesium level will result in an appropriate rise in the calcium level. It is the relationship between the extent of elevation of the calcium and PTH level that must be determined to enhance accurate diagnosis.

Hypophosphatemia occurs in a high percentage of patients with primary hyperparathyroidism. It is uncommon in all other hypercalcemic syndromes except those related to malignant production of PTH-like polypeptides. However, significant weight loss, mild metabolic alkalosis, elevation of the erythrocyte sedimentation rate, and alkaline phosphatase without subperiosteal resorption support a diagnosis of malignant elaboration of a PTH-like polypeptide.

In those patients with primary hyperparathyroidism and rapid bone turnover, the alkaline phosphatase will be elevated. However, it may be elevated as well in liver disease secondary to sarcoidosis, in Paget's disease of bone and in certain patients with malignant bone or hepatic metastasis. Serum protein levels and protein immunoelectrophoresis are also of value in screening hypercalcemic patients for multiple myeloma. Classically, in this disease albumin levels are decreased and γ-globulin levels are increased.

Uric acid levels are elevated in patients with gout that may mimic or coexist with hyperparathyroidism. Uric acid levels are also elevated in patients with multiple myeloma, lymphoblastoma, and other malignancies (i.e., leukemia) that may result in hypercalcemia.

While other laboratory tests are of ancillary help in establishing a diagnosis of primary hyperparathyroidism (urinary cAMP, 1,25–dihroxycholecalciferol determination, and cortisone suppression test), those cited earlier are essential to an adequate diagnosis of this endocrine abnormality.

Operative Approach

When operating upon a patient for primary hyperparathyroidism, certain principles need to be followed. Approximately 85% of parathyroid adenomas are found in normal locations near the thyroid glands. The upper parathyroid glands are more constant in their location, but when these glands become enlarged, they may rotate posteriorly behind the esophagus and extend inferiorly, because of their weight, into the posterior/superior mediastinum. Because the lower parathyroid glands are derived embryologically from the same branchial origin as the thymus, adenomas of these glands may be found within the thymus, and more than one-half of these glands may be in the upper superior mediastinum. Because the location of the adenomas is well defined anatomically, an experienced surgeon will successfully find the offending gland(s) in greater than 95% of patients. Preoperative localization tests are therefore not necessary in the patient undergoing a first neck exploration for suspected hyperparathyroidism.

During the operation, a bloodless field in the neck is essential. It is important to examine both sides of the neck and to try to locate each parathyroid gland. Removal of an obviously enlarged parathyroid gland with others grossly normal will be acceptable for diagnosing a solitary adenoma. After removal of the adenoma, one or more of the remaining parathyroids are biopsied, and a frozen section is obtained to confirm the presence of parathyroid glands. If more than one gland is enlarged, one can assume that hyperplasia is present and a subtotal parathyroidectomy will be performed, leaving one or two well vascularized portions of parathyroid gland in situ. If no abnormalities of the parathyroids can be located initially during the neck exploration, a search of all atypical location sites should be carried out, going as high in the neck as the hyoid bone, along the carotid sheath, within the thyroid lobe itself, and into the anterior and posterior mediastinum by palpation. One should not do a medial sternotomy to look in the lower mediastinum at the time of the first operation.

Secondary and Tertiary Hyperparathyroidism

Secondary hyperparathyroidism (secondary HPT) occurs when there is increased secretion of parathormone and hypertrophy of the parathyroid glands in response to a chronically lowered serum calcium concentration. This situation most commonly occurs in patients with chronic renal failure and is the result of a number of physiologic abnormalities, including hyperphosphatemia due to decreased tubular excretion of phosphate, diminished synthesis of 1,25-dihydroxycholecalciferol by the diseased kidney, skeletal resistance to the action of parathormone, and poor absorption of calcium and vitamin D by the intestinal tract.

Diagnosis of Secondary Hyperparathyroidism

Usually, differentiation of primary from secondary hyperparathyroidism is easily accomplished. Patients with secondary HPT have low or low normal serum calcium levels as opposed to patients with primary HPT, in whom elevated calcium and decreased phosphate levels are the rule. In addition, primary HPT results in increased urinary excretion of both calcium and phosphate, while in secondary HPT the urinary levels of calcium and phosphate are decreased. Occasionally one might see a patient in whom this distinction is not so simple, especially if primary hyperparathyroidism has caused nephrocalcinosis and subsequent renal insufficiency.

Although it is now rare to see significant skeletal disease in primary HPT, it is not at all uncommon for bone disease to dominate the picture of secondary HPT and chronic renal failure (renal osteodystrophy). Renal osteodystrophy may take the form of osteomalacia, osteitis fibrosa cystica, osteosclerosis, or any combination

of the three. Ectopic calcification affecting the arterial tree, skeletal muscles, and other organs may also occur with secondary HPT. The frequency of this complication is thought to be directly related to the product of the serum concentrations of calcium and phosphorus.

Treatment of Secondary Hyperparathyroidism

The initial treatment of secondary HPT associated with chronic renal failure is medical. Attempts to lower serum phosphate levels by dietary restrictions of phosphate and the use of phosphate-binding antacids may be helpful, while serum calcium levels may be supplemented by the addition of calcium to the dialysate bath and oral calcium supplements. The administration of vitamin D metabolites is another adjunctive therapeutic measure. Correction of metabolic acidosis may both improve calcium balance and promote mineralization of bone.

There are four major indications for surgical intervention in secondary HPT: (1) persistent and symptomatic hypercalcemia in prospective renal transplant patients; (2) pathologic fractures; (3) symptomatic HPT including bone pain, ectopic calcification, and intractable itching; and (4) progressive hypercalcemia in patients with functioning renal transplants. The majority of surgeons prefer subtotal (3½ gland) parathyroidectomy as the operative treatment of secondary HPT. However, total parathyroidectomy with autotransplantation of a portion of the glands into the patient's forearm and/or tissue banking of the remaining glands has been advocated by some. This method permits easy removal of additional parathyroid tissue if HPT persists or implantation of portions of the preserved tissue if postoperative hypoparathyroidism develops.

Tertiary Hyperparathyroidism

Tertiary hyperparathyroidism (tertiary HPT) refers to the condition in which secondary HPT appears to have become "autonomous"; i.e., there is persistent HPT in the face of a normal or elevated serum calcium. This situation is often seen after a successful renal transplant has reversed many of the pathophysiologic processes that have led to the development of secondary HPT. However, this parathyroid gland "autonomy" will almost always revert to normal function and patients can be treated medically (oral phosphate administration) until normal parathyroid gland function returns. Rarely, nephrocalcinosis or renal calculi may threaten the function of the transplanted kidney and surgical treatment of tertiary HPT must be entertained in these cases.

Complications of Parathyroid Surgery

The complications of parathyroid surgery are similar to those of thyroid surgery. Hemorrhage, recurrent laryngeal nerve injury, and superior laryngeal nerve injury may occur with equal frequency when exploring the neck for parathyroid disease. Hypoparathyroidism during operations for parathyroid disease occurs in about 25% of patients. However, this is generally transient and permanent hypoparathyroidism rarely occurs. For treatment of these problems, see the section of this chapter dealing with complications of thyroid surgery.

SUGGESTED READINGS

Thyrotoxicosis

Hayek A, Chaman EM, Crawford JD: Long term results of I-131 treatment of thyrotoxicosis in children. *N Engl J Med* 283:949, 1970.

Nofal MM, Beierwaltes WH, Patno ME: Treatment of hyperthyroidism with sodium iodine I-131. *JAMA* 197:601, 1966.

Toft AD, Irving WJ, Sinclair I, McIntosh D, Seth J, Euan HDC: Thyroid function after surgical treatment of thyrotoxicosis. *N Engl J Med* 298:643, 1978.

Thyroid Nodule and Carcinoma

Ashcraft MW, VanHerle AJ: Management of thyroid nodules I and II. *Head Neck Surg* 3:216, 197, 1981.

Block MA: Surgery of thyroid nodules and malignancy. *Curr Probl Surg* 20:135, 1983.

DeGroot LJ, Reilly M, Pinnameneni K, Refetoff S: Retrospective and prospective study of radiation-induced thyroid disease. *Am J Med* 74:852, 1983.

Willems JS, Lowhagen T: Fine-needle aspiration cytology in thyroid disease. *Clin Endocrinol Metab* 10:247, 1981.

Complications of Thyroid and Parathyroid Surgery

Alveryd A: Parathyroid glands in thyroid surgery. *Acta Chir Scan* (Suppl) 389:1-20, 1968.

Holt GR, McMurry GT, Joseph DJ: Recurrent laryngeal nerve injury following thyroid operations. *Surg Gynecol Obstet* 144:567-570, 1977.

Moosman DA, DeWeese MS: The external laryngeal nerve as related to thyroidectomy. *Surg Gynecol Obstet* 127:1011-1016, 1968.

Parathyroid Disease and Hypercalcemia

Campbell DA, Dafoe DC, Swartz RD: Medical and surgical management of secondary hyperparathyroidism. In Thompson NW, Vinik AI (eds): *Endocrine Surgery Update*. New York, Grune and Stratton, 1983, pp 385-402.

Clark OH: Method for diagnosing the cause of hypercalcemia. In Najarian JS, Delaney JP (eds): *Endocrine Surgery*. New York, Appleton-Century-Crofts, 1981, Vol VIII, Book 2, pp 201-209.

Hanley DA: Clinical physiology of parathyroid hormone and vitamin D. In Najarian JS, Delaney JP (eds): *Endocrine Surgery*. New York, Appleton-Century-Crofts, 1981, Vol VIII, Book 2, pp 187-200.

Myers WPL: Differential diagnosis of hypercalcemia and cancer. *Cancer* 27:259, 1977.

Purnell DC, Schalz DA, Smith LH: Diagnosis of primary hyperparathyroidism. *Surg Clin North Am* 57:543, 1977.

Wells SA Jr, Leight GS, Ross AJ: Primary hyperparathyroidism. In Ravitch MM, et al (eds): *Current Problems in Surgery*. Chicago, Year Book Medical Publishers, 1980, Vol 17, pp 400-463.

MEN Syndromes

Sizemore GW, VanHeerden JA, Carney JA: Medullary carcinoma of the thyroid gland and the multiple endocrine neoplasia type 2 syndrome. In Kaplan EL (ed): *Surgery of the Thyroid and Parathyroid Glands*. New York, Churchill Livingstone, 1983.

Vieto RJ, Hickey RC, Samaan NA: Type I multiple endocrine neoplasias. *Curr Probl Cancer* 7:1982.

Skills

THYROID AND PARATHYROID

1. Demonstrate the ability to examine the thyroid gland:
   a. In a patient with a normal thyroid;
   b. In a patient with a Grave's disease;
   c. In a patient with a thyroid nodule.

2. Demonstrate the ability to do indirect laryngoscopy and identify a paralyzed vocal cord.

Study Questions

THYROID

1. In a 35-year-old female presenting with a discrete thyroid nodule:
   a. Outline pertinent points in history taking.
   b. Outline specific features to be looked for in physical exam.
   c. What workup should be done?
   d. Discuss the proper therapeutic approach in this patient.

2. Discuss the risk factors for thyroid malignancy.

3. Discuss the rationale, advantages, and disadvantages of the three methods of treatment of Grave's disease.

4. Discuss the anatomical reasons for the major complications of thyroid surgery.

PARATHYROID

1. In a 40-year-old male presenting with unexpected hypercalcemia on a routine screening blood test:
   a. Outline pertinent points in history taking.
   b. Outline specific features to be looked for on physical exam.
   c. What workup should be done?
   d. Discuss the proper therapeutic approach in this patient.

2. Discuss the intraoperative decision that is necessary in treating primary hyperparathyroidism.

3. Discuss the differences and similarities of the MEN-I and MEN-IIa and -IIb syndromes.

23

Liver

Layton F. Rikkers, M.D., *Jon Thompson, M.D.,*
Merril T. Dayton, M.D., Hollis W. Merrick III M.D.,
and Richard Gusberg, M.D.

ASSUMPTIONS

The student understands the anatomy of the liver.

The student understands the anatomy of portal circulation.

The student understands the pathology of liver cysts and neoplasms.

OBJECTIVES

1. Define portal hypertension and classify its etiology.
2. Describe five clinical manifestations of portal hypertension.
3. List four complications of portal hypertension and diagnostic procedures for each.
4. Outline the treatment methods available for variceal hemorrhage, including the principles for reduction of portal pressure.
5. Describe the medical and surgical treatments for a patient with ascites.
6. Discuss the prognosis for patients with portal hypertension.
7. Describe the presentation and treatment of a patient with hepatic encephalopathy.
8. Compare and contrast the natural histories and diagnostic methods for liver abscesses, neoplasms, and cysts.
9. List the diagnostic methods that differentiate liver abscesses, neoplasms, and cysts.
10. Describe the symptoms and physical signs associated with a liver abscess.
11. Describe the treatment modalities available for liver abscesses, neoplasms, and cysts.

Portal Hypertension

Anatomy and Physiology of the Hepatic Circulation

The liver has a dual blood supply, receiving blood from both the hepatic artery and the portal vein. The portal vein is formed behind the pancreas by the confluence of the superior mesenteric and splenic veins. It is the most posterior structure in the hepatoduodenal ligament (Fig. 23.1). The portal vein bifurcates into right and left branches just before entering the substance of the liver. The left gastric or coronary vein, which drains the lesser curvature of the stomach, enters the portal vein near its origin. The coronary vein is normally a minor branch of the portal vein but becomes a major collateral when portal venous pressure is elevated. The splenic vein lies behind the pancreas for most of its length and is usually joined by the inferior mesenteric vein just prior to entering the portal vein.

The hepatic artery is one of the three major branches of the celiac axis and, as it courses toward the liver, lies medial to the common bile duct and portal vein in the portal triad. Although the hepatic artery contributes only one-third of the blood flow to the liver in normal individuals, it provides approximately 50% of the oxygen supply. The hepatic arterioles are responsive to the usual vasoactive influences such as catecholamines and sympathetic nervous stimulation. In addition, vasodilation of these vessels occurs by autoregulation when hepatic blood flow is decreased in patients with shock or following surgical portal diversion. Changes in portal venous flow are due to vasodilation and vasoconstriction of the splanchnic arterial bed.

Many of the hormones secreted into the portal venous circulation have a role in the regulation of hepatic metabolism. In addition, some hormones, particularly insulin, have trophic effects on the liver and contribute to maintenance of normal liver size, function, and capacity for regeneration.

Etiology and Pathophysiology of Portal Hypertension

Portal hypertension is defined as the elevation of pressure in the portal venous system. It results from either an increase in resistance to portal blood flow, increased flow itself, or a combination of these two factors. Increased resistance to portal flow may be located in the main portal vein itself, within the liver at the presinusoidal, sinusoidal or postsinusoidal level, or in

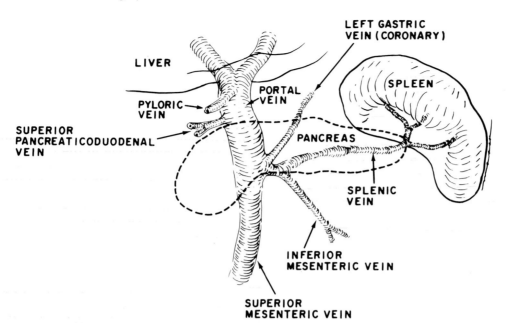

Figure 23.1.   Anatomy of the portal circulation. (From Rikkers LF: Portal hypertension. In Goldsmith HS (ed): *Practice of Surgery, General Surgery*, vol 3, chapter 4, 1981.)

the major hepatic veins (Table 23.1). An example of prehepatic portal hypertension is portal vein thrombosis, which accounts for approximately 50% of cases of portal hypertension in the pediatric age group. Normal hepatic function is maintained in these individuals because hepatic vascular resistance is normal and collaterals develop to maintain portal blood flow to the liver. Schistosomiasis is the most common cause of presinusoidal portal hypertension. Cirrhosis is responsible for over 90% of cases of portal hypertension in the United States. Increased vascular resistance in cirrhosis may occur at the presinusoidal, sinusoidal, and postsinusoidal levels. Individuals with cirrhosis also have an increased splanchnic blood flow. Alcohol is the responsible toxin in approximately 70% of cases. Hepatic vein thrombosis (Budd-Chiari syndrome) is a postsinusoidal cause of portal hypertension that occasionally develops in patients with a hypercoagulable state or idiopathically. The hepatic congestion that occurs may eventually lead to hepatocellular failure and intractable ascites.

Whatever the cause, elevated portal venous pressure is the major stimulus to portal-systemic collateralization. Collaterals form in locations where the portal venous and systemic venous circulations are in close proximity. The major sites of portal systemic collateralization in patients with portal hypertension are shown in Figure 23.2. The most important collateral is the left gastric (coronary) vein that connects the portal vein to the azygos system within the thorax. Increased flow and pressure through this collateral pathway results in gastric and esophageal varices, which may rupture and cause massive upper gastrointestinal hemorrhage. Although all collaterals are distended and under increased pressure, the gastroesophageal varices bleed most commonly. In this location, hydrostatic pressure within the varix probably leads to rupture of the overlying epithelium, which is sometimes only one cell-layer thick.

Complications of Portal Hypertension

Variceal Hemorrhage

Variceal hemorrhage is the most life-threatening complication of portal hypertension. Although many patients with portal hypertension develop esophageal and/or gastric varices, only one-third of the patients ever bleed from varices. The mortality rate secondary to acute variceal hemorrhage ranges from 20–80% and mainly depends on the patient's underlying liver function. Whereas variceal hemorrhage frequently results in death in a patient with advanced and decompensated cirrhosis, individuals with prehepatic portal hypertension rarely die of this complication. Once bleeding occurs, the likelihood of a second episode of variceal hemorrhage exceeds 70% and usually occurs within 6 weeks of the first episode. Although varices

Table 23.1.
Classification of Portal Hypertension

I. Prehepatic
   A. Thrombotic (portal vein thrombosis)
   B. Excessive inflow (arteriovenous fistula)
II. Intrahepatic
   A. Presinusoidal (schistosomiasis)
   B. Sinusoidal (cirrhosis)
   C. Postsinusoidal (veno-occlusive disorders)
III. Posthepatic
   A. Obstructive (Budd-Chiari syndrome)
   B. Cardiac failure

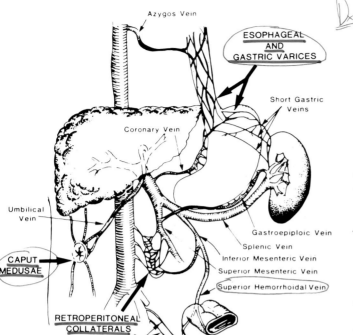

Azygos Vein

ESOPHAGEAL
AND
GASTRIC VARICES

Short Gastric
Veins

Coronary Vein

Umbilical
Vein

CAPUT
MEDUSAE

Gastroepiploic Vein
Splenic Vein
Inferior Mesenteric Vein
Superior Mesenteric Vein
Superior Hemorrhoidal Vein

RETROPERITONEAL
COLLATERALS

middle & inferior
Hemorrhoidal Veins

HEMORRHOIDS

Figure 23.2.   Sites of portal-systemic collateralization. (From Rikkers LF: Portal hypertension. In Goldsmith HS (ed): *Practice of Surgery, General Surgery,* Vol 3, chapter 4, 1981.)

most commonly develop in the esophagus and upper stomach, they may occur at any location within the gastrointestinal tract. However, the site of hemorrhage in over 90% of patients is within 2 cm of the esophagogastric junction.

Diagnosis. Variceal hemorrhage should be suspected when upper gastrointestinal hemorrhage occurs in patients with a history of chronic liver disease, alcoholism, or hepatitis. However, approximately 50% of upper gastrointestinal hemorrhages in patients with known varices arise from lesions other than the varices. The differential diagnosis includes peptic ulcer disease, gastritis, and Mallory-Weiss syndrome. Thus, it is essential that upper gastrointestinal endoscopy be performed during the acute bleeding episode. Because bleeding from varices is often massive, the patient frequently presents with hypotension and hematemesis. Before any attempts at diagnosis are made, it is essential to stabilize the patient. Thus, the appropriate intravenous lines are inserted and blood is typed and cross-matched.

Careful examination of the patient may reveal the presence of spider angiomata, palmar erythema, and gynecomastia, indicating the probable presence of chronic liver disease. The presence of a caput medusa, ascites, or a palpable spleen indicates probable portal hypertension. A history of previously diagnosed chronic liver disease, alcoholism, or hepatitis make varices suspect as the cause of bleeding.

The key for establishing the diagnosis of variceal

hemorrhage is upper gastrointestinal endoscopy, which should be accomplished either in the emergency department or soon after admission to an intensive care unit. Upper GI barium studies should not be undertaken as an initial study in the acute phase as it is less accurate than endoscopy. Gastric lavage with a large bore nasogastric tube is helpful in evacuating blood from the stomach prior to endoscopy. In addition, it will determine whether the upper gastrointestinal tract is the site of hemorrhage in the patient who presents with melena or hematochezia. Varices can be established as the cause of bleeding when the endoscopist observes a bleeding varix or nonbleeding large varices and no other gastrointestinal lesions.

Assessment of portal hemodynamics and vascular anatomy is important both for confirming and diagnosis of portal hypertension and for planning appropriate therapy. This involves measurement of portal venous pressure and visualization of the portal venous system. The most common technique used to estimate portal venous pressure is measurement of the hepatic venous pressure gradient, which is defined as the hepatic venous wedge pressure minus the free hepatic vein pressure. Bleeding from esophageal varices seldom occurs unless this gradient is greater than 12 mm Hg. Selective visceral angiography is the most frequently used method for opacification of the portal venous system and for qualitative estimation of hepatic portal perfusion. Selective injections into the superior mesenteric artery and splenic artery or celiac axis are followed by serial films well into the venous phase with visualization of superior mesenteric, splenic, and portal veins (Fig. 23.3). Angiography is not indicated as an emergency diagnostic test. Direct portography via transjugular or transhepatic approach also permits direct measurement of portal pressures.

Medical Management. Since most patients who present with acute variceal hemorrhage are high risks for emergency surgical therapy, the initial management of these patients is nonoperative. The first priority is restoration of circulating blood volume and reversal or prevention of hemorrhagic shock. Crystalloid, type-specific, and O negative blood should be used until cross-matched negative blood is available. Because blood in the gastrointestinal tract is a potent inducer of encephalopathy, a nasogastric tube should be inserted for administration of a cathartic to clear the gastrointestinal tract of blood. In addition, an agent such as lactulose may be administered to both induce diarrhea (osmotically) and shift the pH to reduce the absorption of ammonia. An antibiotic, such as neomycin, may also be given to reduce bacteria that produce ammonia, a possible etiologic agent in encephalopathy. Once hemorrhage has been controlled, attention should be directed to the treatment of malnutrition, ascites, and encephalopathy if these are present.

Systemic vasopressin may also be used to lower portal pressure by constricting arterioles in the splanchnic circulation, thereby decreasing inflow to the portal ve-

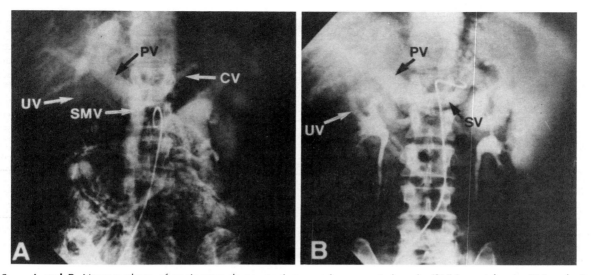

Figure 23.3.   A and B. Venous phase of angiogram demonstrating superior mesenteric vein (SMV), portal vein (PV), splenic vein (SV), coronary vein (CV), and umbilical vein (UV).

nous system. This drug controls active variceal hemorrhage in approximately 50% of patients. Because vasopressin also decreases cardiac output and causes coronary vasoconstriction, it should be avoided in patients with coronary artery disease. Vasopressin may also cause symptomatic mesenteric ischemia in some patients.

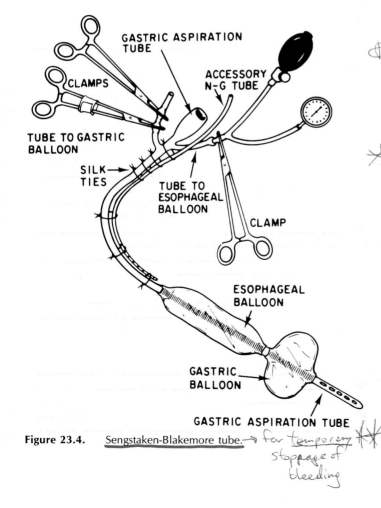

Figure 23.4.   Sengstaken-Blakemore tube.

The most commonly used device for mechanical compression of bleeding esophageal varices is the Sengstaken-Blakemore tube (Fig. 23.4). This triple lumen tube is effective in stopping variceal bleeding in 90–95% of patients. However, unless used according to a strict protocol, there is significant morbidity and mortality associated with balloon tamponade. Complications include: esophageal perforation, ischemic necrosis of the esophagus, asphyxiation secondary to migration of the esophageal balloon, and aspiration. Because recurrent variceal hemorrhage follows balloon deflation in approximately 20–50% of patients, more definitive therapy should be planned for patients who require balloon tamponade.

Esophageal varices may be obliterated nonoperatively by direct injection of a sclerosant into the varices via an endoscope. When applied to actively bleeding patients endoscopic sclerotherapy results in temporary control of hemorrhage in 85–95% of patients. When compared to conventional medical treatment, endoscopic sclerotherapy has been shown to decrease the frequency of recurrent hemorrhage when repeated at intervals of 3–6 months. However, as many as one-half to two-thirds of patients rebleed before varices have been eradicated. Sclerotherapy is being used increasingly for the definitive management of variceal hemorrhage on failed sclerosis of actively bleeding varices where surgical risk is prohibitive; embolization of varices can be done as a temporizing measure through a transhepatic approach to the portal vein and its tributaries.

Surgical Management. Because of the high risk of recurrent hemorrhage, most surgeons believe that a definitive procedure should be performed in individuals who bleed from esophageal varices. The types of operations available include nonshunting (or devascularization procedures) and portal-systemic shunt procedures. Shunt operations decompress either all or a

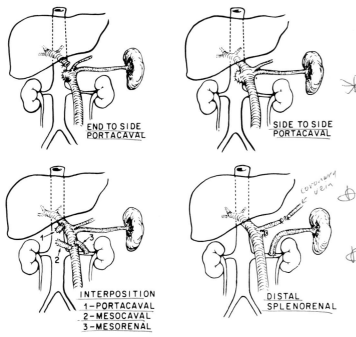

Figure 23.5. Surgical portal-systemic shunts.

portion of the portal venous circulation (Fig. 23.5). Those procedures that divert all portal blood flow away from the liver are termed nonselective shunts, while those that preserve some degree of hepatic portal perfusion are called selective shunts.

The goals of nonshunting operations are to either interrupt collateral pathways to varices or to obliterate varices themselves. Portal blood flow to the liver is preserved with all of these procedures. However, because elevated portal venous pressure is a stimulus to collateralization, reformation of varices and recurrent variceal hemorrhage frequently occur.

The most extensive nonshunting operation is the Sugiura procedure, which consists of splenectomy, proximal gastric devascularization, vagotomy, and pyloroplasty through an abdominal incision, and esophageal devascularization and esophageal transection and reanastomosis through a thoracotomy. A simple, more rapid method of interrupting esophageal collateral pathways is transabdominal esophageal transection and reanastomosis with the end-to-end anastomosis (EEA) stapling instrument, combined with ligation of the coronary vein. However, this procedure has been associated with frequent recurrent hemorrhage. Splenectomy alone minimally lowers portal pressure and recurrent variceal hemorrhage is frequent. Splenectomy *does*, however, prevent variceal hemorrhage in *isolated* splenic vein thrombosis without generalized portal hypertension. This is the most common situation in which a surgical procedure can *cure*, rather than palliate, the portal hypertension.

There are two hemodynamically distinct types of nonselective shunts: the end-to-side portacaval shunt and several varieties of side-to-side portal-systemic shunts. The end-to-side portacaval shunt is con-

structed by division of the portal vein near its bifurcation, with anastomosis of its splanchnic end to the inferior vena cava; the hepatic end of the portal vein is oversewn. This results in a large caliber venous anastomosis that reliably prevents recurrent variceal hemorrhage. However, controlled trials have shown that the end-to-side portacaval shunt minimally prolongs survival when compared to medical treatment alone and that the postoperative course is frequently complicated by debilitating encephalopathy.

The side-to-side portacaval shunt is constructed by direct anastomosis of the portal vein to the inferior vena cava. This shunt diverts the entire portal blood flow and also decompresses the hepatic sinusoids. Because hepatic sinusoidal hypertension is a key factor in the production of cirrhotic ascites, side-to-side portal-systemic shunts effectively relieve ascites as well as prevent recurrent variceal hemorrhage. A side-to-side portal-systemic shunt can also be constructed by placing a prosthetic graft in the portacaval, mesocaval, or mesorenal positions. These interposition shunts are easier to construct than the side-to-side portacaval shunt, but shunt thrombosis is more frequent. An interposition mesocaval or mesorenal shunt is preferable to a portacaval shunt when the upper abdomen is encased in vascular adhesions from prior biliary or other upper abdominal surgery.

The only portal-systemic shunting procedure that consistently preserves portal blood flow to the liver is the distal splenorenal shunt. The distal splenorenal shunt consists of anastomosis of the distal end of the splenic vein to the side of the left renal vein and disconnection of the portal-superior mesenteric venous component of the splanchnic venous circulation from the gastrosplenic component. The objectives of the distal splenorenal shunt are: *(1)* decompression of the gastrosplenic venous circulation, *(2)* preservation of hepatic portal perfusion, and *(3)* maintenance of an elevated portal venous pressure. Because portal perfusion to the liver is maintained, there is a much lower frequency of encephalopathy than following nonselective portal-systemic shunts. Encephalopathy rates following the distal splenorenal shunt range from 10–15%, as compared to 30–50% following nonselective shunts. However, because the high pressure portal venous network is still in juxtaposition to the decompressed gastrosplenic venous system, collaterals eventually reform and portal flow to the liver gradually diminishes with time. Because the distal splenorenal shunt decompresses neither the splanchnic viscera nor the hepatic sinusoids, it is ineffective in relieving ascites; in fact, ascites can be a serious postoperative problem in patients with preoperative ascites who undergo a distal splenorenal shunt.

Selection of the Operative Procedure. The appropriate operation to be performed depends on the status of hepatic hemodynamics, the clinical circumstances, and the experience and skill of the surgeon. The end-to-side portacaval shunt is technically easiest to perform and reliably decompresses the portal venous sys-

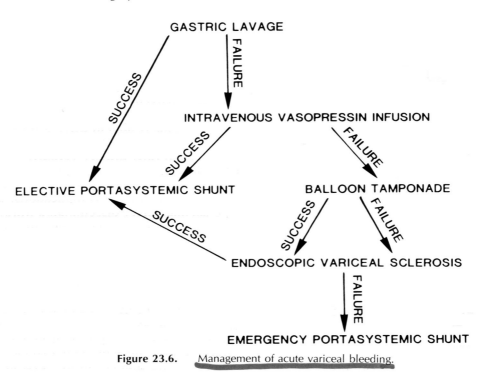

Figure 23.6. Management of acute variceal bleeding.

tem, so it is generally preferred in the emergency situation. A side-to-side portal-systemic shunt is preferred for patients with intractable preoperative ascites in addition to variceal hemorrhage. In patients with evidence of portal blood flow to the liver, compatible anatomy, and easily controlled preoperative ascites, the distal splenorenal shunt is the preferred procedure for control of bleeding esophageal varices. The procedure is generally performed electively but may occasionally be done in the emergency setting when hemorrhage is temporarily controlled by balloon tamponade, allowing time for preoperative angiography. Nonshunting procedures should be used for patients with diffuse splanchnic venous thrombosis and no major portal tributaries available for anastomosis.

Management of Acute Variceal Hemorrhage. An algorithm for management of acute variceal bleeding is shown in Figure 23.6. The sequential use of intravenous vasopressin, balloon tamponade, and endoscopic variceal sclerosis results in control of acute variceal

hemorrhage in over 80% of patients. Emergency surgery is reserved for those few patients who continue to bleed despite aggressive nonoperative treatment. The advantage of this approach is that it allows time prior to surgery for improvement of hepatic functional reserve, which is the major determinant of early postoperative survival. Hepatic reserve is most easily estimated by Child's classification, which consists of two biochemical indices (serum bilirubin and albumin) and three clinical variables (ascites, encephalopathy, and nutrition) (Table 23.2). Approximate operative mortality rates for Child's classes A, B, and C patients are 0–5%, 5–15%, and 20–50%, respectively. Child's class can be significantly improved when an interval of medical management and nutritional support precede elective surgery.

Survival After Variceal Hemorrhage. No matter which treatment is selected, only 40–60% of patients with alcoholic cirrhosis will live for 5 years after the onset of variceal hemorrhage. Operative procedures and endoscopic variceal sclerosis only marginally prolong survival as compared to medical treatment. The relentless progression of liver disease in patients with alcoholic cirrhosis, often secondary to continued alcoholism, is most likely the main factor determining survival. However, a long-term survival of patients with nonalcoholic cirrhosis may be improved following procedures that preserve portal blood flow to the liver (distal splenorenal shunt, nonshunting operations, and endoscopic variceal sclerosis).

Ascites

Ascites frequently complicates portal hypertension, especially when the elevated vascular resistance is at

Table 23.2.
Child's Classification

Criteria	Good Risk (A)	Moderate Risk (B)	Poor Risk (C)
Serum bilirubin (mg/100 ml)	<2.0	2.0–3.0	>3.0
Serum albumin (mg/100 ml)	>3.5	3.0–3.5	<3.0
Ascites	None	Easily controlled	Not easily controlled
Encephalopathy	None	Minimal	Advanced
Nutrition	Excellent	Good	Poor

with frequent estimations of serum electrolytes, blood urea nitrogen, creatinine, and body weight.

The best surgical approach to medically intractable ascites, or ascites that does not respond to medical management, is the peritoneovenous shunt (Fig. 23.7). The peritoneovenous shunt functions as a large lymphatic that returns the ascitic fluid to the vascular compartment. This results in increased cardiac output and renal blood flow, which causes an increase in glomerular filtration rate, urinary volume, and sodium excretion. Although this is a simple technique that can be performed under local anesthesia, complications are frequent. Some of the complications, such as sepsis, hypokalemia, CHF, disseminated intravascular coagulation, and variceal hemorrhage, may be life-threatening.

Portal-Systemic Encephalopathy

Portal-systemic encephalopathy is a psychoneurologic syndrome secondary to hepatocellular dysfunction in combination with portal-systemic shunting. The syndrome may present with diverse symptoms and signs including changes in the level of consciousness, intellectual deterioration, changes in personality, and the characteristic flapping tremor, asterixis. While it may develop spontaneously, it frequently occurs following portal-systemic shunting procedures, especially those that completely divert portal blood flow from the liver.

The exact pathogenesis of portal-systemic encephalopathy remains unclear. The most likely etiology is that intestinal absorption of one or more cerebral toxins either directly bypass the liver or fail to be inactivated by the liver and thereby gain access to the brain. Leading candidate toxins include: ammonia, mercaptans, and γ-aminobutyric acid. Another theory is that the altered plasma profile of amino acids present in patients with chronic liver disease may lead to depletion of normal neurotransmitters and accumulation of false neurotransmitters in the brain. One or more of the following factors is usually responsible for inducing an episode of portal systemic encephalopathy: excess dietary protein, gastrointestinal hemorrhage, infection, metabolic alkalosis, sedatives, azotemia, and constipation. Most of these precipitating factors lead to hyperammonemia, lending support to ammonia as one of the cerebral toxins responsible for the syndrome.

Identification and elimination of any precipitating factors should be the first step in treating portal-systemic encephalopathy. Blood within the gastrointestinal tract should be removed by catharsis, sedatives should be discontinued, infections should be treated with antibiotics and/or surgical drainage, and dietary protein should be restricted. Patients known to be susceptible to encephalopathy should be chronically managed with stool softeners and mild protein restriction (50–60 gm protein per day). If this fails to clear the sensorium, specific pharmacologic treatment should be instituted. Both neomycin, a poorly absorbed antibi-

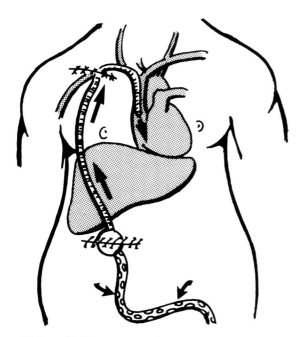

Figure 23.7.   Peritoneovenous shunt.

the hepatic sinusoidal and/or postsinusoidal level. Several factors appear to contribute to the pathogenesis of cirrhotic ascites. Elevated hepatic sinusoidal and intestinal capillary pressure results in transudation of fluid into the interstitial space through porous sinusoidal endothelium. When the liver's capacity for transport of this excess fluid to the lymphatic system is exceeded, ascites results. This third spacing of extracellular fluid results in a circulating volume deficit; secondary mechanisms, such as aldosterone secretion and redistribution of blood flow within the kidney, are set into motion to restore plasma volume. Subsequent expansion of plasma volume then results in further ascites formation.

Ascites may cause significant morbidity and even mortality. Ascites is necessary for the development of the life-threatening complication of spontaneous bacterial peritonitis. The development of tense ascites almost always precedes the onset of the hepatorenal syndrome. Both of these complications are associated with a high mortality rate. In addition, ascites often develops prior to hemorrhage from esophageal varices and may contribute to the magnitude of portal hypertension in these patients.

Ascites can be effectively managed by medical treatment in 95% of patients. The most important elements of medical management are dietary salt restriction (20–30 mEq/day) and diuretic therapy. Because secondary hyperaldosteronism occurs in most patients with ascites, spironolactone is a rational first line diuretic. Spironolactone in combination with salt and water restriction results in an effective diuresis in approximately two-thirds of patients. Other diuretics, such as hydrochlorothiazide or furosemide, may also be added to the regimen. Therapy should be carefully monitored

Table 23.3.
Hepatic Lesions

	Symptoms	Signs	Lab Data	Ultra-sound	Liver Scan	CT Scan	Diagnosis	Treatment
Primary malignancies	Late abdominal pain Weight loss Jaundice	Palpable mass Occasional arterial bruit Friction rub Ascites	↑ AFP (50–80%) ↑ Bilirubin ↑ Alkaline phosphatase	Discrete area of ↑ or ↓ echo	Cold defects(s) Usually single	Area(s) of ↓ attenuation with variable enhancement	Needle or open biopsy	Partial hepatectomy Arterial ligation Chemotherapy
Secondary malignancies	Those of primary malignancy	Palpable mass Friction rub	↑ Bilirubin ↑ LFT's	Multiple areas of ↑ or ↓ echo	Multiple cold defects	Multiple areas of ↑ attenuation with variable enhancement	Clinical diagnosis with/without CT guided biopsy	Treat with chemotherapy for primary neoplasm
Hepatic adenoma	Right upper quadrant pain occuring in females on birth control pills	Right upper quadrant mass May bleed massively	Usually normal	Focal area of ↑ echo Occasional low echo with tumor necrosis	Single cold defect	Single areas of isodense or ↓ attenuation with variable enhancement	Biopsy—may be difficult to differentiate from hepatoma	Discontinue birth control pills and observe Ennuleation Partial hepatectomy when symptomatic
Focal nodular adenoma	Usually asymptomatic right upper quadrant discomfort Not associated with birth control pills	Occasional mass	Normal	Focal areas with normal echo pattern	Decreased, normal or ↑ activity	Nodularity with isodense or ↓ attenuation and variable enhancement	Biopsy	Remove only if symptomatic
Hemangioma	Occasional pain Discomfort	Occasional palpable mass May rupture	Rare coagulopathy (DIC)	Focal area of ↑ echo	Cold defect	Areas of ↓ attenuation that enhance more than normal tissue with contrast	Arteriogram	Excision if symptomatic Radiotherapy Arterial ligation
Cysts	Occasional right upper quadrant discomfort	Occasional mass	Normal	Discrete echo Lucency	Cold defect	Discrete area of ↓ attenuation (low specific gravity)	Ultrasound or CT scan	Usually none Percutaneous or open drainage if symptomatic
Abscess	High fever Right upper quadrant pain	Jaundice Enlarged, tender liver	WBC 20,000 ↑ Alkaline phosphatase ↑ Bilirubin Anemia	Discrete echo Lucency May have some internal echoes	Cold defect	Discrete area(s) of decreased attenuation Possible rim enhancement (low specific gravity)	Right-sided atelectasis air fluid level in liver	Percutaneous or open drainage and antibiotics

otic, and lactulose, a nonabsorbable disaccharide have proven efficacious for the treatment of portal-systemic encephalopathy. Neomycin acts by suppressing bacteria that are responsible for the production of ammonia. Lactulose acidifies the colon and induces a mild catharsis. Lactulose is preferred to neomycin for chronic treatment, as the latter drug may result in ototoxicity and nephrotoxicity. The intravenous and enteral administration of solutions rich in branched-chain amino acids has been proposed for patients with portal-systemic encephalopathy but has not clearly been shown to be of benefit.

Liver Abscess, Neoplasms, and Cysts

Tumors of the Liver

Primary Malignancies

Pathogenesis. Primary hepatic cancer is uncommon in this country, although prevalent in some parts of Africa and Asia. Cirrhosis, hemachromatosis, a_1-antitrypsin deficiency, and history of Thorotrast use predisposes to hepatic malignancy. Infection with chronic hepatitis B virus (HBV) is the main cause, but local factors, such as liver fluke infestations (*Clonorchis sinensis*) in Asia, and ingestion of aflatoxins produced by fungi found in ground nuts and grain, influence the incidence in certain areas of the world. Three main types of hepatic cancer occur: (1) hepatoma, (2) cholangiocarcinoma, and (3) a mixed variety, hepatocholangioma. A distinct variant, fibrolamellar hepatoma, not associated with HBV or cirrhosis occurs in young adults and has a better prognosis. Hepatoblastomas, which resemble the fetal liver, occur in young children. Rarely, sarcomas occur in the liver.

Hepatomas are the commonest type, constituting 80% of primary liver tumors. They occur as: (1) nodular form, consisting of multiple nodules; (2) massive form, usually with a single large lesion; and (3) diffuse form, which infiltrates widely in the liver. Cholangiocarcinomas originate from bile duct epithelium and, therefore, are usually diffuse and spread extensively within the liver tissue. Both types metastasize early and are commonly widespread by the time of diagnosis, as symptoms appear late in the disease.

Clinical Presentation. The clinical course of a patient with primary hepatic malignancy is variable. Abdominal pain, sometimes referred to the right shoulder, distention, weight loss, and jaundice may occur. Often patients complain only of malaise and weakness. Hepatomegaly is present and occasionally an arterial bruit and friction rub over the liver can be detected. Ascites is present in 30% of patients. An abrupt clinical deterioration in a cirrhotic patient may indicate the development of a hepatoma. Massive intraabdominal hemorrhage can occur following intralesional hemorrhage or disruption of a tumor with bleeding into the

Hypersplenism

Portal hypertension is the most frequent cause of secondary hypersplenism (splenomegaly and pancytopenia). Hypersplenism occurs secondary to splenic congestion that results from chronic splenic venous hypertension. Intrasplenic sequestration and destruction of erythrocytes, leukocytes, and platelets leads to anemia, leukopenia, and thrombocytopenia. Hypersplenism occurs in as many as 50% of patients with portal hypertension but is infrequently of clinical significance (platelet count < 30,000/mm³ or WBC count < 1200/mm³). Therefore, splenectomy is rarely required.

peritoneal cavity. Fever and pain may result from tumor necrosis. Obstruction of the portal vein may produce acute portal hypertension and obstruction of the hepatic veins may cause the Budd-Chiari syndrome. Liver failure secondary to replacement of normal liver with tumor is the main cause of death even when extensive metastatic disease is present.

Diagnosis Liver scan, ultrasound, or CT are useful in establishing the diagnosis of hepatic malignancy (Table 23.3). Arteriography is useful to evaluate the extent of disease and assess resectability of the lesion. Hepatomas are usually more vascular than the normal liver and will sometimes demonstrate a marked arterial blush; cholangiocarcinomas are generally less vascular than normal liver. The venous phase of the study may demonstrate venous displacement, occlusion, or esophageal varices. Angiography also aids the surgeon by defining the vascular supply of the tumor. Percutaneous needle biopsies under CT guidance are diagnostic if positive. Occasionally, an open liver biopsy is required but the pathological diagnosis by frozen section is unreliable. a-Fetoprotein (AFP), which is normally present only in the fetus, is elevated in 50–80% of patients with malignant hepatoma. It is also elevated in some testicular tumors and to a lesser degree in acute viral and alcoholic hepatitis and chronic active hepatitis. The serum alkaline phosphatase and bilirubin are commonly elevated.

Treatment. Surgical excision of a nodular hepatoma may cure the patient, but this situation infrequently occurs. However, up to 75% of the liver may be removed if the surgery is for a cure. Cirrhosis is a relative contraindication to resection due to the decreased hepatic reserve and the limited capability of the liver to regenerate. The tumor receives its main blood supply from the arterial circulation whereas the liver parenchyma is principally supplied by the portal vein. Arterial ligation may result in tumor necrosis and has provided transient palliation. Recent experience has shown that good palliation can be obtained by hepatic artery infusion with chemotherapy. The average survival after diagnosis is 6 months. The 5-year survival

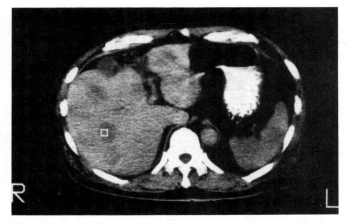

Figure 23.8. CT scan demonstrating multiple hepatic metastases secondary to colon cancer.

after resection is 10%. Fibrolamellar hepatoma has a much better prognosis with a 30% survival following resection.

Metastatic Cancer

The liver is a common site for metastases from cancers of other organs, such as gastrointestinal tract, breast, lung, kidney, uterus, and ovary. More than 95% of patients with liver metastases will have metastases in other organs.

Clinical Presentation. Most patients will have signs and symptoms of the primary tumor. Weakness, anorexia, weight loss, and right upper quadrant pain are commonly present, while ascites and jaundice occur in advanced cases. A large, irregular liver is palpable and a friction rub may be heard.

Diagnosis. Alkaline phosphatase is commonly elevated at an early stage of liver involvement, while bilirubin becomes elevated when the disease is advanced. Large tumors can be detected by liver scan, but the CT is usually preferable because it is more accurate (Fig. 23.8). It is uncommon for an isotope or CT to be positive in the presence of normal liver function tests. The diagnosis of a lesion can be confirmed by a CT-guided liver biopsy or cytology aspiration.

Therapy. Most liver metastases are treated by chemotherapy, which is effective for the primary tumor. Unfortunately, chemotherapy is of limited effectiveness for most tumors. Liver metastases from colorectal carcinoma may be resected for cure if they are confined to a single lobe of the liver. Surgical resection of these metastases results in a 20–25% 5-year survival. If the liver is diffusely involved, hepatic arterial perfusion with high-dose chemotherapy has prolonged survival in some reports. Arterial ligation can offer transient palliation. Overall survival from the time of diagnosis of metastatic cancer to the liver is usually 2–3 months while survival with hepatic metastases from colorectal cancer is 6–7 months.

Benign Tumors

Hemangioma. Hemangioma, which is a cavernous type of vascular tumor, is the most common benign liver tumor. It affects women much more frequently than men. Hemangiomas are usually asymptomatic but occasionally cause pain or a palpable mass when they are greater than 4 cm. Rarely, they may spontaneously rupture, resulting in hemorrhagic shock, or cause high-output cardiac failure. These benign lesions are best diagnosed by CT with intravenous contrast agent enhancement. The clinical course of patients with hemangiomas is usually uncomplicated, but, if symptoms occur, these lesions should be excised if they are confined to a single lobe. Multiple or large lesions can be treated with radiotherapy. If congestive heart failure is present, the clinical condition may be improved by ligation of the hepatic artery.

Hepatic Adenomas. Hepatic adenomas occur primarily in women, are associated with the use of oral contraceptives, and probably have no malignant potential. The lesions may be up to 15 cm in diameter and are multiple in one-third of cases. Patients may present with sudden right upper quadrant pain and/or shock due to spontaneous hemorrhage into the tumor or a rupture into the peritoneal cavity. These complications tend to occur during menses. Hepatic adenomas may present in a less acute manner by causing mild right upper quadrant pain or nausea and vomiting that mimics other acute abdominal diseases. CT or ultrasound are useful for demonstrating a defect in the liver. When symptoms occur, the adenomas should be surgically resected. The lesions may be enucleated, but large lesions may require a partial hepatectomy. Patients with mild symptoms can be followed by CT examination and, if the lesion progresses, resection should be considered. Adenomas have been noted to regress when oral contraception is discontinued. Adenomas may be difficult to differentiate from hepatoma at the time of surgery, either by a gross examination or frozen section.

Focal Nodular Hyperplasia. Focal nodular hyperplasia is a benign condition occurring twice as often in women as men and not associated with use of oral contraceptives. The lesions occur subcapsularly and are usually less than 3 cm in diameter. Larger lesions may cause symptoms and occasionally are multiple. When acute, the lesions demonstrate a characteristic picture of fibrous bands that separate the lesions into lobules. Focal nodular hyperplasia is usually asymptomatic but occasionally causes a right upper quadrant discomfort. These lesions occasionally bleed, enlarge, or result in portal hypertension. They should be removed only if symptomatic.

Cysts of the Liver. Hepatic cysts are usually solitary but may be multiple. One-half of patients with polycystic liver disease also have polycystic kidneys. While cysts are usually asymptomatic, occasionally a large cyst may cause upper abdominal discomfort or be detected as an abdominal mass. A cyst can be diagnosed and treated with percutaneous needle aspiration or surgical drainage if the fluid is clear. A cyst that communicates with the biliary tree should be internally drained into a loop of jejunum. Rarely, a cystadenoma or cyst-adenocarcinoma should be managed by partial hepatic resection.

Hepatic Abscess. A liver abscess may occur secondary to bacterial (pyogenic), parasitic, or fungal infections. Bacterial infections are the most common cause of liver abscess in this country. Pyogenic abscesses may be single or multiple. The single abscess tends to occur more commonly in the right than the left lobe, whereas multiple abscesses are distributed throughout both lobes. Liver abscesses may occur secondary to cholangitis, empyema of the gallbladder, diverticulitis, or appendicitis. An enteric bacterium is frequently responsible. Systemic infections, such as pneumonitis, pyelonephritis, or bacterial endocarditis, may also cause an abscess, usually due to a Gram-positive organism. In 10% of cases a pyogenic abscess has no apparent underlying cause and is termed "cryptogenic."

Clinical presentation. A patient with a liver abscess will often present with high fever and right upper quadrant pain. If the abscess is secondary to biliary disease, jaundice may also occur. However, instead of an acute onset, some liver abscesses may develop in a slow manner over a period of weeks in a previously healthy person. High fevers to 105°F are common and the liver may be enlarged and tender.

Diagnosis. When jaundice is present, it usually indicates a serious infection and is a serious prognostic sign. The white count is commonly elevated to 20,000–30,000/µl and anemia is frequently present. Alkaline phosphatase is commonly elevated even in the presence of normal bilirubin. Many patients will demonstrate right basilar atelectasis and pleural effusion with an elevated and fixed diaphragm. Abdominal films may show only hepatomegaly, but occasionally an air-fluid level may be seen in the liver. Ultrasound and CT of the liver can accurately demonstrate the size, number, and position of the hepatic abscesses.

Treatment. Once the diagnosis has been made, early treatment of liver abscess is imperative. A positive blood culture is strong evidence for a pyogenic rather than amebic abscess. If an amebic abscess is possible, the patient should receive both metronidazole (flagyl) and antibiotics. It is critical to treat hepatic abscesses before the occurrence of complications such as septic shock, progressive impairment of liver function, or dissemination of the infection by rupture into the pleural or peritoneal cavity. Drainage of the abscess by catheter placement under CT guidance accompanied by parenteral antibiotic therapy until drainage stops is successful in curing most hepatic abscesses. Abscesses secondary to another intra-abdominal lesion or those that fail to respond to aspiration require open surgery drainage. At the time of surgery, care is taken to avoid spillage of pus into the abdomen. Samples are taken for culture, sensitivity, and investigation for amebae. The abscess is aspirated and a drain is placed in the cavity and brought out through the abdominal wall.

The overall mortality is approximately 40% and is related to delay in diagnosis of a single abscess and the occurrence of multiple abscesses that are difficult to treat. If treated promptly, the single abscess has a 10% mortality.

Amebic Abscess. Amebic abscess occurs in the absence of amebic dysentery in 50% of cases. The abscess is solitary and usually in the right lobe. Aspiration usually reveals "anchovy paste" material instead of pus. Treatment with metronidazole is usually successful; however, occasionally percutaneous aspiration is utilized to prevent rupture and facilitate resolution. Open drainage is rarely indicated. The mortality for diagnosed amebic abscess is 5%.

Echinococcus Cyst (Hydatid cyst). Enchinococcus infection produces a solitary, often calcified on x-ray, cyst that occurs in the right lobe and causes pain and hepatomegaly. The Casoni skin and the indirect hemagglutination serologic tests are usually diagnostic. If the cyst ruptures into a biliary duct, fever, jaundice, and biliary colic occur. Treatment consists of excision of the cyst with care being taken to avoid rupture as this may cause an anaphylactic reaction and implantation of scolices in the abdominal cavity.

SUGGESTED READINGS

Adson MA, VanHeerden JA, Wagner JS, Ilstrep DM: Resection of hepatic metastases from colorectal cancer. *Arch Surg* 119:647, 1984.

Cello JP, Grendell JH, Crass RA, et al: Endoscopic schlerotherapy versus portacaval shunt in patients with severe cirrhosis and variceal hemorrhage. *N Engl J Med* 311:1589, 1984.

Foster JG: Benign liver tumors. *World J Surgery* 6:25, 1982.

Henderson JM, Warren WD: Current status of the distal splenorenal shunt. *Sem Liver Dis* 3:251, 1983.

Joffe SN: Nonshunting procedures for control of variceal bleeding. *Sem Liver Dist* 3:235, 1983.

Lee NW, Wong JGB: The surgical management of primary carcinoma of the liver. *World J Surg* 6:66, 1982.

Rikkers LF, Soper NJ, Cormier RA: Selective operative approach for variceal hemorrhage. *Am J Surg* 147:89, 1984.

Starzl TE, Keop, LJ, Weil R., Fennell RH, Iwatsuki S, Kano T, Johnson ML: Excisional treatment of cavernous hemangioma of the liver. *Ann Surg* 192:25, 1980.

Warren WD, Millikan WJ Jr, Henderson JM, et al: Ten years of portal hypertensive surgery at Emory. *Ann Surg* 195:530, 1982.

Wellwood JM, Madara JL, Kady B, Haggitt RC: Large intrahepatic cysts and pseudocysts: pitfalls in diagnosis and treatment. *Am J Surg* 135:57, 1978.

Skills

1. Given a patient with portal hypertension, demonstrate the clinical manifestations by physical examination.

2. Given a patient with portal hypertension, estimate the size of the liver and spleen by physical examination.

3. Demonstrate the ability to pass a nasogastric tube in a patient with upper gastrointestinal bleeding.
4. Draw the portal circulation and show the difference between a selective and a nonselective shunt.
5. Develop an algorithm to evaluate a patient with an asymptomatic liver mass.

Study Questions

1. Portal hypertension results primarily from increased resistance to portal flow. Where are the different locations of obstruction to portal flow and what are disease processes that cause obstruction at these locations? How does the location of the portal obstruction affect prognosis?

2. Variceal hemorrhage is the most frequent complication of portal hypertension. The mortality rate from acute variceal hemorrhage ranges from 20–80%. Why is prophylactic shunt surgery not recommended in all patients with esophageal varices? What is the most important factor that influences the outcome from acute variceal hemorrhage?

3. How should the patient with acute variceal hemorrhage be managed initially? Why is it important to perform upper gastrointestinal endoscopy in every patient who presents with upper gastrointestinal hemorrhage and a history of esophageal varices?

4. What are the different types of operations that can be performed for patients who bleed from esophageal varices? What is the difference between selective and nonselective shunt procedures?

5. Ascites can be the source of significant morbidity and mortality. What are the complications that can result from untreated cirrhotic ascites? What is the best approach to medically intractable ascites?

6. How do benign tumors of the liver present clinically? What is the most common type of benign liver tumor?

7. Why is it important to determine the etiology of a liver abscess? What are the different therapeutic modalities that can be used in treating pyogenic liver abscesses?

8. What are the diagnostic procedures that should be performed in evaluating a patient with right upper quadrant pain and suspected liver mass?

9. What is the prognosis of primary hepatic malignancies? What therapeutic modalities can be used in the treatment of these lesions? What are the complications that can occur from liver cancer?

24

The Spleen

James C. Hebert, M.D.
James A. Coil, Jr., M.D.
Ernest E. Moore, M.D.
E. Christopher Ellison, M.D.

ASSUMPTIONS

The student understands the anatomy and embryology of the spleen.

The student understands the hematologic functions of the spleen.

OBJECTIVES

1. Discuss three potential causes of splenic rupture.
2. Outline the clinical examination and use of diagnostic studies in detecting suspected splenic rupture.
3. List five hematologic abnormalities correctable by splenectomy and the indications for surgery in each situation.
4. List the conditions associated with splenomegaly.
5. Discuss the potential adverse consequences associated with splenectomy and discuss methods of reducing these risks.
6. Describe the clinical findings in a patient with a ruptured spleen.

Anatomy and Embryology

General Anatomy and Relationships

The spleen is located in the left posterior upper quadrant under the vault of the diaphragm (Fig. 24.1 and 24.2). Its position is maintained by four suspensory ligaments: the splenophrenic, the splenorenal, the splenocolic, and the gastrosplenic. Normally, these suspensory structures are avascular except for the gastrosplenic ligament, which contains four to six short gastric vessels. Frequently, adhesions exist between the splenic capsule and the omentum or diaphragm. In a normal adult, the spleen weighs between 75 and 150 gm. It is roughly the size of the patient's fist.

Importance of Anatomic Relationships

The spleen's location makes it liable to injury by blunt trauma to the upper abdomen, particularly when posterior fractures of the left ribs occur. As the organ is securely fixed, traction on the supporting ligaments or acquired adhesions may lead to capsular avulsions at points of attachment in both blunt abdominal injuries and by inadvertent manipulation during upper abdominal operations.

Blood Supply

Arterial blood enters the spleen mainly by the splenic artery, a branch of the celiac axis. The artery courses along the superior aspect of the pancreas in a serpentine fashion. The major venous drainage is via the splenic vein, which joins the superior and inferior mesenteric veins to form the portal vein. The splenic vein is located inferiorly and somewhat posterior to the splenic artery. The short gastric arteries and veins as well as the left gastroepiploic vessels provide additional venous drainage.

Accessory Spleens

Accessory spleens (Fig. 24.2) are present in 15–30% of patients in the following areas (in decreasing order of frequency): (1) Hilus of the spleen; (2) splenocolic ligament; (3) gastrocolic ligament; (4) splenorenal ligament; (5) the greater omentum. Although the functional significance of accessory spleens is, as yet, undetermined, it is reassuring to find an accessory spleen prior to complete removal of the spleen for trauma as it may infer immunity competence. Removal of all accessory spleens when operating for hematological disorders is important to assure cure of the disease; therefore, the location and incidence of finding accessory spleens becomes important.

Splenic Function

Hematopoietic Function

During the fifth to the eighth month of embryologic life, the spleen produces both red cells and white cells. The spleen is capable of producing all formed elements

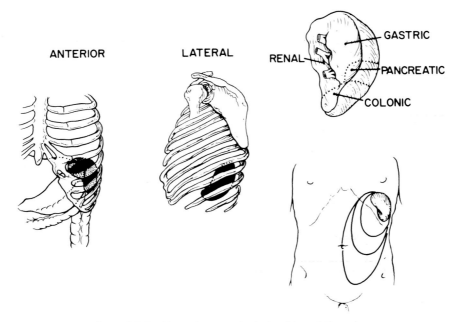

Figure 24.1. Normal external relationships of the spleen.

of blood. In the adult, the spleen does not participate in extramedullary hematopoiesis except in some hematologic and myeloproliferative disorders.

Filtration Function

Red Blood Cells. Abnormal and aged erythrocytes, granulocytes, and platelets, as well as cellular debris, are normally cleared by the spleen. The spleen is capable of discriminating between aged, normal, and abnormal cells. Alterations in the red cell make it sensitive to splenic destruction after 105–120 days. With aging, red cells develop low levels of ATP with loss of membrane integrity. The spleen removes about 20 ml of red blood cells per day. In addition, the spleen's "pitting" function removes nuclear remnants of red blood cells such as Howell-Jolly bodies and other red blood cell inclusions such as Heinz bodies (denatured hemoglobin), Pappenheimer bodies (iron inclusions), and intracellular parasites.

White Blood Cells. The neutrophil has a circulation half-life of 6 hr. The role of the spleen in granulocyte destruction under normal circumstances is uncertain, but in some disease states, granulocytes are sequestered and destroyed.

Platelets. The normal platelet survives roughly 10 days. Although one-third of the platelets are usually stored in the spleen, the specific role of the spleen in platelet removal has not been clearly defined. Splenectomy is frequently followed by a marked increase in platelets in a normal patient.

Reticuloendothelial and Immune Functions

Three additional functions of the spleen include: (1) phagocytosis of particulate antigens; (2) processing an-

tigens and an elaboration of a specific initial antibody response, particularly IgM production; and (3) production of nonspecific phagocytosis promoting peptides, such as tuftsin and properdin, which activates the alternate pathway of the complement system.

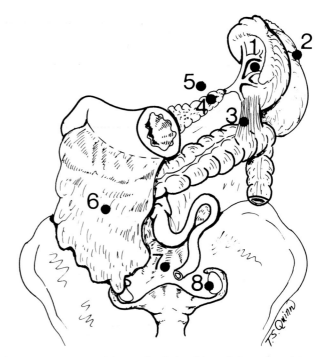

Figure 24.2. Normal internal relationships of the spleen (stomach removed), and location of accessory spleens. **1.** Splenic hilus; **2.** Splenorenal ligament; **3.** Splenorenal ligament; **4.** Tail of the pancreas; **5.** Gastrocolic ligament; **6.** Greater omentum; **7.** Mesentery; **8.** Gonadal.

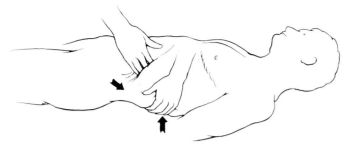

Figure 24.3. Bimanual palpation of the spleen.

General Diagnostic Consideration

Physical Examination of the Spleen

Normal External Relationships. The adult spleen, when normal in size and position (Fig. 24.1), is rarely accessible to abdominal palpation. Its long axis lies immediately behind and parallel to the 10th rib in the midaxillary line. The length of the spleen is approximately 12 cm. Its 7-cm width extends from the 9th to the 11th rib. Splenic percussion and palpation are useful to determine the size of the spleen.

Percussion of the Spleen. The area of splenic dullness is determined by the organ's oblique orientation (Fig. 24.1). It is located in the posterior axillary line and normally does not extend more than 8–9 cm anteriorly. When the exam for splenic dullness is normal, splenomegaly is excluded. The area of splenic dullness may be increased in size by fluid in the stomach and feces in the colon. Thus, the finding is not specific. However, if the area of dullness is enlarged, it should prompt the examiner to make a more careful search for an enlarged spleen on both physical and radiographic evaluation.

Palpation of the Spleen. Palpation of the spleen can be done either bimanually (Fig. 24.3) or by Middleton's method (Fig. 24.4). The enlarged spleen is usu-

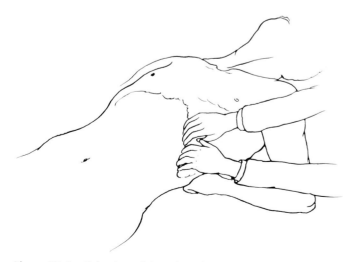

Figure 24.4. Palpation of the spleen by Middleton's method.

Table 24.1.
Classification of Splenomegaly (Based on Degree of Enlargement)

Light Enlargement	Moderate Enlargement	Great Enlargement
Chronic passive congestion	Rickets	Chronic myelocytic leukemia
Acute malaria	Hepatitis	Myelofibrosis
Typhoid fever	Hepatic cirrhosis	Gaucher's disease
Subacute bacterial endocarditis	Lymphoma (leukemia)	Niemann-Pick's disease
Acute and subacute infection	Infectious mononucleosis	Thalassemia major
Systemic lupus erythematosus	Pernicious anemia	Chronic malaria
Thalassemia minor	Abscesses, infarcts	Leishmaniasis
	Amyloidoses	Splenic vein thrombosis
		Leukemic reticuloendotheliosis (hairy-cell leukemia)

ally displaced inferiorly along its oblique axis toward the right iliac fossa. It rarely crosses the midline but may reach the left iliac crest. The enlarged spleen is not tender unless there is: (a) peritoneum inflamed by an infective process; (b) splenic infarction; or (c) splenic trauma with peritoneal blood or a subcapsular splenic hematoma.

A classification, described by Adams, of splenomegaly based on the degree of enlargement of the spleen is helpful to the clinician and is shown in Table 24.1.

Radiographic Evaluation of the Spleen

Objectives. The objective of roentgenographic visualization of the spleen is basically to determine its size or whether the organ has been injured. Five methods are currently available for this purpose: (1) plain abdominal roentgenograms; (2) ultrasonography; (3) technetium-99m liver and spleen scintigraphy; (4) computed tomography (CT); and (5) angiography.

Plain Abdominal Roentgenograms. The abdominal x-ray may be of help in confirming the presence of splenomegaly or indicating splenic injury (Fig. 24.5). Specific abnormal findings include: (1) an elevated, poorly movable left hemidiaphragm with or without a pleural effusion; (2) an enlarged splenic shadow greater than 15 cm in longest diameter; (3) medial displacement of the gastric shadow; and (4) widening of the space between the splenic flexure and the properitoneal fat pad. Routine abdominal x-rays may also demonstrate posterior left rib fractures that would lead one to suspect a splenic injury in the appropriate clinical setting.

Ultrasonography. Abdominal ultrasonography (Fig. 24.6) is a useful technique to determine splenic size and to evaluate the presence of a splenic cyst or abscess. This test is of limited value in trauma because

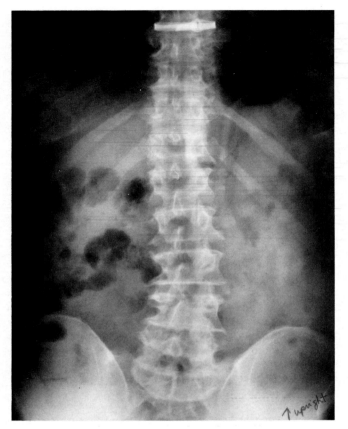

Figure 24.5. Plain film of abdomen showing enlarged spleen. The spleen is a radiopaque shadow in the left upper quadrant.

of associated abdominal wall injury and ileus; i.e., gas within the intestinal tract interferes with visualization of the spleen by ultrasound.

Radionuclide Scan. Radionuclide scan of the spleen using colloidal suspensions of technetium taken up by the reticuloendothelial system (Fig. 24.7) is frequently used to assess splenic size. It has also been used to assess splenic injury. Resolution with this technique is somewhat poor and it is not ideal for splenic trauma; however, it is a good test for determining the size of the spleen and for assessing the presence of functioning splenic tissue such as from splenosis or accessory spleens following splenectomy.

Computed Tomography. CT with and without contrast enhancement is currently the (best) imaging technique to determine both splenic size and the presence of splenic injury (Fig. 24.8). CT allows not only objective evaluation of the spleen, but also an assessment for other intraabdominal problems. Node enlargement, which may accompany some diseases associated with splenomegaly, and detection of other organ involvement in blunt or penetrating trauma are easily identified. In addition, splenic lacerations, subcapsular hematomas and other diseases of the spleen may result in differential densities within the spleen that can be interpreted by a skilled radiologist.

Angiography Angiography of the spleen has two indications: *(1)* splenic vein thrombosis, and *(2)* large primary tumors of the spleen. If splenic enlargement is due to splenic vein thrombosis, arteriography with venous phase is necessary to establish the diagnosis. Hepatic wedge pressures should be obtained simultaneously if the splenic vein is patent. Primary

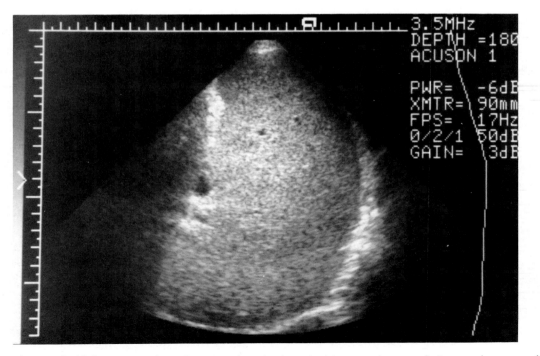

Figure 24.6. Ultrasound of left upper quadrant showing enlarged spleen. In this case splenomegaly is secondary to myelofibrosis.

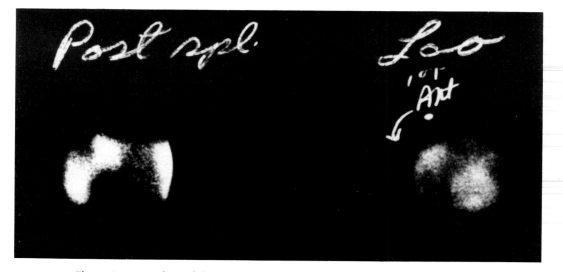

Figure 24.7. Radionuclide scan of the spleen showing a subcapsular hematoma.

tumors of the spleen are rare and tend to be extremely hypervascular. Angiography is therefore recommended to demonstrate primary blood flow as well as collateral circulation prior to splenectomy.

Indications for Splenectomy

Surgical removal of the spleen may be indicated for trauma or for certain hematologic conditions. Table 24.2 lists indications for which splenectomy may be of benefit.

Splenic Trauma

Splenic injury is the most common reason for splenectomy in the United States. Rupture of the spleen

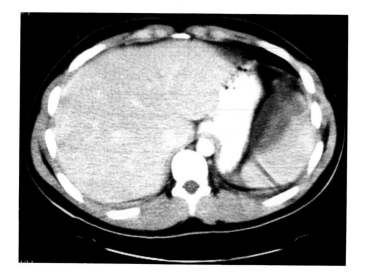

Figure 24.8. CT scan of abdomen showing subcapsular hematoma of spleen as result of infectious mononucleosis.

occurs as a consequence of penetrating or blunt abdominal trauma and from iatrogenic injury during other abdominal operations for other conditions. In selected cases, repair of the spleen or observation of an isolated splenic injury may be appropriate.

Penetrating Splenic Injury

Penetrating injury may involve the spleen. It should be suspected by the trajectory of the wound through the abdominal wall, the flank or the thoracic cavity, particularly below the nipple line. Remember that the diaphragm and upper limits of the abdominal cavity may extend to the nipples during expiration. Isolated splenic injuries rarely occur with penetrating trauma. The organs most often injured include stomach, left kidney, pancreas, and mesenteric vasculature.

Blunt Splenic Injury

Either alone or in combination with other organs, the spleen is the most frequently injured organ following blunt trauma to the abdomen or lower thorax. Isolated splenic injury occurs in only 30% of patients. The most frequently associated injuries include chest (rib fracture), kidney, fracture of the spine, liver, lung, skull and brain, small intestine, colon, pancreas, and stomach.

Operative Trauma

Iatrogenic injury to the spleen occurs during operations on adjacent viscera. The spleen is injured in about 2% of operations involving the viscera of the left upper quadrant. It is usually a traction-type injury with avulsion of a portion of the splenic capsule. Splenectomy always leaves a large cavity in the left upper quadrant that may become filled with blood or fluid and subsequently become infected. This is particularly true if the bowel has been opened as part of the primary opera-

Table 24.2.
Indications for Splenectomy

A. Splenic rupture (repair of the spleen is preferred in certain patients)
  1. Trauma
  2. Spontaneous
  3. Iatrogenic injury
B. Hematologic disorders
  1. Hematolytic anemias
     a. Hereditary spherocytosis
     b. Hereditary elliptocytosis
     c. Thallassemia minor and major (rare)
     d. Autoimmune hemolytic anemia not responsive to steroid therapy
  2. Thrombocytopenia
     a. Idiopathic thrombocytopenic purpura
     b. Immunologic thrombocytopenia associated with chronic lymphocytic leukemia or systemic lupus erythematosus
     c. Thrombotic thrombocytopenic purpura
C. Hypersplenism associated with other diseases
  1. Inflammation
  2. Infiltrative diseases
  3. Congestion
D. Leukemia and lymphoma
E. Other diseases
  1. Splenic abscess
  2. Primary and metastatic tumors
  3. Splenic cysts
  4. Splenic artery aneurysm

Table 24.3.
Types of Splenic Injuries

Type I	Capsular tear or minor parenchymal laceration
Type II	Capsular avulsion with minor parenchymal injury
Type III	Major parenchymal fracture or laceration or through-and-through gunshot or stab wounds
Type IV	Severe parenchymal stellate fracture, crush or bisection, or hilar injury
Type V	Shattered spleen in the patient with multiple injuries

tion. To avoid subphrenic abscess, most surgeons prefer splenic repair to removal after the spleen is injured during another operation.

Spontaneous Rupture

Rupture of the normal spleen without antecedent injury is rare. Spontaneous rupture occurs when the spleen is diseased. Worldwide, the most common cause is malaria, followed by infectious mononucleosis. Spontaneous rupture had been reported in patients with sarcoidosis, acute and chronic leukemia, hairy-cell leukemia, hemolytic anemia, congestive splenomegaly, and polycythemia vera. It is presumed that most of these patients have experienced some form of upper abdominal trauma that was not recognized.

Types of Splenic Injuries

The extent of splenic injury helps determine the type of treatment. Splenic injury may be classified into five types, in increasing order of severity (Table 24.3).

Clinical Presentation and Triage of Splenic Injury

Patients in Whom to Suspect Splenic Injury. Penetrating wounds to the left lower thorax, left abdomen or left flank should lead one to suspect splenic involvement, although any patient with trauma to the trunk could have an injury. Splenic injury should be suspected following blunt injury to the lower chest, abdomen, and flank associated with tenderness in the left upper quadrant and/or ecchymosis and tenderness of

the lateral and posterior left lower chest wall. Kehr's sign (shoulder pain secondary to diaphragmatic irritation) occurs in about one-half the cases. Ballance's sign (fixed dullness to percussion with or without a palpable mass) is seldom identified.

Hemodynamic Presentation. The signs and symptoms of splenic injury vary according to the severity and rapidity of intraabdominal hemorrhage, the presence of other organ injuries, and the interval between the injury and examination.

Hypotension, Narrow Pulse Pressure, Tachycardia, and Distended Abdomen. Patients with splenic injury may enter the emergency room with hemodynamic instability and obvious intraperitoneal bleeding. These patients require fluid resuscitation using either crystalloid solution or blood products and immediate celiotomy with either splenectomy or splenorrhaphy.

Mild Hypotension and Narrow Pulse Pressure, Mild Tachycardia, and Nondistended Abdomen. Frequently the patient will be hemodynamically stable or have mild decreases in blood pressure that respond and stabilize with the infusion of 1–2 liters of crystalloid. He may have tenderness in the upper abdomen or evidence of fractured left posterior ribs (ecchymoses, crepitance, tenderness, and radiologic evidence) that should lead one to suspect splenic trauma. Assessment of these patients should include a rapid search for splenic injury, including plain x-rays and CT scan (preferred) or radionuclide scan. Treatment may include celiotomy with either splenectomy, splenorrhaphy, or observation, depending on the stability of the patient.

Presentation With Hemodynamic Instability or Evidence of Blood Loss Days or Weeks After Injury. Delayed rupture of the spleen may occur after minor or moderate blunt abdominal trauma. Most cases will become clinically evident within 2 weeks of injury. This is probably related to a temporary tamponade of a minor laceration or the presence of a slowly enlarging subcapsular hematoma that eventually ruptures. Initial management depends upon the hemodynamic state.

Algorithm for Diagnosis and Management of Splenic Injury

See page 307.

Operative Treatment of Splenic Injury

The traditional concept of splenectomy for all forms of splenic injury has changed. These changes have re-

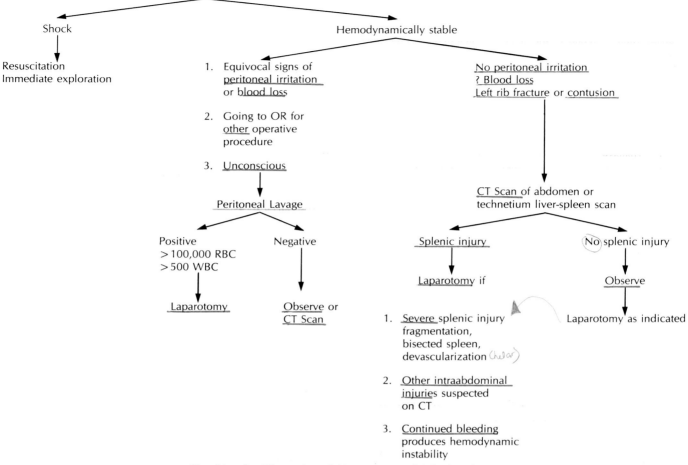

History and Physical Examination

Shock

Hemodynamically stable

Resuscitation
Immediate exploration

1. Equivocal signs of peritoneal irritation or blood loss

2. Going to OR for other operative procedure

3. Unconscious

Peritoneal Lavage

Positive
>100,000 RBC
>500 WBC

Negative

Laparotomy

Observe or CT Scan

No peritoneal irritation
? Blood loss
Left rib fracture or contusion

CT Scan of abdomen or technetium liver-spleen scan

Splenic injury

No splenic injury

Laparotomy if

Observe

1. Severe splenic injury fragmentation, bisected spleen, devascularization (hilar)

2. Other intraabdominal injuries suspected on CT

3. Continued bleeding produces hemodynamic instability

Laparotomy as indicated

Algorithm for Diagnosis and Management of Splenic Injury.

sulted because of the recognition that asplenic individuals, particularly children, are at risk for overwhelming sepsis from encapsulated bacteria. In addition to loss of the spleen's filtering function, which removes particulate antigens and bacteria, splenectomy results in decreased production of IgM and opsonins that assist phagocytosis of encapsulated organisms. Because the spleen can heal with or without surgical intervention and can be safely repaired by available techniques, many surgeons prefer to repair the spleen rather than remove it. In rare cases, particularly in children with no hemodynamic instability and an isolated minor splenic injury (Types I–III) on CT scan or liver-spleen scan, expectant treatment with observation may be an alternative to splenectomy. Nonoperative treatment of children with isolated minor laceration of the spleen should only be undertaken in an ICU situation in which there is an immediately available operating room and when there had been a total blood transfusion requirement of less than 40 ml/kg. A reliable family situation is also important for follow-up. Polyvalent vaccine should be administered. After recovery, the child should avoid contact-type activities for 6–8 weeks and any episodes of abdominal complaints or unusual behavior should be evaluated immediately.

The decision to repair or remove the spleen depends upon a number of factors: (1) the severity of splenic injury; (2) associated injuries; (3) age of the patient; and (4) experience of the surgeon. Splenectomy is required for major lacerations, fragmentation, and hilar injuries. Splenic repair should be possible for most Type I–III injuries. However, in the patients with multiple injuries, splenectomy may be preferred to splenic repair in order to address other or more urgent life-threatening injuries (e.g., patient with widened mediastinum suggesting major aortic injury). Autotransplantation of splenic fragments into the omentum and other anatomic sites is advocated by some although the function of the spleen is questionable.

Disorders of Splenic Function

Overview

Disorders of splenic function may be considered in terms of too little function (hyposplenism and asplenism) or excess function (hypersplenism). Congenital asplenia/hyposplenia is very rare. Splenectomy, therefore, is the most common reason for the asplenic state;

however, other conditions may lead to functional asplenism such as splenic arterial thrombosis or diseases leading to splenic atrophy such as sickle cell disease, celiac disease, systemic lupus erythematosis, ulcerative colitis, thrombocythemia, hyperthyroidism, and thorium-dioxide induced atrophy. The size of the spleen is not related to its hematologic function because hyposplenism may be found with normal or enlarged spleens such as seen in multiple myeloma, sickle cell crisis, acute leukemia, amyloidosis, and sarcoidosis.

Clinically, the most serious problem associated with hyposplenism is the increased susceptibility to overwhelming sepsis by encapsulated organisms. This is secondary to a loss of splenic clearance and impaired antibody production after intravenous challenge of particulate antigens (see complications of splenectomy later in this chapter).

Splenomegaly (anatomic enlargement of the spleen) should not be confused with hypersplenism (excess function of the spleen). Hypersplenism is characterized by cytopenia (anemia, leukopenia, or thrombocytopenia, alone or in combination) and normal or hyperplastic cellular precursors in the bone marrow. These cytopenias result from increased sequestration of cells in the spleen, increased destruction of cells by the spleen, or production of antibody in the spleen leading to increased sequestration and destruction of cells.

Historically, hypersplenism has been divided into primary and secondary types. The concept of primary or idiopathic hypersplenism (hypersplenic syndrome) in the absence of a known cause for splenomegaly is questionable. The number of cases that are now classified as primary has gradually decreased as more information has been acquired concerning the relationship between systemic disease and spleen function.

Three hematologic disorders of splenic function exist in which splenectomy may be helpful: (1) hemolytic anemias, (2) immune thrombocytopenia purpura (ITP), and (3) cytopenias associated with splenomegaly from other diseases (secondary hypersplenism). Assessment of splenic function and the determination of the place for splenectomy in each of these three general categories may be difficult and a specific diagnosis or cause should be systematically sought.

Splenectomy in the Management of Hemolytic Anemia

The most common hemolytic anemia responsive to splenectomy is congenital hereditary spherocytosis, a disorder associated with abnormally shaped red blood cells that leads to increased destruction of the cells. The results of surgery appear to be uniformly good with a very low mortality and morbidity. Although the morphologic characteristics of the red cells are not altered by operation, red cell survival and hematocrit usually reach normal or near normal values postoperatively. Each patient considered for splenectomy is assessed preoperatively for the possible presence of gallstones due to the chronic hyperbilirubin levels. If present, a cholecystectomy can easily be performed at the same

time. An intraoperative search for an accessory spleen should be performed. Splenectomy should be deferred until the patient is at least 5 years old, since the risk of fulminant infection after splenectomy is much higher in young children.

Congenital elliptocytosis, another Mendelian dominant red cell abnormality, also results in a red cell membrane defect. Only a small portion of patients with congenital elliptocytosis develops the clinically significant hemolytic anemia that requires splenectomy.

Thalassemia has several variants. In thalassemia major (homozygous β thalassemia), splenectomy may benefit patients by reducing transfusion requirements, physical discomfort from massive splenomegaly, and the potential for rupture. In the heterozygous type, thalassemia minor, splenectomy is likely to have a greater effect on survival by decreasing transfusion needs and problems associated with iron overload.

Splenectomy is probably not indicated in most cases of sickle cell anemia. Anemias due to enzyme deficiencies, such as pyruvate kinase deficiency and G-6-P-D deficiency, are not responsive to surgery. The procedure is not recommended in these conditions.

Acquired autoimmune hemolytic anemias should be treated initially with steroid therapy; this will usually cause some decrease in hemolysis in the majority of patients. However, sustained remission after complete steroid withdrawal occurs in less than 20% of patients. Prednisone in a dose of 1.0–1.5 mg per kg of body weight is administered for 2–3 weeks; the dose is then gradually reduced over a period of several months or more. Splenectomy is indicated when steroids are ineffective, when high doses are required, and if toxic side effects develop during steroid treatment. Improvement after splenectomy can be observed in up to 60%; however, remissions are not always permanent. Relapses that are not due to regrowth of splenic remnant have been reported as late as 8 years after splenectomy. Splenectomy, in addition to eliminating splenic sequestration of red cells, is frequently followed by evidence of a decrease in antibody production. If complete remission does not occur, there is usually a reduced requirement for steroids postoperatively. In many patients, the direct Coombs test may revert to negative. Utilizing quantitative antibodies studies, it has been estimated that after splenectomy, ten times as much antibody as that needed prior to splenectomy is required to achieve the same degree of hemolysis.

Coombs-negative hemolytic anemia is usually secondary to drugs, toxins, or sepsis; splenectomy is not indicated. However, 2–4% of patients with autoimmune hemolytic anemia will have a negative antiglobulin test. Therefore, occasionally splenectomy is required in patients with hemolytic anemia and a negative Coombs test.

Splenectomy in Thrombocytopenia

Thrombocytopenia may result from a variety of causes (Table 24.4).

In what general classification of thrombocytopenia

Table 24.4.
Classification of Thrombocytopenia

A. Decreased production
   1. Hypoproliferation (toxic agents, sepsis, radiation, myelofibrosis, and tumor involvement of marrow)
   2. Ineffective platelet production (megaloblastic anemia, Guglielmo's syndrome)
B. Splenic sequestration (congestive splenomegaly, myeloid metaplasia, lymphoma, Gaucher's disease)
C. Dilutional loss (following massive transfusion)
D. Abnormal destruction
   1. Consumption (disseminated intravascular coagulation)
   2. Immune mechanisms
      a. Splenectomy sometimes indicated (idopathic thrombocytopenic purpura, chronic lymphocytic leukemia, systemic lupus erythematosus
      b. Splenectomy not indicated (drug-induced thrombocytopenia, neonatal thrombocytopenia, posttransfusion purpura

does the clinician consider splenectomy? Splenectomy is considered only in the idiopathic, immune-mediated thrombocytopenias, those in which an offending drug or other cause cannot be found. These platelet disorders are characterized by the coexistence of low platelet count and normal or increased numbers of megakaryocytes in the bone marrow, in the absence of other hematologic disorders or splenomegaly. Medication history is important, and one must make a particular note of drugs that interfere with platelet function, such as aspirin or other therapeutic agents, that may actually produce thrombocytopenia.

The physical examination of a patient with a suspected bleeding disorder should include a careful search for petechiae. These are pinpoint lesions usually resulting from breakage of small capillaries or increased permeability of the arterioles, capillaries, or venules. These frequently are observed in areas of the body that encounter pressure. Characteristically, they are observed in patients with thrombocytopenia. Purpura represent confluence of petechiae and are also associated with thrombocytopenia. Ecchymoses are extensive purpuric lesions and usually indicate that blood has spread along fascial planes. Ecchymoses are more suggestive of coagulation disorders rather than thrombocytopenia.

Laboratory Tests. If the platelet count is low and coagulation disorders have been ruled out by appropriate laboratory tests, then all medications should be stopped. Antiplatelet antibodies should be determined. Antiplatelet antibodies will be elevated in 85% of patients with idiopathic thrombocytopenic purpura. The bone marrow should be evaluated for megakaryocytes. In disorders of platelet destruction, such as idiopathic thrombocytopenic purpura (ITP) and immunologic thrombocytopenia, the bone marrow will show either normal or increased numbers of megakaryocytes.

Operative Indications. Acute ITP frequently follows an acute infection and has an excellent prognosis in children under the age of 16 years. Approximately

80% of these patients will make complete and permanent spontaneous recovery without specific therapy. Chronic ITP is primarily a disease of young adults, affecting females more often than males. The generally accepted protocol for managing patients with chronic ITP is as follows:

1. An initial 6-week to 2-month period of steroid therapy.
2. If the patient does not respond with an elevation of platelet count, splenectomy is performed.
3. If the patient does respond, steroid therapy is tapered off; and if thrombocytopenia recurs, splenectomy is advised.
4. If there is any manifestation suggestive of intracranial bleeding, emergency splenectomy should be performed.

There is evidence to indicate that patients who had initial response to steroid therapy will respond better to splenectomy. In most series, the results achieved by splenectomy are more impressive than are the responses to steroids. Between 75% and 85% of the total number of patients subjected to a splenectomy respond permanently and require no further steroid therapy.

Patients recently treated with steroids will require a booster dose of cortisone acetate (100 mg intravenously) prior to surgery; this dose should be tapered slowly after the operation. If the platelet counts are below 20,000, platelets should be available for transfusion postoperatively but should not be administered preoperatively. Platelet transfusion is reserved for patients who continue to bleed following splenectomy.

Thrombotic thrombocytopenia purpura (TTP) is a disease of arterials or capillaries characterized by thrombotic episodes and low platelet counts. The pentad of clinical features in virtually all cases consists of fever, purpura, hemolytic anemia, neurologic manifestations, and signs of renal disease. The combination of steroid therapy and splenectomy has been used most frequently; of approximately 300 cases reported, 44 patients survived and 65% of the surviving patients had been treated with steroid therapy and splenectomy. Recently, plasma pheresis has been used with better success than steroids and splenectomy and has become the treatment of choice.

Splenectomy for Hypersplenism Associated with Other Diseases

Definition. A number of clinical syndromes are characterized by selective destruction of various formed elements of the blood. Cardinal features include: (1) splenomegaly; (2) some reduction in the number of circulating blood cells, affecting granulocytes, erythrocytes, or platelets in any combination; (3) a compensatory proliferative response in the bone marrow; and (4) the potential for correction of these hematologic abnormalities by splenectomy. Because the functional compartments of the spleen are intimately interconnected, virtually all causes of splenomegaly may be associated with varying degrees of hypersplenism. Both

Table 24.5.
Diseases Associated with Hypersplenism

A. Infiltrative disease of the spleen
   1. Benign conditions (Gaucher's disease, Niemann-Pick disease, amyloidosis, extramedullary hematopoiesis)
   2. Neoplastic conditions (leukemias, lymphoma, Hodgkin's disease, primary tumors, metastatic tumors, myeloid metaplasia)
B. Congestive disease of the spleen
   1. Portal hypertension
   2. Splenic vein thrombosis
C. Miscellaneous diseases
   1. Felty's syndrome (rheumatoid arthritis, splenomegaly, neutropenia)
   2. Sarcoidosis
   3. Porphyria erythropoietica

infiltrative and congestive forms of splenomegaly may be associated with hypersplenism. Diseases commonly associated with hypersplenism are listed in Table 24.5.

Diagnosis of Hypersplenism. The diagnosis of hypersplenism is suggested by the finding of splenomegaly on abdominal examination. Peripheral blood smear may show pancytopenia, thrombocytopenia, leukopenia, or anemia. Most cases of hypersplenism, however, show pancytopenia. The bone marrow is usually hyperplastic. In cases of myelofibrosis, a bone marrow examination will show increased collagen deposition. Splenic scanning with chromium-labeled, heat-injured erythrocytes may provide information concerning the relative importance of the spleen compared to other reticuloendothelial organs in hemolysis. Further diagnostic approaches to the patient are dictated by the accompanying features such as hematologic findings, lymphadenopathy, portal hypertension, liver dysfunction, or systemic infection.

Splenectomy in the Management of Hypersplenism. Splenectomy is indicated for hypersplenism: (1) if the platelet count is less than 50,000, (2) if the white blood cell count is less than 2000 with or without frequent intercurrent infection, or (3) if there is anemia requiring blood transfusion. In myelofibrosis with myeloid metaplasia as well as other instances of extramedullary hematopoiesis, splenectomy is indicated only when clinical evidence suggests that the compensatory hematopoietic function of the enlarged spleen is outweighed by accelerated sequestration and destruction of red cells.

Hypersplenism associated with congestive splenomegaly due to liver failure and the vascular consequences of portal hypertension requires treatment of the portal hypertension rather than splenectomy. It has been reported that hypersplenism will resolve after appropriate treatment of portal hypertension. Splenectomy as a primary treatment in this setting is contraindicated because it obviates the possibility of doing a selective splenorenal shunt, which is the treatment of choice for most patients with portal hypertension.

If a decision for splenectomy is made, optimal preoperative preparation includes appropriate cell replacement during the intraoperative and postoperative periods. Splenectomy will probably not alleviate the cytopenia completely in most cases. Postoperatively, however, a dramatic increase in the number of platelets may occur and be associated with thrombosis and thromboembolism. This is particularly true in myelofibrosis. Close postoperative monitoring of platelet counts is therefore essential.

Splenectomy in Other Hematologic Diseases

Splenectomy in Leukemia. Although standard textbooks continue to list the role of splenectomy as palliative in the treatment of leukemia, most hematologists avoid splenectomy whenever possible. The advent of successful chemotherapy and the availability of blood component replacement has virtually eliminated splenectomy for leukemia. Hypersplenism remains the only common indication for splenectomy in leukemia. Leukemic reticuloendotheliosis (hairy-cell leukemia) is an indolent progressive form of leukemia. There is progressive hepatomegaly and splenomegaly as the disease progresses and the leukemic cells infiltrate the spleen. Hypersplenism is a common occurrence in this disease and splenectomy is frequently helpful. At one time splenectomy was thought to be an important therapeutic intervention in the treatment of hairy-cell leukemia and was performed routinely. It is now recognized that the survival of patients with leukemic reticuloendotheliosis is not appreciably prolonged by splenectomy and that the risks of the procedure are significant in this patient group. Nevertheless, when hypersplenism or major symptoms become dominant clinical problems, splenectomy is indicated.

Chronic myelogenous leukemia will sometimes lead to massive splenomegaly and splenectomy may be required for the relief of symptoms and, more uncommonly, for hypersplenism. Acute leukemias are not an indication for splenectomy.

Splenectomy in Lymphoma. Staging laparotomy is performed for Hodgkin's disease in order to match treatment with the extent of the disease. The staging classification for Hodgkin's disease is described in Table 24.6. Patients with Hodgkin's disease who have no systemic symptoms and are preoperative stage I, II, or III are candidates for staging laparotomy. Approximately 40% of these patients will have a change in the preoperative staging from the results of the laparotomy. One-third of these patients will be found to have

Table 24.6.
Staging of Hodgkin's Disease

Stage	Description
I	Limited to one lymph node region
II	Two or more regions on same side of diaphragm
III	Disease on both sides of the diaphragm limited to lymph nodes, spleen, and Waldeyer's ring
IV	Disease involving bone, bone marrow, lung, liver, gastrointestinal tract, or any other organ other than lymph nodes, spleen, or Waldeyer's ring

less advanced disease than thought by preoperative test, whereas, two-thirds will be found to have more advanced disease.

Since the purpose of staging laparotomy is to determine the extent of disease in the abdomen, careful systematic examination is required of the surgeon. The sequential steps required in a staging laparotomy include biopsy of both lobes of the liver, splenectomy, and sampling of nodes from each node bearing area (hepatoduodenal, celiac, mesenteric, periaortic, and iliacs). If the patient has had a preoperative CT or lymphangiogram revealing a suspicious node or nodes, then these particular nodes should be sampled. Because the radiopaque contrast material used for lymphangiogram tends to remain in the iliac and periaortic lymph nodes for a considerable length of time, intraoperative plain x-rays may be used to determine if the appropriate nodes have been removed. Often, a bone marrow biopsy is taken from one of the iliac crests.

Staging laparotomy is rarely performed for patients with non-Hodgkin's lymphoma, since the disease does not spread in the orderly progression of Hodgkin's disease. It may be indicated in the presence of recurrent disease, relapse after initial remission, for massive splenic enlargement causing local pressure on abdominal viscera, or with symptomatic hypersplenism.

Complications and Consequences of Splenectomy

In general, mortality from splenectomy is about 6–13% and morbidity is about 5–20%. The most common complications from this procedure follow.

Respiratory Complications (10–48%)

Atelectasis is the most common pulmonary problem after splenectomy. In the early postoperative period, pneumonia and pleural effusion may occur in 10–15% of cases and should lead one to suspect a subphrenic abscess or other complication. Atelectasis will resolve within 2 days in most cases if properly treated with pulmonary physical therapy. Pulmonary problems are the result of a high abdominal incision that may result in reduced respiratory excursions and irritation of the diaphragm.

Hemorrhage (Less Than 1%)

This is a rare complication. It is most frequent in patients having splenectomy for disorders associated with thrombocytopenia. Those in whom the platelet count does not respond to splenectomy are particularly prone to postoperative hemorrhage. Reoperation to gain hemostasis should be considered if there is continued bleeding after correction of coagulation abnormalities or if hemodynamic instability occurs.

Subphrenic Abscess (5–8%)

Removal of the spleen leaves a space in the left upper abdomen that will fill with fluid and blood and may subsequently become infected. It occurs most often after splenectomy for trauma, incidental splenectomy, or the occurrence of postoperative bleeding. This complication is more common is splenectomy was coincident with the opening of the gastrointestinal tract. Subphrenic abscess usually becomes apparent 5–10 days after surgery as evidenced by fever, pain, pleural effusion or prolonged atelectasis, and pneumonia. The placement of prophylactic drains has been shown to increase the risk of subphrenic abscess and they are rarely used.

Injury to Adjacent Structures (1–3%)

The natural attachments of the spleen predispose several adjacent organs to inadvertent injury during splenectomy. Pancreatic injury is the most common, with an incidence of 1–3%. This may take the form of mild postoperative hyperamylasemia, which usually resolves within 10 days, pancreatitis, pancreatic fistula, or pancreatic pseudocyst. The pancreatic injury may be suspected by an elevated serum amylase on the second to fourth day after surgery. Symptoms and signs suggestive of pancreatic injury usually develop 4–5 days after splenectomy and include nausea and vomiting, abdominal distention, pulmonary complications, and abdominal pain.

Injury to the adjacent stomach may occur while the short gastric vessels are being divided. This may lead to development of a subphrenic abscess or a gastrocutaneous fistula. Some surgeons attempt to prevent this complication by avoiding postoperative gastric distention with nasogastric decompression for 48–72 hr, and reinforcing the gastric serosa where short gastric vessels have been avulsed or ligated in close proximity to the gastric wall.

Postsplenectomy Thrombocytosis (40–50%) and Thrombosis (Less Than 5%)

The platelet count increases by 30% between 2 and 10 days after splenectomy. It usually returns to normal within 2 weeks. The incidence of thrombocytosis (platelet count exceeding 400,000 after splenectomy) varies from 40–50%. Theoretically, this increase predisposes the patient to thrombotic complications. The incidence of pulmonary embolism after splenectomy with thrombocytosis is 6%, compared to 0.4% for those without elevations of platelet count. However, there is little evidence to support a correlation between absolute platelet count and thrombosis. Most cases of thrombosis or pulmonary emboli occur in patients with myeloproliferative disorders. At the present time, postoperative treatment with platelet inhibitors, such as aspirin or dipyridamole, seems justified in (1) patients with myeloproliferative disease (e.g., myelofibrosis) with platelet counts greater than 400,000 and (2) after splenectomy for other diseases if the platelet count exceeds 750,000. Treatment should continue at discharge and be stopped when the platelet count returns to normal. Heparinization or chronic coumadin therapy has not proved beneficial and should be avoided.

Postsplenectomy Sepsis (1–4%)

The risk of postsplenectomy sepsis varies with the age of the patient as well as the reason for splenectomy. In otherwise normal <u>children</u>, the potential risk is well established, approximately <u>2–4%</u>. In <u>adults</u>, the incidence is approximately <u>1–2%</u>. Sepsis occurs more commonly in the patient who had splenectomy performed for a <u>hematologic disorder</u>. The overall incidence of postsplenectomy sepsis is 40 times that of the general population and patients are at risk of fatal sepsis any time after splenectomy. <u>Death ensues rapidly</u>, usually <u>24–48 hr after the onset of symptoms</u> and unfortunately <u>antibiotics are usually ineffective</u> in the full-blown syndrome.

Sepsis is most commonly caused by <u>encapsulated</u> organisms. *Streptococcus pneumoniae* (pneumococcus) is the most common agent <u>(50–75%)</u>, followed in decreasing frequency by *Hemophilus influenza*, *Neisseria meningitidis*, β-hemolytic *Streptococcus*, *S. aureus*, *E. coli*, and *Pseudomonas*. Viral infections may occur in some cases and the most common agent is *Herpes zoster*. Certain parasitic infestations, such as <u>babesiosis</u>, which is normally a self-limited infection, may be overwhelming in the splenectomized patient. <u>Malaria</u> can overwhelm the splenectomized host.

<u>Polyvalent pneumococcal polysaccharide vaccines,</u> such as Pneumovax, should be given <u>following</u> either total splenectomy or conservative splenic operations for trauma. Also, patients with splenic trauma who are managed nonoperatively should be vaccinated. Neither the surgeon nor the patient should consider this full protection against overwhelming postsplenectomy sepsis, since both clinical and experimental evidence suggests that splenectomized individuals <u>may not respond to pneumococcal polysaccharide antigens</u>. Children <u>under 2 years</u> of age do <u>not become effectively immunized</u>. Also, pneumococcal types not contained in the vaccine or other bacteria may cause overwhelming sepsis despite the vaccine. Patients undergoing elective splenectomy should be <u>immunized well in advance of splenectomy</u>. The exact timing for administration of Pneumovax is unknown, but <u>greater than 1 week in advance of surgery</u> is probably sufficient. <u>After splenectomy</u>, it is probably wise to <u>wait until the patient is nutritionally intact</u> prior to vaccination.

<u>Long-term antibiotic prophylaxis with oral penicillin</u> (250 mg once or twice daily) is reasonable in the <u>immunologically compromised patient</u> such as renal transplant recipients, those receiving chemotherapy, and perhaps in all children under 6 years of age who have had splenectomy. Lack of compliance, inconvenience, and bacterial resistance are all reasons why this is not definite prophylaxis.

Splenectomized individuals should carry identification to that effect and be instructed to contact their physician at the first sign of any minor infection such as a cold or sore throat. Antibiotics should be started and the patients followed closely.

After <u>removal of the spleen in a normal patient</u>, the <u>white blood cell count will increase by an average of 50% over baseline.</u> In some cases, the number of neutrophils will increase to 15,000–20,000 in the initial postoperative period. The white blood cell count usually <u>returns to normal within 5–7 days</u>. <u>Elevations beyond this period suggest an infectious complication.</u> <u>The peripheral smear of the patient who has had splenectomy</u> will routinely show <u>Howell-Jolly bodies</u> and <u>Pappenheimer bodies</u> as well as <u>pitted red cells</u> on phase microscopy.

SUGGESTED READINGS

Coon WW: Splenectomy for splenomegaly and secondary hypersplenism. *World J Surg* 160:291, 1985.

Coon WW: Splenectomy in the treatment of hemolytic anemia. *Arch Surg* 120:625–628, 1985.

DeFino SM, et al: Adult idiopathic thrombocytopenic purpura: clinical findings and response to therapy. *Am J Med* 69:430, 1980.

Febri PJ, Carey LC: Complications of splenectomy: etiology, prevention, and management. *Surg Clin North Am* 63:1313–1330, 1983.

King DR, Lobe TE, Haase GM, Boles ET: Selective management of the injured spleen. *Surgery* 90:677–682, 1981.

Kinsella, TJ, Glatstein E: Staging laparotomy and splenectomy for Hodgkin's disease. *Cancer Invest* 1:87, 1983.

Oates DD: Splenic trauma. *Curr Prob Surg* 18:341–404, 1981.

Schwartz SI: Splenectomy for thrombocytopenia. *World J Surg* 9:416, 1985.

Singer DB: Post-splenectomy sepsis. In Rosenberg HS, et al (eds): *Perspectives in Pediatric Pathology*. Chicago, Year Book Medical Publishers, 1973, vol 1, pp 285–311.

VanWyck DB: Overwhelming postsplenectomy infection (OPSI): the clinical syndrome. *Lymphology* 16:107–114, 1983.

Williams WJ, et al (eds): *Hematology*, 3rd ed, New York, McGraw-Hill, 1983.

Skills _____

1. Demonstrate the technique to palpate an enlarged spleen.

2. When given a CT scan of the spleen, describe the findings that would indicate a severe splenic injury that might lead to surgical intervention.

3. Discuss the method you would use to perform peritoneal lavage in a patient with suspected splenic trauma.

Study Questions _____

1. A 20-year-old man is involved in a motor vehicle accident. Discuss the approach you would use to determine whether the patient has a splenic injury. Include in your discussion the physical findings, laboratory findings, and

radiographic findings that would suggest a splenic injury.

2. A 6-year-old girl falls out of a tree and injures her left flank and lacerates her spleen. Discuss the indications for nonoperative management of this problem. Discuss the indication for splenectomy. Why would you be hesitant to remove the spleen in a child?

3. An 18-year-old girl notices an enlarged, painless cervical lymph node. Describe your approach to this problem. How would it differ if she were a 60-year-old smoker? Discuss the role of a staging laparotomy in a patient with Hodgkin's disease.

4. A 25-year-old man has gallstones and anemia. Discuss any hematologic diseases that could explain this combination of clinical problems. What composition of gallstones would you expect to find? Discuss the role of splenectomy in a patient with gallstones secondary to splenic sequestration of abnormal red blood cells.

5. A 25-year-old woman notices easy bruisability. How would you evaluate this patient for ITP? Would age of the patient or acuteness of the symptoms influence your approach to this problem? Discuss the indications for medical and surgical therapy of ITP.

25

Diseases of the Vascular System

Bruce L. Gewertz, M.D., *Alan Graham, M.D.,*
Peter F. Lawrence, M.D., John Provan, M.D.,
and Christopher K. Zarins, M.D.

ASSUMPTIONS

The student knows the anatomy of the peripheral arterial and venous circulation.

The student knows the physiology of the clotting mechanism.

The student knows the physiology of neural and pharmacologic control of blood vessels.

OBJECTIVES

ATHEROSCLEROSIS

1. List five risk factors for the development of atherosclerosis.
2. List three specific sites where there is a predilection to develop atheroma and explain why such a predilection exists.
3. List at least two clinical sequelae of atherosclerosis and three ways to retard the atherosclerotic process.

ANEURYSMS

1. Describe the common sites and relative incidence of arterial aneurysms.
2. List the symptoms, signs, differential diagnosis, and diagnostic and management plans for a patient with a rupturing abdominal aortic aneurysm.
3. Discuss the indications, contraindications and risk factors for surgery in chronic asymptomatic abdominal aneurysms.
4. Define and discuss the prevention of the common complications following aneurysm surgery.
5. Compare thoracic, abdominal, femoral and popliteal aneurysms with respect to presentation, complications, (i.e., frequency of dissection, rupture, thrombosis and embolization) and treatment.

PERIPHERAL ARTERIAL OCCLUSIVE DISEASE

1. Describe the pathophysiology of intermittent claudication: differentiate this symptom from leg pain due to other causes.

2. Describe the diagnostic approach and medical management of arterial occlusive disease; include a discussion of the roles of the commonly used noninvasive procedures.
3. List criteria to help differentiate venous, arterial, diabetic and infectious leg ulcers.
4. Describe the operative treatment choices available for chronic occlusive disease of the distal aorta and iliac arteries, superficial femoral/popliteal arteries and tibial and peroneal arteries.
5. List four indications for amputation and discuss clinical and laboratory methods for selection of the amputation site.
6. Describe the clinical manifestations, diagnostic workup and surgical indications for chronic renal artery occlusion.
7. Describe the natural history and causes of acute arterial occlusion and differentiate embolic occlusion and thrombotic occlusion.
8. List six signs and symptoms of acute arterial occlusion and outline its management (e.g., indications for medical versus surgical treatment).

CEREBROVASCULAR INSUFFICIENCY

1. Define and differentiate the following:
   A. Amaurosis fugax
   B. Transient ischemic attacks (TIA)
   C. Reversible ischemic neurological defect (RIND)
   D. Cerebrovascular accident (CVA or stroke)
2. Outline diagnostic methods as well as medical and surgical management of a patient with symptomatic carotid artery disease.
3. List the differential diagnoses and outline a management and treatment plan for patients with TIA.
4. Differentiate hemispheric and vertebrobasilar symptoms.

PULMONARY EMBOLUS, DEEP VEIN THROMBOSIS, AND VENOUS DISEASE

1. Identify the usual initial anatomic location of deep vein thrombosis and discuss the clinical factors

which lead to an increased incidence of venous thrombosis.

2. Identify noninvasive and invasive testing procedures for diagnosing venous valvular incompetence and deep vein thrombosis.
3. Outline the differential diagnosis of acute edema associated with leg pain.
4. Describe five modalities for preventing the development of venous thrombosis in surgical patients.
5. Describe the methods of anticoagulant and thrombolytic administration, evaluation of adequacy of therapy and contraindication to therapy.
6. Describe the clinical syndrome of pulmonary embolus and identify the order of priorities in diagnosis and caring for an acutely ill patient with life-threatening pulmonary embolus.
7. List the indications for surgical intervention in venous thrombosis and pulmonary embolus.
8. Outline the diagnostic, operative and nonoperative management of venous ulcers and varicose veins.

VASOSPASTIC DISORDERS, TRAUMA, AND LYMPHATIC DISORDERS

1. List five underlying diseases or disorders associated with vasopastic changes in the extremities; discuss their diagnosis and treatment.
2. Describe anatomical mechanisms responsible for producing thoracic outlet compression syndrome, appropriate diagnostic studies and surgical treatment.
3. List the indications for arteriography in a patient with a possible arterial injury to the extremities.
4. Given a patient with recent trauma, outline the physical findings, diagnostic plan and treatment for suspected arterial injury.
5. Define lymphedema praecox, lymphedema tarda, primary lymphedema, secondary lymphedema.
6. Explain the pathophysiology of lymphedema and discuss its treatment.

DIAGNOSTIC RADIOLOGY IN VASCULAR DISORDERS

1. Describe the indications and risks for arteriogram and venogram.
2. Define and discuss transluminal angioplasty, citing the indications for this procedure.
3. Discuss the methodology, use and reliability of perfusion scans and ventilation scans.

Arterial Disease

Atherosclerosis

The risk factors for the development of atherosclerosis include cigarette smoking, hypertension, hypercholesterolemia, diabetes mellitus, obesity, sedentary lifestyle, personality traits (Type A personality), hereditary factors, and elevated heart rate. The first four factors are of greatest importance and appear to be cumulative in effect. Thus the greater number of risk factors a patient has, the greater the likelihood of developing atherosclerosis.

Although these risk factors are systemic in nature and atherosclerosis is a generalized disease, its clinical presentation is characterized by extensive plaque formation in specific localized sites that produce clinical symptoms. The term _arteriosclerosis_ generally refers to involvement of the small arteries while _atherosclerosis_ refers to aortic or large vessel lesion formation. However, in practice the terms are frequently used interchangeably.

The most common sites of clinically important atherosclerosis are the coronary arteries, carotid bifurcation, and lower extremity arteries. Arterial bifurcations and branching points throughout the body are common sites of plaque formation; hemodynamic factors, such as hypertension, fluctuations in wall shear stress, low flow velocity, and turbulence, may account for the localization patterns. Contrary to common teaching, at the carotid bifurcation plaque forms along the lateral wall of the carotid sinus where there is relatively slow flow, low wall shear stress, and stasis. It is postulated that there is increased contact time between atherogenic factors in the blood (e.g. lipids) and the vessel wall at this site. In the lower extremities, slow blood flow related to relative inactivity and the effects of smoking on the vessel wall have been specifically implicated as risk factors. It appears that smoking is a greater risk factor for peripheral atherosclerosis (nine times the normal population) than coronary atherosclerosis (four times the normal population).

The common clinical sequelae of atherosclerosis include (1) myocardial infarction or angina pectoris due to coronary atherosclerosis, (2) transient ischemic attacks or strokes due to carotid bifurcation atherosclerosis, and (3) intermittent claudication, foot-rest pain, or gangrene due to peripheral atherosclerosis. Less common clinical presentations are due to atherosclerosis of the renal arteries and mesenteric arteries. Can you predict what the presenting symptoms in these patients might be? Symptoms are due to either gradual progressive stenosis from an enlarging plaque or sudden occlusion due to thrombosis of the vessel. Clinical sequelae are much more severe with sudden occlusion, which does not allow the development of collateral arterial channels; with gradual progression of the disease and narrowing of the vessel wall, the collaterals are able to circumvent the stenosis to some extent. Plaque ulceration often becomes a nidus for thrombus formation or platelet deposition; distal embolization of this material may produce acute ischemic events (Figs. 25.1 A–C).

Slowing of the atherosclerotic process can only be achieved by modification of risk factors. Control of hypertension clearly has a beneficial clinical effect by reducing the progression of plaque accumulation. Reduction of serum lipid levels, especially low density

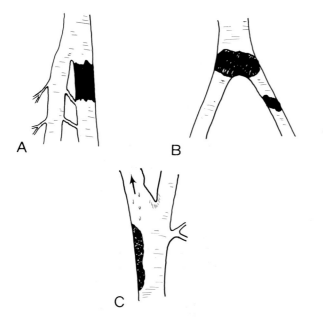

Figure 25.1. A, Symptoms of chronic occlusion of main vessel are mitigated by the development of collateral arterial channels that refill the vessel distal to the occlusion. **B,** Sudden occlusion of a major vessel (secondary to an embolus or a thrombus) is often poorly compensated because collaterals are not sufficiently developed. **C,** Ulcerative arterial lesions may cause symptoms from embolization of atherosclerotic debris or thrombi.

lipoproteins, has been shown to decrease coronary artery plaque formation. Cessation of smoking will slow the progression of coronary and peripheral atherosclerosis.

Reduction in the stressful lifestyle is felt to be of benefit, and exercise has been shown to reduce heart rate and increase high density lipoproteins (HDL) levels. While control of blood glucose is important, there is little objective evidence that precise control prevents the secondary vascular complications of diabetes.

Aneurysms

Pathogenesis

An aneurysm is defined as a dilation of an artery to more than twice its normal diameter. Vessels may dilate eccentrically and assume a saccular appearance or dilate diffusely to form a fusiform aneurysm. Aneurysms are further classified by the extent of involvement of the arterial wall and the mechanism of formation. "True" aneurysms reflect congenital or acquired weakness of the entire vascular wall and are composed of all three major layers of the blood vessel, including adventitia, media, and intima. "False" aneurysms are usually secondary to traumatic disruptions of the artery and are covered only by a thickened fibrous capsule. The most common causes for true aneurysms are acquired atherosclerosis or rare congenital diseases such as Marfan's syndrome and fibromuscular dysplasia. "False" aneurysms usually follow untreated

vascular injuries secondary to penetrating (gunshot or stab wounds) or blunt injury, or failed vascular operations in which the suture or vessel wall degenerates, such that the prosthetic graft is no longer closely held to the native artery. The term "mycotic" aneurysm is used for the very rare aneurysm that is infected, irrespective of causative agent (bacteria or fungus).

Atherosclerosis is the most common cause for aneurysm formation. It is postulated that the atherosclerosis involves and ultimately weakens the wall, causing the artery to dilate. The sites of aneurysm formation parallel those areas most frequently involved with atherosclerotic occlusive disease—the infrarenal abdominal aorta and other major bifurcations of the arterial system such as the common femoral, popliteal, and carotid arteries.

Clinical Presentation

The clinical presentation of aneurysms include (1) rupture, (2) embolization, and (3) thrombosis. Dissection per se is generally not a complication of abdominal aortic or peripheral aneurysms but refers to a specific pathology usually seen in the thoracic aorta. Rupture is more common in larger aneurysms, as wall stress is directly related to the intraluminal pressure (p) and the radius (r) and inversely correlated with wall thickness (stress = $p \times r$/thickness). The turbulence and reduced velocity of flow in the aneurysm sac results in thrombosis along the outermost portion of the aneurysm. Distal embolization (downstream migration of clot) or sudden occlusion can result from thickening of this intraluminal thrombus. Aneurysms of peripheral extremity vessels, such as the femoral, popliteal, and axillary arteries, are more frequently associated with embolization or thrombosis and rarely rupture.

Diagnosis

The diagnosis of both aortic and peripheral aneurysms can be made by a carefully conducted physical examination in most patients. When there is doubt about the existence or size of an aneurysm (frequently due to a patient's obesity), then other diagnostic tests are used. Ultrasonography is the least expensive and is a reliable technique to determine the aneurysm size. A computed tomography (CT) scan can also be useful, particularly for aneurysms that extend above the renal arteries or are difficult to evaluate with ultrasound, although it is more expensive than ultrasonography. A plain x-ray may identify aneurysms that are calcified. Aortography is not a good method to determine the presence or size of an aneurysm, although it is frequently used prior to surgical repair to assess the quality of vessels proximal and distal to the aneurysm, where a bypass graft may be placed.

Treatment

The predilection for *aortic aneurysms* to rupture suddenly prior to other clinical symptoms makes these lesions life threatening, whereas *peripheral aneurysms,* excluding those involving the carotid artery, are usually limb threatening. Hence, detection of an asymptomatic aortic aneurysm should be taken seriously, with consideration of treatment prior to rupture. There is no medical therapy for an aneurysm, although some clinicians aggressively treat hypertension to reduce the risk of rupture (there is little clinical research evidence to support this approach). Most clinicians feel that an infrarenal aortic aneurysm greater than 5 cm in diameter (as documented by CT scan or ultrasound) is an indication for surgery in good-risk patients. This is based on epidemiologic data that suggests that such aneurysms have approximately a 30% risk of rupture within 3 years. Furthermore, with elective mortality of aneurysm resection at as low as 2%, such patients can be returned to a normal life expectancy for age-matched controls with comparable cardiac disease. Operative risk is increased by (1) severe pulmonary disease, (2) severe ischemic heart disease, and (3) renal dysfunction; age per se is not a significant risk factor. Operation involves graft replacement of the involved aorta and/or iliac vessels. These procedures are more complicated if the portion of aorta at or above the renal arteries needs to be replaced. Fortunately, the vast majority (95%) of aortic aneurysms are confined to the infrarenal aorta.

More urgent consideration must be directed toward patients with either *symptomatic* or *ruptured* aneurysms. Symptoms of aneurysm expansion include back or abdominal pain unrelated to exercise. Aneurysm rupture is suggested by the classic triad of (1) abdominal or back pain, (2) pulsatile abdominal mass, and (3) shock. An aneurysm that is symptomatic is associated with a much higher risk of rupture than an asymptomatic aneurysm (30% in 1 month versus 30% in 3 years) and should be resected urgently.

A ruptured aneurysm requires immediate, emergency operation to avoid the nearly 100% mortality associated with delay in diagnosis and therapy. For this reason, any patient with signs or symptoms consistent with a ruptured aneurysm (especially severe pain and hypotension) needs immediate operation. Minimal, if any, diagnostic studies are indicated other than the documentation of a pulsatile abdominal mass. With such an aggressive approach, the mortality of ruptured aneurysms has been lowered to less than 25% in some centers, when the procedure is begun prior to anuria and massive blood loss.

Complications

The complications of aortic surgery are more frequent in high risk patients and those unstable prior to operation. The most serious problems include perioperative renal failure, colonic ischemia, and myocardial infarction. Renal failure can usually be avoided by generous intraoperative and postoperative fluid replacement to counter large extravascular fluid accumulations in the retroperitoneal tissues. In the presence of cardiac disease, effective fluid management may require careful monitoring of pulmonary capillary pressure by

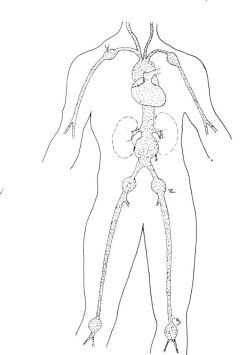

Figure 25.2. Common sites for the development of atherosclerotic aneurysms include the infrarenal abdominal aorta as well as the femoral, popliteal, and axillary arteries. Peripheral aneurysms are frequently bilateral and multiple.

Swan-Ganz catheter. Because the inferior mesenteric artery is nearly always involved in the aneurysm, colonic blood flow depends on collateral circulation from the superior mesenteric artery and celiac axis. Patients with stenoses or occlusions of the latter two vessels may require reimplantation of the inferior mesenteric artery into the aortic graft to avoid infarction of the left colon. Hypotension prior to surgery predisposes a patient to colonic ischemia. The prevalence of coronary artery disease and the increased peripheral resistance caused by temporary aortic occlusion during graft placement may necessitate intraoperative infusion of vasodilators to lessen left ventricular work and minimize the risk of intraoperative myocardial infarction.

An uncommon but lethal late complication of prosthetic aortic grafts is erosion of the graft into the third or fourth portion of the duodenum, which lies immediately adjacent to the proximal aortic suture line ("aortoduodenal fistula"). This results in graft infection and often catastrophic upper gastrointestinal hemorrhage. Suspicion of this complication should be raised anytime a patient with an aortic graft is evaluated for occult gastrointestinal blood loss. Frequently several bleeding episodes of small or moderate quantity ("herald bleeds") occur prior to the episode of exsanguinating hemorrhage. Management of aortoenteric fistulae requires graft removal and extraanatomic bypass.

Peripheral aneurysms (femoral and popliteal) are frequently bilateral and multiple and are associated with occult aortic aneurysms in nearly 50% of the cases (Fig. 25.2). The risk of thrombosis and embolism are such that any popliteal, axillary, or carotid aneurysm should be strongly considered for operation. It is incumbent on the clinician to search for other aneurysms when a patient is found to have a peripheral aneurysm. Treatment of peripheral aneurysms requires bypass of involved segments with prosthetic grafts (in femoral or axillary aneurysms) or saphenous vein grafts (in carotid or popliteal aneurysms).

Aortic dissections result from a tear in the intima and the separation or "dissection" of the intima from the media by the pulsatile column of blood. These lesions almost always begin in the thoracic aorta but may progress distally to the abdominal aorta and compress or "exclude" the vascular supply to the intestines, kidneys, or spinal cord. Dissections may also involve the ascending aorta with obstruction of the coronary artery ostia, producing myocardial infarction or dilation of the annulus of the aortic valve and acute aortic (valve) insufficiency. Dissections occur almost exclusively in hypertensive patients who present with acute severe chest pain radiating to the back. Diagnosis is confirmed by CAT scan and angiogram. Treatment of acute dissection is often limited to blood pressure control and careful observation for intestinal or renal ischemia. Surgical treatment is reserved for patients with these complications or enlargement of a chronic dissection. Abdominal aortic aneurysms almost never dissect in this fashion.

Peripheral Arterial Occlusive Disease

Lower Extremity Ischemia

Clinical Presentation.   The clinical manifestations of peripheral arterial occlusive disease of the lower extremities are intermittent claudication, rest pain, skin ulceration, gangrene, and impotence. The physical findings associated with these symptoms include reduced or absent pulses, dependent rubor, blanching of the skin on elevation, atrophy of skin appendages, and hair loss. Intermittent claudication arises from the term claudicatio, which means to limp. It is a clinical syndrome of pain or fatigue in large muscle groups that occurs with exercise and is relieved by rest. In such patients, the circulation is adequate at rest, but arterial occlusion prevents the augmentation of blood flow necessary for exercise. As a consequence, muscle metabolism is impaired and the acidic products of anaerobic metabolism accumulate in the muscle and cause pain. Patients rest for several minutes and the pain subsides. Aortoiliac occlusive disease is associated with claudication in the hips and buttocks as well as impotence; superficial femoral artery obstruction commonly causes calf claudication alone. The level of claudication is always below the level of the arterial obstruction.

The natural history of untreated claudication is generally benign; in the classic Framingham study there was only a 5% risk of major amputation for gangrene within 5 years if claudication was treated conserva-

tively. It is noteworthy that a full 20% of these patients died from cardiac disease and stroke during the same 5-year period.

The presence of rest pain indicates a much more severe degree of ischemia than claudication. Typically, the patient experiences pain in the toes and forefoot during the night which causes him to awaken from sleep. Temporary relief is obtained by dangling the affected leg over the side of the bed or getting up and walking. These maneuvers increase cardiac output and restore hydrostatic pressure that can slightly augment the perfusion pressure in the legs. Nocturnal cramps in the calf muscles can usually be distinguished from rest pain by the location of the pain and the absence of advanced ischemic changes in the skin.

The outlook for patients with rest pain is far worse than that for patients with claudication. The lack of sleep and constant pain can cause deterioration of personality, especially in older patients. In addition, if left untreated, nearly 50% of patients with rest pain will require amputation for intractable pain or gangrene.

Cutaneous ulcers may be the first evidence of peripheral vascular disease. Although the underlying cause of these lesions is severe ischemia from arterial occlusive disease, the inciting event is often minor skin trauma. Arterial ulcers must be distinguished from ulcers caused by venous disease and diabetes unassociated with arterial occlusive disease. Each type of ulcer has certain clinical and physical characteristics, and therapy is directed at correcting the underlying etiology.

The ischemic arterial ulcer is most commonly found on the toes, heel, dorsum of the foot, or lower third of the leg. The pain is severe, persistent, and worsens at night. The ulcer itself is generally "punched out" with a pale or necrotic base.

Venous ulcers are located in the "gaiter" distribution around the ankle, especially the medial and lateral malleoli. They are less painful, more diffuse and shallow, and usually have some evidence of granulation tissue at the base. The presence of arterial ulcers implies a very high risk of subsequent gangrene and is generally considered an indication for arterial reconstructive surgery. The treatment of venous ulcers, on the other hand, is almost always conservative, as will be outlined below.

Diabetic ulcers are usually located in the plantar or lateral aspect of the foot. They resemble arterial ulcers in shape but are characteristically painless. They are a direct result of the neuropathy of diabetes. Due to injury to autonomic, motor, and sensory nerves, the skin becomes dry, the shape of the foot changes, and patients do not feel the mechanical irritation of the skin that leads to skin breakdown. Since arterial occlusive disease is frequently associated with diabetes, the arterial circulation must be critically evaluated in all diabetics presenting with a foot ulcer.

Dry and wet gangrene can be differentiated clinically. Digits are affected initially, but progression to the forefoot is not unusual. Dry gangrene represents mummification of tissue without active purulent tissue and

ankle/brachial reflex < 0.4
severe arterio occlussis
disease (rest pain, gangre

25 : Diseases of the Vascular System   **319**

cellulitis. Small amounts of infection superimposed on a severe chronic ischemic state can progress very rapidly to wet gangrene. Wet gangrene indicates active infection with cellulitis and purulent tissue planes. This is an indication for aggressive treatment to prevent ascending infection: urgent debridement of the infected tissue, antibiotics, and revascularization of the extremity.

Severe occlusive disease of the aortoiliac segment is often associated with impotence, since arterial inflow to the penis is compromised by the reduction in internal iliac artery blood flow. Erection is attained by increasing arterial inflow to the corpora cavernosa. Obstruction to venous outflow helps maintain an erection. In advanced cases, patients may present with the classic *Leriche syndrome* including impotence, buttock atrophy, and claudication from distal aortic occlusion.

Diagnosis. The evaluation of a patient with peripheral arterial occlusive disease is based on a thorough clinical examination, noninvasive vascular testing, and angiography. A careful history and physical examination will usually suggest the diagnosis of peripheral vascular occlusive disease. The complaints of changes in skin color and temperature, claudication, and rest pain are characteristic of the disease process. Physical findings include a loss of hair on the extremities, thinning of the skin, atrophy of muscles, loss of distal pulses, and skin ulcerations or gangrenous changes. An astute clinician can usually both diagnose and localize the level of disease. Noninvasive tests are employed after the clinical examination to confirm the presence of occlusive disease, identify the level and severity of the disease, and assess whether angiography will be required. *Doppler U/S*

The hand-held Doppler ultrasound instrument has made measurement of lower extremity blood pressure possible and allowed an objective means of assessing lower extremity perfusion. The basis of the Doppler ultrasound is the Doppler effect. The Doppler probe emits ultrasound waves in the range of 2–10 MHz. This is scattered by the moving red blood cells within the blood vessel producing a frequency shift that is picked up by the receiving crystal of the Doppler probe. This frequency shift is proportional to blood flow velocity.

To measure the blood pressure in the legs, a blood pressure cuff is placed at the ankle and inflated while blood flow in the dorsalis pedis or posterior tibial artery are auscultated with the Doppler probe. Inflation of the cuff above systolic pressure causes obliteration of the Doppler signal; systolic blood pressure is best recorded as the cuff is deflated and flow resumes. Because the systemic blood pressure may fluctuate, causing variations in the ankle pressure, it is useful to compare the ankle pressure to the brachial pressure (usually expressed as an ankle/brachial index). Patients without occlusive disease have ankle/brachial pressure indices of 1.0, whereas patients with more severe manifestations of arterial occlusive disease, such as rest pain or gangrene, have ankle/brachial pressure indices of 0.4 and less. Normal ankle pressures usually can identify patients with lower extremity pain due to nonvascular causes such as spinal stenosis or arthritis. Although some patients have calcified vessels that cannot be compressed by blood pressure cuffs, leading to a false elevation of the ankle pressures, the resting ankle/brachial index is the most accurate indicator of the presence or absence of vascular disease. It is reproducible and can be followed to identify progression of disease. It must be recognized that blood flow can be detected by Doppler at very low levels of circulation; patients may have frank gangrene of their foot even though some audible Doppler signals are heard at the ankle.

Because patients with claudication develop symptoms only with exercise, stress testing is a useful means for documenting the degree of walking impairment. Patients with normal circulation have no diminution of the ankle blood pressure following exercise. In patients with claudication, there is a substantial drop in ankle pressure with exercise; ankle pressure returns to normal with rest.

Doppler detectors also provide an electrical signal proportionate to the velocity of the flow in the blood vessel being studied. The shape of the waveform reflects the status of the vessel (Fig. 25.3). Normally a *triphasic* waveform is seen; with the development of a proximal stenosis, the waveform becomes *biphasic*. As the stenosis becomes more severe, the peak of the wave

Doppler U/S

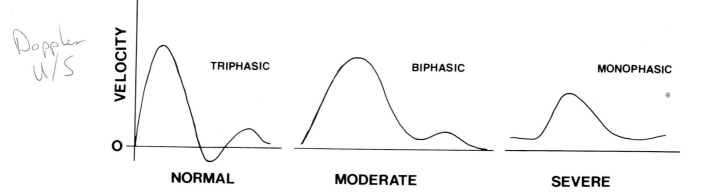

Figure 25.3. The Doppler ultrasound instrument can provide an analog display of blood flow velocity (waveform). With progressive occlusion the waveform changes from "triphasic" to "biphasic" to "monophasic."

form is blunted and the waveform widens to become *monophasic.*

If a patient is found to have arterial occlusive disease that may be amenable to surgery, then angiography is used to delineate precisely the nature and extent of disease. The infrarenal aortic inflow must be completely assessed, including biplanar projections to avoid missing a proximal lesion. Adequate visualization of the distal arterial tree, including the foot arch, is mandatory for a correctly planned distal bypass. The complications and techniques of angiography will be discussed later.

Treatment.   A number of medical and surgical options are available for the treatment of peripheral occlusive disease. Patients with claudication that does not severely limit their lifestyle have a good long-term outlook; only 5% come to major amputation in a 5-year period. Because these patients are often smokers, hypertensive, or hyperlipidemic, control of these risk factors is important and may slow the progression of disease. A daily exercise program of walking or bicycle riding will help stimulate collateral circulation and increase walking distance. This may be the only treatment necessary.

Medical therapy for peripheral vascular disease has also included agents that vasodilate vessels and lower the viscosity of blood. Vasodilators are ineffective and should not be used, although rheologic agents such as Pentoxifylline may be useful in some patients.

Transluminal balloon angioplasty is a percutaneous method of dilating arterial stenoses or recanalizing occluded vessels. The procedure is usually performed in the angiography suite after completion of diagnostic angiography. Patient selection is important and clinical criteria similar to those used to select patients for operation should be used. Dilation of vessels that appear significant on angiography but produce minimal or no symptoms is inappropriate and must be avoided. The best candidate for transluminal angioplasty has stenosis with severe symptoms due to an isolated, hemodynamically significant lesion of the iliac or proximal superficial femoral artery. Other favorable clinical situations include short segment superficial femoral artery occlusions or stenoses of previously placed venous bypass grafts.

Transluminal angioplasty employs a catheter with a balloon of predetermined maximum diameter at its tip. The catheter is passed through the obstructing lesion under x-ray guidance. Inflation of the balloon disrupts the plaque and stretches the arterial wall, resulting in enlargement of the lumen.

Results from angioplasty depend on the site dilated, the length of the stenosis, whether a complete obstruction is being dilated, the degree of calcification in the plaque, and the tortuosity of the vessel. In the iliac region, over 90% of lesions can be successfully dilated with a 70% 2-year patency. Angioplasty of the superficial femoral arteries has less impressive results. Initial success rates of 75% fall to approximately 50% at 2 years, depending on patient selection.

Endarterectomy is the standard operative treatment for carotid bifurcation atherosclerosis but has a more limited usefulness in the treatment of peripheral vascular occlusive disease. Carotid plaques are very localized, whereas lower extremity atherosclerosis usually is extensive with no discrete starting or end points. Some patients with localized aortoiliac disease are candidates for aortoiliac endarterectomy, although bypass proce-

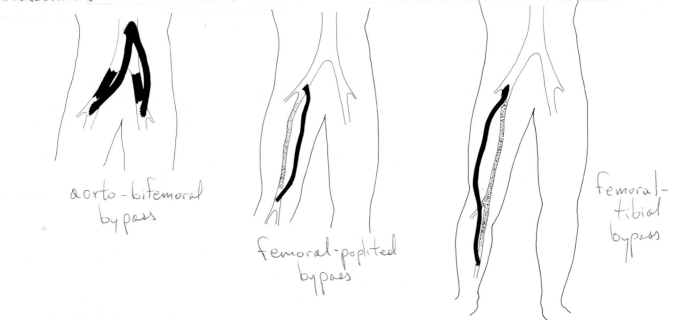

Figure 25.4.   Depending on the site of occlusion, various bypass procedures may be utilized. Pictured are aorto–bifemoral, femoral-popliteal, and femoral-tibial bypasses.

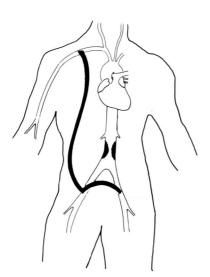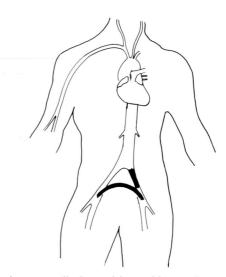

Figure 25.5. Alternative bypass procedures include such "extraanatomic" procedures as axillo-femoral-femoral bypass for aortoiliac occlusive disease and femoral-femoral bypass for unilateral iliac occlusion. *for high-risk operative pts.*

dures are much more commonly performed. Most surgeons employ local endarterectomy in the common femoral artery and profunda femoris arteries at the time of anastomosis of bypass grafts.

Bypass procedures are the standard operative treatment for lower extremity peripheral occlusive disease. Procedures can be divided into "inflow" and "outflow" procedures depending upon the level of obstruction. Inflow procedures refer to those used for aortoiliac obstructions and outflow procedures refer to those used for superficial femoral and popliteal artery obstructions. Certain basic surgical principles must be followed to obtain the best results. Adequate flow into the graft must be assured and it is imperative that the distal anastomosis is placed on a vessel that has an adequate caliber to maintain graft patency (Fig. 25.4).

The most common operative procedure for aortoiliac obstructions is the aortobifemoral bypass graft. In this operation, a prosthetic graft is sutured to the infrarenal aorta proximally and the common femoral arteries distally. In the presence of a superficial femoral artery obstruction, the profunda artery can be used as the primary outflow bed.

Aortofemoral bypass grafting is a stable and durable operation; the 5-year patency rate is greater than 90% and perioperative mortality is low (<2%). Should such operations fail, they do so because of progression of distal disease rather than failure of the procedure itself.

Immediate complications of aortobifemoral grafts are due mainly to technical problems. Problems include postoperative retroperitoneal hemorrhage, early graft thrombosis, groin hematomas, lymphatic leaks, and intraoperative distal embolization. Long-term complications include thrombosis, graft infection, pseudoaneurysm formation, and aortoduodenal fistula.

Patients who require bypass of an aortoiliac lesion, but are too ill to withstand an aortobifemoral graft, may be treated by axillofemoral or femorofemoral bypass grafts. These extraanatomic operations are designed to relieve inflow obstruction but do not require entering the abdomen. Thus, they are safer for high-risk patients and can be used to bypass the aorta in the presence of intraabdominal infection. Unfortunately, these grafts fail more frequently than aortobifemoral grafts due to their longer course and the risk of external compression in subcutaneous tunnels. For this reason, extra-anatomical grafts should be considered only when aortofemoral grafts or local endarterectomies are not feasible (Fig. 25.5).

Claudication or severe ischemia of the legs in the absence of aortoiliac disease is due to obstruction of the superficial femoral artery or popliteal artery and its branches. A preoperative angiogram visualizes the distal arterial tree and allows selection of the proximal and distal extent of the femoral-distal bypass necessary to restore adequate flow. The patient's own saphenous vein is the best conduit to use for these grafts; veins can be removed and reversed so valves are "open" or used in the in situ position after cutting each valve individually. If the saphenous vein has been used for another procedure or is not suitable for bypass, then prosthetic materials such as polytetrafluoroethylene (PTFE) and treated umbilical veins can be inserted. These prosthetic materials do not have the longevity of the saphenous vein but have acceptable results.

Limb salvage rates for these "outflow" procedures at 5 years are roughly 75% for femoropopliteal bypass grafts and 50% for femoral tibial bypass grafts. Limb salvage rates are usually 15% higher than the patency rates of the grafts. The long-term success of each bypass graft depends on the inflow, the type of conduit used, the outflow bed, and the technical aspects of the procedure. Thrombosis is the most serious early complication and is usually caused by technical error or inadequate outflow for the graft. Prompt thrombectomy or, in selected cases, local thrombolysis and recognition of any underlying technical problem will usually restore patency of the graft.

Chronic Intestinal Ischemia

Clinical Presentation. The principal symptoms of chronic intestinal ischemia include abdominal pain and weight loss. In most patients, pain occurs within 2 hours of meals. While the character of the pain varies from a persistent epigastric ache to more severe colic, nearly all patients with true ischemia describe reproducible postprandial symptoms.

Weight loss results from a purposeful limitation of ingested food, as most patients soon find that the intensity of postprandial pain correlates with the volume of food ingested. It now appears that this "food fear," unassociated with intestinal malabsorption, accounts for the nutritional disturbances experienced by these patients. Although motility disorders and mucosal abnormalities are occasionally observed, these latter mechanisms probably play only small roles in the clinical presentation.

Because of the typical age of presentation (greater than 45 years of age) and the general muscle wasting, diagnoses of primary visceral malignancy or carcinomatosis are often suggested. In fact, carcinoma of the pancreas is probably the single most important differential diagnosis.

Diagnosis. The diagnosis of chronic mesenteric ischemia is based on an accurate history and precise arteriographic studies. A single obstructive lesion in either the celiac axis, superior mesenteric artery, or inferior mesenteric artery rarely results in clinically significant ischemia. In symptomatic patients, tandem stenotic lesions or occlusion of two of these vessels is most common. To make the diagnosis, arteriograms should show (1) hemodynamically significant lesions of at least two of the three major visceral arteries and (2) evidence of collateral circulation appropriate for the specific lesions. Aortic orifice stenoses cannot be evaluated arteriographically without lateral and oblique projections to complement the standard anterior/posterior views (Fig. 25.6).

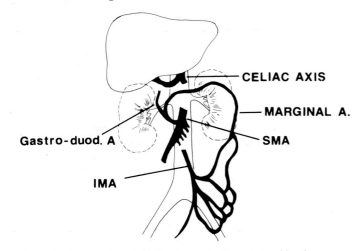

Figure 25.6. The intestinal circulation is characterized by three main vessels: the celiac axis, the superior mesenteric artery (SMA), and the inferior mesenteric artery (IMA). Collaterals connect these major vessels such that chronic occlusion of one vessel is well compensated.

∴ at least 2 vessel occlusion is required to produce chronic intestinal ischemic symptoms.

Treatment. Revascularization is indicated if all of the following conditions are met: (1) no evidence of other gastrointestinal pathology including malignancy or peptic ulcer disease; (2) persistent weight loss and postprandial pain; and (3) arteriograms consistent with visceral ischemia. Under these conditions, a technically successful operation can be expected to result in symptomatic improvement in a majority of patients. Furthermore, there is some evidence that revascularization can prevent catastrophic mesenteric infarction, which occurs with major changes in cardiovascular function or progression of atherosclerotic lesions.

Surgical procedures include both endarterectomy of orifice stenoses and bypasses using autologous veins or prosthetic grafts. The decision to perform more than one bypass or endarterectomy depends on the individual circumstances. Most patients experience sufficient improvement of intestinal blood flow with a single vessel reconstruction; however, some experienced surgeons routinely perform multiple bypasses to minimize the necessity of reoperation, should one of the grafts fail.

Renovascular Hypertension

Occlusive lesions of the renal artery are the most common cause of surgically correctable hypertension. Stenoses can result from atherosclerosis, fibromuscular dysplasia, or post-traumatic subintimal dissections. It has been suggested that renovascular hypertension accounts for 3–5% of the hypertensive population. In view of the continued improvements in surgical technique, the most difficult problems lie in specifically defining the risks and benefits of screening procedures for the large number of hypertensive patients.

Clinical Presentation. The presentation of renovascular hypertension depends on the underlying disease process. Patients with atherosclerotic lesions of the renal artery may present with cardiac or cerebrovascular complications of their poorly controlled hypertension. These patients are less likely to experience the sudden onset of severe diastolic hypertension that characterizes patients with dysplastic lesions of the renal artery. Fibromuscular dysplasia is the most common cause of renovascular hypertension in pediatric patients, occurring in males and females with an equal frequency. Dysplastic lesions in young adults are more frequently seen in females (Fig. 25.7).

Diagnosis. Renal scans, split renal function studies, and intravenous urography have been used as screening studies to separate patients with renovascular hypertension from the general hypertensive population. The high incidence of false-negative results limits reliance on these studies. Urograms may contribute to the diagnosis of renal ischemia by revealing: (1) decreased size of one kidney, (2) ureteral notching from collateral blood supply, or (3) delayed nephrogram with hyperconcentration of dye. Most importantly, urography can exclude primary renal disease. Experience suggests that arteriography with selective views of each

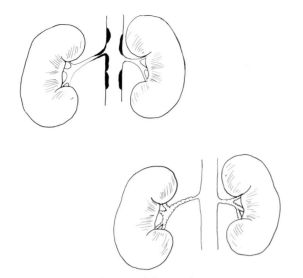

Figure 25.7. Stenotic lesions of the renal artery may cause renovascular hypertension by activation of the renin-angiotensin axis. Atherosclerotic lesions occur at the origin of the renal artery, while lesions of fibromuscular dysplasia commonly involve the more distal renal arteries toward the branches of the vessel.

renal artery is the *only* true screening study. Additional techniques, such as pharmacoangiography, can enhance visualization of collaterals and better define the true hemodynamic and functional significance of a given stenosis.

Early enthusiasm for the diagnostic accuracy of renal vein renin ratios (RVRR > 1.4) has been replaced by the realization that bilateral disease and the formation of collaterals return such ratios toward unity. To determine better which patients will be cured or improved by renal revascularization, many clinicians assess renin secretory activity. This is expressed as a renal systemic renin index (RSRI) that is calculated. Documentation of ipsilateral renin hypersecretion (RSRI > 0.48) and contralateral renin suppression (RSRI ~ 0) can predict "cure" of renovascular hypertension following successful surgery. Patients demonstrating both ipsilateral and contralateral renin hypersecretion are unlikely to be more than "improved" following successful renal artery repair. Unreliable renin determinations may result from subtle changes in sodium intake or an inability to discontinue hypertensive medications safely before venous sampling.

Treatment. If a hemodynamically significant renal artery lesion can be documented, arterial reconstruction should be strongly considered in: *(1)* all pediatric patients, *(2)* adults requiring adrenergic blocking agents for adequate blood pressure control, and *(3)* any patient with a documented decrease in renal function.

Procedures include endarterectomy for atherosclerotic lesions or aortorenal bypass utilizing autologous vein and artery or prosthetic material. An alternative technique, percutaneous transluminal "balloon" angioplasty, is effective especially in fibromuscular dysplastic lesions. It is least effective for patients with lesions within 10 mm of the vessel origins.

Results. Current experience with fibromuscular disease in pediatric patients and young adults suggests that more than 95% of patients can be cured or improved with revascularization. Most centers experience less than a 5% failure rate; graft occlusions in the immediate postoperative period occur in less than 1%. More than 90% of patients with atherosclerosis localized to the main renal artery experience beneficial results, although unfavorable results including graft failure occur in 5%. The poorest response to surgery is noted in those patients with generalized atherosclerosis. In addition to a higher operative mortality rate, 25–30% of these patients have an unfavorable response.

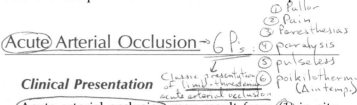

Acute Arterial Occlusion

Clinical Presentation

Acute arterial occlusion may result from *(1)* in situ thrombosis of preexistent occlusive disease, *(2)* arterial emboli, *(3)* vascular trauma, or *(4)* thrombosis of an aneurysm. Patients with in situ thrombosis may describe a history of claudication or rest pain that has recently and suddenly accelerated. Arterial emboli, vascular trauma, and aneurysmal thrombosis are usually not associated with previous vascular symptoms but also occur suddenly. When the occlusion is sudden and not associated with prior development of collateral vessels, then the symptoms tend to be more severe.

The classic presentation of a limb-threatening acute arterial occlusion includes *(1)* pallor, *(2)* pain, *(3)* paresthesias, *(4)* paralysis, *(5)* pulseless, and *(6)* poikilothermy (change in temperature). The skin temperature change is usually limited to the portion of the limb well beyond the occlusion. For example, with femoral artery occlusion the level of ischemia may not extend much above the knee because of collateral blood flow circumventing the femoral occlusion and providing some circulation to the thigh.

Internal organs, especially the intestines, kidney, and brain, are also subject to sudden arterial occlusion resulting in loss of function and infarction. Unfortunately, the manifestations of ischemia are not as obvious as those seen in the extremities and the diagnosis is often delayed, resulting in disastrous consequences.

Venous acute deep thrombosis may also present with limb pain: onset of the pain is not sudden but occurs gradually over 6–12 hr. Usually the skin of the involved limb is somewhat darker with prominent venous distension, in contrast to the pallor associated with arterial occlusion. Swelling is far more common in venous occlusion. Often episodes of iliofemoral or axillary vein thrombosis are induced by long periods of flexion at the hip or shoulder joints accompanied by relative dehydration ("effort thrombosis").

Arterial thrombosis occurs at anatomic sites favored by atherosclerosis, especially the infrarenal aorta, femoral, and popliteal vessels. A history of claudication and stigmata of arterial occlusive disease, such as loss of secondary skin characteristics, suggest preexistent stenoses.

The great majority of emboli originate in the left heart. Emboli arise most commonly from atrial fibrillation and mural thrombus from transmural myocardial infarction. These thrombi can be dislodged when cardioversion is performed within 2 weeks of myocardial infarction. Rheumatic mitral stenosis can also result in atrial fibrillation and perivalvular emboli. Endocarditis, specifically of nonbacterial origin, is also a frequent cause of emboli. This should be considered in patients with a history of radiation exposure and neoplastic disease. Thoracic or abdominal aortic aneurysms may also be responsible for the distal embolization of atheromatous debris or mural thrombi.

The most frequent site of embolic occlusion is the femoral artery. Other common sites of impaction of emboli include the axillary arteries, popliteal arteries, iliac arteries, and aortic bifurcation. The superior mesenteric artery is the most common visceral blood vessel affected.

Management

Preoperative care consists of immediate anticoagulation with intravenous heparin. Contraindications to heparin include a new neurologic deficit, gastrointestinal bleeding, head injury, or other potential site of bleeding. It is important to replace volume deficit carefully with the knowledge that many of these patients have underlying cardiac disease. Base deficits should be assessed and appropriately replaced with sodium bicarbonate. Pharmacologic support should be considered when severe cardiac disease is present. Additional agents that may be helpful following acute arterial occlusion include dextran and mannitol. Dextran tends to enhance the electronegativity of both the red blood cell and the vessel wall and, by this mechanism, decreases thrombosis distal to the occlusion. Mannitol reduces cellular swelling by drawing fluid out of the intracellular compartment to the extracellular compartment by its direct osmotic effect. This is of particular importance immediately following restoration of blood flow, when ischemic cells swell due to poor function of the energy-dependent sodium pump. Mannitol also provides an osmotic diuresis that can ameliorate the nephrotoxic effects of myoglobin from ischemic muscle. Recent evidence also indicates that mannitol may reduce cellular injury by acting as a free-radical scavenger for the ischemic muscle.

If there is any question about the viability of the limb affected by acute arterial occlusion, immediate embolectomy or thrombectomy should be considered. Delays can result in severe muscle ischemia and ultimate amputation. Arteriography is not essential in the diagnosis and treatment of embolic occlusions, although it is often helpful in cases of sudden thrombosis of preexistent occlusive disease. If a limb remains clearly viable despite arterial occlusion, anticoagulation alone may be appropriate in some high-risk patients and local catheter infusion of thrombolytics may be considered in others.

The surgical approach is directed at both curing the cause and opening distal flow at the site of the occlusion. Thrombosis unassociated with embolization usually requires some form of bypass graft or endarterectomy to avoid repeated episodes of thrombosis. Results are variable and depend on the extent of occlusive disease and the duration of ischemia. In embolic occlusion, thrombectomies can be performed through peripheral vessels using specialized balloon catheters (Fogarty® catheters). While this can be done under local anesthesia, many surgeons feel that an intubated patient is better oxygenated and less anxious than a patient managed with local anesthesia. Careful and complete thrombectomy should be performed both proximally and distally. The distal thrombectomy is essential, as nearly one-third of patients with arterial occlusions have discontinuous thrombus past the point of occlusion. The thrombus or embolus should be inspected following removal because the configuration of the thrombus wall is often the best hint of its origin. If the thrombus/embolus has a rubbery appearance or does not fit the contour of the artery where it was found, then it probably is an embolus from another site. Treatment for the embolic source can then be determined.

After restoration of flow it is important to examine the extremity carefully to determine whether tissue damage and edema have produced a compartment syndrome from increased pressure. If so, a fasciotomy is necessary to relieve compartmental pressure and avoid compression of both arterial and venous vessels in the limb.

Unfortunately, the mortality rate for acute arterial occlusion remains relatively high. This can be attributed to the advanced age of patients suffering in situ thrombosis and emboli and the severity of coincident myocardial disease. The most frequent causes of death are myocardial infarction and pulmonary embolus. In cases of embolic arterial occlusion, postoperative anticoagulation must be pursued. Without anticoagulation, emboli recur in roughly one-third of patients within 30 days. With the use of heparin and warfarin postoperatively, the recurrence rate decreases to less than 10%.

Cerebrovascular Insufficiency

Carotid Artery Disease

The primary blood supply to the anterior and middle cerebral arteries are the paired internal carotid arteries. Obstructive or ulcerative lesions in these arteries may lead to symptoms of cerebrovascular insufficiency. Presentations vary from short-lived neurologic deficits to profound strokes with fatal outcomes.

Pathogenesis. The mechanisms of ischemia include low flow distal to severely stenotic atherosclerotic plaques and emboli from roughened intimal lesions discharging platelets or debris; often both processes coexist. Decreases in cerebral blood flow occur when hy-

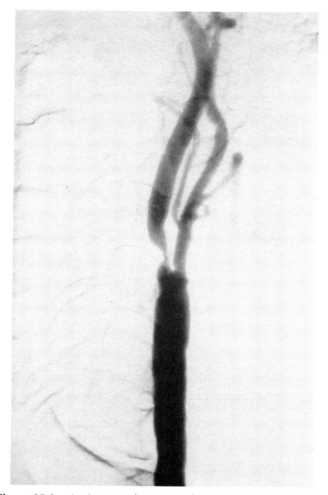

Figure 25.8. Angiogram of an internal carotid artery stenosis in a patient demonstrating symptoms of chronic decrease in cerebral blood flow.

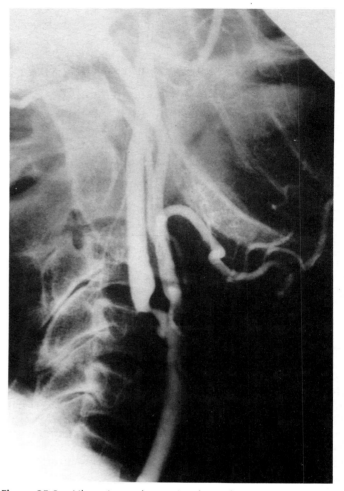

Figure 25.9. Ulcerative and stenotic atherosclerotic lesion at bifurcation of carotid artery in a patient suffering transient ischemic attacks.

potension or low cardiac output is combined with carotid artery disease or when a stenotic carotid artery suddenly thromboses. In the former cases, neurologic deficits occur in so-called "watershed" areas between the perfusion territories of main cerebral arteries where collateral flow is marginal. While sudden thrombosis of a carotid artery may result in a massive cerebral infarction, collateral circulation from the contralateral carotid artery and the basilar artery may prevent any symptoms ("silent" occlusion). The neurologic deficit following single or multiple emboli depends on the site of impaction. It is noteworthy that similar repetitive neurologic deficits may be caused by either (1) recurrent ischemia of watershed areas or (2) impaction and lysis of intermittent emboli directed by consistent anatomic and hemodynamic factors (Figs. 25.8, 25.9).

Etiology. Atherosclerosis is the most common cause for symptomatic extracranial and intracranial lesions of the carotid arteries and other major vessels supplying the brain. Atherosclerotic lesions are characteristically localized in areas of high turbulence at the bifurcation of the carotid artery in the neck. Associated lesions may occur at the intrathoracic origin of the vessels of the aortic arch and the intracranial carotid siphon. Other less common causes for carotid disease include fibromuscular dysplasia, trauma, and Takayasu's arteritis.

Clinical Presentation. It is useful to classify cerebrovascular symptoms by the timing and severity of the deficits.

Transient ischemic attacks (TIA) are short-lived often repetitive changes in mentation, vision, motor, or sensory function that are completely reversed within 24 hours. Since TIAs often involve the middle cerebral artery distribution, patients frequently present with contralateral arm, leg, and facial weakness. A specific type of TIA involves transient ipsilateral monocular blindness (*amaurosis fugax* or "fleeting blindness"), due to emboli to the ophthalmic artery. Longer lasting episodes (up to 72 hours) that still result in no permanent neurologic deficit are termed *reversible ischemic neurologic deficits (RIND)*. A cerebral infarction (stroke or *cer-*

ebrovascular accident [CVA]) results in permanent neurologic deficits and nonviable brain tissue that can usually be documented by CAT scan. Neurologic recovery is quite variable and may be complete, but the time course of recovery (weeks or months) clearly distinguishes infarcts from TIA or RIND. Atherosclerotic carotid artery disease is not the only disease responsible for these clinical presentations. TIAs can also be caused by migraines, seizure disorders, brain tumors, intracranial aneurysms, and arteriovenous malformations.

The severity of the neurologic deficit is determined by the volume and location of ischemic brain. The most commonly involved area is the perfusion territory of the middle cerebral artery (the parietal lobe), which is the main outflow vessel of the carotid artery. Hypoperfusion of the middle cerebral artery causes contralateral hemiparesis or hemiplegia, especially in the upper extremity, and paralysis of the contralateral lower part of the face ("central seventh nerve paralysis"). Associated findings include some degree of hypesthesia (decreased sensation) on the paralyzed side and a contralateral homonymous hemianopsia (visual field deficit). Difficulty with speech (aphasia) is noted if the dominant hemisphere is involved. The left hemisphere is dominant in nearly all right-handed people and roughly 50% of left-handed people.

Patients with ischemia of the brain tissue supplied by the anterior cerebral artery present with contralateral monoplegia, usually more severe in the lower extremity. Posterior cerebral artery ischemia may result from carotid artery occlusive disease but is also related to obstruction of both vertebral arteries or the basilar artery. Dizziness or syncope may be accompanied by visual field defects, palsy of the ipsilateral third cranial nerve, and contralateral sensory loss.

Diagnosis of Cerebrovascular Disease. Many patients with asymptomatic extracranial carotid disease first present with cervical bruits secondary to turbulent flow near the stenotic vessel. Bruits from carotid artery stenoses are high pitched and localized to the angle of the jaw. Unfortunately, even experienced examiners frequently cannot distinguish carotid bruits from turbulence in other cervical blood vessels. In addition, as many as 50% of symptomatic ulcerations may be unassociated with stenoses and hence not present with bruits. Finally, when a stenosis becomes very severe (>85% of luminal area) the intensity of the bruit may decrease and disappear.

Noninvasive tests have been developed to characterize extracranial carotid disease better without the risk of arteriography. Indirect noninvasive tests include oculoplethysmography (OPG) and directional supraorbital Doppler examination. OPG measures volume changes in the eye with each heart beat. Since the ophthalmic artery is the first intracranial branch of the internal carotid artery, a severe stenosis in the carotid artery would delay the ipsilateral pulse volume recording. Supraorbital Doppler examination is based on the observation of reversed flow in the supraorbital vessels

with severe internal carotid artery occlusive disease. The decrease in distal internal carotid artery pressure changes blood flow from the normal pattern outward through the ophthalmic artery to retrograde perfusion; that is, blood flows inward providing collateral blood flow to the middle cerebral via periorbital branches of the external carotid. The OPG is potentially inaccurate in bilateral disease and/or obstruction of the ophthalmic artery; in addition, none of the indirect tests can identify nonstenotic ulcerations.

Direct tests use ultrasound techniques (Duplex scan) to image the extracranial vessels. Bilateral disease can be reliably identified. Furthermore, the nature of the plaque (soft, calcific, or ulcerated) and its precise location (common versus external versus internal carotid) can be determined.

The definitive study of the extracranial carotid system remains arteriography. Although both intravenous and arterial contrast injections may be used, arterial injections are usually needed for clear definition of disease. Arteriography is appropriate in all symptomatic patients and in asymptomatic patients with high grade stenoses or ulcers identified by noninvasive tests.

Treatment. Medical therapy for cerebrovascular disease is directed at control of risk factors (such as hypertension and hyperlipoproteinemia), anticoagulation with heparin and warfarin, and administration of antiplatelet drugs such as aspirin and dipyridamole. The latter two therapies help prevent sudden thrombosis of stenotic lesions and inhibition of platelet activation on ulcerative lesions. Anticoagulation and antiplatelet therapy are most commonly used in patients with ulcerative nonstenotic lesions or severe intracranial disease, where surgical therapy would not change the natural history of the disease.

Carotid endarterectomy is indicated in patients with transient ischemic attacks associated with stenosis or ulceration of the ipsilateral carotid artery. This approach is based on the 10% incidence of stroke each year after a TIA. Endarterectomy is also indicated in selected patients with completed strokes and carotid disease, since recurrent strokes occur in up to 50% of these patients. Operation is usually delayed a minimum of 4–6 weeks following the stroke to decrease perioperative morbidity.

The proper treatment of asymptomatic patients with stenotic carotid lesions remains controversial. Many clinical studies have documented an increased incidence of cerebrovascular symptoms in these patients, although the incidence varies widely from 10–30%. In general, operation may be appropriate in selected asymptomatic patients with low operative risk and those undergoing major surgical procedures that may predispose to hypotension and stroke.

In experienced hands, the morbidity and mortality for carotid endarterectomy is less than 2%. Recurrent lesions may occur in up to 10%, so long-term followup is necessary. Restenosis within 2 years usually represents intimal hyperplasia, while later presentations reflect recurrent atherosclerosis.

Vertebrobasilar Disease

The classic syndrome of vertebrobasilar insufficiency ("*subclavian steal syndrome*") is associated with subclavian or innominate artery occlusive disease. This syndrome occurs when an occlusive lesion proximal to the origin of the vertebral vessel decreases perfusion pressure in the distal subclavian artery. The vertebral artery then functions as a collateral pathway for the arm. During arm exercise, flow is reversed in the vertebral artery; as a consequence basilar artery blood flow and perfusion pressure are decreased. Symptoms of posterior cerebral and cerebellar ischemia are common especially if concurrent flow limiting carotid lesions are present (Fig. 25.10).

The typical presentation of a patient with subclavian steal syndrome includes arm claudication, light-headedness, syncope, and nausea correlated with exercise. Supraclavicular bruits are frequently heard and blood pressure in the involved subclavian artery is usually reduced by at least 40 mm Hg. Because of the different anatomy of the arch vessels, left-sided involvement is far more common.

In patients with associated carotid artery disease, carotid endarterectomy alone may relieve symptoms of vertebrobasilar insufficiency by increasing collateral flow to the posterior cerebral artery and cerebellum. However, in most symptomatic patients with subclavian steal, the most commonly performed procedure is *carotid-subclavian bypass*, which restores normal blood flow to the subclavian artery and antegrade perfusion to the vertebral artery.

Venous Disease and Pulmonary Embolus

Anatomic Considerations

Venous drainage of the lower extremity is accomplished through the superficial and the deep venous systems. The superficial venous system is composed of the greater and lesser saphenous veins and their tributaries; the deep venous system is composed of large veins that run beside the major named arteries of the lower extremity (i.e., the common iliac, internal and external iliac veins, as well as the common femoral, superficial femoral, and profunda femoral veins parallel the arteries of the same name). The anterior tibial, posterior tibial, and peroneal veins are almost always paired (venae comitantes) such that in the calf there are six primary deep veins in contrast to three primary arteries. There are multiple bicuspid valves in the superficial, deep, and communicating veins. The superficial and deep venous systems communicate through perforating veins that direct blood from the superficial to the deep system with venous valves. Incompetence of valves and perforating veins due to inflammation or distension allows retrograde flow from the deep system to the superficial system and can result in varicosities and ulcerations.

The muscle compartments in the calf are important in venous circulation, since muscle contraction in-

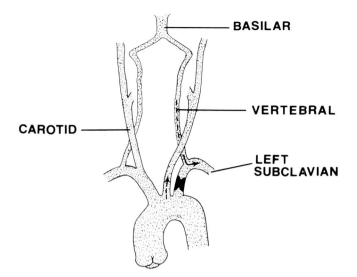

Figure 25.10. Diagrammatic illustration of subclavian steal syndrome. Proximal occlusion of left subclavian artery results in retrograde flow of blood via left vertebral artery, "stealing" blood from basilar circulation. This results in transient dizziness and syncope with arm exercise.

creases pressure in the compartment, thereby forcing blood back to the heart. This muscular pump is an important mechanism in preventing both chronic edema and deep vein thrombosis. Postoperative deep vein thrombosis probably results from inaction of this muscle pump when patients are paralyzed and under anesthesia.

Deep Venous Thrombosis

The clinical situations that lead to deep venous thrombosis (DVT) were first described by Virchow and include endothelial injury, stasis, and hypercoagulability. Bony and soft tissue trauma to the legs are the most common cause of endothelial injury; there is evidence that stasis and venous distention also injure the endothelium. Slow flow and stasis are seen with prolonged bed rest, congestive heart failure, and obesity. Hypercoagulable states are common in patients with neoplasms and account for the high incidence of venous thrombosis in these patients. Patients with prior deep vein thrombosis may have a combination of endothelial injury and stasis, and are therefore also considered "high risk."

Prevention of Deep Vein Thrombosis. Deep venous thrombosis with pulmonary embolus is one of the most common and feared complications following major surgery, due to a combination of stasis, hypercoagulability, and trauma that occurs in the perioperative period. Therefore, surgeons have had a great interest in methods of preventing DVT.

Modalities for preventing the development of venous thrombosis in surgical patients include early ambulation following operation, elevation of the foot of the operating room table to promote venous drainage, compression boots to facilitate venous flow during the operation, and perioperative anticoagulation using low-dose heparin or aspirin.

Diagnosis. The diagnosis of deep venous thrombosis progresses through clinical suspicion and physical examination to be confirmed by noninvasive testing and venography. The physical findings of calf tenderness, swelling of the leg or ankle, and Homans' sign (calf pain with dorsiflexion of the foot) are suggestive, but not sufficiently accurate, to confirm the diagnosis of deep vein thrombosis. In fact, the accuracy of diagnosis based on clinical and physical examination alone is only 50%; therefore, more objective diagnostic studies need to confirm DVT prior to treatment. In addition to deep vein thrombosis, the differential diagnosis of acute edema associated with leg pain includes congestive heart failure, trauma, ruptured plantaris tendon, acute or chronic arterial insufficiency (due to dependency of the leg to relieve the pain), infection, lymphangitis, lumbosacral strain and sciatica, muscle hematoma, and renal failure.

Noninvasive diagnostic procedures can increase diagnostic accuracy to approximately 95%. The most commonly used tests utilize the Doppler ultrasound probe to listen directly to venous flow; indirect tests, including impedance plethysmography and phleborheography, supplement the Doppler exam. ^{125}I-Fibrinogen scanning also can be used to detect calf vein thrombosis. Recently duplex scanning has been used to visualize the clot in veins and diagnose DVT and may supplant other noninvasive procedures. If noninvasive diagnostic tests are not definitive, venography should be performed; it is the "gold standard" against which all other studies are compared.

Treatment. The treatment of acute deep venous thrombosis is anticoagulation, accomplished with an intravenous loading dose of aqueous heparin (125 units/kg), followed by a continuous infusion of heparin such that the partial thromboplastin time is prolonged to twice normal. This usually requires 800–1200 units of heparin per hour. Long-term anticoagulation is begun in 5–7 days and achieved with sodium warfarin (Coumadin), which is administered at a dose to prolong the prothrombin time to approximately 1.5 times normal, or 18–20 seconds. Contraindications to anticoagulant therapy include a bleeding diathesis, such as gastrointestinal ulceration, recent stroke or arteriovenous malformations in the brain, recent surgery, hematologic disorder (such as hemophilia), Rendu-Osler-Weber syndrome (hereditary telangiectasia), and bone marrow depression due to chemotherapy.

Heparin and Coumadin anticoagulant therapy prevents continued propagation of existing thrombus. It does not lyse thrombus that may have formed in the deep venous system. Fibrinolysis can be achieved through the endogenous plasminogen system or may be stimulated by administering exogenous streptokinase or urokinase. Although this therapy is very effective in achieving thrombolysis, hemorrhage is a major complication. Intracranial bleeding is of particular concern and great care must be taken in selecting patients for this form of therapy.

The indications for surgical intervention in venous thrombosis are very limited. Even in situations of complete ileofemoral thrombosis with massive edema *(phlegmasia cerulea dolens),* venous thrombectomy has limited usefulness because of the high rethrombosis rate.

Postphlebitic Syndrome

The postphlebitic syndrome results from valvular incompetence in the veins of the deep venous system. The clinical manifestations are chronically swollen legs with hyperpigmentation and venous stasis ulcerations in the "gaiter" (around the ankle) zone. This syndrome usually follows an episode of deep venous thrombosis, although patients are frequently unaware of prior DVT. When thrombus forms in the deep venous system, it is gradually lysed by the fibrinolytic system and often recanalizes, although there is usually residual scar tissue within the vein. This may entrap the valves, leaving them shortened, fibrotic, and incompetent. Venous valvular incompetence allows retrograde flow from the deep veins, through the perforators, and into the superficial veins; the swelling and skin changes are a direct result of the increased venous pressure. Hence, treatment is geared toward reduction of edema and pressure by elevation of the legs and the use of external support such as elastic stockings or medicated boots (UNNA boot).

Venous ulceration should be treated with elastic support and elevation. If an isolated incompetent perforator is demonstrated venographically at the base of an indolent venous ulcer, ligation is appropriate. While skin grafting of venous ulcerations is necessary occasionally, good external support and wound debridement is usually sufficient to heal most venous stasis ulcers.

Varicose Veins

Primary varicose veins are due to valvular incompetence in the greater saphenous vein, particularly at the junction of the greater saphenous vein with the common femoral vein. Primary varicose veins are often familial and cause symptoms of discomfort over the veins and fatigue in the legs after standing. Patients with primary varicose veins have *no* ankle edema or ulcers and have no abnormality of the deep venous system. *Secondary varicose veins* arise because of abnormalities in the deep venous system, often due to a prior episode of deep venous thrombosis, with valvular destruction and incompetent perforating veins.

Selected patients with primary varicose veins can be helped by ligating and stripping the veins. However, patients with secondary varicose veins due to abnormalities of the deep venous system should only undergo stripping if the deep venous system is patent and the patient has venous stasis ulcers that have not responded to nonoperative therapy. In general, varicose veins should be treated nonoperatively. Ligation and stripping of a greater saphenous vein that is minimally diseased is undesirable because the saphenous vein is of great value for arterial reconstructions, including coronary artery bypass grafts.

Pulmonary Embolism

Pulmonary embolism results from migration of venous clots to the pulmonary arteries. Clots may originate in any peripheral vein, especially the iliac, femoral, and large pelvic veins.

Patients with pulmonary embolism may present with no specific clinical findings or with massive cardiovascular collapse and death. The classic findings of pleuritic chest pain and hemoptysis are rarely found in patients with pulmonary embolism. When such findings are present, they usually indicate pulmonary infarction; the pain is due to a pleuritic reaction to the infarct. Dyspnea is the most common clinical finding, while dyspnea and hypoxia are frequently seen. Right heart strain on ECG is frequently seen in massive pulmonary embolus. However, since most patients with pulmonary embolism may be free of symptoms and signs, pulmonary embolism cannot be ruled out on the basis of normal clinical findings.

The definitive diagnosis of pulmonary embolism is made by ventilation perfusion lung scan or pulmonary arteriogram. If the chest x-ray and ventilation scan are normal, then a wedge-shaped or lobar defect on perfusion scan indicates a high probability of pulmonary embolism. However, if either the chest x-ray or ventilation scan is abnormal, perfusion scanning is not reliable. While pulmonary angiography remains the definitive test, emboli may lyse within 2–7 days. Hence, a normal pulmonary angiogram 1 week after the suspected clinical event does not rule out the occurrence of pulmonary embolism.

The primary therapy of pulmonary embolism is heparin anticoagulation; the rationale for therapy is prevention of subsequent emboli. Patients with massive pulmonary emboli with hemodynamic instability and acute elevation of pulmonary artery pressure should be supported and oxygenated. If hypotension and hypoxia persist despite intubation and vasopressors, pulmonary embolectomy may be considered. This is the so-called Trendelenburg operation and involves direct surgical removal of the pulmonary embolus. Unfortunately, morbidity and mortality exceeds 80% for this operation, emphasizing that prevention of pulmonary embolus is the best therapy. For multiple pulmonary emboli with markedly elevated pulmonary artery pressures, fibrinolytic therapy may also be considered. When patients have a contraindication to anticoagulation or develop recurrent emboli while on anticoagulation, then a mechanical device (filter) can be placed in the inferior vena cava to catch emboli.

There is no direct relationship between clot size, cardiopulmonary dynamics, other risk factors, and survival of acute pulmonary embolism. Multiple small emboli may result in cardiovascular collapse as well as massive emboli.

Amputations

The goal of arterial reconstructions is salvage of ischemic extremities. On occasion, though, reconstruction is not possible, or ischemia and infection are too far advanced, leaving amputation as the only option. In addition to rest pain and gangrene, other indications for amputation include trauma and neoplasm. An amputation is virtually never performed for venous disease without coexisting arterial insufficiency. In general, the more distal the amputation, the better the rehabilitation potential. Unfortunately, the inadequacy of skin blood flow in patients with advanced ischemia may limit the level of amputation.

Toe, transmetatarsal, and Symes (ankle) amputations are preferable if blood supply is adequate, because patients can ambulate without much training and without prostheses. Unfortunately, in diabetics and patients with advanced peripheral vascular occlusive disease, such amputations are associated with a high failure rate. It is generally accepted that a midfoot perfusion pressure (as measured by Doppler probe and cuff) should exceed 50 mmHg to be confident of healing of these distal amputations, although some amputations may heal at lower levels.

In the presence of an occluded and unreconstructible superficial femoral artery, a below-knee amputation is often the most suitable procedure. If perfusion pressures exceed 50 mmHg at the popliteal artery, or when ankle/arm pressure ratio is greater than 0.6, healing can be expected in more than 75% of below the knee amputations. Even if blood flow is barely detectable by

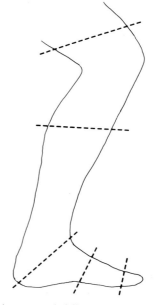

Figure 25.11. Schematic of differing amputation levels including toe, transmetatarsal, ankle (Symes), below-the-knee (BKA), and above-the-knee (AKA). Amputation level is dictated by the degree of ischemia. The general principle includes salvage of as much length of the leg as possible. Therefore, the surgeon performs the most distal amputation that will be accompanied by primary healing of the skin incisions.

Doppler at the popliteal artery, below the knee amputation is worth performing, since walking with a below-knee prosthesis requires far less energy expenditure than that associated with above the knee prostheses.

Above the knee amputations are necessary for very advanced ischemia involving the skin around the knee and the posterior muscles of the calf. Often above the knee amputation is selected for high risk or bedridden patients, although transferring from wheelchairs and beds is far easier with a functional knee joint preserved by a below the knee amputation (Fig. 25.11).

In addition to selecting the proper level of amputation, meticulous surgical technique must be exercised to avoid injury to marginally viable tissue. Skin must be treated gently and dissection must be sharp and precise. The mortality and morbidity of amputation is generally high, due to the frequently associated cerebral and coronary artery vascular disease, as well as complications such as aspiration pneumonia and pulmonary embolus. For these reasons, early and aggressive physical therapy is employed to hasten mobilization of these patients.

Arteriovenous Malformations

Arteriovenous malformations result from abnormal embryologic development of the maturing vascular spaces, producing pathologic arteriovenous connections involving small and medium-sized vessels. There is an equal male-to-female ratio, with the lower extremities involved two to three times as frequently as the upper extremities. Although the lesions are present at birth, most are identified only in the second and third decade as they gradually enlarge. A thrill is often present over the fistula and the affected limb may be hypertrophied, but pain is rare. In large arteriovenous malformations, skin ulceration and bleeding can be troublesome complications. Rarely congenital arteriovenous fistulae produce cardiac enlargement and failure due to the increase in cardiac output.

The management of symptomatic and localized congenital arteriovenous malformations is surgical. However, treatment of large or diffuse lesions can be extremely difficult and is associated with a high recurrence rate. An alternative is percutaneous intraarterial embolization of the main "feeding" artery to decrease the amount of blood shunted from arterioles to venules.

Acquired arteriovenous fistulae are also abnormal communications between arteries and veins but usually result from iatrogenic injuries or penetrating trauma such as gunshot or knife wounds. The arterial injury decompresses into the vein, and a permanent connection may then be the result. Frequently these fistulae are associated with a false aneurysm and involve large vessels. A palpable thrill or bruit may be present as well as local warmth. Venous hypertension and venous stasis changes will occur if the arteriovenous fistula is long-standing. Can you predict the changes that occur in pressure and flow in the artery and vein proximal and distal to a fistula?

All acquired arteriovenous fistulae should be repaired, to prevent the development of complications such as cardiac failure, local pain, aneurysm formation, limb length discrepancy, and venous hypertension. Spontaneous closure of a posttraumatic arteriovenous fistula is rare. Operative intervention requires complete dissection and separation of the involved vessels and appropriate vascular repair. An alternative form of treatment for some acquired arteriovenous fistulae is catheter-directed occlusion using detachable balloons or other embolic agents.

Vasospastic Disorders and Thoracic Outlet Syndrome

Episodic digital vasospasm involving the hands and feet was first described by Maurice Raynaud in 1862. Presently the term *Raynaud's syndrome* is used to define cold- or emotion-induced episodic digital ischemia. Up to 90% of patients are female and 50% have an associated autoimmune disease such as scleroderma, lupus erythematosus, rheumatoid arthritis, and Sjogren's syndrome. A subpopulation appears to have a work-related syndrome caused by the use of vibratory machinery. Unilateral Raynaud's syndrome is more common in males, and may be due to proximal large vessel arterial disease.

While the clinical aspects may vary, the classic Raynaud attack consists of three distinct phenomena. Cold exposure initially results in profound vasospasm and blanching of the digits. After 15 min, this is followed by cyanosis, presumably from venous filling with delayed venous emptying. Later digits and hands become hyperemic as vasospasm lessens and flow to the digits is restored.

The diagnosis of Raynaud's syndrome is made from the history and can be confirmed by an ice immersion test. Coexistent symptoms of connective tissue disorders frequently can be elicited; laboratory tests, such as sedimentation rate, complement assay, and antinuclear antibody assay, often will confirm the immunologic disorders associated with the syndrome.

Treatment consists of discontinuing any medications that cause reduced cardiac output or vasospasm, and may be associated with Raynaud's syndrome, such as ergotamines, birth control pills, and β-blockers. Other pharmacologic agents can be used to decrease the tendency toward vasospasm. Presently, calcium channel blocking agents are most commonly used. Surgical sympathectomy has not been shown to be an effective treatment. Revascularization of an ischemic extremity may markedly improve Raynaud's symptoms in patients with arterial occlusive disease.

Symptoms that mimic a vasospastic disorder may occur in the *thoracic outlet syndrome*. This syndrome is also encountered in young and middle-aged females. Symptoms are caused by compression or irritation of the brachial plexus and, to a much lesser extent, the subclavian artery as they pass through the thoracic outlet and the costoclavicular space.

Anatomic causes of the syndrome include: *(1)* an elongated transverse process of the seventh cervical vertebra; *(2)* a fully developed cervical rib; *(3)* congenital bands in the outlet related to the cervical rib, middle scalene muscle, or anterior scalene muscle; and *(4)* a narrowed costoclavicular space, often due to a previously fractured rib or clavicle with callus formation.

Paresthesias of the arm and hand reflect neurologic compression and are much more frequent than arterial symptoms. When arterial symptoms do occur, they include coldness of the hand and arm, pallor, and muscle fatigue. In rare instances, stenosis of the subclavian artery may cause emboli to the hand.

Evaluation of these patients involves a detailed history and thorough physical examination to document localized scalene muscle tenderness and radicular phenomena. The Adson test (disappearance of the radial pulse on abduction and external rotation of the shoulder), said to be indicative of thoracic outlet syndrome in the early literature, is now regarded as totally unreliable. Cervical spine x-rays should be obtained to identify cervical ribs or bands. Nerve conduction velocity across the outlet have proved to be of little value in most cases. Angiography is recommended only if a harsh bruit is present or embolization is suspected.

Once the diagnosis has been confirmed, nonsurgical treatments, including postural training, should be attempted. If symptoms persist, surgical decompression of the outlet is warranted. The most frequently applied procedure is resection of the first thoracic rib, removal of any cervical ribs, and division of the anterior scalene muscle.

Vascular Trauma

Blood vessels may be injured directly by penetrating trauma, including stab wounds and gunshot wounds, and blunt trauma, especially fractures of the long bones. In high speed collisions involving motor vehicles or aircraft, vessels may be partially or totally disrupted by the shearing stress of sudden acceleration and deceleration. While patients with arterial injuries may present with obvious signs, such as external hemorrhage or absence of distal pulses, often the signs of vascular injury are subtle. Hemorrhage may be occult and confined to soft tissue or body cavities. Other findings indicative of vascular injury include acute arteriovenous fistulae (associated with "to-and-fro" murmurs or palpable thrills), neurologic deficits and paresthesias (due to nerve compression by adjacent hematomas), or organ-specific deficits reflecting obstruction of the main arterial supply (e.g., cerebral infarction with carotid artery injuries). It must be remembered that injury to the endothelial surface ("intimal flaps") may not cause thrombosis for hours or days and hence cannot be diagnosed by physical examination until such a complication occurs. A common misconception is that a patient with an arterial injury must have a reduced or absent distal pulse; this *only* occurs if the injury is hemodynamically significant.

Immediate diagnosis and treatment of arterial injuries is indicated to avoid excessive blood loss and restore extremity or organ blood flow. If the diagnosis is missed on initial evaluation, late complications may be much more difficult to treat. These late complications include pseudoaneurysms or false aneurysms when small lacerations in vessels gradually enlarge and expand, high volume arteriovenous fistulae with arterial and venous insufficiency and high output cardiac failure, and delayed thrombosis from untreated intimal flaps or dissections.

The poor reliability of physical diagnosis in accurately assessing the location and extent of vascular injury mandates arteriography when penetrating trauma occurs in proximity to blood vessels, even if no overt signs of injury are present. Because of the tremendous concussive energy of high velocity missiles, extensive damage can result even from "near misses." Specific types of blunt trauma (especially dislocation of knees and elbows) are so frequently associated with arterial contusions and intimal disruption that arteriography is prudent.

While the consequences of venous injury are not as severe as arterial trauma, venous laceration must be considered in any patient presenting with evidence of excessive blood loss and no arterial lesion on angiography. Venography can usually confirm and localize the injury. Venous injury also predisposes to the development of deep venous thrombosis.

Immediate vascular repair may be as simple as ligation or lateral suture. However, in some cases, bypass grafts may be necessary to resect the contused vessel completely. In such situations it is preferable to utilize autologous vein from an uninjured extremity, since this graft material has a high patency rate and low infection rate, even in the face of contamination. Repair of a concomitant major venous injury in an extremity results in a higher patency rate for the arterial repair.

Lymphatic Disorders

The lymphatic system serves a number of functions, including drainage of proteins and extracellular fluid that are lost from the capillary circulation and removal of bacteria and foreign materials. Lymphedema occurs in situations of impaired lymph transport and transcapillary fluid exchange. In these situations, production of lymph continues at a constant rate, but drainage is inadequate and protein-rich fluid accumulates. The high osmolality of the lymphatic fluid attracts even greater amounts of extracellular fluid.

Primary lymphedema is classified into *(1) congenital lymphedema,* when the edema is present at birth; *(2) lymphedema praecox,* when edema starts early in life, usually between 10 and 15 years of age; and *(3) lymphedema tarda,* when the onset is after the age of 35. Lymphangiographic appearances further divide primary lymphedema into hyperplasia (usually associated with lymphedema tarda), if numerous large dilated lymphatic vessels are present, and hypoplasia (usually associated with lymphedema praecox), if lymphatics are few in number and small in caliber. *Acquired lymphedema* occurs after recurrent infection, radiation, surgical excision, or neoplastic invasion of regional lymph nodes.

Patients often present with diffuse enlargement of extremities ("milk leg") and localized inflammation. The lymphangitis is a direct result of edema impairing local tissue defenses. With time, the soft "pitting" edema becomes "woody" in character as progressive fibrosis of the connective tissue occurs.

Treatment consists of both medical and surgical management, neither of which can cure the process. Proper support hose, avoidance of prolonged standing, bed elevation at night, diuretics, and meticulous foot care to minimize lymphangitis are the primary medical therapies. Lymphangitis must be treated aggressively with antibiotics, elevation, and bed rest. Patients with recurrent inflammation should be considered candidates for continuing antibiotic therapy. Patients with long standing acquired lymphedema are at risk for developing *lymphosarcoma* and should be examined frequently.

Surgical intervention should be considered only if medical management totally fails. Surgical approaches fall into two categories: reconstruction of lymphatic drainage (lymphangioplasty) or excision of varying amounts of subcutaneous tissue and skin. Unfortunately, results of surgery remain quite disappointing.

Diagnostic Radiology in Vascular Disorders

Arteriograms (also called angiograms) and venograms (also called phlebograms) are invasive procedures and should be employed cautiously. Specific indications for each procedure are discussed previously in this chapter. These studies are generally performed to localize disease, *not* to diagnose it. The history, physical exam, and noninvasive lab studies should be adequate to manage a patient medically in most situations. Contrast studies are the "roadmap" for the surgeon once the vascularization is decided upon. The most commonly used technique for arteriography involves puncture of a peripheral artery with passage of an intravascular catheter for selective injection of arteries (Seldinger technique). The femoral artery is frequently used although axillary and brachial arteries are also employed. Lower extremity venograms are performed by cannulating a foot vein and then injecting contrast. Recently some arteriograms have been performed with intravenous injection of contrast agent and serial computer-aided images of the relevant arteries (intravenous digital angiograms). Contrast agent loads may be slightly higher, which increases nephrotoxicity; imaging is often not as sharp as that seen with arterial injection. However, the avoidance of an arterial puncture may be desirable in patients with advanced arterial occlusive disease.

The principal complications of arteriography include bleeding around the puncture site, thrombosis at the puncture site due to an intimal flap caused by passage of the catheter, hypersensitivity reaction to the iodinated dye, and contrast-related renal toxicity, especially in diabetics. Bleeding may be immediate or delayed and may result in later appearance of a pseudoaneurysm. The initial presentation of local bleeding includes paresthesias in the involved limb due to compression of adjacent nerves. Thrombosis usually occurs within 6 hours of the arterial puncture but may occur days later. Surgical exposure with closure of the puncture site and repair of the injured intima are appropriate and should be performed urgently to avoid later complications.

In patients with known hypersensitivity to iodinated contrast, steroids and antihistamines can be administered before the procedure to decrease the incidence and severity of reactions. All patients should be questioned carefully as to previous allergy prior to undergoing arteriograms or venograms. Hydration before and after arteriography is important in all patients. Judicious use of diuretics has also been shown to decrease nephrotoxicity.

Venograms are less risky procedures. A low incidence of phlebitis ($<3\%$) can be expected if the injected contrast is dilute and is flushed from the veins with heparinized saline after the study is completed. Newer nonionic contrast agents are associated with a decreased incidence of post venography thrombophlebitis.

SUGGESTED READINGS

Atherosclerosis

Ross R: The pathogenesis of atherosclerosis—an update. *New Engl J Med* 314:488–500, 1986.

Aneurysms

Anton GE, Hertzer NR, Beven EG, O'Hara PJ, Krajewski LP: Surgical management of popliteal aneurysms. Trends in presentation, treatment and results from 1952 to 1984. *J Vasc Surg* 3:125–134, 1986.

Crawford ES, Crawford JL, Safi HJ, Coselli JS, Hess KR, Brooks B, Norton HJ, Glaeser DH: Thoracoabdominal aortic aneurysms: preoperative and intraoperative factors determining immediate and long-term results of operations in 605 patients. *J Vasc Surg* 3:389–404, 1986.

Lawrie GM, Crawford ES, Morris GC Jr, Howell JF: Progress in the treatment of ruptured abdominal aortic aneurysm. *World J Surg* 4:653–660, 1980.

Chronic Peripheral Arterial Occlusive Disease

Boyd AM: The natural course of arteriosclerosis of the lower extremities. *Angiology* 11:10–14, 1960.

Cronenwett JL, Warner KG, Zelenock GB, Whitehouse WM Jr, Graham LM, Lindenauer SM, Stanley JC: Intermittent claudication. Current results of nonoperative management. *Arch Surg* 119:430–436, 1984.

Diehl JT, Cali RF, Hertzer NR, Beven EG: Complications of abdominal aortic reconstruction. An analysis of perioperative risk factors in 557 patients. *Ann Surg* 197:49–56, 1983.

Reichle FA, Rankin KP, Tyson, RR, Finestone AJ, Shuman C: Long-term results of 474 arterial reconstructions for severely ischemic limbs: a fourteen year follow-up. *Surgery* 85:93–100, 1979.

Rush DS, Gewertz BL, Lu CT, Ball DG, Zarins CK: Limb salvage in poor-risk patients using transluminal angioplasty. *Arch Surg* 118:1209–1212, 1983.

Szilagyi DE, Elliott JP Jr, Smith RF, Reddy DJ, McPharlin M: A thirty-year survey of the reconstructive surgical treatment of aortoiliac occlusive disease. *J Vas Surg* 3:421–436, 1986.

Acute Arterial Occlusive Disease

Dale WA: Differential management of acute peripheral arterial ischemia. *J Vas Surg* 1:269, 1984.

Cerebrovascular Insufficiency

Pessin MS, Hinton RC, Davis KR, et al: Mechanisms of acute carotid stroke. *Ann Neurol* 6:245–252, 1979.

Thompson JE, Talkington CM: Carotid surgery for cerebral ischemia. *Surg Clin N Am* 59:539–553, 1979.

West H, Burton R, Roon AJ, Malone JM, Goldstone J, Moore WS: Comparative risk of operation and expectant management for carotid artery disease. *Stroke* 10:117–121, 1979.

Pulmonary Embolus, Deep Vein Thrombosis, and Venous Disease

Coon WW: Epidemiology of venous thromboembolism. *Ann Surg* 186:149–164, 1977.

Huss RD, Raskob GE, Hirsh J: Prophylaxis of venous thromboembolism. An overview. *Chest* 89:374S–383S, 1986.

Vasospastic Disorders and Thoracic Outlet Syndrome

Porter JM, Rivers SP, Anderson CJ, Baur GM: Evaluation and management of patients with Raynaud's syndrome. *Am J Surg* 142:183–189, 1981.

Roos DB: The place for scalenectomy and first-rib resection in thoracic outlet syndrome. *Surgery* 92:1077–1085, 1982.

Diagnostic Radiology

Hessell SJ, Adams DF, Abrams HL: Complications of angiography. *Radiology* 138:273–281, 1981.

Skills

The student can perform a complete examination of the vascular system.

1. Demonstrate the use of a unidirectional doppler to:
   A. Auscultate the femoral, popliteal, and pedal arteries.
   B. Auscultate the femoral, popliteal, and axillary veins.
   C. Measure the systolic blood pressure in the arm and ankle.

2. Describe the technique used to puncture a femoral artery for a sample of blood, including necessary equipment and potential complications.

3. Auscultate a carotid artery in a patient with a carotid bruit and describe the bruit in detail.

4. Given a patient with an abdominal aortic aneurysm, measure the size and extent of aneurysm, and compare the measurements with those produced by ultrasound.

5. Given a patient with ischemic rest pain in the foot, demonstrate the physical findings, including dependent rubor, pallor on elevation, and delayed capillary refill.

6. Given a patient with chronic arterial insufficiency, locate and grade all pulses in the extremity.

Study Questions

1. A 55-year-old executive presents with a 7-cm pulsatile mass in the epigastrium unassociated with symptoms. What are the best tests to confirm the diagnosis of abdominal aortic aneurysm? What is the prognosis of a 7-cm abdominal aortic aneurysm? What are the indications and complications of surgical therapy?

2. A 24-year-old man suffers a gunshot wound to his right groin. There is minimal external bleeding. How would you care for the patient? In specific, what diagnostic tests would be indicated? Operation would be appropriate under what circumstances? What are the late complications of untreated vascular injuries?

3. A 34-year-old female complains of acute shortness of breath 5 days after a cholecystectomy. Physical exam reveals only right leg swelling. What diagnostic tests would be needed to define the pathology?

4. A 68-year-old patient presents with sudden onset of left arm weakness that resolves in 1 hr. A bruit is heard in the right cervical area. What noninvasive and invasive diagnostic tests would be indicated to assess the degree of extracranial and intracranial occlusive disease? What are the accepted indications for carotid endarterectomy?

5. An 18-year-old woman complains of chronic right leg swelling without ulceration. How would you determine the etiology of her swelling? What is the differential diagnosis of unilateral leg swelling? How is lymphedema managed?

6. Discuss the evaluation and management of a patient with primary and secondary varicose veins. How would your management change if the patient developed an ulcer in the "gaiter zone"?

7. A 40-year-old man develops paresthesias of the ulnar aspect of the left arm when he raises his arm above his head. How would you evaluate this patient? What is the differential diagnosis of this type of symptom? What are the medical and surgical options for a patient with thoracic outlet syndrome?

26

Transplantation

Mitchell Goldman, M.D.
Thomas G. Peters, M.D.
Bruce Jarrell, M.D.
Steven Leapman, M.D.

ASSUMPTIONS

The student understands the anatomy and physiology of the urinary, pancreatic, pulmonary, hepatic, and cardiac systems.

The student understands the function of the immune system and its role in the rejection of foreign tissue.

OBJECTIVES

1. List the organs and tissues which are currently being transplanted; give the graft survival statistics for organs from related living and cadaver donors.
2. List the criteria for establishing death for the purpose of organ and tissue donation.
3. Given a potential donor, list the acceptable and exclusionary criteria for the donation of each organ and tissue.
4. List the current forms of immunosuppression for transplantation and describe their mechanics of action and specific complications.
5. List the common methods of gaining access to the circulation for the purpose of hemodialysis, chemotherapy, or nutrition; list the advantages and disadvantages of each.
6. Define the following: autograft, isograft, allograft, xenograft, orthotopic, and heterotopic.
7. Describe methods of organ preservation during the interval from harvest to transplantation for kidney, liver, pancreas, heart; list acceptable preservation time intervals.
8. Distinguish between "hyperacute", "accelerated acute", "acute", and "chronic" rejection with regards to pathophysiology, time interval from transplant, histology and prognosis.

Transplantation

The concept of tissue replacement or transplantation is based on the idea that patients with end-stage dis-

ease of critical organs can be kept alive beyond the useful life of these organs and tissues. During the first half of the 20th century, the failure of any organ essential to life was uniformly fatal. However, technology to sustain life despite transient organ failure was slowly developed; early dialysis for acute renal failure and refining of respirators for respiratory insufficiency are two examples. The experimental techniques of organ and tissue transfer were tried in man, mostly in the form of kidney transplantation and skin grafting. The early attempts at kidney transplantation failed because the understanding of immunology did not evolve as rapidly as did the idea of organ replacement. Currently, because of improved understanding of immunology and of organ and tissue preservation, end-stage failure of several organs essential to life no longer dooms the patient to an imminently fatal course; now the techniques of organ transplantation can be successfully applied in many cases. In addition, tissues not vital to life such as cornea, bone, skin, and dura are currently transplantable and have improved the quality of life of numerous individuals.

Organ and Tissue Donation

Organs and tissues for transplantation may come from either cadaver donors or from living relatives. Even though grafts from living related donors may be advantageous because of increased graft survival, ready availability, and immediate graft function, cadaveric donors continue to be the major source of graft tissues for transplant centers. Only kidney, segmental pancreas, and bone marrow grafts can be taken from living relatives; all other organs and tissues are usually procured from a cadaveric donor. Recognition of a potential cadaveric donor is the initial step leading to organ donation. Solid organs can only be transplanted if they have been perfused by an intact cardiovascular system until the time of retrieval; therefore, any patient with normal cardiac function, who has been pronounced "brain dead," is a potential donor. The diagnosis of *brain death* must be made prior to organ harvest. This is usually done by the primary care physician or a neurospecialist. Donors are previously healthy individuals who have sustained irreversible central nervous system injury, either from trauma, cerebrovascular accident, central nervous system tumors, or cerebral anoxia. Contraindications to donation include most chronic medical problems, pre-existing hypertensive cardiovascular disease, malignancy other than primary brain tumors, cardiac arrest resulting in prolonged warm ischemia of organs, and uncontrolled infection. Additionally, the presence of HIV antibody precludes organ donation. The President's Commission for the study of Ethical Problems in Medicine and Biochemical and Behavioral Research agreed upon a definition of brain death and endorsed criteria that serve as guidelines. These guidelines are separated into clinical criteria and confirmatory objective studies. Clinical criteria indicate that the individual is totally unresponsive to stimuli (Table 26.1). Clinical situations that mimic complete unresponsiveness include barbiturate or morphiate overdose, or profound hypothermia, and they must be excluded. Confirmatory studies, while not mandatory, serve to support the diagnosis of brain death. Evaluation of the potential donor requires serial observation over a period of 6–24 hr. During this time, referral by the primary hospital staff to the transplant center is initiated.

For specific organs and tissues, age may be a relative contraindication to organ donation, and acute or chronic diseases affecting certain organs may exclude them from consideration. A history of hepatic disease excludes liver donation, and a history of hepatitis B will exclude most organ and tissue donation.

Pre-existing renal disease excludes kidney donation while diabetes mellitus precludes pancreatic donation. Cardiac trauma, coronary artery disease, pneumonia, or donor age over 35–40 years excludes cardiac and heart-lung donation. Minimal hypertension is a relative contraindication to kidney donation. Severe hypertension is an absolute contraindication to cardiac or renal donation. A laboratory screen is useful to determine organ acceptability (Table 26.2).

Consent for organ or tissue donation is obtained through a signed donor card, a drivers license, a consent statement, a will, or by permission of the next of kin or suitable legal guardian. In medicolegal situations involving medical examiners, permission may also be required from both the medical examiner and the legal guardian. The optimal situation regarding organ donation occurs when the family has previously discussed and agreed upon organ donation. Once the donor is declared brain dead, treatment is directed towards optimizing organ function. Ventilation is maintained with a mechanical respirator and arterial blood gases monitored. Because many closed head injury patients are purposely dehydrated to decrease cerebral edema, vigorous rehydration may be necessary. If vigorous hydration with crystalloid or colloid is inadequate to maintain perfusion, a vasopressor, dopamine or dobutamine, is used. Vasoconstrictors are avoided

Table 26.1.
Criteria to Determine Cessation of Brain Function

Clinical	Confirmatory Tests
1. Absence of spontaneous respirations	1. Disconnecting respirator
2. Absence of pupillary light reflex	2. Electroencephalogram (EEG)
3. Absence of corneal light reflex	3. Radionuclide brain scan
4. Absence of oculocephalic or oculovestibular reflex	4. Cerebral angiography
5. Unresponsiveness to stimuli	
6. Known cause for condition	
7. Duration of condition over time	
8. Known irreversibility	

because of the vasospastic effect on renal and splanchnic beds. Donors developing massive diuresis from diabetes insipidus may require Pitressin. Although oliguria is often corrected with hydration, diuretics (furosemide or mannitol) may help initiate and maintain urinary output. Monitoring of cardiac and pulmonary function is imperative in the case in which a heart, heart-lung or lung donor is considered. Bone, skin, dura, fascia, and eye donors need not have a functioning cardiovascular system and can be procured up to 12 hr after the cessation of cardiac and respiratory function.

Organ Preservation

Effective preservation of whole organs after harvest from the donor ensures the success of cadaveric transplantation by providing time for distant transplant centers to retrieve the needed organs, to perform precise tissue typing and crossmatching between donor and recipient, to prepare the recipient, and to enhance national and international organ sharing programs. The most critical steps in solid organ preservation are rapid

Table 26.2.
Laboratory Studies Used to Determine Acceptability of Organs for Transplantation

Lab Study[a]	Evaluated Organ
Electrocardiogram (ECG)	Heart, Heart-Lung
Chest x-ray	Heart, Lung, Heart-Lung
CPK with MB bands	Heart, Heart-lung
BUN, creatinine	Kidney
Glucose	Pancreas
Liver function tests	Liver
Blood, urine, sputum culture	All
Hepatitis screen	All
RPR/VDRL	All
HIV	All

[a] CPK, creatine phosphokinase; VDRL, serologic test for syphilis.

Table 26.3.
Current Preservation Methods and Durations

Organ	Preservation Method	Typical Solution	Useful Duration
Kidney	Ice slush	Hyperosmotic Hyperkalemic	24–48 hr
	Hypothermic pulsatile preservation	Colloid solution	72 hr
Heart	Ice slush	Crystalloid with/ without cardioplegia	4 hr
Liver	Ice slush	Hyperosmotic Hyperkalemic	9–12 hr
Pancreas	Ice slush	Hyperosmotic Hyperkalemic or silica gel plasma	24 hr
Heart-lung Lung Eyes	Donor transported to transplant center		
Scleral grafts	Frozen	With/without glycerin	Several months
Cornea	Refrigerated Cryopreserved	MK medium	3–14 days Several months
Skin	Cryopreserved Lyophilized	Glycerine, DMSO	Indefinitely
Skeletal tissue	Cryopreserved Lyophilized	Glycerine, DMSO	Indefinitely

organ cooling and sterile storage in a cold environment (Table 26.3).

Kidney, heart, liver, and pancreas are routinely flushed in situ with a cold solution in order to stop metabolism rapidly. In general, hyperosmotic (325–420 mOsm/liter) or hyperkalemic solutions are used. In some situations, a colloid is added. The organs are subsequently removed, packed in sterile containers and placed in ice. Hypothermic (7–10° C) continuous pulsatile perfusion with a colloid solution is used in clinical renal preservation to extend preservation time. Cryopreservation with cryoprotectants, such as glycerine and dimethylsulfoxide (DMSO), and lyophilization are useful in preserving skin, skeletal, and scleral tissues. Nutrient media and normothermic or hypothermic preservation may be used with cornea, skin, cartilage, and bone. Heart-lung and lung donors are currently transported to the transplant center, as immediate implantation is necessary to ensure a functional graft.

Immunology

Transplantation involves a surgical procedure that transfers tissue from one site to another site in the same individual or between different individuals. Classification of transplants is based on genetic relationship and on position in the body. An *autograft* is tissue transferred from one site of the body to another in the same individual such as a skin graft removed from the leg and placed on a wound elsewhere. An *isograft* is tissue that is transferred between genetically identical individuals such as a renal transplant between monozygotic twins. An *allograft* is tissue transplanted between genetically dissimilar individuals of the same species such as a cadaver donor renal transplant. A *xenograft* is tissue transferred between individuals of different species such as porcine skin grafted onto human burn victims. An *orthotopic* graft (orthograft) is an organ placed at the normal anatomic position. It usually necessitates native organ removal, as in cardiac transplantation. *Heterotopic* grafting involves organ placement at a site different from the normal anatomic position, as in renal transplantation.

The success of a transplanted graft depends upon the degree of genetic dissimilarity between the organ and the host, and the effectiveness of the immunosuppressive means used to alter host response. In vitro testing can identify favorable donor-recipient genetic combinations. In addition, the discovery of new immunosuppressive agents has resulted in better graft survival, fewer and less severe rejection episodes, and less risk of infection, leading to an improved outlook for patients requiring transplantation.

Immune competence in man is primarily based upon preformed humoral antibody responses. Antibodies are immunoglobulins produced primarily by B lymphocytes responding to foreign antigen. Antibodies may be present at birth (ABH blood group antibodies) or may be acquired. For successful transplantation, *ABO blood group compatibility* is required for organs expressing ABO antigens (kidney and heart). If ABO blood group directed antibodies are present in the blood infusing an organ containing one or more of these antigens, antibody-mediated killing of the endothelium results in thrombosis and organ necrosis. Acquired antibodies directed against human leukocyte antigens (HLA system) may form as a result of blood transfusions, pregnancy, or previously transplanted organs. These antibodies are complement dependent and are cytotoxic to tissue with similar surface antigens. Recipient serum must be tested for the presence of these antibodies by a microcytotoxicity test using lymphocytes of the donor as target antigens. If recipient antibodies are present, lymphocyte killing takes place (positive crossmatch). If certain organs are transplanted in the presence of a positive crossmatch, circulating antibodies attach to the donor organ endothelium and, in the presence of complement, destroy the organ. The presence of incompatible ABO blood groups or preformed complement-dependent antibody directed toward donor tissue usually are a contraindication to transplantation.

The genetic loci for both humoral and cellular immune responsiveness are located on the short arm of the sixth chromosome. These loci are responsible for two classes of histocompatibility molecules. Class I antigens are single chain polypeptides and are cataloged as HLA, B, or C. These antigens are present on all nucleated cells and are inherited in an autosomal codominant fashion. The sub loci are genetically transferred as haplotypes on a single segment of chromosome. Thus, a recipient shares one of two haplotypes with each parent. Following Mendelian genetics, a recipient has a 25% chance of sharing two haplotypes, a 50% chance of sharing one haplotype, and a 25% chance of not sharing a haplotype with a sibling. Unrelated individuals randomly share similar antigens. Class I antigens play an important role in the antigen recognition phase of cellular immunity. They are detected by a serologic test using lymphocytes and a known panel of antisera in a complement-dependent microcytotoxicity test. In living related donor kidney transplants, these antigens have a very strong correlation with graft success.

Class II antigens are glycoproteins that consist of two polymeric chains, each containing a common subunit. These antigens are present on B lymphocytes, dendritic cells, endothelial cells and monocytes. There are currently several series within this HLA locus including the HLA-D locus and the HLA-Dr locus. The antigens are responsible for the cellular arm of the immune response and are defined by the mixed lymphocyte culture test (MLC). The MLC is a strong predictor of success in living related renal transplants. It requires 5–7 days to perform and is, therefore, not useful in cadaver transplants, especially cardiac, liver, and pancreatic transplants. The HLA-Dr locus correlates with the D locus and can be evaluated by a serologic test. In renal transplants, Dr-matched cadaver donor transplants have an approximately 20% advantage in graft success when compared to Dr-unmatched transplants. Since heart, liver and lung transplants require cadaveric donors, and since preservation time is significantly shorter than in renal transplantation, ABO matching and crossmatching are the tests performed most often prior to transplantation. In some instances, even crossmatching has been disregarded when an emergency transplant is performed. Pancreatic transplants, when a living, related donor is being used, are generally evaluated using an MLC reaction. Bone, skin, dura, and other cryopreserved or lyophilized tissues generally do not require typing and crossmatching prior to transplantation, as it seems that they have very weak immunogenic activity after preservation. There are reports of better results with corneal transplants after HLA matching.

Immunologic Events Following Transplantation

Rejection, the immunologic attempt to destroy foreign tissue following transplantation, is a complex and incompletely understood event. Four types of clinically identified rejection occur and are classified by the time of occurrence and by the immune mechanism involved.

Hyperacute rejection occurs minutes to several hours following graft implantation. The organ becomes flaccid, cyanotic, and, in the case of the kidney, anuric. Histologically, polymorphonuclear leukocytes are packed in the pericapillary area and endothelial necrosis with vascular thrombosis is present. Hyperacute rejection is associated with the presence of preformed antibodies directed toward either ABO blood group or HLA antigens. It rarely occurs today because crossmatching and blood group matching are performed.

Accelerated acute rejection occurs during the first several days following transplantation. In the kidney it is characterized by oliguria and may be accompanied by disseminated intravascular coagulation, thrombocytopenia, and hemolysis. The organ becomes swollen and congested. Histologically, extensive arteriolar necrosis and perivasculitis are present. Immunologically, it is felt to represent a second set of anamnestic responses mediated by both antibodies and lymphocytes. Usually the antibody crossmatch is negative but may become positive following the rejection. When a preformed antibody is present, it may be at a low or undetectable level such that a pretransplant crossmatch would be negative. This type of rejection is rare and there is no effective treatment.

Acute rejection occurs in up to 90% of cadaver donor transplants and may even occur in well-matched living, related donor transplants. Acute rejection is clinically characterized by organ failure. Microscopically, there is T lymphocyte infiltration into vascular and interstitial spaces. In the kidney, glomeruli are often spared relative to other regions. In the heart, the infiltrate is generally pericapillary and is associated with interstitial edema and myonecrosis. In the liver, the infiltrate is often in the area of the vascular triad. This type of rejection is treatable with increased doses of immunosuppressant; if it is reversed, the patient has an excellent chance of retaining the graft. Repeated acute rejections may ultimately damage the organ.

Chronic rejection is a slow, progressive immunologic destruction over a period of months to years, characterized by vascular intimal hyperplasia, lymphocytic infiltration, and atrophy and fibrosis of renal, cardiac, or hepatic tissue. Immunologically, chronic rejection is mediated by both humoral and cellular elements through poorly understood mechanisms and is unaltered by increased immunosuppression.

Immunosuppressive Drug Therapy

Even in a perfectly matched living related renal transplant, immunosupression is necessary to prevent rejection (Table 26.4). All immunosuppressive drugs have the common side effect of diminution of resistance to infection. Not only are the usual bacterial infections common, but opportunistic infections, such as fungal and viral infections including cytomegalovirus and other herpes viruses, are more prevalent. Immunosurveillance against tumors is also impaired resulting in a 10–100-fold increased incidence of tumors, especially lymphomas.

Table 26.4.
Immunosuppression Methods in Renal Transplantation

Pharmacologic	Biologic	Other
Azathioprine	Blood transfusion	Radiation
Cyclophosphamide	Antilymphocyte	a. Total body
Cyclosporine	serum or globulin	b. Selected port
Methylprednisolone	Antithymocyte	c. Graft
	globulin	
Sodium succinate	Monoclonal OKT$_3$	Splenectomy
Prednisone		Plasmapheresis
		Thoracic duct drainage

Azathioprine is the drug first used routinely in clinical renal transplantation. It is an antimetabolite and is metabolized to its active form, 6-mercaptopurine, by the liver. Its principle action is inhibition of nucleic acid synthesis, thus inhibiting T lymphocyte differentiation. The usual dose is 1–3 mg/kg of body weight orally, and this dosage must be continued for the life of the organ graft. Its major side effect is bone marrow suppression manifested by leukopenia or thrombocytopenia that may be corrected by reduction of dose. Hepatitis has also been attributed to azathioprine.

Prednisone or its equivalent is used in nearly all whole organ transplants in combination with either azathioprine or cyclosporine. Its mechanism of action is not fully known, but it is a nonspecific inhibitor of both cell-mediated and humoral immunity. It is administered in varying doses ranging from 0.5–2 mg/kg of body weight per day initially and tapered to lower doses over several months after transplantation. It is also used in high doses in the treatment of acute rejection. Complications specific to steroids include the development of peptic ulcer disease, cataracts, aseptic necrosis of the joints, colonic perforation, and Cushing's syndrome.

Antilymphocyte globulin is a material prepared by immunizing an animal, such as a horse, with human lymphocytes. Specific antilymphocyte sera are being developed using monoclonal antibodies. In humans, antilymphocyte globulin is directed specifically toward T lymphocytes, reducing the peripheral blood T lymphocyte level to less than 1% from the normal 60–70% of circulating lymphocyte level. Some centers have demonstrated a protective effect when given prophylactically at the initiation of transplantation, but its most effective use appears to be in treatment of acute rejection, eliminating the toxicity associated with high dose steroid therapy. Antilymphocyte globulin is associated with a modest increase in viral infections, particularly cytomegalovirus, and anaphylaxis may occasionally result from the presence of preformed antibodies directed toward horse, rabbit or goat antigens. Monoclonal antibodies, made from hybridomas of mouse myeloma cells, have been successfully used in the treatment of rejection and, most recently, as prophylaxis against rejection in cardiac transplants. OKT$_3$, a monoclonal antibody against the T cell receptor, has been extremely successful in abrogating steroid-resis-

tant rejection. *Cyclophosphamide* is an alkylating agent which blocks the development of immunoblasts and the differentiation of T and B lymphocytes. It is not often used in transplantation. It is, however, useful in patients who develop severe hepatotoxicity from azathioprine therapy. Myelosuppression and hemorrhagic cystitis are complications associated with cyclophosphamide.

Cyclosporine is an undecapeptide which blocks the production and the secretion of interleukin 2, a T cell growth factor elaborated by helper T cells exposed to foreign HLA-D antigen. It prevents the proliferation and maturation of cytotoxic T lymphocytes responsible for graft rejection. The dose may range from 5–15 mg/kg tailored to trough blood levels monitored by radioimmunoassay or by high pressure liquid chromatography. Cyclosporine is a potent immunosuppressive drug in renal, hepatic, pancreatic, heart, and heart-lung transplantation, improving graft survival by 10–30% and is used in combination with a much reduced dose of steroids. It is associated with significant "acute and chronic" nephrotoxicity which may be minimized by regulating serum levels. However, some patients must be taken off the drug because of significant renal impairment. In renal transplantation, it may be clinically difficult to distinguish nephrotoxicity from acute rejection. Renal biopsies are performed but are often not diagnostic because the classic cellular infiltrate of rejection is not always present. Other side effects are hirsutism, gingival hyperplasia, hypertension, hyperkalemia, hepatotoxicity, and breast fibroadenomas. The incidence of lymphoma and other neoplasms is similar to that of other immunosuppressive drugs.

Blood transfusions given prior to a first cadaver renal transplant or prior to a cardiac transplant are associated with a 20% increase in graft survival. The transfusion effect may represent active enhancement. Prior to renal transplantation routine blood transfusion for patients awaiting transplant is often followed. Transmission of hepatitis and presensitization to HLA antigens resulting in a small percentage of patients having difficulty in crossmatching may result. In living, related renal transplants, donor-specific transfusion is effective in single haplotype, highly reactive, MLC, living, related pairs with a 90% overall 1-year renal allograft survival.

Kidney Transplantation

End-stage renal failure therapy commonly involves the chronic use of either hemodialysis or peritoneal dialysis to maintain life. The principle of dialysis is simple: on one side of the semipermeable membrane is the extracellular fluid of the patient; on the other side of the membrane is material that is to be discarded. Products of normal metabolism not excreted by the failed kidney accumulate in the extracellular fluid, are passed through the semipermeable membrane to the dialysate solution, and are artificially excreted. Hemodialysis requires connection of the patient's vascular space to a

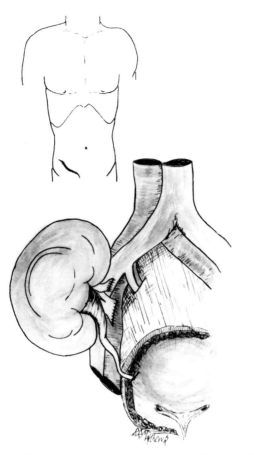

Figure 26.1. The heterotopic human renal allograft in the right extraperitoneal iliac fossa. The renal artery and vein anastomoses are end-to-side, respectively, to the external iliac artery and vein. A tunneled ureteroneocystostomy allows entirely normal micturition.

dialysis machine. In acute situations, large cannulae are inserted into the venous circulation by femoral or subclavian vessels. For chronic hemodialysis, permanent access to the circulation involves connecting an artery to a vein, in an easily accessible and reusable area, such as the radial artery and cephalic vein at the wrist or brachial artery and cephalic vein just above the anteromedial elbow joint. A vascular conduit of polytetrafluoroethylene, dacron, or bovine arterial grafts may be placed in a subcutaneous tunnel with one end sewn to an artery and the other to a vein to provide the large caliber fistula for hemodialysis. In peritoneal dialysis, access to the peritoneal membrane requires a transabdominal indwelling catheter that can be used for infusion and drainage of dialysate fluid. Most hemodialysis and peritoneal catheter placement procedures are performed under local anesthesia. Postoperative complications involve infection of synthetic or foreign material as well as clotting or aneurysm of the vascular access, dysfunction of the peritoneal dialysis catheter, and peritonitis. The large numbers of patients on chronic dialysis (over 50,000 in the United States) attest to the efficacy of the surgical procedures that permit dialysis therapy.

A patient with end-stage renal failure from any cause may be a transplant candidate regardless of the type or duration of dialysis support. The acceptable age range for kidney recipients varies from 1–60 years, although infants and those over age 60 have been successfully transplanted. The patient should be free of infections and should be free of cancer for at least 5 years. Patients with localized cancers such as skin cancer may be transplanted after successful excision. Other chronic disease processes must be minor, self-limiting, or under control; for example, the patient with known coronary artery disease should be optimally treated and demonstrate cardiovascular stability before undergoing renal transplantation.

Kidney transplantation is nearly always a heterotopic allograft, placed in the extraperitoneal iliac fossa (Fig. 26.1). The renal artery and vein are sewn to a corresponding iliac vessel and the ureter is implanted in the urinary bladder. Technical variations are common and include intra-abdominal graft placement in infants and small children, as well as donor-to-recipient, ureter to ureter anastomosis instead of transplant ureter to recipient bladder ureteroneocytostomy.

Treatment of the renal transplant recipient involves methods used for any operative procedure as well as those specific to the patient receiving a transplant. Ambulation, diet, and medication orders are much the same as for patients having operations such as herniorrhaphy or appendectomy. Early postgraft care involves hourly monitoring of vital signs and urine output. When urine volume exceeds 500 ml hourly, attention to serum electrolytes aids appropriate fluid replacement. Immunosuppression for renal transplantation varies from center to center. Acute rejection is common and is treated by modification of the immune response to prevent graft loss while allowing for suitable host defense mechanisms to allay severe, acute infections. Signs and symptoms of acute rejection include increasing serum creatinine, proteinuria, hypertension, fever, decreasing urine output, and occasionally low-grade abdominal pain. Usually several days of intravenous Solumedrol® therapy are given. Acute rejection in renal transplantation is generally reversible.

The results of kidney transplantation have improved since 1975. Functional graft survival of 70–80% for cadaveric kidneys and 95% for living, related donor organs at 1 year is now common. In addition, patient survival now exceeds 95% at 1 year. Death due to infection has fallen drastically. These improvements are due to better preparation of the end-stage renal failure patient with refined dialysis techniques, blood transfusions, and pharmacologic measures, and to recognition of the limits of antirejection therapy. Overuse of immunosuppressive therapy does not result in better graft survival and is detrimental to patient survival. Renal allograft loss requires return to dialysis, but often second and subsequent renal allografts are performed successfully.

Complications of renal transplantation fall into two categories; complications of the transplant itself, and nonrenal complications (Table 26.5). Both types of complications have early and late components. Early

Table 26.5.
Complications of Renal Transplantation

	Early	Late
Renal	Massive diuresis	Ureteric stenosis
	Ureter anastomotic leak	Vascular anastomotic
	Hemorrhage	stenosis-aneurysm
	Lymphocele	Recurrent primary re-
	Rejection	nal disease
	Rupture	
Nonrenal	Infection	Infections
	Myocardial infarction	Progressive athero-
	Peptic ulcer disease	sclerotic vascular
	Thromboembolic disorders	disorders, hyper-
	Steroid-induced acne	tension
		Diabetes mellitus
		Aseptic joint necrosis
		Cataract
		Cushings syndrome

complications of kidney transplantation include excessive diuresis, urinary leak or fistula, hemorrhage, vascular anastomotic leak or thrombosis, formation of perigraft lymphocele, graft rupture, and severe rejection. Late complications related to the graft include stenosis of the ureter or renal artery and recurrent disease in the kidney transplant. The latter problem, most common with focal glomerular sclerosis and systemic diseases such as diabetes, is fortunately infrequent (less than 5%). Perigraft infection occurs both early and late. Nonrenal complications occurring early are infections or cardiovascular events, such as postoperative myocardial infarction, cerebrovascular accident, and deep vein thrombophlebitis. Late problems unrelated to the kidney include infection, peptic ulcer disease, aseptic joint necrosis, cataracts, diabetes mellitus, hypertension, liver disease, and the risk of neoplasia that accompanies immunosuppression. Kidney transplant recipients are generally treated prophylactically for ulcer disease by a surgical approach or given an H_2 receptor blocker after transplantation. Infections are the most commonly encountered complications. They may

Table 26.6.
Indications for Liver Transplantation

Adult	End-stage liver failure from
	Primary biliary cirrhosis
	Sclerosing cholangitis
	Budd-Chiari syndrome
	Ethanol abuse (no alcohol prior 12 months)
Child	Progressive liver or metabolic failure from
	Biliary atresia
	α_1-antitrypsin disease
	Wilson's disease
Adult and child	Life-threatening or end-stage liver failure from
	Hepatitis
	Acute, irreversible toxic liver damage
	Primary hepatic tumor confined to liver

be common infections, such as pneumococcal pneumonia or they may be unusual, such as a necrotizing fasciitis from a rare fungus. Organisms which cause clinical infection in the immunosuppressed host include cytomegalovirus (mouth and gastrointestinal tract), common bacteria, fungi, and protozoa such as *Pneumocystis carinii*.

While complications do occur, kidney transplantation remains the model of solid organ replacement therapy. Currently done in over 6000 patients annually in the United States, results of kidney transplantation from both cadaver donors and living related donors are improving. The advent of cyclosporine and refined use of other immunosuppressive agents have made kidney transplantation a safe and effective method for treating end-stage renal failure.

Liver Transplantation

The patient who is considered a liver transplant candidate has a life expectancy of 1 year or less, is between 1 and 55 years of age, and is free of extrahepatic malignancy and infection. Transplantation is best carried out prior to the onset of terminal events associated with end-stage liver failure. The patient who is in and out of hepatic coma is a poor candidate for liver transplantation because metabolic problems, including coagulopathy, often preclude a successful operation. The patient who has known significant liver disease but has not reached terminal phases has an excellent chance of surviving the procedure. Specific indications for liver transplantation include chronic active hepatitis, sclerosing cholangitis, primary biliary cirrhosis, and the Budd-Chiari syndrome (Table 26.6). Certain centers are replacing livers when a primary hepatic cancer is confined to that organ, while others will not accept such cases in the belief that patients with malignancy are poor candidates for any organ replacement therapy. The use of liver transplantation for alcoholic cirrhosis has produced good results in compliant patients.

Liver transplantation uses the whole liver from a cadaver donor and is nearly always an orthotopic graft. Removal of the recipient native liver begins while the donor liver is being removed. Once native hepatectomy is completed, the new liver is implanted by sewing the suprahepatic vena cava to the cuff of the remaining suprahepatic vena cava, and performing an infrahepatic vena caval anastomosis (Fig. 26.2). The hepatic artery is sewn to the hepatic artery of the recipient, and the donor portal vein is sewn to the recipient portal vein. Biliary drainage is commonly achieved by duct-to-duct anastomosis in the adult and Roux-en-Y choledochojejunostomy in the child.

Patient and graft survival in liver transplantation is approaching 85% at 1 year for patients who are operated on before the terminal phases of their disease. In patients in hepatic coma, survival statistics for both the operation and the postoperative period are poor. Less than one half of these patients live to 1 year beyond the time of transplant because of the complicated

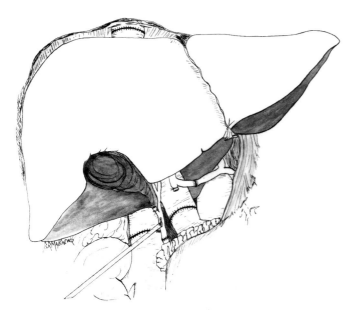

Figure 26.2. The orthotopic human hepatic allograft. End-to-end vascular anastomosis connects donor and recipient hepatic artery, portal vein, and vena cavae in both supra- and infrahepatic locations. The common bile duct-to-duct anastomosis shown is that most commonly in use.

course following major surgery in the face of acutely life threatening hepatic failure. The complications of liver transplantation include perioperative complications of hemorrhage, bleeding disorders, vascular thrombosis, and leaks or strictures of the biliary tract. Perihepatic infection and transient organ system failure, including respiratory, renal and cardiac, often accompany the post-transplant course. Acute rejection does occur but usually is less frequent and milder than rejection seen in kidney transplantation. Cyclosporine has been more successful in preventing liver rejection than it has been for other organs. Late complications of liver transplantation include stenosis of the biliary tree, recurrent hepatitis, ongoing chronic rejection, and toxicity from cyclosporine or other immunosuppressive drug therapy.

Heart and Heart-Lung Transplantation

The indication for heart transplantation is end-stage cardiac failure in a patient who is less than 55 years old and is expected to die from heart disease within 6 months. The patient must be free of infection and malignant neoplasm and must have a chance for full rehabilitation. Currently, diabetics are excluded from cardiac transplantation. Specific indications for heart transplantation include idiopathic cardiomyopathy, viral cardiomyopathy, ischemic cardiac disease, postpartum cardiac disease, terminal cardiac valvular disease, and hypertensive cardiomyopathy. In general, cardiac transplantation is most often performed in adults, since congenital cardiac problems are usually amenable to operative correction. A heart-lung transplant is performed when severe pulmonary vascular disease accompanies cardiac disease.

The usual cardiac transplant is an orthotopic allograft. The recipient heart is removed and the donor heart is sewn into place by attaching the left and right atria of the donor heart to the residual left and right atria of the recipient. The pulmonary artery and aortic anastomoses are completed (Fig. 26.3). The heart is resuscitated and allowed to take over support of the recipient. In some centers, heterotopic grafts are performed. Heterotopic grafts allow the recipient's own heart to remain as a safety net in case the donor heart is rejected.

The outcome of cardiac transplantation has improved over the course of the last two decades. With the use of cyclosporine and endomyocardial biopsy for the diagnosis of rejection, the 1-year graft and patient survival is 80%. Rejection can be diagnosed only by an endomyocardial biopsy that is obtained through a centrally-placed venous access line. The small number of heart-lung transplants performed currently does not allow a projection of statistical survival. However, approximately 70% of the currently performed grafts survive for 1 year.

The complications of cardiac transplantation are largely those of infection and rejection with ensuing progressive cardiac failure. In heart-lung transplants a restrictive fibrosis of the lung has also been described. Early postoperative problems in addition to infection

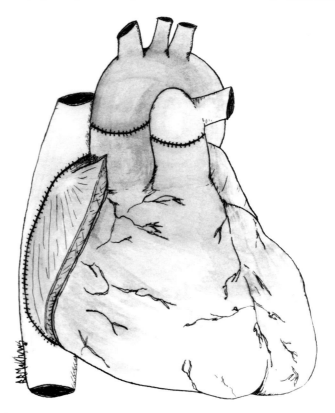

Figure 26.3. The orthotopic human cardiac allograft. The left and right atria of the graft are sutured to the posterior-most atrial walls, which remain intact in the recipient. End-to-end anastomoses of the pulmonary artery and aorta are completed prior to resuscitating the transplanted heart and terminating cardiopulmonary bypass support.

include respiratory, renal, and cerebrovascular complications. Later problems seem limited particularly to chronic rejection of the allograft as well as the long term effects of immunosuppressive therapy. Accelerated coronary artery disease occurs in some patients and may be related to chronic rejection. Retransplantation for this problem has been performed as well as percutaneous transluminal angioplasty.

Pancreas Transplantation

Pancreas transplantation has been performed in patients with complications of severe diabetes. Done largely for the patient who has progressive diabetic vascular disease that will lead to the loss of limb or loss of vision, pancreas transplantation has also been deemed appropriate in many patients with decreasing renal function secondary to renal diabetic angiopathy. A functioning pancreatic allograft allays the progressive destruction that severe diabetes mellitus causes in cardiovascular, renal, ophthalmic, and other tissues. Islet cell transplantation is not currently effective.

Partial and whole organ pancreatic transplantation using a variety of techniques has been performed with many technical problems. The current method most widely applied in pancreas transplantation uses the tail of the pancreas transplanted either at the iliac vessels or in the femoral triangle. The splenic artery and vein are used for revascularization. The duct is either obliterated or the proximal part is anastomosed to a jejunal segment. The duodenum is anastomosed to the bladder. In the latter technique, urinary amylase, serum glucose, and insulin levels may be followed to diagnose rejection.

The complications of pancreatic transplantation include perigraft infection and hemorrhage, vascular thrombosis, rejection, and pancreatic enzyme secretion resulting in tissue digestion. Of those recent pancreatic transplants done since the advent of cyclosporine, more than two-thirds have functioned for 1 year or more. Although graft loss from technical causes is fairly high in pancreatic transplantation, graft loss appears to be primarily due to rejection, because the pancreas is a highly immunogenic organ. When the duodenum has been anastomosed to the bladder, balanitis and metabolic disorders have been the most frequent additional complications.

Other Organs

Currently allografts of bone marrow, parathyroid tissue, bone, skin, and lung have been occasionally successful. The use of cyclosporine, especially for lung and bone marrow transplantation, has allowed these procedures to gain promise. The development of small intestinal transplantation is proceeding in the laboratory; so far the clinical application of this therapy has been uniformly unsuccessful. Allografts of skin, bone, fascia, dura, endocrine organs, eyes and blood vessels are used clinically in a variety of situations or are being investigated in several centers.

SUGGESTED READINGS

Black PMcL: Brain death. *New Engl J Med* 299:338–344, 393–400, 1978.

Calne RY: Liver grafting. *Transplantation* 35:109–111, 1983.

Cohen DJ, Loertscher R, Rubin M, Tilney NL, Carpenter CB, Strom TB: Cyclosporine: a new immunosuppressive agent for organ transplantation. *Ann Internal Med* 101:667–682, 1984.

Copeland JG, Mammana RB, Fuller JK, Campbell DW, McAleer MJ, Sailer JA: Heart transplantation four years' experience with conventional immunosuppression. *JAMA* 251:1563–1566, 1984.

Evans RW, Manninen DL, Garrison LP, Hart LG, Blagg CR, Gutman RA, Hull AR, Lowrie EG: The quality of life of patients with end-stage renal disease. *New Eng J Med* 312:553–559, 1985.

Morris PJ: *Kidney Transplantation Principles and Practice.* New York, Academic Press—Grune & Stratton, 1979.

Simmons RL, Finch ME, Ascher NL, Najarian JS: *Manual of Vascular Access Organ Donation and Transplantation.* Springer-Verlag, New York, 1984.

Spees EK, Sanfilippo F, Goldman MH, Peters TG, Reitz BA, Vaughn WK: A comparison of kidney, heart, and other organ procurement and sharing—The SEOPF experience. *Heart Transpl* 2:212–218, 1983.

Sutherland DER: Minnesota experience with 85 pancreas transplants between 1978 and 1983. *World J Surg* 8:244–252, 1984.

Wilson SE, Owens ML: *Vascular Access Surgery.* Chicago, Year Book Medical Publishers, 1980.

Study Questions

1. A 45-year-old male is involved in a motor vehicle accident in which he suffered a closed head injury. He may be a potential organ donor. How would you determine whether he is an acceptable donor? What are brain death criteria? What organs or tissues may be transplanted?

2. A multiple organ donor is available. What immunologic matching should be done for the following organs or tissues: kidney, liver, pancreas, heart, lung, bone, and skin? Explain the methods of preservation and the limits of preservation for each organ or tissue.

3. A person would like to receive a living, related renal transplant from one of his four siblings. What matching tests are done? How is the donor evaluated? What are the graft survival statistics for cadaver and living, related transplants?

4. What are the recipient criteria for cardiac, pancreatic, and hepatic transplantation?

5. Discuss the types, mechanisms of action, uses and complications of the various immunosuppressive agents available.

6. A 35-year-old female has a creatinine clearance of 8 ml/min. What are the options for the treatment of her end-stage renal disease?

27 Malignant Diseases of the Skin

Nicholas P. Lang, M.D., *Harold I. Freeman, M.D.,*
J. M. Stair, M.D., R. D. Degges, M.D.,
C. Thompson, M.D., H. Garner, M.D.,
G. F. Baker, M.D., Kent C. Westbrook, M.D.,
and Peter C. Haines, M.D.

ASSUMPTIONS

The student understands the anatomy of the skin and subcutaneous tissue.

The student understands the anatomy and function of the immune system.

The student understands the pathologic difference between benign and malignant nevi.

OBJECTIVES

1. List the predisposing factors for and four categories of melanoma.
2. List four signs and symptoms of a malignant nevus.
3. Outline the steps for confirming a diagnosis and the extent of malignant melanoma.
4. On the basis of the extent of a malignant nevus, differentiate the malignant potential and prognosis.
5. Outline the local, regional, and systemic therapies for malignant melanoma.
6. Describe the etiology and incidence of basal and squamous cell carcinomas.
7. Discuss the clinical characteristics, treatment methods, and prognosis for basal and squamous cell carcinomas.

Nearly every individual has from nine to fifteen freckles, moles, or other abberrations of the skin. While the most common malignant tumor in the United States is a skin cancer, it is impractical to remove every lesion from every individual. Fortunately, the vast majority are benign and in many cases the lesions are only of cosmetic importance. Many patients, however, raise questions about the malignant potential of these skin lesions and whether they should be removed. It is for this reason that every physician be aware of the characteristics associated with malignant lesions of the skin in order that appropriate therapy be instituted in a timely fashion. The general characteristics of malignant lesions are listed in Table 27.1 and should be committed to memory.

Basal Cell and Squamous Cell Carcinomas

Etiology and Incidence

There is a growing awareness in the United States of the importance of physical fitness. The potential benefits of exercise in reducing the risks of serious cardiovascular disease has lead to increased numbers of joggers and participants in other physically active sports. However, concomitant with the desire to increase physical fitness is a preoccupation with the maintenance of a youthful and attractive appearance. A "healthy" suntan often is equated psychologically with body youthfulness, sensuality, and success. Unfortunately, just as the link between cigarette smoking and carcinoma of the lung has been firmly established, there is clear evidence that cancer of the skin has, as one of its etiologies, chronic exposure to sunlight.

Approximately 300,000 new cases of nonmelanoma

Table 27.1.
Characteristics of Malignant Skin Lesions

1. Change in pigment (darker or lighter)
2. Rapid growth
3. Bleeding
4. Crusting
5. Serous exudate
6. Loss of skin appendages, hair follicles, etc.
7. Satellite nodules
8. Regional lymphadenopathy
9. Raised border
10. Central ulceration
11. Pain, itching, or other discomfort
12. Inflammatory areolae
13. Rubbery texture

skin cancers are diagnosed annually, compared to 14,000 cases of melanoma. Thus, roughly one-third of all new cancers in man are skin cancers, and the vast majority are either squamous or basal cell carcinomas. These figures represent a 15–20% increase over the incidence reported only a decade earlier according to the National Cancer Institute. Of the two most common lesions, basal cell carcinoma (BCC) predominates (80%) over squamous cell carcinoma (SCC) (20%) in incidence. Fortunately, these nonmelanoma neoplasms have cure rates as high as 97% with present therapeutic modalities. However, approximately 1,600 people die annually from nonmelanoma-derived skin cancers. If one considers that the skin is the most easily accessible portion of the body for diagnostic observation, and that early diagnosis of skin malignancies facilitates treatment and cure, it behooves the physician to be able to recognize these tumors and their potentially premalignant precursors clinically in order to institute prompt therapy. Although skin cancers may remain curable as they increase in size, the cosmetic and functional deformity resulting from the excision of a large tumor, may make reconstruction of the defect a formidable challenge (Figs. 27.1–27.5). Furthermore, while BCC rarely metastasize, large SCC clearly have metastatic potential.

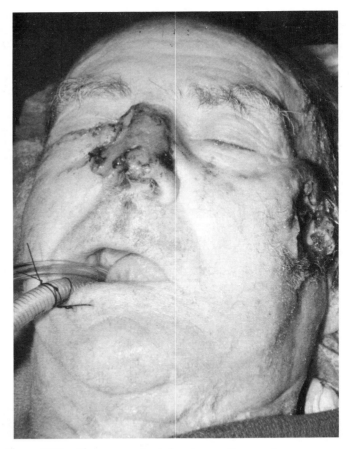

Figure 27.2. The same patient showing another synchronous squamous cell cancer of the nose eroding through the entire nasal skin and portions of the cartilage.

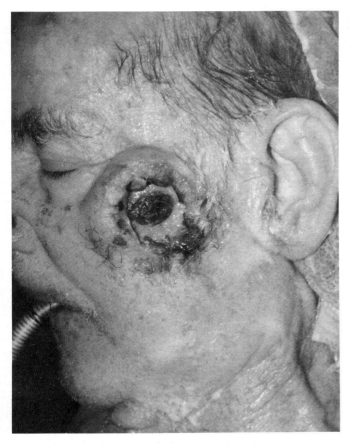

Figure 27.1. Approximately 79-year-old male with large neglected squamous cell carcinoma of the left cheek. The tumor extends in depth almost to the periosteum of the zygomatic bone.

A variety of etiologic factors have been implicated in the development of basal and squamous cell carcinomas. The most frequently associated factor is solar radiation, especially ultraviolet light in the spectrum of 290–320 nm. Thus, physicians practicing in areas of greatest solar exposure tend to encounter a larger group of patients with basal and squamous carcinomas. The cumulative effect of the radiation induces irreversible epidermal damage and the tumors are often observed in association with other skin changes caused by solar radiation: wrinkling, telangiectasias (dilated blood vessels), actinic keratosis (erythematous, gritty-surfaced lesions), and solar elastosis (yellowish papules). Given the relationship to sun exposure, it is not surprising that approximately 80–90% of the tumors are located in the head and neck area and the backs of hands.

Genetic and ethnic factors as reflected in skin complexion play an important predisposing role in the development of SCC and BCC. Fair-skinned caucasians with light hair and eye color are at greater risk than those with darker pigmentation. These tumors are unusual in black patients. Melanin may, therefore, afford a protective function to the potential damage induced by solar radiation. Another example of genetic influence is the condition xeroderma pigmentosum, which

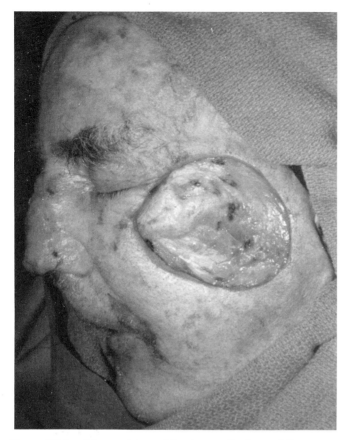

Figure 27.3. After excision of the tumor. Portions of the zygoma can be seen in the area near the lateral aspect of the eye.

using the x-ray equipment without appropriate protection, and in patients who were once treated for benign skin conditions, such as acne with x-radiation.

Basal Cell Carcinoma

Clinical and Histopathologic Characteristics. Basal cell carcinoma arises from the basal layer of germinating cells of the skin epithelium or from epthelial appendages such as hair follicles or sebaceous glands. Generally, the lesions grow slowly and are nonaggressive. However, if the tumor is left untreated, it will destroy normal tissues in its growth path, including cartilage. Another characteristic of the tumor is its tendency to spread microscopically a significant distance beyond the visible lesion. Although a number of descriptive forms have been proposed based on appearance, only three major varieties will be discussed here.

Nodular basal cell carcinoma: The typical early lesion begins as a smooth, dome-shaped, round, waxy, or pearly appearing papule (Fig. 27.7). It may take as long as 1 year to double in size. It may have telangiectasias on the surface that bleed readily when traumatized. As the tumor enlarges, the center tends to undergo necrosis forming a central ulcer with invasion into deep structure (Fig. 27.8). The tumor is then referred to as a ''rodent ulcer'' and becomes more difficult to irradicate. If the tumor is not adequately treated, it may erode into the deep structures including the skull, orbit, or brain.

Pigmented basal cell carcinoma: This lesion is similar to the nodular form, except that it contains melanocytes

is a rare genetically transmitted disease characterized by faulty DNA repair of ultraviolet damage. Patients with this abnormality eventually develop numerous cutaneous neoplasms (Fig. 27.6).

The incidence of tumor increases with age. Most patients are over 65 years old at the time of diagnosis. There is a three-to-one predominance of these tumors in men, possibly related to employment patterns requiring greater sun exposure. Certain chemicals, such as arsenicals, are associated with skin cancers and the first demonstration of a specific cause for cancer is credited to Pott in 1775 when he showed a relationship between soot and carcinoma of the scrotum in chimney sweepers. SCC, also called epidermoid carcinoma, may arise in chronic burn scars. Marjolin (1828) described the process of malignant ulceration in burn scars and hence these lesions are commonly referred to as Marjolin's ulcers. Carcinomas developing in burn scars are aggressive tumors, and can be rapidly lethal. Epidermoid carcinoma may also develop within chronic draining skin sinuses and fistulas, as seen, for example at the site of a chronic osteomyelitis infection. These tumors also tend to be highly malignant.

Although less commonly observed today, radiation is another physical agent responsible for the production of malignant skin tumors, usually SCC. This phenomenon is particularly true for dentists and physicians

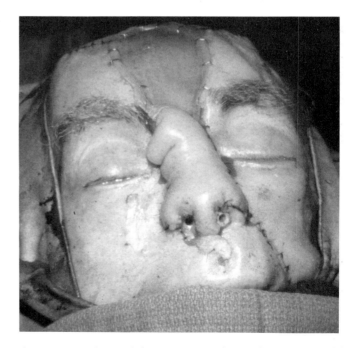

Figure 27.4. The nasal skin was removed, as well as portions of the nasal cartilages. The nose was reconstructed with a forehead flap and left nasolabial flap. The resulting forehead defect was covered with a split thickness skin graft and the cheek defect was repaired also with a skin graft.

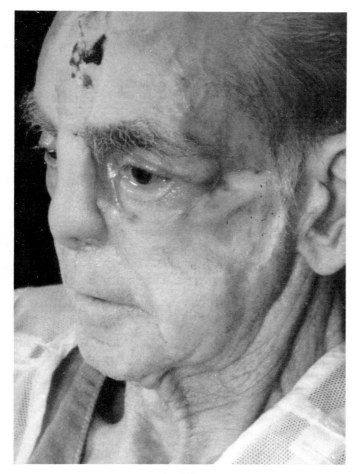

Figure 27.5. Patient's appearance approximately 1 month after completion of his reconstruction.

Treatment. Effective therapy of both basal and squamous cell carcinomas centers on two major principles; confirmation of the diagnosis histologically and complete removal or destruction of the tumor. With small lesions (0.5 cm or less), after obtaining histological confirmation by needle biopsy many dermatologists recommend treatment with cryotherapy (freezing the tumor), or curettage (using sharp spoon-like instruments to remove the bulk out of the tumor). Radiation therapy and radium implants are no longer used. The disadvantages of the above treatment modalities is that complete excision is not guaranteed, as tissue surrounding the tumor is destroyed and not examined microscopically. Most surgeons recommend surgical excision for the management of basal cell carcinomas. To insure complete tumor removal, a 1-cm margin of normal tissue is included in the resected specimen. A 0.5-cm margin is minimal for a lesion close to a critical anatomic feature such as the eyelid. With a morphea-like or fibrosing tumor a 1.5-cm margin is preferable. At the time of excision the specimen is carefully labeled to let the pathologist know how the specimen is oriented (i.e., superior margin, anterior, etc.). A diagram of the position of the specimen with regard to other surrounding structures is also useful. Careful frozen sections are performed on the resected tumor and, if

that import a dark brown or blue-black color. Understandably it may be confused with melanoma.

Morphea-like or fibrosing basal cell carcinoma: In this case the tumor assumes an indurated, yellowish plaque with ill defined borders, over which the skin remains intact for a long period of time. The skin actually looks shiny and taut because of the intense fibroblastic response the tumor induces giving it a "scar-like" appearance (Fig. 27.9). This variety is less common than the nodular form and is more often initially overlooked. The margins of this form of basal cell carcinoma are very difficult to identify because the tumor cells invade normal tissue well beyond the visible margin.

Histologically, the tumor consists of masses of darkly stained cells that extend downward from the basal layer of epithelium into the dermis and subcutaneous tissue. The peripheral nuclei have palisading configuration.

Basal cell carcinoma rarely show rapid early growth. In fact, there is no pain or discomfort and the patient will defer seeking medical attention until the lesion is quite well advanced. Alternatively, the patient may first seek care because of troublesome bleeding from the tumor when it is traumatized while shaving the face.

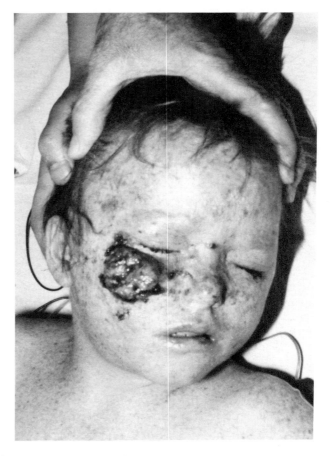

Figure 27.6. Four-year-old child with xeroderma pigmentosum. A large squamous cell carcinoma is present on the right cheek.

the margins are clear of tumor, the surgical wound is either closed primarily, skin grafted, or a flap is turned to provide coverage. In the event that there is uncertainty about the margin of the specimen, either additional tissue is sent for frozen section, or if the wound is large, it may be dressed sterilely to await the result of permanent sectioning prior to skin grafting or coverage with a flap. The reason for postponing closure is to prevent the harvest of either an insufficient graft or flap if additional resection is necessary.

Prognosis. With adequate surgical excision approximately 95% of patients should be cured. Recurrence at the site of tumor removal is usually due to tumor cells left at the margins. However, 20% of individuals with a single basal cell carcinoma will develop a second lesion within 1 year. Forty per cent of those individuals who have had multiple tumors can be expected to develop an additional BCC within 1 year. It would seem, therefore, that certain patients experience a field change within the skin that gives them an increased susceptibility to the further development of BCC tumors. Therefore, after tumor resection in all patients with basal cell cancers it is imperative to continue follow-up of the patients at 6-month to 1-year intervals.

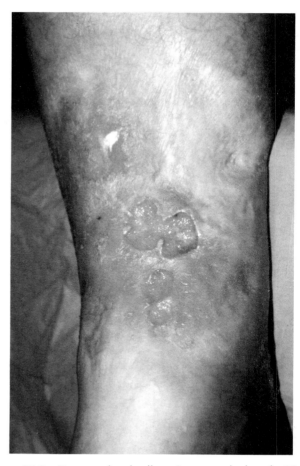

Figure 27.8. Recurrent basal cell carcinoma on the leg of a 63-year-old-male demonstrating the ulcers that form as the lesion penetrates more deeply, outstrips its blood supply, and then undergoes central necrosis.

Squamous Cell Carcinoma

Clinical and Histopathologic Characteristics. Squamous cell carcinoma differs from BCC in a number of ways, the most important of which is the potential for metastatic spread. Usually, the lesions reach considerable size before metastases occur, but this potential necessitates careful examination of the lymphatic drainage of the area at the time of the initial physical examination. Approximately 75% of SCC occur in the head and neck with the lower lip being the most frequent site. The tumor may arise de novo, or from an area with preexisting skin damage, burn scars, chronic ulcers, osteomyelitic sinuses, or chronic granulomas. It has also been seen in chronic discoid lupus erythematous scars. Any chronic nonhealing ulcer of the leg that is increasing in size and not responding as expected to appropriate therapy should be biopsied in four quadrants to rule out SCC. Bowen's disease is a skin condition characterized by chronic scaling and occasionally a crusted, purplish, or erythematous raised lesion. This entity is considered carcinoma-in-situ that has not yet broken through the epidermal-dermal junction. It may, over a period of time, become a frankly invasive squamous cell carcinoma.

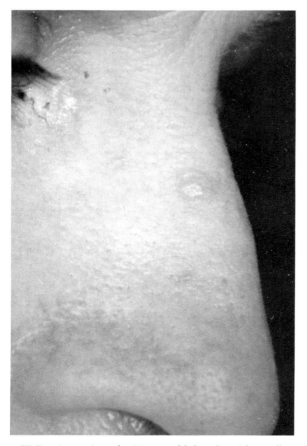

Figure 27.7. Approximately 50-year-old female with small, early, basal cell carcinoma on the lateral bridge of the nose. This lesion was simply elliptically excised with clear margins.

It is not entirely clear how often metastatic spread occurs from SCC, although considering all SCC tumors, the rate of metastases is probably low (approximately 1–2%). It is known, however, that tumors arising from thermal injury, draining osteomyelitic sinuses, chronic ulcers, and Bowen's disease tend to metastasize much more often than tumors arising in solar damaged skin. It has been observed that tumors arising de novo or in actenically damaged skin that penetrate a distance of 8 mm or greater from the surface are most likely to metastasize.

Clinically the tumor arises as an erythematous firm papule on normal or sun-damaged skin. It grows relatively slowly and is, at first, difficult to distinguish from a hyperkeratotic lesion. The key warning feature is a thickening or induration extending some distance beyond the lesion itself. As the tumor enlarges, it forms a nodule with central ulceration surrounded by firm induration. Beneath the area of ulceration is a whitish or yellowish necrotic base. When this is removed, a crater-like defect remains (Fig. 27.10). It does not have the "pearly" raised margins of a basal cell tumor (Fig. 27.7). Often these tumors have crusts or scabs over them from repetitive trauma, bleeding, or leakage of the serous exudate (Fig. 27.11). As with BCC, the SCC lesions may enlarge and erode through adjacent tissue and can cause considerable destruction (Fig. 27.12).

Microscopically, the tumors consist of irregular nests

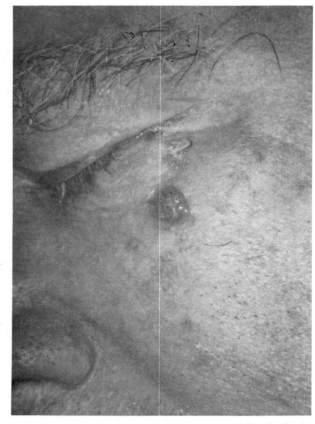

Figure 27.10. Small squamous cell carcinoma of the cheek of a 56-year-old white male. Note the ulcer-like appearance.

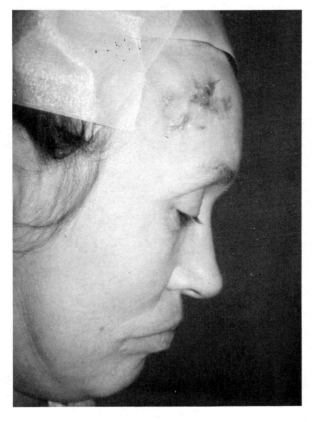

Figure 27.9. Large morphea-type basal cell carcinoma of the forehead with fibrous tissue reaction giving it a scar-like appearance.

of epidermal cells that infiltrate the dermis to varying depths and reveal varying degrees of differentiation. The more differentiated the tumor, the greater the number of "epithelial pearls" (keratinous material) seen in the depths of the tumor.

Treatment. The considerations for therapy of these lesions are essentially the same as in basal cell carcinomas. The standard margin for resection is 1 cm, and the same criteria apply for skin grafting and flap coverage. The major difference is in the consideration of whether lymph node dissection should be performed concurrently with excision of the primary lesion.

Prognosis. The prognosis for small lesions is excellent, as it is with basal cell carcinoma, with a cure rate of 95%. In larger lesions that penetrate the subcutaneous tissue the risk of nodal metastasis increases substantially. Once lymph node involvement has occurred, the prognosis is poor. Two-thirds of patients with squamous cell carcinoma may succumb to this lesion once the disease has penetrated into the subcutaneous tissue. Nearly all patients with lymph node involvement eventually die of their disease. Followup in patients with excised squamous cell carcinomas should be as rigorous as in the patient with basal cell carcinoma. The patient should be examined for local recurrence, evidence of regional nodal metastasis and new lesions at least every 6 months. In those patients with large

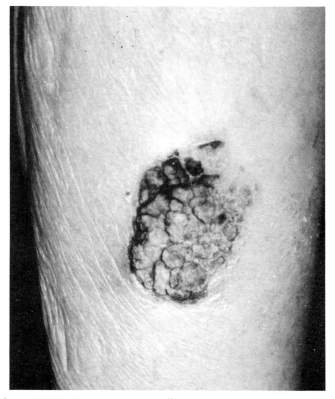

Figure 27.11. Large squamous cell carcinoma of the leg covered by a crust of congealed serous fluid and blood. When these crusts are removed the underlying lesion bleeds considerably.

lesions and the potential for metastases, repeated examinations on a monthly basis for 1 year and then every 3–6 months thereafter is recommended.

Melanoma

Embryology of Melanocytes.

Melanocytes are derived from neural crest tissue. The cells migrate during early gestation to the skin, uveal tract, meninges, and ectodermal mucosa. Melanocytes reside in the skin in the basement layer of the epidermis and elaborate melanin pigment under a variety of stimuli.

The number of melanocytes per unit area of skin surface does not correlate with the propensity to develop melanoma. Melanocyte density in caucasians and blacks is about the same for any skin site. Differences in skin pigmentation are determined by the melanosome-pigment package passed out of the melanocyte, by way of its dendritic process, and phagocytized by surrounding keratinocytes. These cells then migrate up to the epidermis giving the phenotypic patterns and degrees of skin coloration observed in people.

Epidemiology and Etiology of Melanoma

The etiology of melanoma is not known for certain at this time; however, 50–60% of melanomas can be

demonstrated to arise from or near benign nevi. The triggering event for malignant transformation is not known. Benign nevi are extremely common and very few ever become malignant. The one exception is the congenital giant hairy nevus, also termed the bathing trunk nevus, which undergoes malignant transformation to melanoma in 10–30% of these lesions that are untreated.

Familial malignant melanomas have been described and account for 3–6% of all melanomas. Up to 44% of patients who develop multiple primary melanomas have family histories of this tumor. Familial melanomas tend to occur at a younger age than sporadic cases. Three to five per cent of patients who have developed a melanoma will develop a second primary melanoma. These patients have a risk calculated to be 900 times that of the population at large.

A third recognized risk factor for hereditary melanoma is the dysplastic nevus syndrome. Several kindreds with familial melanoma have been character-

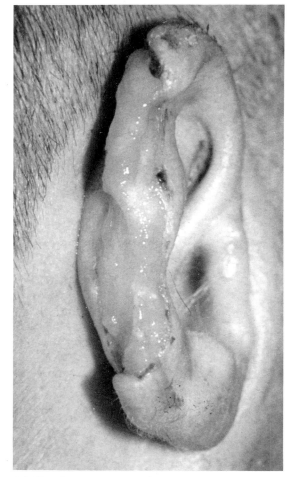

Figure 27.12. Posterior aspect of an ear eroded by squamous cell carcinoma extending into the ear cartilage. This patient presented to the emergency room giving a history of having his ear bitten by a dog. Careful examination of the lesion raised the index of suspicion for a skin malignancy. A frozen-section biopsy at the time of operation confirmed this lesion as SCC.

ized by large premalignant nevi predominantly in the horse-collar distribution over the upper trunk. Genetic predisposition to malignant melanoma is also carried by the hereditary syndrome xeroderma pigmentosum.

Several studies have indicated an increased incidence of melanoma toward the equator. These studies have been done both in New Zealand and in Australia as well as in the United States. Melanomas are known to occur with increased incidence on the lower legs of females and the trunk of males. While these data suggest that sunlight exposure has a role in melanoma etiology, they cannot explain the occurrence of melanoma in areas of the body with minimal sunlight exposure.

The incidence of melanoma is increased in people with light complexion and blue eyes. This is seen most clearly in Australia and New Zealand where the incidence of melanoma in the Celtic population is the highest in the world: 14 per 100,000 in men and 17 per 100,000 in women. These figures compare to 4–5 per 100,000 in the United States. All of these factors seem to influence the development of melanoma. However, no single explanation is satisfactory for all of the locations and frequencies of melanoma.

Significance and Incidence of Melanomas

Malignant melanoma seems to increase in frequency as the distance to the equator is decreased. Eighty-eight per cent of head and neck cutaneous melanomas occur outside the protected area (hair-bearing scalp). Approximately one-quarter of cutaneous melanomas occur in the head and neck area. Because the head and neck comprise only 9% of the total body surface area and approximately one-half of this is covered with hair, this is the highest incidence of melanoma for any anatomic site. This suggests but does not prove a solar etiology for melanoma in this area. The site distribution of malignant melanoma in black people is strikingly dissimilar from that in whites. In Uganda approximately 70% of melanomas are found on the

plantar surface of the foot in blacks compared to only 6% in whites. Likewise, 8% of melanomas in Uganda occur in the nasopharynx, an extremely rare site in the white population. Melanoma accounts for approximately 1% of the cancers in the United States and about the same proportion of cancer deaths. It represents only 5% of cutaneous neoplastic growths; however, its malignant potential is more aptly represented by the fact that melanoma results in 74% of the deaths from skin cancer.

The prevalence of melanoma is 22,000 cases per year. The age-adjusted incidence is 4.2 per 100,000 population. The incidence among blacks is 0.8 per 100,000 while that among whites is 4.5 per 100,000. There is an age variation in the incidence with a progression from 0.4 cases per 100,000 in the 10–19-year-old age group up to 16 cases per 100,000 in the over-80 age group. In addition, statistics collected on the incidence of melanoma demonstrate clearly an increase in the incidence of this disease with an apparent doubling of occurrence approximately every 15 years. This increase does not appear to be due to more complete reporting or to an alteration in the pathologic criteria for diagnostic inclusion. The increase in incidence is accompanied by a parallel rise in mortality.

Classification of Melanoma

As many as eleven types have been described excluding ocular lesions. For our purposes in this chapter, melanoma will be classified as lentigo maligna melanoma, superficial spreading melanoma, nodular melanoma, acral lentiginous melanoma, and other.

Lentigo maligna melanoma is the term used for melanoma that occurs in a Hutchinson's freckle. This type of melanoma is characterized by a long period of development and by the fact that it tends to occur on the face, head, and neck of older people. The median age at diagnosis is about 70 years. This type of melanoma constitutes 10–15% of cutaneous melanomas and is the

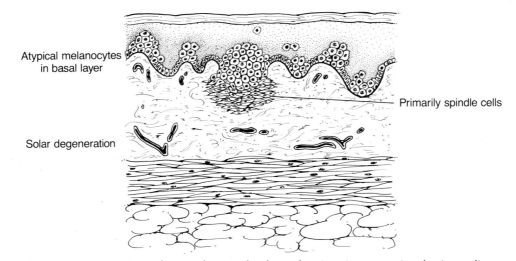

Figure 27.13. Lentigo maligna melanoma develops when invasion occurs in a lentigo maligna.

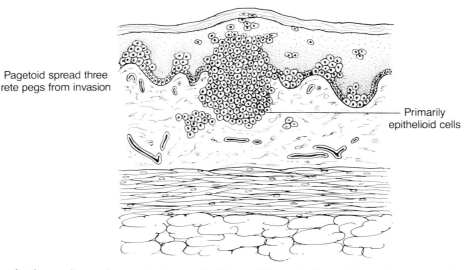

Pagetoid spread three rete pegs from invasion

Primarily epithelioid cells

Figure 27.14. Superficial spreading melanoma is characterized by radial growth (Pagetoid spread) and vertical growth (invasion).

most benign of the cutaneous melanomas (Figs. 27.13, 27.16). This commonly occurs in areas heavily exposed to the sun. Females seem to be more frequently affected than males. The lesions are large, flat, and tan or brown in color. As the vertical growth phase begins to develop, the lesion will become focally elevated. The basic tan-brown pattern of the radial growth phase persists during this period. The elevation may be either lighter or darker in color than the surrounding radial growth phase. The rarity of rose and pink colors in the radial growth phase distinguishes lentigo maligna melanoma from superficial spreading melanoma.

Superficial spreading melanoma accounts for approximately 70% of all cutaneous melanomas. It is intermediate in malignancy. This tumor affects the sexes equally with the legs being the site most commonly affected in females and the back most commonly affected in males. The peak incidence for the occurrence of superficial spreading melanoma is the fifth decade (Figs. 27.14, 27.17). As in the lesion previously discussed, there are both radial and vertical growth phases. The radial growth phase of superficial spreading melanoma is characterized by melanoma cells within the epidermis and papillary dermis and by a host response of inflammatory cells, fibroblasts, and new blood vessel formation. The radial growth phase of superficial spreading melanoma is more obviously elevated than the radial growth phase of lentigo maligna melanoma. The vertical growth phase in superficial spreading melanoma seems to develop more rapidly than in lentigo maligna melanoma and is heralded by the appearance of a palpable nodule. The vertical growth phase seems to be the source of metastatic disease and, depending on the depth of invasion, can produce metastasis in up to 85% of the cases. Early superficial spreading melanoma lesions are a haphazard combination of colors, usually tan, brown, blue, and black. Most lesions also contain areas of rose and pink colors. The common characteristics of variation in color, marginal notching, and loss of skin creases dis-

tinguish this lesion from the more common intradermal junctional nevus. More advanced lesions will have palpable nodularity indicating development of a vertical growth phase and may be surrounded by satellite nodules. Many of these tumors may contain white sections that represent areas of spontaneous regression.

Nodular melanoma is the most malignant type. It constitutes about 12% of all cutaneous melanomas. Nodular melanoma occurs twice as often in males as in females (Figs. 27.15, 27.18). This is made up almost exclusively of a vertical growth phase. The host cellular response is generally less than that seen with other types of melanoma. Clinically, these lesions tend to develop quickly and have a palpable nodular component in their earliest development. The color of nodular melanoma is blue-black. The variability in coloration and margins seen with the superficial spreading melanoma is rare in the nodular type.

Acral lentiginous melanoma occurs on the palms, soles, and in the subungual locations. This melanoma has some of the growth characteristics of both superficial spreading and nodular melanoma. The exact prognostic significance of these different characteristics has not been determined in a large series of cases. Acral lentiginous melanoma (Fig. 27.19 A, B), however, seems to be worse in prognosis than superficial spreading melanoma but not so severe as nodular melanoma. This melanoma is characterized by both a radial and a vertical growth phase. In the subungual location, the radial growth phase may simply be a streak in the nail associated with irregular tan-brown staining of the nail bed. In addition to the types listed above, melanoma may arise in a giant hairy nevus, in the oral, vaginal, or anal mucous membrane, in a blue nevus, in a visceral organ, and occasionally presents as a metastatic lesion without a demonstrable primary.

Staging of Malignant Melanoma

In the past 15 years, a better understanding of the growth and development of the primary melanoma le-

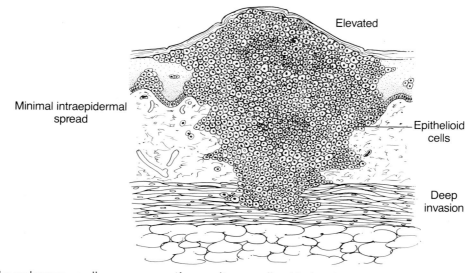

Elevated

Minimal intraepidermal spread

Epithelioid cells

Deep invasion

Figure 27.15. Nodular melanoma usually appears as uniform malignant cells with deep invasion and little intraepithelial growth.

sion has allowed surgeons to design treatment tailored to the characteristics of the primary lesion and to predict outcome on the basis of these characteristics. Two features of the tumor that seem most important in determining prognosis are the radial and vertical growth phases. Three of the four common varieties of melanoma (lentigo maligna, superficial spreading, and acral lentiginous melanoma) are characterized by an indolent radial growth phase that may last for several years. The radial growth phase is characterized by abnormal melanocytes extending centrifugally in the epidermis with minimal invasion of the papillary dermis. In su-

perficial spreading melanoma these large epithelioid cells occur in nests and as an intradermal component at least three rete pegs away from the area of invasion. These cells have relatively uniform nuclei with an abundance of dusky cytoplasm. The vertical growth phase consists of malignant cells that invade into the dermis for variable distance. There may be cells that vary in appearance from one cluster to another. A lymphocyte infiltration is fairly common around these invading cells.

W. H. Clark (1) developed a system of microstaging for primary melanoma that is based on the level of invasion of the tumor. Level I lesions are confined to the epidermis; at level II, they invade the papillary layer of the dermis; at level III, they reach the junction of the

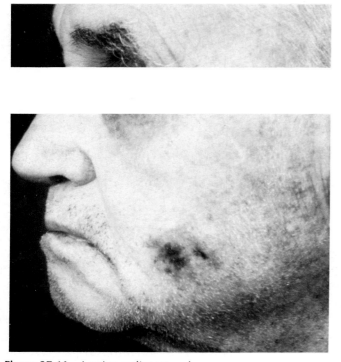

Figure 27.16. Lentigo malignant melanoma.

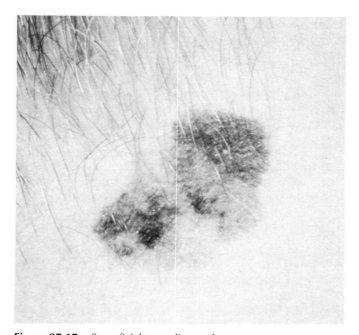

Figure 27.17. Superficial spreading melanoma.

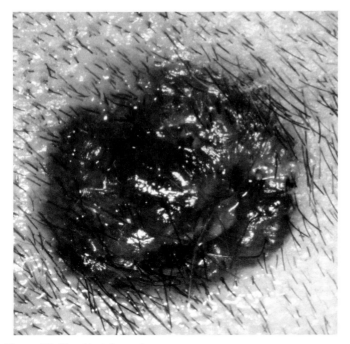

Figure 27.18. Nodular melanoma.

papillary and reticular layers; at level IV, they invade the reticular dermis and, at level V, the subcutaneous fat. Survival is related to the depth of invasion: it is best for level I and worst for level V lesions. A disadvantage of this system is that different pathologists may interpret the levels of invasion variably (Fig. 27.20).

Because of weakness in the Clark microstaging system, Breslow (2) proposed the use of an ocular micrometer to measure the thickness of the tumor in millimeters at the deepest point of its vertical growth. This system allows a more objective evaluation and easier comparison among pathologists. The thicker the tumor, the worse the prognosis (Fig. 27.20).

This tumor can spread via both the lymphatic and the blood route. The lymphatic spread can present as in-transit metastases or as enlarged nodes. The former result from melanoma cells being trapped between the primary tumor and regional lymph nodes. This produces a region of the cutaneous metastases located more than 3 cm from the primary site. Mechanical blockage of afferent lymph drainage by either metastatic disease or lymph node dissection is felt to be the cause of these in-transit metastases.

While regional lymph nodes may serve as a filter for metastatic melanoma cells, they by no means stop all metastatic cells. Once melanoma becomes metastatic, it has a striking trophism for small bowel mucosa and distant cutaneous sites. The most common cause of gastrointestinal bleeding in a patient with melanoma is small bowel metastases. These same metastases can also cause obstruction and intussusception. The lung, liver, and brain are other common metastatic sites.

The TNM (tumor-node-metastasis) system combines information from the Clark and Breslow systems as well as the status of lymph nodes and distant metastases to give a comprehensive staging of these patients (Table 27.2).

Diagnosis of Malignant Melanoma

There are eight lesions that are occasionally confused with cutaneous melanoma. Each of these can frequently be differentiated by an expert on a clinical basis. However, if there is any question, a histologic examination will provide the necessary confirmatory evidence. *Junctional nevi* generally appear during the early years of life and are particularly apparent during adolescence. They may vary in size from a few millimeters to several centimeters. They are light to dark brown in color with a flat, smooth surface and irregular edges. *Compound nevi* are usually brown or black with a raised nodular surface frequently containing hair. They are usually less than 1 cm in size and can occur in all age groups. *Intradermal nevi* can be very large al-

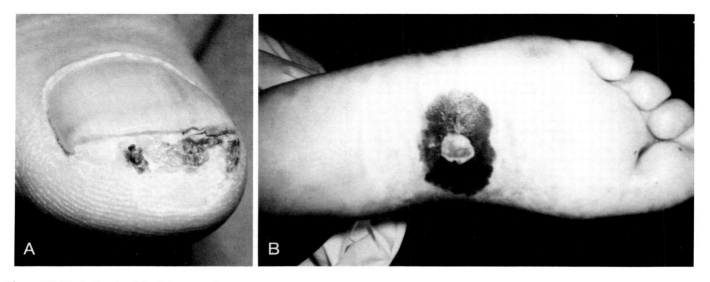

Figure 27.19. A, B, Acral lentiginous melanoma.

Table 27.2.
TNM Classification

Primary Tumor (T)

TX No evidence of primary tumor (unknown primary or primary tumor removed and not histologically examined).

T0 Atypical melanocytic hyperplasia (Clark level I); not a malignant lesion.

T1 Invasion of papillary dermis (level II) or 0.75-mm thickness or less.

T2 Invasion of the papillary-reticular-dermal interface (level III) or 0.76–1.5-mm thickness.

T3 Invasion of the reticular dermis (level IV) or 1.51–4.0-mm thickness.

T4 Invasion of subcutaneous tissue (level V) or 4.1-mm or greater thickness, or satellite(s) within 2 cm of any primary melanoma.

Nodal Involvement (N)

NX Minimum requirements to assess the regional nodes cannot be met.

N0 No regional lymph node involvement.

N1 Involvement of only one regional lymph node station; node(s) movable and not over 5 cm in diameter, or negative regional lymph nodes and the presence of less than five in-transit metastases beyond 2 cm from the primary site.

N2 Any one of the following: (1) involvement of more than one regional lymph node station; (2) regional node(s) over 5 cm in diameter or fixed; (3) five or more in-transit metastases or any in-transit metastases beyond 2 cm from the primary site with regional lymph node involvement.

Distant Metastasis (M)

MS Not assessed.

M0 No known distant metastasis.

M1 Involvement of skin or subcutaneous tissue beyond the site of primary lymph node drainage.

M2 Visceral metastasis

Stage Grouping

Stage IA	T1, N0, M0
Stage IB	T2, N0, M0
Stage IIA	T3, N0, M0
Stage IIB	T4, N0, M0
Stage III	Any T, N1, M0
Stage IV	Any T, any N, M1, or M2
	Any T, N2, M0

American Joint Committee on Cancer, Manual for Staging of Cancer pp. 34–35, J.B. Lippincott 1983.

though they are usually less than 1 cm in diameter. Their color varies from light to dark brown and they may have a raised warty or smooth surface. The presence of coarse hairs serves to distinguish them from other nevi. *Blue nevi* are smooth blue or blue-black lesions less than 1 cm in size with well defined regular margins. They commonly occur on the face, dorsum of the feet and hands, and the buttocks. They are rarely associated with malignant melanoma. *Basal cell carcinomas* are most common in middle-aged persons. The pigmented basal cell tumor usually has a blue-black coloration with raised edges and capillary neovascularity. Initially, the lesion will be smooth but can become ulcerated. *Seborrheic keratoses* are occasionally black in color. They usually are 1 cm in size or larger and typically appear as raised, warty, and greasy in consis-

tency. They have the appearance of being "stuck" onto the skin. *Dermatofibroma* is occasionally dark brown in color. It usually is smooth, slightly raised, and without hairs. It typically grows very slowly and never becomes malignant. *Subungual hemorrhage* is usually sudden in onset and will be sharply defined beneath the nail bed. By comparison, melanoma will be of gradual onset and characterized by poorly demarcated streaks extending along the axis of the nail. The diagnosis of hemorrhage can be confirmed by puncturing the nail and evacuating the blood. With the passage of time, the entire subungual hemorrhage will migrate distally with clearing of the nail bed. Subungual melanoma, however, is a persistent lesion.

Many of the features of cutaneous melanoma permit clinical diagnosis prior to biopsy. The key to making the diagnosis of lentigo maligna and superficial spreading melanoma is irregularity. There is an irregularity of coloration, of border, and of surface. Taken together these characteristics allow the experienced clinician to diagnose the majority of melanomas. Patients, however, present with many other types of pigmented lesions that require diagnosis. Although it is possible to be quite certain about some pigmented lesions, there are many others that require biopsy for histologic examination before planning therapy. The nodular melanoma does not have the border variability seen in the lentigo maligna and superficial spreading melanoma. However, it does have the variability of color and does present as a raised nodule. The coloration, thickness, and rapid growth permit easy clinical diagnosis.

Accurate microstaging of melanoma is so important in the management of this disease that the person performing the biopsy must present the pathologist with adequate and satisfactory material. The pathologist cannot be expected to reconstruct the lesion from multiple fragments of tissue about which he has no information regarding orientation. It is the responsibility of the physician performing the biopsy to maximize its value by direct communication with the pathologist, proper handling of the tissue after its removal, and proper planning of the biopsy. If possible, a biopsy should consist of complete excision of the lesion with a small margin of normal tissue so the pathologist can accurately stage the lesion. If for some reason this is not feasible, the second choice is to perform an incisional biopsy. The biopsy must include the thickest portion of the lesion so the pathologist will correctly stage the lesion.

Treatment

The two questions regarding local therapy concern the proper width of excision and the proper depth of excision. Current recommendations are 2-cm lateral margins for most lesions; the old recommendation of 5-cm lateral margins in every direction is not only unacceptable, but is not feasible in certain locations. The depth of the excision in most cases should extend through the subcutaneous tissue to the level of the underlying fascia. Excision of fascia with the lesion contributes little to the protection of the patients from the spread of melanoma.

There is general agreement that, if regional lymph nodes are clinically palpable (clinical stage III), a regional node dissection should be performed. There is also agreement that, if these nodes are not palpable and the primary lesion is less than 0.76 mm thick (clinical stage IA), a regional node dissection is not indicated since the incidence of metastatic disease from such lesions is extremely low. There is a great deal of controversy regarding the management of regional lymph nodes in other cases of stage I and II melanoma. Some authorities recommend node dissections only if regional nodes become palpable on follow-up; others recommend prophylactic dissections depending on the thickness and other characteristics of the primary lesion.

The management of distant disease is determined primarily by the location and the symptoms. Metastatic disease to the brain is usually handled by either radiation therapy alone or a combination of surgical removal plus whole brain radiation. Pulmonary nodules, if few in number, may be resected but this is not generally practiced. These patients usually receive chemotherapy. Distant spread on an extremity that involves in-transit metastases can be managed by a regional form of therapy, regional limb perfusion (utilizing a chemotherapeutic agent, such as L-phenylalanine mustard, and hyperthermia). This can frequently give a satisfactory result with salvage of the extremity and prolongation of the patient's life. This treatment is beneficial only if the disease is confined to that extremity. Dimethyl-triazeno-imidazole-carboxamide (DTIC) is the most active single agent for the treatment of metastatic melanoma. It has also been tried in combination with other agents. An optimistic response rate would be approximately 20% combining both complete and partial responses. At this time there is no effective chemotherapy for either primary or metastatic melanoma.

Most patients with recurrent metastatic melanoma should be treated on protocol so that data collection could continue and treatment be improved.

Radiation is rarely used as the single treatment for melanoma; however, it is used for the treatment of metastatic disease, such as whole brain radiation following brain metastasis. The development of new fractionation methods with higher single doses given less frequently has increased the response from 35% up to 75%. This improvement has made radiation therapy useful in the management of patients with metastatic disease.

Results of Treatment

In stage I and II (disease limited to the primary site) both the Clark and Breslow systems of microstaging allow us to subdivide patients into different risk categories for recurrent disease and eventual death (Table 27.2). In general, the risk of recurrence following excision of a primary melanoma is extremely low if the melanoma is less than 0.76 mm in thickness. On the other hand if the melanoma has a thickness of 4 mm or greater, the probability of recurrence of the disease and death of the patient is extremely high. Overall 5-year survival rate of patients in stage I and II is about 75%.

In stage III (disease spread to the draining lymph nodes), the presence of metastatic disease in the regional lymph nodes is an ominous prognostic sign. This clear demonstration that the melanoma has the potential to spread beyond the primary site decreases the disease-free 5-year survival rate to the 20–40% range. This prognosis is made even worse as the number of involved lymph nodes increases.

In stage IV (disease spread to distant sites), average survival for patients in this category is 6 months. Patients with only skin and lymph node metastases do better (median survival 14 months) than patients with

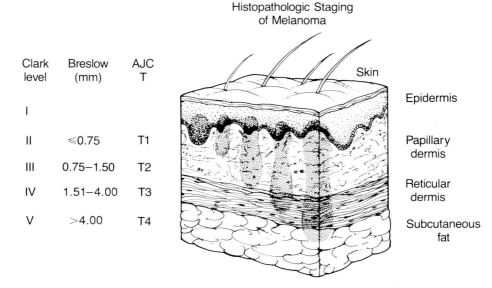

Figure 27.20. The Clark and Breslow classifications are both used in the American Joint Committee (AJC) staging system.

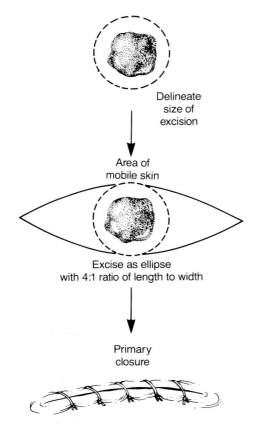

Delineate
size of
excision

↓

Area of
mobile skin

Excise as ellipse
with 4:1 ratio of length to width

↓

Primary
closure

Figure 27.21. Scalpel excision is used for smaller lesions with primary closure.

visceral metastases (median survival 4 months). A recent review by Balch et al. (3) shows five factors that seem to affect prognosis in melanoma. These are pathologic stages (I, II), ulceration, surgical treatment, thickness, and primary site location (upper extremities versus others). While these data were developed from a retrospective analysis of a large group of patients, clinicians in general agree that these factors are important in predicting the outcome for a patient with melanoma.

Excisional Biopsy. A biopsy should be considered any time a patient has the following symptoms: color change, size change, itching, bleeding, or oozing; or the following signs: irregular color, nodularity, scab formation, ulceration, or irregular notched margins. If possible, excisional biopsy is preferred because the entire lesion is available for step-section histopathological analysis to determine depth of penetration. This information is extremely critical for the further management of the patient. Prior to beginning local anesthesia, the physician should outline an ellipse around the lesion with 2–4-mm margins. The long axis of the ellipse should be placed in such a way that therapeutic reexcision of the site can be easily performed. In general, the long axis of the ellipse should be directed toward the node bearing area. In addition, the physician should confirm to his satisfaction that the planned defect can be easily closed without undue tension. Once

the ellipse has been outlined, a field block type of local anesthesia should be administered with a single injection at either end of the ellipse infiltrating into normal tissue rather than into the tumor. Full-thickness skin and subcutaneous tissue should be excised as part of the biopsy. Once bleeding points have been controlled, the skin should be reapproximated using alternating simple and vertical mattress stitches to give a smooth straight closure (Fig. 27.21). If size or location of the primary site prevents excisional biopsy, then an incisional biopsy should be performed.

Incisional Biopsy Prognosis is not compromised by the use of incisional biopsy as long as definitive therapy is applied in a reasonable period of time. Selection of the biopsy site is critical because of the bearing of tumor thickness on prognosis. Any incisional biopsy must include some of the thickest part of the pigmented lesion to allow correct microstaging. Placement of the incisional biopsy should be in such a way as to not compromise definitive surgical therapy. Field block anesthesia should be used with a single puncture near the site of the planned biopsy in normal skin so that the infiltration is in normal skin and underneath rather than into the melanoma. The normal skin involved in the biopsy site should be reapproximated. Many authors recommend leaving the biopsy defect in the pigmented lesion open to avoid introducing melanoma cells into the subcutaneous tissue by the passage of the needle.

Melanoma is increasing in frequency. It is much less common than basal cell or squamous cell carcinoma, but is the cause of 74% of the deaths from skin cancer. The risk factors for melanoma are easily identified by even the lay person. Consequently, early detection is a reasonable goal. This should result in improved cure rates. Questions still remain regarding the treatment of certain groups of stage I and II melanoma. These are being addressed by randomized prospective trials. The physician has a responsibility to assist the patient with early diagnosis, correct staging, and treatment. This will ensure maximum benefit from the health care system for the patient.

REFERENCES

1. Clark HW Jr, From L, Bernardino FA, Mihm MC: The histogenesis and biologic behavior of primary human malignant melanomas of the skin. *Cancer Res* 29:705, 1969.
2. Breslow A: Thickness, cross-sectional areas and depth of invasion in the prognosis of cutaneous melanoma. *Ann Surg* 172:902, 1970.
3. Balch CM, Murad TM, Song S-J, Ingalis A, Halperen NB, Maddox WA: A multi-factorial analysis of melanoma: prognostic histopathological features comparing Clark's and Breslow's staging methods. *Surgery* 86:343–351, 1979.

SUGGESTED READINGS

Ariel IM: *Malignant Melanoma.* New York, Appleton-Century-Crofts, 1981.
Beahrs OH, Myers MH (eds): *Manual for Staging of Cancer,* 2nd Edition. American Joint Committee on Cancer. Philadelphia, J.B. Lippincott, 1983.
Bellet RE, Mastragelo MJ, Berd D, McGuire HC: Primary cutaneous

melanoma. In Kahn SB, Love RR, Sherman C, Chakravorty R (eds): *Concepts in Cancer Medicine,* 2nd ed. 1983; New York, Grune & Stratton, 1983, pp 545–555.

Freidman HI, Cooper PH, Wanebo HJ: Prognostic and therapeutic use of microstaging of cutaneous squamous cell carcinoma of the trunk and extremities. *Cancer* 56:1099–1105, 1985.

Goldsmith HS: Melanoma—an overview. *Cancer* 29:194, 1979.

Haynes HA, Mead KW, Goldwyn RM: Cancers of the skin. In DeVita VT, Hellman S, Rosenberg SA (eds): *Cancer Principles and Practice of Oncology,* 2nd ed. Philadelphia, Lippincott, 1985, pp 1343–1370.

Immerman SC, Scanlon EF, Christ M, Knox KL: Recurrent squamous cell carcinoma of the skin. *Cancer* 51:1537–1540, 1983.

Mastrangelo MJ, Baker AR, Katze HR: Cutaneous melanoma. In Devita VT, Hellman S, Rosenberg SA (eds): *Cancer Principles and Practice of Oncology,* 2nd ed. Philadelphia, J.B. Lippincott, 1985, pp 1371–1422.

Mysliborski JA: Cutaneous neoplasms. *NY State J Med* 80 (11):1716–1720, 1980.

Shiu MH, Chu F, Fortner JG: Treatment of regionally advanced epidermoid carcinoma of the extremity and trunk. *Surg Gynecol Obstet* 150:558–562, 1980.

Sober AJ: Diagnosis and management of skin cancer. *Cancer* 51:2448–2452, 1983.

Skills

1. Demonstrate the ability to perform an adequate and satisfactory biopsy of a suspicious nevus that will permit the staging of a malignant melanoma if found.

2. Indicate physical features and symptoms of a nevus that make it suspicious for a malignant melanoma.

Study Questions

1. Describe the management of a 50-year-old farmer who presents with a 1-cm nodule with raised borders and a shallow central ulcer over the dorsum of his left hand. Discuss the management of similar lesion over the bridge of his nose.

2. A 47-year-old man sustained a burn over his left pretibial area at age 15. Since then the area has intermittently shown signs of a sore that bleeds easily and scabs but has never completely healed. Discuss the management of this patient.

3. A 62-year-old man who is a chronic pipe smoker has developed a flat, white, plaque-like lesion on his lower lip. Describe the diagnostic evaluation of this patient.

4. Discuss the etiologic theories related to melanoma and how these should be considered in preventing the development of this cutaneous malignancy. Consider the same question with regard to basal and squamous cell carcinomas.

5. Discuss the differences between the growth phases of the various types of melanoma and how these relate to prognosis.

6. A 25-year-old blonde, blue-eyed woman is found to have a black, pruritic nevus on her right leg that is highly suspicious for a malignant melanoma. Review the risk factors for melanoma that would and would not be pertinent to her case.

7. Outline the presentations of malignant melanoma that comprise its several classifications and include a differential diagnosis of lesions with which it can be confused.

8. Compare microstaging systems on the basis of the vertical growth of malignant melanoma and relate them to the TNM classification.

9. An excisional biopsy of a small nevus on the left knee of a 45-year-old man has revealed the presence of a nodular malignant melanoma that measures 1.2 mm in vertical depth. Two lymph nodes are palpable in the man's left groin. What is the surgical treatment for this situation? The patient presents 3 months later with a focal right-sided neurologic deficit. The remaining physical examination, including blood work and chest radiographs, are negative for abnormalities. What are the treatment options in this situation? If occult gastrointestinal hemorrhage with partial small bowel obstruction develops, what are the treatment options?

10. A 40-year-old man had primary excision of a malignant melanoma on his left leg 6 months ago. Margins of the specimen were considered free of malignant cell involvement. He presents now with occult blood in his stool and evidence of partial small bowel obstruction. Outline the steps in the evaluation of metastatic disease.

Malignant Diseases of the Lymphatics and Soft Tissue

E. Stan Lennard, M.D., *William B. Farrar, M.D.,*
Charles L. Huang, M.D., William M. Rambo, M.D.,
and Jeffrey Schouten, M.D.

ASSUMPTION

The student understands the anatomy and physiology of the lymphatic system.

OBJECTIVES

1. List the signs and symptoms in the clinical staging and diagnosis of lymphoma.
2. Describe the surgeon's role in the staging of lymphoma.

3. Identify the different types of sarcoma.
4. Discuss the differences between "sarcoma" and "carcinoma" and their clinical staging.
5. List the characteristics of a sarcoma that may be found by physical examination and outline the diagnostic approaches to determine its extent.
6. Outline the medical and surgical treatment modalities for sarcoma and discuss the relative value of each.

Hodgkin's and Non-Hodgkin's Lymphomas

Lymphomas are defined as malignancies arising in the lymphoreticular components of the reticuloendothelial system. Collections of lymphoid cells occur in lymph nodes, the white pulp of the spleen, Waldeyer's ring, the thymus gland, and lymphoid aggregates in the submucosa of the respiratory and gastrointestinal tract (Peyer's patches). The two major subgroups of malignant lymphomas are Hodgkin's disease (accounting for one-fourth of all lymphomas) and the non-Hodgkin's lymphomas. Lymphomas have been classified based upon immunohistopathologic standards (International Working Formulation, Table 28.1). Lymphomas may originate from B cells, T cells, histiocytes, or other lymphoid cells.

Hodgkin's Lymphoma

The initial description of Hodgkin's disease was reported in 1832 by Thomas Hodgkin. The most common presentation of Hodgkin's disease is asymptomatic cervical lymphadenopathy. Systemic symptoms (B symptoms) are defined as fever, night sweats, or weight loss greater than 10% of the body weight. An unusual symptom reported by some patients is pain at the site

of disease associated with alcohol intake. Hodgkin's disease may be localized or disseminated at the time of presentation. Patients may present with signs and symptoms secondary to mass effect from mediastinal or retroperitoneal disease.

The incidence of Hodgkin's disease is characterized by a bimodal curve with peaks in young adulthood and the elderly age group. The average age of a patient with Hodgkin's disease is 32 years of age. The etiology of Hodgkin's disease is unknown although various theories have been postulated including an infectious etiology associated with a viral infection, particularly the Epstein-Barr virus. There is also a suggestion of a heredity factor. The cellular origin of Hodgkin's disease is also uncertain but it may be derived from either T cells or macrophages.

Hodgkin's disease has been categorized histologically by the Rye classification system into four categories: lymphocyte predominant, nodular sclerosis, mixed cellularity, and lymphocyte depleted (Table 28.2). The histologic categorization is based upon the relative proportion of neoplastic cells to the reactive component of the tumor. Histologically, Hodgkin's disease appears as a tumor composed predominantly of a large *reactive* background with a few malignant mononuclear cells

Table 28.1.
The International Working Formulation of Non-Hodgkin's Lymphoma

Low Grade
  A. Malignant lymphoma
     Small lymphocytic consistent with chronic lymphocytic leukemia
     Plasmacytoid
  B. Malignant lymphoma, follicular
     Predominantly small cleaved cell
        Diffuse areas
        Sclerosis
  C. Malignant lymphoma, follicular mixed, small cleaved and large cell
        Diffuse areas
        Sclerosis

Intermediate Grade
  D. Malignant lymphoma, follicular
     Predominantly large cell
        Diffuse areas
        Sclerosis
  E. Malignant lymphoma, diffuse
     Small cleaved cell
        Sclerosis
  F. Malignant lymphoma, diffuse
     Mixed, small and large cell
        Sclerosis
        Epithelioid cell component
  G. Malignant lymphoma, diffuse
     Large cell
        Cleaved cell
        Noncleaved cell
        Sclerosis

High Grade
  H. Malignant lymphoma
     Large cell, immunoblastic
        Plasmacytoid
        Clear cell
        Polymorphous
        Epithelioid cell component
  I. Malignant lymphoma
     Lymphoblastic
        Convoluted cell
        Nonconvoluted cell
  J. Malignant lymphoma
     Small noncleaved cell
        Burkitt's
        Follicular

Miscellaneous
  Composite
  Mycosis fungoides
  Histiocyte
  Extramedullary plasmacytoma
  Unclassifiable
  Other

Table 28.2.
Histopathologic Types of Hodgkin's Disease

Classification (Rye)	Relative Frequency (%)
Nodular sclerosis	50
Mixed cellularity	37
Lymphocyte predominance	5
Lymphocyte depletion	8

dominant group has the best prognosis followed by the nodular sclerosis subgroup. The most common histologic type is nodular sclerosis.

Staging and Preoperative Evaluation

The critical factor in determining therapy for patients with Hodgkin's disease is an accurate and thorough staging evaluation. The staging of Hodgkin's disease is based on the Ann Arbor system that is reproduced in Table 28.3. Thus, all patients undergo a thorough evaluation including a complete physical examination with particular attention to the peripheral lymph nodes. A chest x-ray is also required. The next stage in the evaluation is an *excisional* biopsy of an abnormal lymph node; preferentially cervical or axillary nodes should be biopsied as opposed to inguinal lymph nodes. The next step in the workup after histologic diagnosis should be an evaluation of the retroperitoneal lymph nodes, as well as examination of the bone marrow. A CT scan or lymphangiogram may be obtained to evaluate the retroperitoneal lymphatics.

The staging laparotomy plays a critical role in the evaluation of most patients with limited stage Hodgkin's disease at the time of diagnosis (stage I, II or III). Visceral organ involvement (bone marrow, pulmonary, or liver) is an indication for systemic chemotherapy. Splenic involvement classically does *not* cause splenomegaly, Therefore, splenectomy is necessary for an adequate staging evaluation of the spleen. Additionally, a significant *false-positive* and *false-negative rate* exists for

Table 28.3.
Ann Arbor Staging Classification for Hodgkin's Disease

Stage	Findings
I	Involvement of a single lymph node region (I) or a single extra lymphatic organ or site (I^E)
II	Involvement of two or more lymph node regions on the same side of the diaphragm (II) or localized involvement of an extralymphatic organ or site (IIE)
III	Involvement of lymph node regions on both sides of the diaphragm (III) or localized involvement of an extralymphatic organ or site (IIIE) or spleen (III^S) or both (III^{SE})
IV	Diffuse or disseminated involvement of one or more extralymphatic organs with or without associated lymph node involvement. The organ(s) involved should be identified by a symbol:

A, Asymptomatic
B, Fever, sweats, weight loss > 10% of body weight

and multinuclear giant cells (Sternberg-Reed cells). The Sternberg-Reed cell is a large multinucleated cell with mirror-image nuclei, each containing a prominent nucleolus. The histologic classification has some impact on prognosis, and it is felt that the lymphocyte pre-

both the lymphangiogram and the CT scan, thus mandating laparotomy for histologic evaluation of abdominal and retroperitoneal lymph nodes. The staging laparotomy includes a splenectomy and biopsy of the splenic hilar, celiac, portahepatis, mesenteric, paraaortic, and iliac lymph nodes; these are all examined separately. A bilateral wedge-and-needle biopsy of the liver is also performed. The ovaries in premenopausal women are sutured to the presacral fascia in the midline to allow for radiation sparing. Clips are placed to mark the splenic hilar region as well as each ovary to assure that ovarian migration does not occur after repositioning.

Treatment

The treatment of Hodgkin's lymphoma is determined by the stage (Table 28.4). Radiotherapy is recommended for limited stage disease and chemotherapy is recommended for advanced disease. Chemotherapy has significantly altered the prognosis of patients with Hodgkin's disease in that it is curative even in patients with widespread disease in over 50% of the cases. The most commonly used chemotherapeutic regimen is the MOPP regimen (nitrogen mustard, vincristine, procarbazine, and prednisone). The other commonly used regimen includes a combination of adriamycin, bleomycin, vinblastine, and decarbazine (ABVD); this regimen may be alternated with the MOPP regimen. Radiation is administered in doses of 3000–4000 rads to areas of nodal involvement as well as adjacent nodal bases.

Prognosis

The prognosis for patients with Hodgkin's disease in general is excellent (Table 28.4). Risk factors include the stage of disease at the time of treatment, as well as the histology. However, with adequate staging and therapy, 80% of patients with Hodgkin's disease are cured. Secondary malignancies remain a significant risk for patients with Hodgkin's disease. This risk is increased significantly if combined chemotherapy and radiotherapy are administered.

Non-Hodgkin's Lymphoma

Non-Hodgkin's lymphomas are classified into two basic categories, nodular and diffuse. These represent a large spectrum of malignancies of the lymphoepithelial system.

Patients may also present with signs and symptoms secondary to disseminated disease, depending upon the extent of visceral organ involvement. Other dramatic presentations include the superior vena cava syndrome, acute spinal cord compression syndrome, and meningeal involvement.

The treatment of non-Hodgkin's lymphoma is variable and dependent upon the individual histologic sub-

Table 28.4.
Treatment and Prognosis in Hodgkin's Disease

Stage	Therapy	5-Year Survival (% estimated)
Stages IA, IIA, and IIIA	Radiation	90–95
Stages IIB and IIIB	Radiation and/or chemotherapy	60–70
Stage IVA	Chemotherapy	80
Stage IVB	Chemotherapy	50

type and stage evaluation. Staging for the evaluation of patients with non-Hodgkin's lymphoma usually includes a bone marrow aspiration and biopsy and an abdominal CT. In general, staging laparotomy is not indicated due to the high incidence of systemic involvement. Patients are staged by the Ann Arbor Classification like patients with Hodgkin's disease (Table 28.3).

Combination chemotherapy and radiation therapy have been useful in the treatment of patients with certain types of lymphoma. Diffuse histiocytic lymphoma appears to be the most curable with combination chemotherapy.

Radiotherapy is useful in localized non-Hodgkin's lymphoma, although this is an uncommon presentation. Radiation therapy is also used to treat specific complications related to mass effect. These would include the superior vena cava obstruction, ureteral obstruction, or spinal cord compression.

Special Surgical Considerations

Non-Hodgkin's lymphomas may arise from nodal or extranodal sites. Diffuse histiocytic lymphomas can arise in the gastrointestinal tract, most commonly in the stomach. The tumor originates in the submucosal layer of the stomach and may be missed by a mucosal biopsy. Characteristically, patients present with complications due to upper gastrointestinal bleeding, altered gastric motility, or obstruction. The upper gastrointestinal series usually shows a thickened stomach wall with loss of motility and enlarged mucosal folds. Surgical resection is indicated for most patients both to resect the local tumor as well as to perform an adequate staging evaluation. The surgical procedure should include a liver biopsy as well as lymph node biopsies and splenectomy, depending upon the individual patient. Following surgical resection, treatment is indicated for patients with disease extending outside the gastric wall or involving the spleen, liver, or lymph nodes. The options include local radiotherapy or systemic chemotherapy. The primary treatment of patients with gastric lymphoma by chemotherapy *without* resection has been associated with a high incidence of gastric bleeding and perforation due to rapid tumor lysis. Therefore, it is recommended that all patients undergo resection prior to systemic treatment.

Sarcoma

Soft Tissue Sarcomas

Somatic tissues are derived from embryonic mesoderm. These "soft tissues" are found in organs and structures throughout the body. They are ubiquitous but predominate in organs of locomotion, connective, and support tissues. Neoplasms arising in these tissues are usually referred to as soft tissue tumors; if malignant, however, the term sarcoma (derived from the greek word "sarkoma" meaning fleshy growth) is used to describe the growth. Although most sarcomas arise from structures/tissue derived from mesoderm, some may arise from epithelium that may have its origin from any of the three germ layers: ectoderm, endoderm, or mesoderm.

Malignant neoplasms of soft tissues are classified according to their tissue of origin (Table 28.5). Benign soft tissue tumors are common, infrequently produce symptoms, and therefore, are not usually a problem for the patient. Excision may sometimes be necessary, however, for either cosmesis or symptoms, such as pain.

Because visceral structures contain supporting and connective tissue, sarcomas may be found in any structure or organ. The majority, however, occur in the extremities and trunk (Table 28.6). In this section, emphasis will be on peripheral tumors. However, statements made regarding peripheral sarcomas apply equally to retroperitoneal and centrally situated tumors except for the following:

1. Complete extirpation may prove more difficult due to proximity and involvement of vital structures, e.g., retroperitoneal tumors (Fig. 28.1).
2. Radiation may be severely limited for the same reason as above (Fig. 28.1).
3. Satisfactory cosmetic results may be difficult to achieve especially with head and neck tumors.

Incidence

Soft tissue sarcomas are relatively uncommon, comprising less than 1% of all malignancies diagnosed annually in the United States. In children under 15 years of age, however, this figure rises to about 6%, and in this age group ranks fifth as a cause of cancer death. Approximately 5000–6000 new cases of soft tissue sarcoma are diagnosed every year in the United States and about one-half of these patients will eventually die of their tumor. Death results from uncontrollable local recurrence invading adjacent tissue/structures or metastasis to the lungs and other less common sites, e.g., liver and bone. There does not appear to be any predilection with respect to race or sex. There is, however, the aforementioned peak in children under 15 years of age, and also an increased incidence in adults in the fifth decade.

Table 28.5.
Soft Tissue Tumors and Their Tissue of Origin

Tissue	Benign	Malignant
Fibrous tissue	Fibroma	Fibrosarcoma
Adipose tissue	Lipoma	Liposarcoma
Striated muscle	Rhabdomyoma	Rhabdomyosarcoma
Smooth muscle	Leiomyoma	Leiomyosarcoma
Synovial mesothelium	Mesothelioma	Synovial sarcoma
Blood vessels	Angioma	Angiosarcoma[a]
Lymph vessels	Lymphangioma	Lymphangiosarcoma
Peripheral nerve	Neuroma	Malignant neurolemmoma, schwannoma

[a] See text for discussion of Kaposi's sarcoma.

Epidemiology

There are no proven epidemiological factors in patients suffering from soft tissue sarcomas. Some investigators have suggested a genetic predisposition or an increased incidence in patients with genetically transmitted disease, e.g., intestinal polyposis, Gardner's syndrome and von Recklinghausen's disease. Firm evidence to support these theories is as yet still lacking.

Etiology

Patients often associate a recent traumatic incident with the discovery of a tumor. There is, however, no confirmed etiological basis for what appears to be a fortuitous relationship. Animal experiments have shown that certain carcinogens and even viruses may produce sarcomas, but again there is no convincing evidence that such is the case in humans.

Certain preexisting conditions appear to increase the incidence of sarcoma development, e.g., chronic lymphadematous extremities, granulating wounds, burn scars, and tissues subjected to high-dose irradiation. The occurrence of sarcomas in situations described above is so infrequent that it is thought by most that soft tissue sarcomas occur de novo.

Classification

Prior to the late nineteenth and early twentieth centuries very little, or no distinction, was made between

Table 28.6.
Soft Tissue Sarcoma Sites and Frequency

Site	Frequency (%)
Lower extremity	
Above knee	30
Below knee	10
Upper extremity	20
Trunk	20
Head and neck	10
Retroperitoneal	10

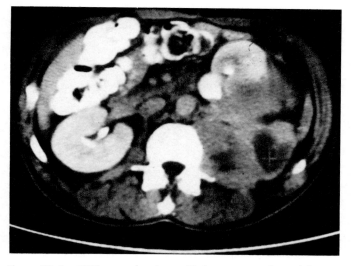

Figure 28.1. CAT scan of patient with large retroperitoneal liposarcoma arising from left psoas muscle. Note the invasion of kidney and vertebrae, and areas of necrosis within tumor.

neoplastic conditions of soft tissues and other non-neoplastic conditions, such as infections. With the progressive improvement and accuracy of histopathologic examination, great strides were made in differentiating neoplastic from non-neoplastic conditions. It was not until 1940, however, that Stout and Lattes classified the sarcomas according to their cells of origin. Today, more than 50 different histological types of soft tissue sarcomas are recognized.

It might appear at first glance that a classification of soft tissue sarcomas based on histologic origins would be reasonably straightforward; unfortunately, this is not the case. It is not unusual for a particular tumor to contain cells at varying stages of differentiation at any given time. It should be noted also that tissue culture studies indicate that sarcomas have the potential for dedifferentiation into any of the other soft tissue elements. Not infrequently, both factors make classification of sarcomas based on histologic origin very difficult. In these circumstances, pathologists may be forced to use the less desirable terms ''spindle cell sarcoma'' or ''sarcoma of unknown histiogenesis.'' The use of electromicroscopy may sometimes be helpful in identifying the cell of origin of some soft tissue sarcomas; however, the early expectations of this means of identification have been disappointing. More recently, another method of classification of sarcomas by histopathologic grading has been developed. This system deemphasizes the identification of the cell of origin and emphasizes the number of mitoses present per high power field in a given tumor. This method not only provides a means of grading the tumor but also provides an estimate of prognosis. This concentrated effort by pathologists and surgeons to grade soft tissue sarcomas accurately is critical when decisions are being made in the management and treatment of patients.

Histologic grade of primary tumors are assigned as follows:

Grade I—well differentiated,
Grade II—moderately differentiated,
Grade III—poorly differentiated.

Other cellular characteristics and morphologic features of sarcomas considered in assessing grade are degree of cytologic differentiation, degree of cellularity, loss of polarity, and formation of extracellular substances. It is important to understand that *the single most important prognostic factor in the management of sarcomas is the histologic grade of the primary lesion.*

Soft tissue sarcomas are staged by histopathologic grade and the additional criteria of tumor size, regional lymph node involvement, and metastatic status. The Task Force on Soft Tissue Sarcoma of the American Joint Committee for Cancer Staging has adopted four parameters: G, histopathologic grade; T, tumor size; N, lymph node involvement; and M, distant metastasis. These parameters provide a well recognized and accepted staging system (Table 28.7).

Points of Interest in the Natural History of Soft Tissue Sarcomas

1. Soft tissue sarcomas frequently appear to have a pseudocapsule through which extensions of

Table 28.7.
American Joint Committee (AJC) Staging System for Sarcomas of Soft Tissue

Staging Parameter	Description
Histologic grade of malignancy (G)	
G¹	Low
G²	Moderate
G³	High
Primary tumor (T)	
T¹	Tumor < 5 cm
T²	Tumor = 5 cm
T³	Tumor that grossly invades bone, major vessels, or major nerves
Regional lymph nodes (N)	
N⁰	No histologically verified metastases to regional nodes
N¹	Histologically verified regional lymph node metastasis
M⁰	No distant metastasis
M¹	Distant metastasis

Conventional Terminology Stage	AJC Equivalents			
	G	T	N	M
IA	1	1	0	0
IB	1	2	0	0
IIA	2	1	0	0
IIB	2	2	0	0
IIIA	3	1	0	0
IIIB	3	2	0	0
IIIC	1–3	1–2	1	0
IVA	1–3	3	0–1	0
IVB	1–3	1–3	0–1	1

the malignant tumor invade surrounding tissues/structures.

2. Soft tissue sarcomas tend to invade locally along anatomic planes, i.e., nerve fibers, fascial planes, blood vessels, and muscle bundles.

3. The poor prognosis in soft tissue sarcomas is the result of aggressive invasion into nearby structures/tissue and a tendency for early hematogenous dissemination.

4. Soft tissue sarcomas spread to regional lymph nodes infrequently.

5. Distant metastasis is usually to the lungs (Fig. 28.2).

6. Metastases are infrequently detectable at the time of diagnosis of the primary tumor and then usually only for large, high-grade lesions.

7. Eighty per cent of all local recurrences following surgery occur within 2 years.

8. Distal lesions result in better cure rates than proximal lesions.

9. Local excisions result in local recurrence rates of 50% as opposed to 20% for radical excision or amputation.

10. When feasible, pulmonary resection is recommended for pulmonary metastasis.

11. Eighty per cent of all patients who develop disseminated disease will do so within 5 years after primary tumor resection.

12. *Overall* 5-year survival of patients with soft tissue sarcoma is approximately 50%.

13. Prognosis in terms of 10-year survival decreases with advancing stage. Stage I tumors have about 80% survival rate; stage II, stage III, and stage IV tumors have survival rates of 60%, 25%, and 3%, respectively.

14. Death of the patient results from uncontrollable local recurrence or metastasis to lung, liver, or other sites.

Signs and Symptoms

Most malignant soft tissue tumors are relatively slow growing and do not cause symptoms until they become large. Symptoms are usually produced by compression of nearby structures, i.e., nerves, lymphatics, or vessels, the most common presentation being that of a patient complaining of a painless lump or mass. As these lesions not infrequently arise in the depths of large anatomic compartments, e.g., thighs and buttocks, they may reach very large proportions before the patient becomes aware of their presence and seeks medical advice, a factor that significantly influences management and prognosis (Figs. 28.3, 28.4, 28.5).

Diagnosis

Early detection of soft tissue malignancies requires a *high index of suspicion* by both patient and physician.

Clinical evaluation of any patient begins with the history. In the case of a lump or mass, a careful and complete history is taken directing attention to such factors as past trauma, possible infections, and genetic factors. The physical examination must include an accurate and detailed assessment of the mass in question; i.e., the site and position (anatomic compartment) of the mass, consistency and size of the mass, the depth of the mass with respect to the skin (subcutaneous, intramuscular), mobility of the mass, multiple or single, discrete or diffuse, increased local warmth, and tenderness. Despite the fact that it is uncommon for sarcomas to metastasize by lymph channels to regional nodes, about 2–3% will spread in this manner, so it is

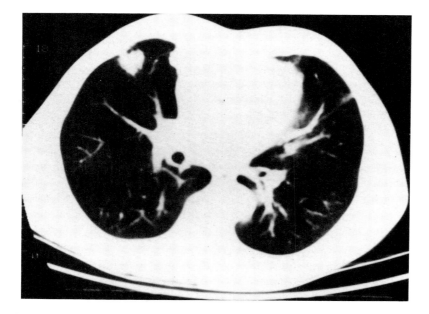

Figure 28.2. CAT scan of patient with lung metastasis from retroperitoneal sarcoma.

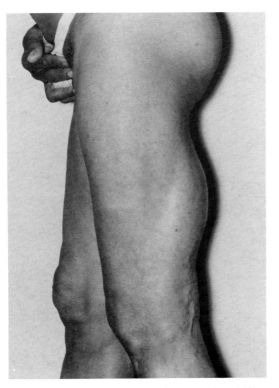

Figure 28.3. 56-year-old patient with large painless thigh mass (lateral view). The final diagnosis was liposarcoma.

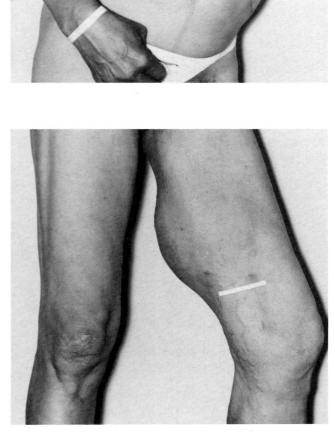

Figure 28.4. Same patient as Figure 28.3, medial view.

essential that regional nodes are examined carefully in every case.

After careful physical examination, the size of the mass, the extent of the mass, and the relationship of the mass to surrounding structures and normal anatomy is cofirmed with various investigatory techniques (x-rays, tomograms, and CT scans). On occasion xerography, arteriography, lymphangiography, and bone scans may be necessary. Arteriograms are especially useful when the suspicious mass is compressing or involving a major vessel. Finally, it must be stated that the above investigations not withstanding, the sine qua non of diagnosis of sarcomas is the *biopsy*. Many soft tissue tumors are benign and because there are no pathognomonic clinical signs or symptoms that one may use to distinguish between benign and malignant lesions, it must be obvious that the final court of appeal remains the histopathologic assessment of the tumor mass.

A biopsy specimen is essential for diagnosis but it also provides information required by the physician in planning appropriate therapy and allows him/her to predict the outcome with a fairly reasonable degree of accuracy.

Sarcomas grow in a three-dimensional manner taking the path of least resistance and compressing surrounding tissue. This latter phenomenon gives the impression of the tumor being encapsulated. It cannot be emphasized strongly enough that the surrounding tissue has simply formed a pseudocapsule and microscopic extensions of malignant tissue that project be-

yond the pseudocapsule aggressively invade surrounding tissues/structures. Because of this propensity to extend and invade, the method of biopsy of suspicious soft tissue masses becomes of paramount importance. Because the biopsy site must be removed when definitive surgery is performed, *the biopsy incision must be carefully orientated and located* to prevent compromise of the eventual surgical procedure.

From the foregoing, it will be obvious that attempting an excisional biopsy of a suspicious lump should not be undertaken lightly. Small lesions (less than 3 cm in diameter) may be managed by excisional biopsy when the surgeon feels he/she can be assured of excising the entire lesion including any extension of malignant tissue.

"Aspiration biopsy" and "needle biopsy" are sometimes used in selected cases; however, the small amount of tissue obtained with these methods frequently makes histopathologic diagnosis and grading difficult, if not impossible.

The most often used and most reliable method of obtaining tissue samples is "incisional biopsy." Using this method, minimum disruption of tissue planes can be achieved and a generous sample (always helpful to the histopathologist) can be obtained. Biopsy incisions for extremity lesions are usually placed longitudinally, while at other sites the incisions are orientated parallel to the long axis of the main muscle mass. The likeli-

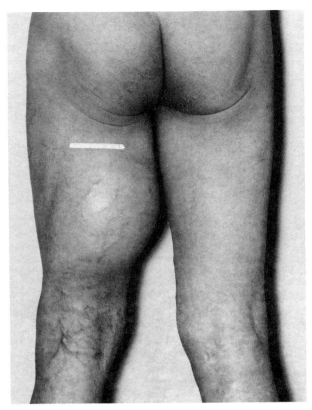

Figure 28.5.   Same patient as Figure 28.3, posterior view.

hood of developing skin flaps to cover defects when definitive surgery is performed must be anticipated and provision made for this eventuality when planning the location of the biopsy incision.

Routine work-up for a patient with a suspected sarcomatous mass should include the following:

1. A careful history and complete physical examination,
2. Chest x-rays,
3. Soft tissue radiograph of the mass including the area in which it is situated,
4. CT scan (Fig. 28.6) or ultrasound of the lesion and the area in which it is situated,
5. Full-chest CAT scans or full-chest tomograms,
6. A complete blood chemistry with a sequential multichannel autoanalyzer (SMA12) to detect any blood chemistry abnormality.

In addition to the above, in appropriate situations, arteriography or bone scans may be necessary. Lymphangiograms may be required in patients suffering from high-grade synovial sarcomas and rhabdomyosarcomas of the extremities because these lesions tend to metastasize via the lymphatics and involve regional nodes.

Treatment

There are numerous approaches to the management of soft tissue sarcomas; however, complete surgical excision with a wide margin of normal tissue still remains the basis for present day treatment of malignant soft tissue tumors.

During the late 1940's, simple excision of soft tissue sarcomas was practiced with a recurrence rate in the neighborhood of 85–95%. After it was realized that more extensive resection was required to remove microscopic extensions of malignant tissue, the recurrence rate was reduced to approximately 25% by radical resection. Not unexpectedly, where feasible, amputations with adequate proximal margins free from tumor (distal extremity lesions) reduced the recurrence rate even further to 10–15%. This improvement in local control, disease-free interval, and survival rate was offset by the considerable loss of function and cosmetic disability in patients who were managed by radical excision or amputation. Treatment modalities were sought that provided eradication of the primary tumor and microscopic extensions with a minimum of cosmetic and functional disability. Today, the modalities adopted in the management of soft tissue sarcomas include surgery alone, surgery combined with radiation, surgery combined with radiation and intraarterial chemotherapy, radiation alone, and systemic chemotherapy in conjunction with one or other of the aforementioned. Although the efficacy of the various modalities of treatment has not yet been fully established, suffice it to say that more conservative surgery combined with radiation therapy appears to be producing results equal to, if not in some cases better than, the traditional approach of radical surgery.

Surgery

The goal of the surgeon is to make sure that complete local excision is carried out at the time of the initial procedure. The three-dimensional spread of sarcomas must be taken into account and if necessary, entire muscle compartments including the origin and insertion of muscle groups, adjacent fascial planes and adjacent structures may have to be excised in order to encompass the spreading growth. Distal tumors may be managed by amputation, but even in these instances, it may be necessary to sacrifice the origin of muscles or muscle groups. For example, a large, high-grade, below-knee sarcoma would probably require an above-knee amputation to include the origins of the muscles of the leg. The *overall* recurrence rate for soft tissue sarcomas treated by surgery alone is about 85% for local excision, 50% for muscle group and compartment excision, and as one would expect with amputation, the recurrence rate drops to about 35%.

Radiation Therapy

Radiation when used alone, without surgery, results in a local recurrence rate of between 75–85%. Used in conjunction with surgical excision, either preoperatively or postoperatively, results are considerably improved and a local recurrence of 10–30% is achieved, depending on the location of the primary lesion. By removing the gross tumor mass surgically and destroying microscopic disease by radiation, a more conser-

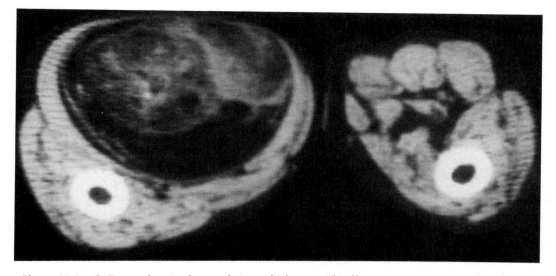

Figure 28.6. CAT scan showing large soft tissue thigh mass. This fibrosarcoma was proven by a biopsy.

vative surgical approach may be adopted. A reduction in cosmetic deformity and functional loss is thus achieved, depending on the location of the primary lesion. Currently, this combined approach appears to be the most effective therapy in the management of soft tissue malignancies.

Chemotherapy

Sarcomas are relatively insensitive to chemotherapeutic agents; however, newer agents and combinations of agents are producing responses that appear promising. Further work and evaluation of adjuvant therapy is needed before more can be said of this modality of treatment. The drug adriamycin, when used for patients who have disseminated or recurrent sarcoma not amenable to surgery, frequently produces temporary relief.

Follow-up

Patients who have been treated for soft tissue sarcomas must be followed extremely carefully. Monthly physical examinations with x-rays and CAT scans when appropriate are required for the first year. The length of time between check-ups may be extended during the second and third years but continued careful long-term followup is mandatory.

Kaposi's Sarcoma

Kaposi's sarcoma, a rare type of skin cancer, was seldom seen in the United States until recently. Angiosarcomas include malignant tumors of blood and lymphatic tissue and although the etiology and pathogenesis of Kaposi's sarcoma has not been entirely elucidated, it is usually included in this group of malignances. The tumor is more common in Jews, Italians, and Africans and is most often seen in the skin of the lower extremity. Less frequent sites are the trunk

and upper extremity. Beginning as a small purple macule or papule, the lesion slowly spreads until it eventually progresses to multiple sites. Further spread takes place proximally along veins and lymphatics, and if via the latter pathway, edema of the limb may result from obstruction of regional lymph nodes. In advanced cases, visceral involvement of the GI tract, liver, and spleen may occur. Other common sites of metastasis are distant lymph nodes and the lung.

Biopsy of Kaposi's sarcoma usually shows undifferentiated mesenchymal cells arranged along vessels in a sheath-like manner. As these tumor cells are pleuripotential endothelial cells, plasmacytes, reticulum cells, fibroblasts, and histiocytes may be found in the specimen.

With small localized lesions, surgical excision or local radiation is effective. In more advanced cases, chemotherapeutic agents produce responses in about 50% of patients with early disease and 20% of patients with advanced-stage disease. The agents used are vinblastine or a combination of doxorubicin, bleomycin, and vinblastine.

In the past 5–6 years, over 9000 cases of a heretofore unrecognized syndrome has been diagnosed in the United States. The fundamental defect in this disease is an impaired cellular immune mechanism that results in the increased incidence of severe opportunistic infections and neoplasms, Kaposi's sarcoma being one of the latter. The syndrome of AIDS (acquired immune deficiency syndrome) is reported in certain high risk groups, e.g., homosexuals, drug abusers, hemophiliacs, and persons who have received blood transfusions. An infective agent, a virus, is the cause of the syndrome. The virus in question has been identified as the human immunodeficiency virus (HIV). Non-AIDS-related Kaposi's sarcomas are less aggressive than AIDS-related Kaposi's sarcomas. The former may respond to radiation therapy or combination chemotherapy as stated above. AIDS-related Kaposi's sarcomas on the other hand usually result in death from uncontrolled spread of the tumor or complications of the defective immune condition. Of the over 9000 cases of AIDS diagnosed in the United States, about 35% will develop Kaposi's sarcoma. Other cancers that have been reported in AIDS patients are B-cell lymphoma (occurring in 3% of cases), Hodgkin's disease, plasmacytoma, Burkitt's lymphoma, and T-cell non-Hodgkin's lymphoma.

SUGGESTED READINGS

Anderson T, Chabner BA, Young RC, et al: Malignant lymphoma. I. The histology and staging of 473 patients at the National Cancer Institute. *Cancer* 50:2699–2707, 1982.

Das Gupta TK, et al: The role of chemotherapy as an adjuvant to surgery in the initial treatment of primary soft tissue sarcomas in adults. *J Surg Oncol* 19:139–144, 1982.

DeVita VT Jr: The consequences of the chemotherapy of Hodgkin's disease. *Cancer* 47:1–13, 1985.

DeVita VT Jr, Hellman S: Hodgkin's disease and the non-Hodgkin's lymphoma. In DeVita VT Jr, Hellman S, Rosenberg SA (eds): *Cancer Principles and Practice of Oncology.* JB Lippincott, Philadelphia, 1982, pp 1331.

DeVita VT Jr, Hellman S, Rosenberg SA (eds): *Cancer: Principles and Practice of Oncology.* Philadelphia, JB Lippincott, 1985.

DiGiovanna JD, et al: Kaposi's sarcoma. Retrospective study of 90 cases with particular emphasis on the familial occurrence, ethnic background and prevalence of other diseases. *Ann Intern Med* 86:693–700, 1982.

Friedman-Klein AE, et al: Disseminated Kaposi's sarcoma in homosexual men. *Am J Med* 71:779–783, 1981.

Grieco MB, Cady B: Staging laparotomy in Hodgkin's disease. *Surg Clin North Am* 60:369–379, 1980.

Hoppe RT, Coleman CN, Cox RS, et al: The management of Stage I–II Hodgkin's disease with irradiation alone or combined modality therapy: the Stanford experience. *Blood* 59:455–465, 1982.

Lindell MM, et al: Diagnostic technique for the evaluation of the soft tissue sarcoma. *Semin Oncol* 8:160–171, 1981.

The Non-Hodgkin's Lymphoma Pathologic Classification Project: National Cancer Institute sponsored study of classifications of non-Hodgkin's lymphomas. Summary and description of a working formulation for clinical usage. *Cancer* 49:2112–2135, 1982.

Rosenberg SA, et al: The treatment of soft-tissue sarcomas of the extremities. Prospective randomized evaluations of (1) limbsparing surgery plus radiation therapy compared with amputation and (2) the role of adjuvant chemotherapy. *Ann Surg* 196:305–315, 1982.

Suit HD: Soft tissue sarcomas, the role of radiation therapy. *Hosp Prac* July 1982:114–120.

Suit HD, et al: A clinical and pathological staging system for soft tissue sarcomas. *Cancer* 40:1562–1570, 1977.

Sutow WW, et al: Chemotherapy of sarcomas—a perspective. *Semin Oncol* 8:201–214, 1981.

Trotter MC, Cloud GA, Davis M, et al: Predicting the risk of abdominal disease in Hodgkin's lymphoma. *Ann Surg* 201:465–469.

Skills

LYMPHOMA

1. In a patient who complains of weight loss, fever, and night sweats, demonstrate the ability to inspect and palpate all peripheral lymph nodes in the body.

2. Describe the performance of an excisional lymph node biopsy in the posterior cervical lymphatic chain.

SARCOMA

1. Demonstrate the ability to localize a soft tissue mass to skin, subcutaneous tissue, or muscle on physical examination and to characterize it by size, consistency, temperature, and tenderness.

Study Questions

LYMPHOMA

1. A 30-year-old man presents with complaints of fever, sweating at night, and a 15-pound weight loss. What aspects of the physical examination are of particular interest? What special laboratory examination(s) are indicated? If cervical lymphadenopathy is present, identify the appropriate surgical procedure to be performed. What tests are required to evaluate inaccessible, deep lymph nodes in the body? What are the steps in a staging laparotomy?

2. A 25-year-old woman presents with right axillary lymphadenopathy. Three rubbery nodes are palpable and are movable and nontender. What are important aspects of this patient's physical examination to consider potential etiologies for this adenopathy? An excisional biopsy is performed to harvest an abnormal lymph node. What is the procedure for evaluating this node?

3. Specify indications for radiotherapy in non-Hodgkin's lymphoma.

4. A 45-year-old man developed a significant upper gastrointestinal hemorrhage, requiring the transfusion of 6 units of blood. An ulceration is seen in the distal antrum on upper endoscopy. Would you expect endoscopic mucosal biopsies to be productive? An upper gastrointestinal series obtained 2 days later revealed a thickened gastric antral wall with prominent rugal folds. Do you consider this patient an operative candidate? If so, what procedures should be accomplished at the operation? What would be risks of preoperative systemic chemotherapy?

SARCOMA

1. Describe the embryologic origin of soft tissue tumors called sarcomas. What age group(s) are affected most commonly by sarcomas? What regions of the body are most frequently involved? What is the usual cause of death?

2. Outline the grades of primary sarcomas, including cellular characteristics and morphologic features. What is the single most important grade feature in the management of sarcomas? What feature of soft tissue sarcomas is the principal determinant of a poor prognosis?

3. What is the sine qua non of diagnosis of sarcomas? Characterize the microscopic features of the pseudocapsule that account for the high local recurrence rate. What are the disadvantages of aspiration and needle biopsies of soft tissue sarcomas?

4. What is the principle in the surgical treatment of sarcomas to minimize the risk of local recurrence and to maximize the chance of a cure? What is the advantage to the patient of combining surgical excision with irradiation? What is the role of chemotherapy in the treatment of sarcomas?

5. Characterize clinical and histopathological features of Kaposi's sarcoma. What are the modes of treatment? What is the relation of Kaposi's sarcoma to AIDS?

Appendix

Strategies for Effective Learning and Retention in a Surgery Clerkship

Debra A. DaRosa, Ph.D.
Richard Bell, M.D.
Judith G. Calhoun, Ph.D.

OBJECTIVES
1. Define four major behaviors and strategies effective in optimizing learning.
2. Apply a self-directed learning approach to daily patient assignments.
3. Employ a basic search strategy for accessing information efficiently and methodically.
4. Self-assess clinical case presentation skills.

Surgery will always be a bit more practical, more clinical, and more urgent, because of the personal nature of the surgeon's commitment to his patient, and the crystal clear nature of the result. The medical student and society at large recognize surgery as a natural, ancient, and essential part, not only of the undergraduate curriculum, but of the background and knowledge of every physician. (F. D. Moore)

The purpose of the surgery clerkship is not to teach details of the operative procedure or techniques. Its purpose is to teach critical diagnostic and evaluation skills as well as basic surgical principles. A surgery clerkship is an ideal and unique opportunity to develop critical diagnostic and evaluation skills, gain a basic understanding of surgical principles, hone the technical facility necessary to various clinical procedures, and learn the basic principles of sterile technique, wound care, fluid and electrolyte management, nutrition, and critical care. Regardless of the chosen discipline, all physicians will be involved with patients in need of surgical care. Therefore the surgery clerkship is an extremely important learning experience, particularly for those pursuing nonsurgical careers (1).

As we progressed through society's educational system, starting in kindergarten, we listened, read, and studied. We were largely passive recipients of information. We were tested and retested. If we listened, read, and studied, we did well on tests and were considered "good" students. The tests predicted our grades, which reinforced this passive cyclical learning process. Doing well on examinations was the "end all" and primary reason for learning. In the clinical clerkship years, tests can no longer be the primary reason for learning. Tests are still benchmarks of progress that reflect the knowledge base, but most pen and pencil tests tell us nothing about the ability to apply that knowledge base to patient problem solving. Although it may be difficult, it is critical that this attitude and learning approach, successfully employed for years, be quashed. Tests are important, but the results will not tell students if they are clinically competent.

The clinical learning approach in a clerkship involves the ability to answer questions based on what the student knows, but also the ability of the student to articulate questions based on what he or she does not know. Students need to learn to identify their own deficiencies through self-evaluation, as well as the subjective evaluation of faculty, residents, and colleagues, and not look to psychometric measures alone as reflections of performance. These can serve as excellent supplements to judgments but should not be used, as in our earlier educational experience, as indications of abilities to be a "good" doctor.

As Abernathy and Abernathy state (2), knowing the "right question" and how to find its answer is the key to clinical surgery for both a clerk and the most experienced practitioner. There are two mediums for learning surgery: the first is based on experiential acquisition of knowledge and skills and the second is based on didactics and reading resources. The first requires long hours of observing, trying, and trying again. Learning on a surgical service requires getting involved with the patients and the surgical team, on rounds, in the operating room, and in the clinics. The second medium requires sharp listening, reading comprehension, and retention skills. The ability to articulate questions, based on what one observes, listens, or reads, that trace the thought process a surgeon uses when thinking through a problem will not only be the key to success as a surgical clerk, but also as a life-long learner.

This chapter provides guidelines for effective learning for those entering the clinical years. The approach taken to learning directly influences recall and retention. This chapter outlines and summarizes strategies for effective learning in a clinical environment, based on adult educational principles and theory. It outlines a guideline for optimizing learning on the surgical service, describes a self-directed learning approach and a basic information search strategy, and presents an approach for organizing and self-assessing case presentation skills.

Optimizing Learning

Both students and faculty can impact the quality and efficacy of learning activities. Faculty need to be proficient at designing and developing quality learning experiences and evaluation methodologies. Students need to extend faculty efforts by being active participants in the learning process and the management of their own self-development and assessment skills. Specific student strategies that can be used to optimize learning include the following:

Be Motivated

Motivation is a critical condition for learning, as it reflects attitude, industry, and assertiveness in mastering curricular goals and objectives. These attributes are the ones most highly valued in students on a surgical clerkship. Surgical faculty look for this degree of interest and independence in surgical clerks and as a rule reward students for it. Surgical patients and their diseases will provide opportunities for you to motivate yourself. Students should not, however, wait for such opportunities. Students need to remember that more will be learned and retained by doing (active learning) than simply by listening to someone speak (passive learning). Assertiveness is important. Students should ask faculty, for example, if they could follow on rounds, observe in clinic, or demonstrate a specific technique. Most faculty like to see students seeking opportunities to learn. Assertive learning demonstrates interest and intellectual curiosity, which are characteristics frequently evaluated by faculty and later reported to residency program directors in letters of recommendation.

Although most medical students are motivated learners, the basis for this learning drive must be kept in its proper perspective. Examination scores, grades, honors, and high subjective ratings are unquestionably important, but students should ultimately be striving to meet their learning needs and not just pass tests or gain recognition. Educational research has not been able to consistently demonstrate a relationship between examination scores [including the Medical College Admissions (MCAT) or National Board of Medical Examiners (NMBE)] and clinical performance. Therefore good test scores, although critical to compete for AOA, honors, or residency positions, do not mean students have filled all learning voids. When asked a question or encountered with a problem for which additional information is needed, clerks should demonstrate motivated behavior by pursuing the necessary resources and reporting the findings to the situation or individual initially presenting the problem or question. In the long run, it is the clerk who goes the second mile who stands out, as well as maximizes learning opportunities.

Identify the Intent of the Instruction and Learning Activities

By determining what is expected from the learning situation, students will be better prepared to guide their learning activities and strategies. Mager (3) stated: ''If you're not sure where you're going, you're liable to end up somewhere else—and not even know it.''

This guidance can most readily be obtained by critically reviewing the written goals and objectives for the clerkship, if such are provided. If they are not, faculty should be asked to identify their expectations of students and the criteria for acceptable levels of performance. Whether written in detail or globally stated, understanding the instructional goals and objectives is essential for facilitating the integration of instructional content and process, meeting evaluation demands, and promoting the efficient use of time.

The operating room is a learning environment unique to surgery. There might be a slight variation in perspective among the attending physicians about the intent of instruction for students in the operating room. Most faculty agree, however, that while residents should arrive knowledgeable of the general operative technique and principles and the conduct of specific operations, medical students should come to the operating room knowledgeable of the following:

1. The disease for which the operation is performed, e.g., pathophysiology underlying the clinical setting, treatment or modification of the pathologic process by operation, alternative methods of therapy, clinical signs and symptoms, prognosis, and potential complications of the procedure.
2. Applicable basic sciences, i.e., physiology, anatomy, and pathology (4).

Medical students (especially on a surgical rotation) must contend with a major problem rampant in medical education, information overload. Students will be extremely busy during their clerkship, but they need to take responsibility for establishing a proper balance between bedside and book learning. Extensive reading assignments limit the time available for thinking about what is being read. Students are forced to memorize what they can to pass multiple choice examinations. Finding time for reading, much less the time to think critically, can be a major problem for the surgical clerk whose hours are stretched among rounds, the operating room, ward activities, and countless other duties. Often it is advisable to first scan the printed material to assess the scope and then write a general outline. This will establish an organized mental ''filing system.'' If hurriedly read or ''crammed,'' the information will not be retained in a recallable format. As each section is read, associate the new information with what you already know, emphasizing similarities and differences. This process is called ''positive transfer.'' Cramming may successfully serve short-term recall needs but will not store the information in long-term memory for future use.

Students are not encouraged to read textbooks from cover to cover, as retention is slight. Acquisition of organized knowledge is better accomplished by applying what is read to clinical situations, as learning is then reinforced. Material that is read for information related to a patient problem or case is better retained, as the information is actively relevant and applicable.

This is not to suggest that students should not read randomly in textbooks. It is important to keep up with reading, regardless of patient availability. It is not, however, a worthwhile time investment to read when overtired or when the ability to concentrate and think about what is being read is limited. Students should reserve quiet time for reading within reasonable time limits. These time limits vary among individuals. Some students can concentrate better by reading, for example, at several different 30-minute intervals throughout the day, while others, with high-concentration abilities, can read with reasonable retention at one setting for a longer period. These limitations are often realized during those times when students have reread the same paragraph more than once and are still not registering the information. Individuals need to determine the time of day that best suits their reading style. Some students find early mornings a more productive time to read, while others prefer different periods of the day. This scheduling may conflict with other uncontrollable time demands, but it doesn't hurt to be aware of times when one is more alert and perhaps in a better state of mind for concentrating.

If learning objectives are not provided with an extensive reading assignment, the instructor should be asked to help focus studying by pointing out what in the readings is critical or important in order not to miss the ''forest for the trees.'' Generally surgical students need to concentrate on the areas of anatomy, pathophysiology, diagnosis, indications for surgical intervention, and potential complications. It is the resident who must understand the details of operative procedures. The surgical clerkship introduces the student to surgical disease; it does not teach surgical technique (5).

Studying should not be limited to instructional objectives. Students need to go beyond the objectives when possible and seek additional information to ensure a comprehensive understanding of the subject area.

Not knowing what is expected in terms of interaction or performance while in the emergency room, outpatient clinic, the operating room, or elsewhere is common for students during their first clinical rotations. Students need to take responsibility for their own learning and *ask* residents or faculty for direction. Surgical clerkships, like others, are limited in time. Plodding along without specific learning objectives deprives the student of valuable learning opportunities. Different residents and faculty may have varying student expectations. Being perceptive and flexible in this regard is critical. Learning these differences and approaching learning activities accordingly will serve the student's best interests.

Seek Appropriate Learning Activities

Learning is the student's responsibility. It is important to discriminate and carefully select among the many instructional methods and resources available to resolve knowledge or skill voids. Students should choose those methods and materials that match their individual learning styles, time constraints, and desired levels of skill and performance. The student who learns better through visual presentations and repetition should seek out slide-tape or video presentations and/or computer simulations to augment the printed materials provided for a particular learning situation. If written materials are preferred, students should identify or ask for additional references and related readings that may be applicable and helpful. Students need to challenge themselves by seeking out real world, relevant activities that involve actual problem-solving activities rather than passive participation. Requesting additional cases related to what is being studied is also advisable. First-hand experience is highly effective in aiding retention.

As clerks become more successful and self-confident, they should ask peers or faculty to observe and constructively comment on practice and application activities. For instance, when suturing skill is first addressed, performance can be enhanced if the various techniques as covered in the textual material are practiced with a number of different surfaces before actually demonstrating the skill. When relatively proficient, comments can be requested from a peer or a helpful faculty member, soliciting both the good and bad aspects of performance.

There are various written resources also helpful to the surgery clerk. Abernathy and Abernathy's book of questions typically asked on rounds, in the operating room, and on oral examinations is an excellent self-learning exercise (2). Stillman's book on general surgery is another excellent instructional resource that includes a set of well-tested multiple choice questions allowing for reinforcement of the newly acquired information by its immediate use in deductive reasoning on patient management issues. Stillman recommends consulting the chapter related to a newly encountered patient matching that condition (4).

Be Receptive to Faculty Feedback and Evaluation

Students need to be particularly attuned to feedback and evaluation. It is not unusual to have completed a write-up, a technical procedure, or a four-hour period in an outpatient clinic without an expert opinion as to the specifics of what was done well or poorly. Most faculty are not consistent or detailed in providing student feedback as they contend with busy daily schedules, yet feedback helps in evaluating one's progress. Studies have shown that without informational feedback, errors of commission and omission are repeated and eventually become habitual. Students should *not* assume that they are correct unless told otherwise. Requesting faculty or residents to review and discuss a completed write-up or observe a procedure is acceptable, and in fact to be urged, if feedback is not regularly provided. Without feedback, proper learning cannot be reinforced. Sufficient external feedback will also sharpen self-assessment skills, which are a key source of reinforcement.

Self-Directed Learning

Self-directed learning is a continual process of asking oneself questions and resolving them. This learning approach requires that students accept primary responsibility for learning and utilize instructors as facilitators of learning. The success of this method is premised on the fact that students bring a good deal of useful prior learning and experience to any situation. Students are in the best position to identify their own learning voids. The self-directed learning approach is concerned not only with what is learned, but how it was learned, in light of future professional tasks as a lifelong self-reliant learner (6). This approach is an active experiential approach to learning, which enhances retention of information.

Effective self-directed learning skills are critical to learning in the surgery clerkship. Preparation is often the key. Before observing a patient in the operating room, students should read about the patient's problem or observe available videotapes and become familiar with the anatomy, relevant pathophysiology, and basic surgical principles. Students should reflect on what they already know in these areas and identify what else needs to be known. Learning will be reinforced in the operating room and provide a basis of knowledge for relating to the experience. Assertively seek as much information as is feasible within the time and procedural constraints of the operation. After the operation, questions concerning postoperative management, psychosocial care, or other relevant information needs should be thought through and resolved by consulting additional sources of information.

The surgical clerkship is not designed to teach the student to be a physician or to take responsibility for the patient's total care. Learning is the student's primary objective. With this in mind, consider the following approach. When assigned a new patient, complete a brief history and physical examination in order to construct a list of possible diagnoses. The next step is to identify the important problems or learning issues. Using this basic foundation, the student should leave the patient for a short time and seek additional information based on the developed problem list. With this additional data base, the student can return to complete the history and physical examination with the patient. This will provide for a more informed, organized, and focused inquiry and examination method. An alternative approach is to conduct a thorough history and physical examination, make a list of possible hypotheses, and then leave the patient to research the necessary information. As similar clinical problems are encountered, the workup process will become methodical and efficient. Eventually this approach will imitate the pattern of an experienced physician.

The concept of responsible self-directed learning is extremely important to the surgical student in the transition from classroom to clinical training. As a junior member of a patient care team, the student must learn how to resolve self-initiated questions in order to make sound clinical judgments. To accomplish this, the student must determine what he or she already knows about a patient's problem, what needs to be known, and where the sources to fill the information void can be found. These information-seeking skills enable students to become independent, self-directed learners in medical school and throughout their medical careers.

Becoming a responsible, self-directed learner is an important element in achieving and maintaining clinical competence. Medical students cannot possibly learn during their formal training all they will ever need to know; they must, therefore, equip themselves with the skills necessary to access the myriad resources that can supply information pertinent to their identified learning needs.

Information Seeking Skills

Studies have shown that the necessity for specific, standard diagnostic or therapeutic information dominates the daily information needs of medical students, residents, and physicians (7). Generally information is wanted the same day as the need arises. Results indicated that books, usually in personal libraries, are the most frequently used resource. The strategy used by most clinicians for information seeking is based on convenience and habit. The major implication of this research is that the tendency is for physicians to respond to information problems via known pathways, which are probably established early in a medical career. Therefore students should be introduced to available information resources that are most useful and efficiently accessed. A basic information search strategy can prevent frustration and assist students to access answers to questions methodically and efficiently.

One approach to searching for information is the deductive strategy, or going from general to more specific resources. The first step is to glean background information by consulting general or specialty textbooks. Textbooks can provide comprehensive and succinct background information that can prompt a search for more up-to-date information. It is critical to use *recent* textbooks, since their content is quickly outdated. Even some information in the latest editions may be outdated before it is published. Reviewing textbooks, however, can provide searchers with a basic overview, key words, and references that can assist in the pursuit of additional data through such resources as *Index Medicus*.

Index Medicus is the major biomedical literature index. An index provides titles of published articles catalogued according to headings or descriptors but does not include abstracts or other descriptions of the articles. Its citations to the journal literature include approximately 3000 journals. *Index Medicus* is published monthly and cumulated annually in the *Cumulated Index Medicus.* Each monthly volume includes an author and subject index, as well as a very helpful section entitled ''Bibliography of Medical Reviews.''

The ''Bibliography of Medical Reviews'' in *Index Medicus* can save searchers a great deal of time, especially when searching the literature for research purposes. A review article is a comprehensive, focused article on a specific topic referencing all pertinent and related articles in the recent biomedical literature. The ''Bibliography of Medical Reviews'' references review articles separately and is found in the beginning of each monthly and annual issue.

The ''Medical Subject Headings'' (frequently referred to as MESH) is the guide to using *Index Medicus* and is found in the January issue. It can guide the searcher to the appropriate vocabulary in *Index Medicus.* MESH is arranged into two sections: an alphabetic listing and a hierarchical or ''tree'' structure. The tree listing shows how each term fits into the scheme of the overall picture of what is being searched. Using trees, one can search for an exact term, one that is broader, or one that is narrower, depending on what amount of information is available. The trees simply break subjects into categories and subcategories for the purpose of organization. For example, category C-19 concerns the endocrine diseases, a general category. The subcategory on breast disease is C-19.146. This is further subdivided into specific components of breast disease, i.e., fibrocystic disease of the breast (C-19.146.378). In looking for fibrocystic diseases, the category C4.182.289 is also listed. This number refers to other categories where this particular topic can be cross-referenced. While the numbers have no specific significance in the actual retrieval of references, they are important in finding the key word or related terms under which topics may be found in *Index Medicus.* References to articles appear in *Index Medicus* under the most specific MESH term available. It is worth the time to sit down with a librarian and learn how to utilize MESH. This small time investment can save future hours and headaches.

Thus one basic search strategy is to use a deductive approach by reviewing basic texts, then *Index Medicus,* and finally journal articles. Occasionally, however, other resources may be needed.

It can take up to six months from the time an article is published until it becomes referenced in *Index Medicus.* Students can review *Current Contents* to locate pertinent, newly published articles. This resource, published by the Institute for Scientific Information, organizes current published articles by listing each article's title in a subject index based on key words. Its use as a tool for searching the literature on a specific topic is limited; however, it is useful for seeing what types of articles are being printed. This is a very good resource for keeping current on what is being published in specific areas of interest.

When conducting a complicated search involving two or more topics, a computer search can be an effi-cient resource. The MEDLARS system is a computerized system that references medical literature in numerous data bases. MEDLARS searches are conducted through most medical libraries; the librarian conducting the search can help determine which data bases and key words are pertinent to information needs.

Another option is to check the reference list at the end of a textbook chapter related to the subject of interest. Although probably outdated, searchers can find current articles from older articles. For example, assume a journal article by John C. Schuster was referenced at the end of a textbook chapter concerning the use of CEA to monitor colon cancer recurrences, a subject on which more information is needed. The reference in the textbook cites it was written in 1970, which means the information is outdated. A review of the citation section of the *Social Science Citation Index* can provide the names and references of authors who recently cited the Schuster article in their published paper(s). This provides sources for updated information published on the topic of interest.

There are numerous other resources available, including audiovisuals such as movies, audiotapes, or slide-tape shows, which can be accessed through a library catalogue or from personnel in the library multimedia section. Other resources include *Spivak's Manual of Problems in Internal Medicine,* which provides disease descriptions with key articles; syndrome dictionaries providing information on syndromes named for individuals; *Excerpta Medica,* which publishes abstracts on American and foreign journal articles; and other abstracting resources such as *Biological Abstracts, Chemical Abstracts,* and *Psychological Abstracts.*

Once the articles are located, the reader's task has just begun. Articles are published for a variety of reasons, and it is often helpful to determine why the one the student is reading was printed. Many articles are anecdotal accounts, usually concerning case reports of rare conditions or unusual manifestations of a disease. New ideas, surgical techniques, or articles concerning product evaluations are readily available, generally to serve as marketing tools for the manufacturer, rather than to provide scientific information. Frequently the student will be confronted with the publication of a collected series of patients with similar problems or diseases. The student must be careful in drawing conclusions that may relate to his or her patient, or even in accepting the conclusions proposed by the author. Learning to critically evaluate the medical literature is a lifelong process, but the following considerations may help the student who is reading an article.

Comparative analysis (e.g., one form of treatment versus another, drug A versus drug B) should be randomized, prospective, and double blinded. Conclusions drawn based on historical controls may not be valid. For example, an article that proposes that the incidence of infection after penetrating abdominal trauma is lower with drug A based on experiences with similar patients 10 years ago is certainly suspect. Considering the improvements in prehospital care, resuscitation, and the development of trauma centers in the past 10 years, the reduced infection rate may not be attributed to the drug alone. While drug A may have contributed to the results, drug B or C may have produced a similar result, or perhaps even better. The conclusion should not be that drug A is indicated but that the prophylactic antibiotics may be useful. The extent of the contribution of drug A to the improved result, in this case, remains unanswered.

Similar populations for comparison should be chosen. This is perhaps the most difficult aspect of clinical research. Diseases often present with varied spectrums, severity, and in association with other medical conditions. The researcher should have made every possible attempt to control for these differences by categorizing the populations studied based on clinical staging, sex, age, and associated health factors. Often this is not possible in clinical practice, but randomization of treatment is not accomplished if efforts to control these variables are neglected. Each subject in the trial should have the same chance of receiving treatment A or B, thus avoiding inadvertent selection based on known or unappreciated bias. Those individuals who are responsible for the care of the patient and those who evaluate the results should be blinded as to which type of treatment was given. This prevents the introduction of bias in the analysis of the results. Double blinding may not be possible when one compares surgical alternatives, but every effort should be made to honestly appraise the results.

Few of us are experts at statistical analysis, but the reader of scientific articles should have a basic understanding of biostatistics. One must determine if the numbers used in the study are large enough to draw general conclusions. An analysis of the incidence of spontaneous fistulae formation in 10 patients with Crohn's disease would be meaningless. Furthermore, one must determine the difference between clinical and statistical significance. In many cases, populations of greater than 1000 may be required to show statistical significance. If such is the case, then clinical significance, despite the statistics, may have little relevance. Many larger medical centers have biostatisticians who can provide guidance in this area.

The student should also question whether the populations being studied are analogous to those seen in the institution where the student is working. A small community hospital may see a different population than a large, inner-city, charity institution. The etiology of upper gastrointestinal bleeding in a Veterans Hospital may be quite different than the etiology in a community hospital. Comparison of the results of treatment or even the natural history of the disease may not be appropriate.

The student must also ask if the conclusions follow the facts presented. This aspect of literature analysis may require the greatest insight. Without training or research experience, it is often impossible for the novice to question the methodology used, but one can ask if the conclusions seem reasonable or perhaps too extreme to be credible.

Orientation to the Patient
  Social
  Medical (chronic, major past problems)
  Chief complaint (description, duration)
  History source (relation, reliability)

Major Active Problem(s) (MAP)
  Date of onset
  Where patient presented
  New or old problem
  Duration/persistence
  Character (quality, intensity, frequency, location, radiation)
  Chronology of problem
  Relation to other events (time of day, activities, rest, food, position, response to palliation, response to provocation)
  Associated symptoms
  Previous evaluations and their outcomes
  Previous therapy and response
  Significant negatives (symptoms, relation to other events, prior medical history)

Family History

Social History

Past Medical History, Medication, Allergies
  Active problems summarized (onset, status, treatment)
  Inactive problems listed
  Medication (generic name, dosage, recent changes)
  Medical allergies and type of response

Edited Review of Systems

Physical Examination (PE)
  General appearance
  Vital signs
  Positive PE findings related to MAP
  Significant negative PE findings

Laboratory and Radiological Data
  Lab data needed for diagnosis/management
  Radiological data needed for diagnosis

Differential Diagnosis and Plan
  Differential diagnosis for each MAP
  Differential diagnosis related to relevant data
  Plan for each MAP

Figure A.1. Major Components of Case Presentation (From Anderson, WA, Bridgham, RG, Alquire, PC, Mayle, JE: Improving Medical Students' clinical case presentation skills. Presented at the annual meeting of the American Educational Research Association, New Orleans, April, 1984.)

Surveys have shown that verbal exchanges with colleagues are a common source of information (8, 9). This was found to be especially true of younger physicians (10). While verbal communication is a quick mechanism for accessing information, it should be viewed with some caution. Greene states that the value of colleagues as an information source is great but that one needs to consider the limitations and pitfalls of depending on verbal interaction alone. He also points out the dangers to which inaccurate and/or incomplete information can lead (11). It may therefore be advisable to request an article from a colleague being consulted that can provide additional information on the subject.

	QUALITY OF PERFORMANCE							
	Unacceptable		Borderline		Satisfactory		Superior	
PRESENTATION SKILLS	1	2	3	4	5	6	7	8
Presents with minimal prompting from notes; doesn't read from record.	1	2	3	4	5	6	7	8
Uses precise, accurately pronounced terminology.	1	2	3	4	5	6	7	8
Presents in a manner that holds attention.	1	2	3	4	5	6	7	8
SUCCINCTNESS	1	2	3	4	5	6	7	8
Completes within the time alloted.	1	2	3	4	5	6	7	8
Includes only data needed to understand the patient's problem and its management.	1	2	3	4	5	6	7	8
Presents findings without equivocation or irrelevant description of how gained.	1	2	3	4	5	6	7	8
ORGANIZATION	1	2	3	4	5	6	7	8
Presents each section as a unit; doesn't hop around.	1	2	3	4	5	6	7	8
Presents information in appropriate order; doesn't withhold important orienting information.	1	2	3	4	5	6	7	8
Presents data organized by their relation to an active problem or to a diagnostic hypothesis.	1	2	3	4	5	6	7	8
PROBLEM DEFINITION	1	2	3	4	5	6	7	8
Describes and prioritizes problems appropriately.	1	2	3	4	5	6	7	8
Defines the etiology and ramifications of major problems.	1	2	3	4	5	6	7	8
Summarizes problems in a complete problem list.	1	2	3	4	5	6	7	8
REASONING IN DIAGNOSIS AND MANAGEMENT	1	2	3	4	5	6	7	8
Includes all reasonable possibilities in the differential diagnosis.	1	2	3	4	5	6	7	8
Adequately discusses the differential diagnosis.	1	2	3	4	5	6	7	8
Identifies important considerations in the workup and management of the case.	1	2	3	4	5	6	7	8
OVERALL QUALITY OF PREPARED PRESENTATION	1	2	3	4	5	6	7	8

Comments:

Figure A.2. Part II of the Michigan State University Rating Form for Case Presentations (From Anderson, WA, Bridgham, RG, Alquire, PC, Mayle, JE: Improving Medical Students' clinical case presentation skills. Presented at the annual meeting of the American Educational Research Association, New Orleans, April, 1984.)

Being an effective learner requires efficient information-seeking skills that enable an individual to find responses to self-directed questions and critically review these responses. The use of the medical literature is a skill that can be mastered, despite the myriad of published information. For most undergraduates, the printed word will become the most important link with ongoing medical education after graduation. Students need to invest time, either independently or through an elective, learning about resource access and availability. It will prove to be an investment yielding both short- and long-term payoffs and aid in the processes required of an efficient life-long learner.

Case Presentation Skills

Although medical students are called on daily to present an oral summary of a patient's clinical case, they rarely receive formal training in giving these presentations. Frequently cited problems include their inability to properly organize the case presentation, present relevant information in a concise manner, and present the case in a smooth, professional manner (12).

Two studies identified the critical features and qualities of an effective clinical case presentation. By-products of these studies included rating forms for valid and reliable assessment by faculty and students of clinical case presentation skills. Clinical faculty from the Michigan State University Department of Medicine identified nine essential components of a case presentation to be used by students in preparing a clinical case presentation (12). These nine major components and their related subcomponents are listed in Figure A.1. This form is appended for use in organizing case presentations. Figure A.2 provides a rating mechanism for assessing case presentations.

A review of this checklist and others (13) indicates students should perform the following to ensure effective presentation of clinical cases.

1. Carefully study and review the case to ensure familiarity, understanding, and related knowledge of all major components and subcomponents.
2. Organize the presentation to flow coherently from section to section in an appropriate order.
3. Be succinct and focused; include only the relevant data that is needed to understand the patient's problem and its management.
4. Specifically define and summarize completely all essential problems and reasonable possibilities in relation to both the differential diagnosis and the management of the case.
5. Display professional presentation skills: maintain eye contact, talk rather than read to the audience, use proper voice projection to hold audience attention, provide meaningful summarization where appropriate, allow participant interaction, and provide carefully developed adjunctive materials.

If the elements included on the sample checklist are utilized for self-evaluation during the design and development of the presentation, whether it is a patient case presentation or an oral presentation to other health providers, the quality of the final presentation should be greatly enhanced.

Summary

There are numerous behaviors and learning strategies based on research findings concerning adult edu-

cation that can optimize learning while on the surgery clerkship. These include demonstrating motivation and industry, identifying the intent of instruction and various clinical learning activities in order to combat being victims of unspecified levels of expectations, seeking out situations or individuals that provide for applying and practicing what has been learned, and initiating self, faculty, and resident evaluation and feedback.

Self-directed learning skills are critical to the student in transition from the classroom to the hospital. Students must learn to address a patient's problems by identifying what they know, what needs to be known, and how to use efficient information-seeking skills to acquire the information needed.

Case presentation skills will be required throughout medical school and residency. Learning to self-assess these skills will enable students to improve case presentations as they graduate through their medical education career.

Paying attention to how you learn will assist in managing the myriad information requiring mastery prior to graduation. The chapters in this book employ a sound learning approach by detailing learning objectives and including self-assessment mechanisms to test recall and application abilities. Although this text differs in approach from its academic cousins, it provides for a useful and practical learning experience.

REFERENCES

1. Zelenock GB: Basic surgical clerkships. In: *Medical Education: A Surgical Perspective*. Chelsea, MI, Lewis, 1986, pp 151–170.
2. Abernathy C, Abernathy B: *Surgical Secrets*. Philadelphia, Hanley & Belfus, 1986.
3. Mager RF: *Preparing Instructional Objectives*. Belmont, CA, Fearon, 1962.
4. Turnage RH: *Medical Education: A Surgical Perspective*. Chelsea, MI, Lewis, p 53, 1986.
5. Stillman RM: *General Surgery Review and Assessment*. New York, Appleton-Century-Crofts, 1983.
6. Barrows HS: Problem-based, self-directed learning. *JAMA* 250:3077–3080, 1983.
7. Northup DE, Moore-West M, Skipper B, Teaf SR: Characteristics of clinical information-searching: investigation using critical incident technique. *J Med Educ* 58:873–881, 1983.
8. Weinberg AD, Ullian L, Richards WD, Cooper P: Informal advice and information-seeking between physicians. *J Med Educ* 56:174–180, 1981.
9. Fineberg HV, Gabel RA, Sosman MB: Acquisition and application of new medical knowledge by anesthesiologists. *Anesthesiology* 48:430–436, 1978.
10. Neufeld VR, Woodsworth AA: Survey of physician self-education patterns in Toronto. II. Use of journals and personal filing systems. *Can Libr J* 29:215–222, 1970.
11. Greene NM: Gossip and the acquisition of knowledge. *Anesth Analg* 57:519–520, 1978.
12. Anderson WA, Bridgham RG, Alguire PC, Mayle JE: Improving medical students' clinical case presentation skills. Presented at the annual meeting of the American Educational Research Association, New Orleans, April, 1984.
13. Blane CE, Calhoun JG: Objectively evaluating student case presentations. *Invest Radiol* 20:121–123, 1985.

Index